Synbiotics in Metabolic Disorders

This book explores the potential role of prebiotics, probiotics, and synbiotics in managing various metabolic disorders, chronic diseases, and metabolic syndromes. The initial chapter provides an overview of metabolic disorders, including their classification, symptoms, and underlying causes. Additionally, the chapter discusses the intricate signaling pathways and mechanisms through which prebiotics, probiotics, and synbiotics interact with the human body in relation to type-2 diabetes, obesity, phenylketonuria, and hemochromatosis. Additionally, this book highlights the potential impact of probiotics and synbiotics on oxidative stress, inflammation, lipid metabolism, and blood pressure. Furthermore, this book focuses on the gut–brain axis and how synbiotics may influence neurotransmitter metabolism. With an emphasis on the gut–microbiota axis, this book presents a compelling narrative that explores the rationality behind synbiotic use and offers a glimpse into future perspectives for managing metabolic disorders effectively. This book is intended for researchers in the fields of nutraceuticals, nanomedicine, endocrinology, nutrition, gastroenterology, and metabolic medicine who are working in the field of probiotics, prebiotics, and symbiotics for the treatment of metabolic disorders.

Synbiotics in Metabolic Disorders

Mechanisms, Therapeutic Potential, and Future Perspectives

Edited by
Neeraj Mishra, Sumel Ashique, Arshad Farid, and Ashish Garg

CRC Press
Taylor & Francis Group
Boca Raton London New York

CRC Press is an imprint of the
Taylor & Francis Group, an informa business

Designed cover image: Shutterstock

First edition published 2025
by CRC Press
2385 NW Executive Center Drive, Suite 320, Boca Raton FL 33431

and by CRC Press
4 Park Square, Milton Park, Abingdon, Oxon, OX14 4RN

CRC Press is an imprint of Taylor & Francis Group, LLC

ISBN: 9781032702414 (hbk)
ISBN: 9781032702421 (pbk)
ISBN: 9781032702438 (ebk)

DOI: 10.1201/9781032702438

Typeset in Times
by codeMantra

Contents

Contributors

Debojyoti Adak
Department of Regulatory Affairs
Quest Vitamins, Middle East FZE Dubai, United Arab Emirates

Thomas Adelina
Department of Medicinal Chemistry and Pharmacognosy, School of Pharmacy
Catholic University of Health and Allied Sciences
Mwanza, Tanzania

Mohit Agrawal
School of Medical & Allied Sciences
K.R. Mangalam University
Gurugram, India

Asad Ahmad
Faculty of Pharmacy
Integral University Lucknow
Lucknow, India

Mohammad Ahmad
Faculty of Pharmacy
Integral University Lucknow
Lucknow, India

Sohail Ahmad
Gomal Center of Biochemistry and Biotechnology
Gomal University
Dera Ismail Khan, Pakistan

Usama Ahmad
Faculty of Pharmacy
Integral University Lucknow
Lucknow, India

Md. Khokon Miah Akanda
Department of Pharmacy
University of Asia Pacific
Dhaka, Bangladesh

Juber Akhtar
Faculty of Pharmacy
Integral University Lucknow
Lucknow, India

Arthur Amule Anyole
Department of Pharmaceutical Sciences, Faculty of Medicine
Mbarara University of Science and Technology
Mbarara, Uganda

Yusuf Asad
Biomedical Engineering Program, Department of Electrical and Computer Engineering
North Dakota State University
Fargo, North Dakota

Sumel Ashique
Department of Pharmaceutical Sciences
Bengal College of Pharmaceutical Sciences & Research
Durgapur, India

Innocent Ayesiga
Ubora Foundation Africa
Kampala, Uganda

Muhammad Badar
Gomal Center of Biochemistry and Biotechnology
Gomal University
Dera Ismail Khan, Pakistan

Badruddeen
Faculty of Pharmacy
Integral University Lucknow
Lucknow, India

Mithun Bhowmick
Department of Pharmaceutical Sciences
Bengal College of Pharmaceutical Sciences & Research
Durgapur, India

Pratibha Bhowmick
Department of Pharmaceutical Sciences
Bengal College of Pharmaceutical Sciences & Research
Durgapur, India

Phool Chandra
Teerthanker Mahaveer College of Pharmacy
Teerthanker Mahaveer University
Moradabad, India

Hema Chaudhary
School of Medical & Allied Sciences
K.R. Mangalam University
Gurugram, India

Delafrique Deogratias
Department of Pharmaceutical Sciences, Faculty of Medicine
Mbarara University of Science and Technology
Mbarara, Uganda

Maria Faraz
Gomal Center of Biochemistry and Biotechnology
Gomal University
Dera Ismail Khan, Pakistan

Arshad Farid
Gomal Center of Biochemistry and Biotechnology
Gomal University
Dera Ismail Khan, Pakistan

Mohammad Abdul Faseeh
Department of Biopharmaceutics
Quest Vitamins, Middle East FZE, Dubai, United Arab Emirates

Sana Fatima
Gomal Center of Biochemistry and Biotechnology
Gomal University
Dera Ismail Khan, Pakistan

Nandani Goyal
Department of Nutrition and Nutraceutical
Dr Reddy`s Laboratories Limited
New Delhi, India

Prakash Chandra Gupta
School of Pharmaceutical Sciences
Chhatrapati Shahu Ji Maharaj University
Kalyanpur, India

Fazal Haq
Institute of Chemical Sciences
Gomal University
Dera Ismail Khan, Pakistan

Shabnoor Iqbal
Department of Pharmacology
University of the Free State
Bloemfontein, South Africa

Anas Islam
Faculty of Pharmacy
Integral University Lucknow
Lucknow, India

Aarzoo Jangra
Department of Food Technology
SRM University Delhi-NCR
Sonepat, India

Yash Jasoria
School of Medical & Allied Sciences
K.R. Mangalam University
Gurugram, India

Roomah Javed
Gomal Center of Biochemistry and Biotechnology
Gomal University
Dera Ismail Khan, Pakistan

Braize Ben Kagimu
Department of Pharmaceutical Sciences, Faculty of Medicine
Mbarara University of Science and Technology
Mbarara, Uganda

Ivan Kahwa
Department of Pharmacy, Faculty of Medicine
and
Pharm-Bio Technology and Traditional Medicine Centre of Excellence
Mbarara University of Science and Technology
Mbarara, Uganda

Monika Kaushik
Amity Institute of Pharmacy
Amity University Madhya Pradesh
Gwalior, India

Alamgir Khan
Gomal Center of Biochemistry and Biotechnology
Gomal University
Dera Ismail Khan, Pakistan

Mohammad Irfan Khan
Faculty of Pharmacy
Integral University Lucknow
Lucknow, India

Muhammad Ajmal Khan
School of Medicine
University of Maryland
Baltimore, Maryland

Muzammil Ahmad Khan
Gomal Center of Biochemistry and Biotechnology
Gomal University
Dera Ismail Khan, Pakistan

Akash Kumar
Department of Food Technology
SRM University Delhi-NCR
Sonepat, India

Ashok Kumar
Department of Internal Medicine
University of Kansas Medical Center
Kansas City, Kansas

Mukesh Kumar
Department of Food Technology
Guru Jambheshwar University of Science and Technology (GJUS&T)
Hisar, India

Sanjesh Kumar
Department of Pharmacology
Institute of Pharmaceutical Research, GLA University Mathura
Mathura, India

Yusuf Kyejjusa
Department of Chemistry and Biochemistry, Faculty of Science
Islamic University in Uganda
Mbale, Uganda
and
Department of Chemistry, Faculty of Science
University of Lahore
Lahore, Pakistan

Prathap Madeswaraguptha
Amity Institute of Pharmacy
Amity University Madhya Pradesh
Gwalior, India

Subhajit Mandal
Department of Pharmacology
P.G. Institute of Medical Sciences
Chandrakona, India

Sanzia Mehjabin
Department of Pharmacy
Varendra University
Rajshahi, Bangladesh

Popat Mohite
AETs St. John Institute of Pharmacy and Research
Palghar, India

Muhammad Muzammal
Gomal Center of Biochemistry and Biotechnology
Gomal University
Dera Ismail Khan, Pakistan

Shaista Naz
Gomal Center of Biochemistry and Biotechnology
Gomal University
Dera Ismail Khan, Pakistan

A. H. M. Nazmul Hasan
Department of Pharmacy
University of Asia Pacific
Dhaka, Bangladesh

Denis Odongo
Department of Pharmaceutical Sciences, Faculty of Medicine
Mbarara University of Science and Technology
Mbarara, Uganda

Joash Okoboi
Department of Biochemistry, School of Health Sciences
Soroti University
Soroti, Uganda

Timothy Omara
Department of Chemistry, College of Natural Sciences
Makerere University
Kampala, Uganda

Radheshyam Pal
Department of Pharmacology
Pandaveswar School of Pharmacy
Pandaveswar, India

G. M. Masud Parvez
Department of Pharmaceutical and Biomedical Sciences, College of Pharmacy
University of Georgia
Athens, Georgia

Kamla Pathak
Faculty of Pharmacy
Uttar Pradesh University of Medical Sciences
Saifai, India

Rashmi Pathak
Department of Pharmacy
Invertis University
Bareilly, India

Bhupender Prajapati
Shree S. K. Patel College of Pharmaceutical Education and Research
Ganpat University
Mehsana, India

Jhilam Pramanik
Department of Food Technology
William Carey University
Shillong, India

Abhijeet Puri
AETs St. John Institute of Pharmacy and Research
Palghar, India

Priyanka Ray
Department of Pharmaceutics, Guru Nanak Institute of Pharmaceutical Science & Technology
Sodepur, Kolkata, India

Neetu Sachan
Maharana Pratap College of Pharmacy
Mandhana Kanpur
Kanpur, India

Wasim Shah
Department of Life Science, University of Science and Technology of China
Anhui Province, China

Himanshu Sharma
Teerthanker Mahaveer College of Pharmacy
Teerthanker Mahaveer University
Moradabad, India

Nisha Sharma
School of Pharmaceutical Sciences
Chhatrapati Shahu Ji Maharaj University
Kalyanpur, India

Aditya Singh
Faculty of Pharmacy
Integral University Lucknow
Lucknow, India

Sudarshan Singh
Office of Research Administration
and
Department of Pharmaceutical Sciences, Faculty of Pharmacy
Chiang Mai University
Chiang Mai, Thailand

Bhagavathi Sundaram Sivamaruthi
Office of Research Administration
Chiang Mai University
Chiang Mai, Thailand
and
Innovation Centre for Holistic Health, Nutraceuticals, and Cosmeceuticals
Faculty of Pharmacy, Chiang Mai University
Chiang Mai, Thailand

Navaneetha Krishnan Subramaniyan
Department of Pharmaceutical Chemistry, Dr. Kalam College of Pharmacy
Thanjavur, India

Vijayaraj Surendran
Department of Pharmaceutical analysis, Dr. Kalam College of Pharmacy
Thanjavur, India

Farzad Taghizadeh-Hesary
ENT and Head and Neck Research Center and Department
The Five Senses Health Institute, School of Medicine, Iran University of Medical Sciences
Tehran, Iran
and
Clinical Oncology Department
Iran University of Medical Sciences
Tehran, Iran

Amin Ullah
Department of Health and Biological Sciences
Abasyn University Peshawar
Peshawar, Pakistan

Swarnakshi Upadhyay
School of Pharmaceutical Sciences
Chhatrapati Shahu Ji Maharaj University
Kalyanpur, India

Murugesan Vanangamudi
Amity Institute of Pharmacy
Amity University Madhya Pradesh
Gwalior, India

S. Venishaa
Department of Nanoscience and Technology
Bharathiar University
Coimbatore, India

About the Editors

Dr. Neeraj Mishra has been working as a Professor at Amity Institute of Pharmacy, Gwalior, since July 2019. He has around 20 years of teaching and research experience. He has more than 100 publications of international and national repute on recent concepts of novel drug delivery systems, oral delivery of synbiotics, localized drug delivery, and targeted and controlled drug delivery of nanocarriers and microparticles for the treatment of breast, colon, and neurodegenerative disorders. He has also edited 10 books and authored 25 book chapters. He has been granted three international patents and two Indian patents. Dr. Mishra is the recipient of the "Distinguished Professor Award" 2019 from DST-NSTMIS, SPAICS, Indore, and M.P. in September 2019. Dr. Mishra has also received the "Outstanding Scientist Award" 2020, 6th International Scientist Awards on Engineering, Science, and Medicine, 20–21 June 2020, Chennai, India. Dr. Mishra has received the "Distinguished Professor Award" 2021 from the Indian Pharmaceutical Association, MP State Branch, Indore. Dr. Mishra has received the "Best Academician Award" in the Indian Pharmacy Graduate Association, M.P. State International Conference held on May 6, 2023, at DAVV Auditorium, Indore, India.

Dr. Sumel Ashique has been working as an Assistant Professor at the Department of Pharmaceutical Sciences, Bengal College of Pharmaceutical Sciences & Research, Durgapur 713212, West Bengal, India. He has 3.5 years of teaching experience and has published more than 50 research studies and review articles in internationally and nationally accredited, reputed journals. He has been working in targeted drug delivery, nanotechnology, and gut microbiome. He has also been granted 5 patents from IP and Australia, and has authored more than 20 book chapters. He has edited 5 books under CRC Press, Springer, Wiley, and Taylor-Francis Publisher.

Dr. Arshad Farid is a distinguished academic and researcher with a prolific career spanning over 15 years in teaching and research. He is currently serving as an Assistant Professor in the Gomal Center of Biochemistry and Biotechnology at Gomal University, Pakistan. He completed his Ph.D. in Biotechnology from the Centre of Biotechnology and Microbiology (COBAM), University of Peshawar, Pakistan. His remarkable achievements have garnered him international recognition, as evidenced by his selection for the British Council-Charles Wallace Fellowship program for the academic year 2022–2023. In 2007, he was also awarded a prestigious scholarship to the University of Glasgow, UK, funded by the Higher Education Commission (HEC) of Pakistan. He has authored or co-authored more than 70 research papers and has been granted nine patents.

Dr. Ashish Garg obtained a B.Pharm. in 2011 and a M.Pharm. in 2013 from Guru Ramdas Khalsa Institute of Science and Technology, Pharmacy, Jabalpur, M.P., India. He has pursued his Ph.D. from SRK University, M.P. He has over 10 years of experience in both teaching and research. He has authored more than 100 research and review articles published in national and international journals of high repute. Additionally, he has edited ten books and been awarded three patents and one design patent. He is presently working as an Associate Professor in the Department of Pharmaceutics at Guru Ramdas Khalsa Institute of Science and Technology, Jabalpur, Madhya Pradesh, India.

1 An Introduction on Metabolic Disorders

Yash Jasoria, Mohit Agrawal, and Hema Chaudhary

1.1 INTRODUCTION

An imbalance in the body's distribution and metabolism of macronutrients, such as proteins, lipids, and carbs, is referred to as a metabolic disease. Metabolic disorders can arise when abnormal chemical interactions disturb the body's normal metabolic function. It can alternatively be described as an inherited single gene aberration, most of which are autosomal recessive. Weight gain, type 2 diabetes mellitus (T2DM), and inflammatory bowel disorders are among the metabolic conditions that are most prevalent globally. A genetic abnormality that results in an insufficient amount of an enzyme is known as an inherited metabolic disease. Inborn errors of metabolism are the term used to describe these disorders, of which there are several kinds. When the pancreas or liver are not functioning correctly, metabolic disorders can also arise (Zakir et al., 2022). Individuals who have problems with the metabolism of tiny molecules may first exhibit acute sickness. Every kid experiencing a sudden illness in which an underlying metabolic issue might be present should have basic laboratory testing completed. Slowly progressing encephalopathies and systemic symptoms are typically seen in patients with metabolic abnormalities affecting a whole organelle. A variety of bodily fluids include chemicals that can be utilized to assess the effectiveness of therapy as well as serve as indications of the existence and advancement of certain metabolic diseases (Guerrero et al., 2018). Genetics, dietary modifications, physical activity, and aging have all been connected to the current epidemics of metabolic diseases, which include obesity, T2DM, liver lipid problems, and metabolic syndrome. The prevalence of these metabolic disorders is rising quickly, but there is also strong evidence that other environmental variables could also be involved (Heindel et al., 2017).

1.2 LIST OF METABOLIC DISORDER

1.2.1 Obesity

There are health hazards linked to obesity. In adults, the prevalence of obesity was a little over 36% in 2011, whereas in children, it was 17%. In comparison to males (34.3%), women (38.3%) had a greater prevalence of obesity. There was no discernible sex difference among all the youngsters (Ogden et al., 2015). The hypothesis that exposure to environmental pollutants has a role in the rising prevalence of obesity, and diabetes has been the subject of much discussion. A symposium on the present level of knowledge on these important public health concerns was arranged by the NIEHS Division of the National Toxicology Program. Multiple exposures to the environment and T2DM were shown to be linked, according to an assessment of the body of research. Additionally, there was evidence for the "developmental obesogen" theory, which postulates that exposure to chemicals may change the way adipocytes differentiate or how brain circuits that control food behavior develop, hence raising the risk of obesity. The effects may be most evident if one follows a diet heavy in fat, carbs, or calories is followed later in life along with the growing exposure. There is relatively little data on the relationship between type 1 diabetes and exposure to environmental chemicals(Thayer et al., 2012). In the European Union (EU), diabetes and obesity are on the rise. It is becoming more widely acknowledged that endocrine-disrupting chemical (EDC) exposure has a role, separate and apart from physical exercise and nutrition (Legler et al., 2015). Numerous studies and acknowledgments indicate that throughout the last several decades, the prevalence of diabetes has grown in both low- and middle-income nations and high-income countries. Diabetes's global impact is unknown, especially in low- and middle-income nations (Seuring et al., 2015).

Mammalian populations have experienced significant and persistent increases in body weight, similar to what has happened to human populations. This is true even in the absence of the factors that are generally thought to be the main causes of the obesity epidemic in humans due to their effects on diet and physical activity (Klimentidis et al., 2011).

According to Trasande et al. (2012), there are many metabolic systems that bisphenol A exposure can affect. This implies that exposure to bisphenol A at levels relevant to the environment may cause an increase in body mass and consequently lead to obesity in humans. Adult studies have recently looked into this idea. The skyrocketing costs of health care associated with treating co-morbidities associated with obesity-related conditions include dyslipidemia, hyperglycemia, hypertension, liver and gallbladder disorders, insulin resistance, and T2DM (Legler et al., 2015). Obesity is also associated with neurological problems, cancer, and obstructive sleep apnea. Determining the causes of obesity has therefore grown to be a significant public health concern (Heindel et al., 2017).

DOI: 10.1201/9781032702438-1

1.2.2 Type 2 Diabetes

Diabetes is another form of metabolic disease, which is characterized by elevated blood sugar levels brought on by deficiencies in either or both of the actions or production of insulin. Long-term harm, malfunction, and failure of several organs, including the kidneys, eyes, nerves, heart, and blood vessels, are linked to diabetes's persistent hyperglycemia (American Diabetes Association, 2010). Some of the elements that lead to the decrease in insulin action known as insulin resistance include an increase in inflammatory signaling, the activation of endoplasmic reticulum (ER) stress pathways, and the direct damage that excess lipids and other metabolic fuels bring to organs and tissues. A metabolic component to the malfunctioning of β-cells observed in T2DM is addressed. The typical increase in pyruvate cycling caused by glucose is inhibited by excessive lipid exposure (Muoio and Newgard, 2008). Diabetes type 2 has been associated with several environmental exposures. Evidence was also presented in support of the "developmental obesogen" theory, which suggests that chemical exposure may change how the brain develops circuits that control eating habits or the differentiation of adipocytes, which raises the risk of obesity. During later life, the effects may be most apparent if a diet heavy in calories, carbohydrates, or fat is combined with the growing exposure (Thayer et al., 2012).

Diabetes is expected to affect 2.8% of people globally in 2000 and 4.4% of people globally in all age categories by 2030. Between 2000 and 2030, there were 171 million more people worldwide estimated to have diabetes. Although diabetes affects males more frequently than women, more women than men have the disorder. By 2000 and 2030, the number of people living in cities in emerging nations is expected to double. It appears that the rise in the percentage of adults over 65 is the most significant demographic shift affecting diabetes prevalence worldwide (Wild et al., 2004).

One of the main controllable risk factors for T2DM is obesity. Obesity and diabetes are linked to a higher risk of death, especially from cardiovascular disease (CVD). Increased rates of type II diabetes, dyslipidemia, hypertension, acid reflux disease, and several cancers have also been associated with being overweight. The high proportion of obese people with diabetes suggests that more should be done to reduce obesity because it can be changed to reduce the chance of developing diabetes. In addition to treating obesity medically and surgically, these initiatives should focus on obesity prevention. One of the biggest studies on purposeful weight loss among diabetes is the look AHEAD experiment (Nguyen et al., 2011).

1.2.3 NAFLD and Hyperlipidemia

The non-alcoholic fatty liver disease, or "NAFLD," refers to a buildup of fat in the liver that is not brought on by chronic liver disease or heavy alcohol consumption. Steatosis, fibrosis, and finally cirrhosis are the stages of this spectrum sickness that advance. One of the hallmarks of steatohepatitis is hepatocellular membrane damage and inflammation. Among young people, NAFLD is one of the most frequent causes of persistent liver disease (Anderson et al., 2015).

Clinically, dyslipidemia, hypertriglyceridemia, insulin resistance, high blood pressure, and/or T2DM are common in people with NAFLD, and they are all risk factors for CVDs. In actuality, NAFLD is rather common in people who have elements of MetS. More than 76% of people with T2DM, for example, have been observed to have NAFLD. Furthermore, NAFLD is present in more than 90% of individuals who are extremely obese and undergoing bariatric surgery. NAFLD patients have many risk factors for CVD, which makes CVD-related mortality one of the primary causes of death for these individuals. The incidence of NAFLD was determined using a selected group of studies that monitored healthy nondrinkers for the development of NAFLD at baseline but did not have NAFLD. We included longitudinal studies of NAFLD patients to evaluate the effects of hepatocellular carcinoma (HCV) on NAFLD outcomes, including liver-related mortality, cardiac mortality, and total mortality. Histological progression was determined using liver samples (Younossi et al., 2016).

1.2.4 Metabolic Syndrome

The metabolic syndrome is a group of metabolic disorders that includes insulin resistance, glucose intolerance, obesity, dyslipidemia, hypertension, and hyperinsulinemia (Dallongeville et al., 2004). More than one in four persons in the US suffers from the metabolic syndrome, which has become epidemically common in contemporary culture. More than 20 years ago, it was believed that insulin resistance was a major factor in the development of the metabolic syndrome. There has been a great deal of conversation about the part that insulin resistance plays in the metabolic syndrome. Atherosclerosis, cholesterol gallstones, and increased biliary cholesterol production can all result from insulin resistance alone, in addition to glucose intolerance. This contends that, contrary to what some experts have said, the metabolic syndrome is more than just a group of problems that need to be taken into account and managed separately. In actuality, the metabolic syndrome is a condition in which a common pathophysiological disturbance—insulin resistance—is the cause of many, but not all, of its components (Haas and Biddinger, 2009).

1.3 THE ROLE OF GENETICS IN METABOLIC DISORDERS

1.3.1 Role of Genetics Factors in Obesity

The "obesogenic environment" and alterations in lifestyle that have led to more availability to calories and less energy expenditure have been emphasized in the hunt for explanations of the current obesity pandemic. Long acknowledged are the genetic components of obesity, but genetics is also playing a bigger role in this relatively quick transformation in the population. Analysis of genetic components in unprecedented depth has been made possible by the technological revolution in genotyping that has coincided with the obesity pandemic. This includes examining the role of several genetic factors in more prevalent types of obesity, as well as single genes that cause unusual forms of the disease (Waalen, 2014). A genome-wide association research and a Metabochip meta-analysis of body mass index (BMI), a metric frequently used to quantify adiposity and define obesity in up to over 3 lakh individuals, were employed in an examination into the genetic foundations of obesity (Locke et al., 2015). As per Speliotes et al. (2010), 2.8 million single nucleotide polymorphisms (SNPs) in a maximum of 123,865 people were demonstrated to be associated with BMI, so serving as genetic markers for predisposition to obesity. Up to 125,931 more individuals had focused follow-up on 42 SNPs. identified 18 new loci ($P<5\times10^{-8}$) connected to BMI, one of which contains a copy number variation near GPRC5B, and verified the existence of 14 previously identified loci linked to obesity susceptibility. MC4R, POMC, SH2B1, BDNF, and other critical hypothalamic regulators of energy balance map in close proximity to the incretin receptor GIPR. Further insights into the regulation of body weight in humans may come from examining genes found in recently related loci.

Very few types of obesity are known to have single gene mutations or chromosomal abnormalities, such as those causing Prader–Willi and Bardet–Biedl syndromes. These types of obesity are often signs of genetic diseases. It is hypothesized that additional environmental variables might alter these genetic predispositions because many individuals who contain genetic variations associated to elevated BMI are not fat (Goldstone and Beales, 2008).

1.3.2 Role of Genetic Factors in Diabetes

Genetic factors influence diabetes type 1 and type 2. The highly polymorphic HLA class II genes that control the immune system are located in a region on chromosome 6 that accounts for more than half of the inherited susceptibility to insulin-dependent diabetes mellitus. Diabetes susceptibility and resistance are predicted by alleles of HLA-DQβ, according to an analysis of the DNA sequences of diabetics. Additionally, the autoimmune response to the islet cells that produce insulin is characterized by residue 57 of the β-chain, which is a component of the DQ molecule (Todd et al., 1987). For more than 30 years, clinical indicators, diabetes-associated autoantibodies, family history, and genetic risk factors have been used to describe people with T1D. More than 20 additional genetic variations linked to type 1 diabetes have been found through whole-genome research (Vehik et al., 2013).

More than 90% of cases of the illness are T2DM, which is rapidly increasing in both prevalence and incidence around the world. Diabetes type 2 is an incurable condition brought on by a confluence of hereditary and environmental factors. A significant genetic component to T2DM is also suggested by a wealth of research (Lyssenko and Laakso, 2013). According to the findings of twin studies, the heritability of T2D is thought to vary from 30% to 70%. Nearly 70 loci for T2D have been found by genome-wide association studies (GWASs) since the development of high-throughput genotyping methods. On the other hand, the impact of a single locus on T2D is quite small, and the heredity of T2D appears to be partially accounted for by all observed loci. Geneticists are becoming mystified about T2D, which was formerly referred to as their nightmare or headache. Investigative work is currently being done to try and unravel this riddle by finding unusual or low-frequency genetic variations with greater impacts. Another problem is that it is very impossible to connect genetic variations linked to disease pathogenesis since most genetic variants found by GWAS are found in non-coding areas of the genome (Hara et al., 2014).

1.3.3 Role of Genetic Factors in Lipid Disorder Metabolism

It is uncertain that both heredity and environment affect blood lipid levels. Age appears to have less of an impact on some blood lipids than on others due to hereditary variables. Though its impact on other blood lipids and apolipoproteins appears to be smaller in the elderly, early infancy seems to have a significant role in predicting total cholesterol levels later in life (Heller et al., 1993). It is uncertain how much heredity and environmental factors affect blood lipid levels. Age appears to have less of an impact on some blood lipids than on others due to hereditary variables. Though its impact on other blood lipids and apolipoproteins appears to be smaller in the elderly, early infancy seems to have a significant role in predicting total cholesterol levels later in life. A large-scale, nationally representative population-based sample survey was used to demonstrate the strong connections between blood lipids and the polymorphisms and haplotypes in ITGB3, PON1, and APOE across the three principal racial/ethnic groupings in the US population. Essential components that influence plasma lipoprotein concentrations may shed light on the molecular processes controlling blood lipid and cholesterol levels (Chang et al., 2010).

A deficiency in low-density lipoprotein receptor (LDLR) endocytosis unique to a particular cell type is the hallmark of autosomal recessive hypercholesterolemia. Individuals with this illness have decreased liver LDLR-mediated absorption of low-density lipoproteins (LDL), but normal fibroblast function is unaffected (Garuti et al., 2005).

Dyslipidemia is a clinical condition commonly observed as the primary risk factor for cardiovascular ailments. Dyslipidemias have a substantial hereditary component, even though secondary variables may contribute to their clinical presentation. The genes encoding for proteins that interact with the LDLR, such as APOB, PCSK9, and

LDLRAP1, as well as the gene for the receptor itself, are commonly responsible for familial hypercholesterolemia (Ramasamy, 2016).

Abnormally low levels of lipoproteins containing apolipoprotein-B (apoB) are the hallmark of the autosomal dominant disorder familial hypobetalipoproteinemia (FHBL). Chromosomes 10 and 3p21 include loci linked to FHBL, or it can result from mutations in APOB, PCSK9, or ANGPTL3. There should be additional genes involved, though. The apoB-containing lipoproteins' kinetic characteristics and the PCSK9 and APOB genes' aberrant sequences were found in FHBL patients at a sizable hospital. While the other two showed lower rates, three individuals showed greater rates of apoB production, both synthetically and catabolically. PCSK9 (R46L, A53V, I474V, D480N*, and E498K*) and apoB (N441D*, Y1395C, P2712L, D2285E*, I2286V, T3540S*, and T3799M*) genes showed a large number of polymorphisms, some of which had not been previously described, in the FHBL patients. Hepatic ultrasonography changes in just one of the four probands were indicative of hepatic steatosis. In short, from a metabolic and genetic standpoint, FHBL in the absence of shortened apoB is a diverse illness. Although it is not a necessary cause of steatosis, hypobetalipoproteinemia is a risk factor (Gutiérrez-Cirlos et al., 2016).

1.3.4 Role of Genetic Factors in NAFLD

Inadequate lipid management by hepatocytes induces fibrogenesis, carcinogenesis, and inflammation, which largely contribute to the pathogenesis of NAFLD. Epidemiological, familial, and twin studies have demonstrated strong heritability for NAFLD, which is presently the most prevalent cause of liver damage in wealthy countries. The primary genetic factor influencing the amount of fat in the liver is the ubiquitous PNPLA3 variation I148M, which inhibits the remodeling of hepatocellular lipid droplets (Dongiovanni and Valenti, 2016). African Americans, who have the lowest risk of NAFLD, have an allele of PNPLA3 that has been linked to a reduced hepatic fat level. Therefore, polymorphism in PNPLA3 is linked to interindividual and ancestry-related variations in hepatic fat accumulation and NAFLD susceptibility (Romeo et al., 2008). Hepatic fat buildup, which is typically linked to systemic insulin resistance, is one of the primary features of NAFLD. NAFLD can deteriorate in the presence of NASH and ultimately result in cirrhosis and HCV. The way that NAFLD progresses and becomes vulnerable is mostly determined by genes. The primary two genes responsible for interindividual variations in hepatic steatosis and susceptibility to progressive NASH are now PNPLA3 I148M and TM6SF2 E167K (Dongiovanni et al., 2015).

1.4 A REVIEW OF THE HORMONES AND TISSUES THAT REGULATE METABOLISM

Obesity, which is on the rise, has been related to a number of factors, including genetics, hypothalamic malfunction, intestinal gut flora, and a rise in the consumption of high-energy meals. Heart attacks, high blood pressure, T2DM, and a number of malignancies are all made more likely by obesity. Failure of the homeostatic processes that control hunger, food intake, and energy balance may result in the consumption of a calorie-dense diet that causes and maintains obesity. The bacteria in the stomach that aids in food digestion and the hypothalamus, which regulates energy requirements, hunger, and fullness, are the primary causes of obesity development. Insulin secretion, glucose homeostasis, insulin regulation, and the pathobiology of obesity and T2DM are all influenced by a wide range of factors, including cholecystokinin, leptin, brain-derived neurotrophic factor, long-chain fatty acid coenzyme A, endocannabinoids, and the vagal neurotransmitter acetylcholine. As a result, interactions occur between the hypothalamus, pancreas, liver, and stomach. It is evident from these data that managing obesity necessitates a multifaceted strategy (Das, 2010). The only proven treatment for obesity at this time that can help people permanently lose weight is bariatric surgery. On the other hand, weight increase typically occurs after pharmaceutical treatments for obesity. While the precise processes underlying sustained weight reduction after bariatric surgery are still being investigated, certain gut hormones have been linked to the phenomenon. In order to assist the CNS manage food intake, gut hormones filter information about nutrition and energy status that is sent from the stomach to it. Glucagon-like peptide-1, pancreatic polypeptide, oxyntomodulin, cholecystokinin, peptide YY, and pancreatic polypeptide all reduce hunger in different but complementary ways, whereas ghrelin increases food intake (Suzuki et al., 2011).

Endocrine-immune interactions play a critical role in a reciprocal regulatory system that, when obese, produces an increasingly vicious cycle that promotes chronic adipose inflammation and metabolic dysfunction, in the lean state adopting a "virtuous cycle" with an anti-inflammatory "flavor." The complex structure of this tissue is highlighted by studies demonstrating both gain and loss of function, which implicate many leukocyte subpopulations in the etiology of WAT inflammation associated with obesity (Exley et al., 2014).

Ghrelin, a hormone produced by peripheral sources, could have a crucial part in the complex relationship between stress, mood, and food intake. Research is gradually elucidating the neural circuitry behind this interaction. More and more research are showing a link between environmental risk factors like obesity and mental illnesses including stress, anxiety, and depression. The only orexigenic hormone that is known to promote appetite from the periphery is ghrelin. Stress-induced food reward behavior has been linked to elevated plasma ghrelin levels, and ghrelin may have a significant function in this process. Additionally, it has been shown time and time again that atypical sadness or chronic stress is associated with a higher consumption of calorie-dense "comfort foods," which is one of the main causes of the rising obesity incidence (Schellekens et al., 2012). The endocannabinoid system's primary role is to modulate food reward. The endocannabinoid system in the brain is an electrical signaling pathway made up of endogenous ligands for cannabinoid receptors. Endocannabinoid action drives up appetite and promotes energy storage as fat in adipose tissue via improving palatability. Both "wanting" and "liking," which are often referred to as appetitive (orienting toward food) and consummatory (hedonic appraisal of food after consumption), are components of food reward (Jager and Witkamp, 2014).

According to Volkow et al. (2013), there are some similarities between drug addiction and fat. Both diseases may be characterized as ones in which the importance of a certain kind of reward (drugs or food) is overemphasized in comparison to other rewards, and even higher than it should be. Many brain functions, including insult motivation, conditioning, self-control, stress reactivity, and interoceptive awareness, are impacted by disrupted dopaminergic pathways in obese and drug-addicted individuals.

1.5 ROLE OF OXIDATIVE STRESS IN METABOLIC DISORDERS

Metabolic disorders have been associated with dyslipidemia, insulin refractoriness, insufficient insulin production, glucose intolerance, and chronic inflammation, in additional to causing improper cellular physiology and cellular redox imbalance. Numerous diseases, such as diabetes, arthritis, cancer, and cardiovascular problems (as seen in Figure 1.1), are significantly more likely to occur in an environment with high oxidation. The body's chronic inflammatory status is also influenced by it. By activating redox signaling pathways and changing the gene expression of inflammatory markers, the elevated oxidative stress (OS) associated with obesity and metabolic disorders can exacerbate and prolong inflammatory conditions, resulting in a vicious cycle (Yadav et al., 2016). However, a number of research indicate that OS and chronic inflammatory diseases occur before metabolic problems, while their consistency varies. OS is characterized by an overabundance of reactive oxygen species (ROS) and oxidative free radicals, which are the outcome of an imbalance between the oxidative and anti-oxidative systems of cells and tissues. Overexposure to ROS can cause cellular dysfunction, energy metabolism loss, altered cell signaling and cell cycle regulation, decreased biological activity, immune activation, and inflammation. Generic mutations, cellular transport mechanisms, proteins, lipids, and nucleic acids are among the targets of ROS attack. Moreover, signs of nutritional stress, such as those caused by a high-fat, high-carb diet, include elevated lipid peroxidation products, protein carbonylation, a compromised antioxidant system, and lowered glutathione (GSH) levels. Numerous chronic medical conditions emerge as a result of these alterations, which initiate a pathogenic environment (Rani et al., 2016).

Pregnancy-related metabolic illnesses, such as hypertensive disorders of pregnancy (HDP) and gestational diabetes mellitus (GDM), are leading causes of morbidity and death in both expectant mothers and infants. The types of hypertensive disorders that occur during pregnancy include hemolysis, increased liver enzymes, low platelet count (HELLP), white hypertension, mask hypertension, chronic hypertension, and preeclampsia (PE). Although the cause of HDP is yet unclear, one of the key pathophysiological mechanisms of the illness is thought to be OS. Many research works have linked OS to high blood pressure. The development of hypertension is caused by blood vessel constriction resulting from an imbalance of ROS in the vascular walls. Chronic dopaminergic disorders (HDP) and GDM are likewise linked to OS (Phoswa and Khaliq, 2021).

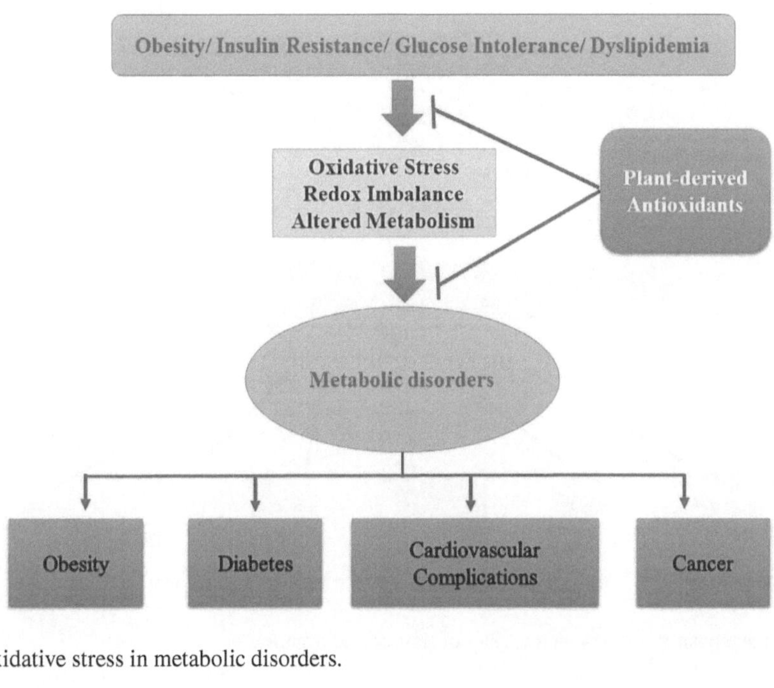

FIGURE 1.1 Role of oxidative stress in metabolic disorders.

Metabolic diseases are linked to a process that causes oxidation of LDL. OS can occur in lipoproteins for several causes. T2DM and high blood pressure are linked to this set of risk factors, even if the syndrome's notion is hotly contested. Numerous metabolic illnesses have been revealed to be significantly influenced by insulin resistance. Atherosclerosis and T2DM are associated with an increased risk of lipid profile abnormalities, such as increased susceptibility to lipid peroxidation (Manzoor et al., 2022).

Bone and mineral metabolism changes as a result of diabetes mellitus. Bone fractures are more common in diabetic bone disease, which also lowers quality of life and prolongs fracture recovery. Not all of the best treatments are available for these conditions, and it's unclear what pathways lead to their consequences. An elevated level of OS can lead to diabetic osteopenia (Hamada et al., 2009).

1.6 THERAPEUTIC MANAGEMENT OF METABOLIC DISORDERS

Growing research over the last 10 years has shown that one of the key factors influencing metabolic diseases including T2DM and obesity is the gut flora. The bacterial composition of the body can be significantly altered (dysbiosis) by an obesity-causing diet. This can lead to pro-inflammatory pathways and metabolic endotoxemia, which can ultimately induce insulin resistance and cardiometabolic diseases. Through many methods, including direct effects on the mucosal barrier and surrounding cells, probiotic supplementation may be beneficial in the prevention and treatment of obesity, inflammation, and other related metabolic diseases. These actions may particularly limit chronic inflammation (Le Barz et al., 2015). Possible effects on the host that may result from the cell walls, metabolites, and/or postbiotics of probiotics, including immunomodulation, antioxidant defense, anti-obesogenic effects, hypocholesterolemia, antidiabetic effects, and anti-inflammatory properties. Additionally, it has positive effects on a variety of tissues and organs shown in Figure 1.2. In order to manage inflammatory, obesity, T2DM, and OS-associated disorders, probiotics and their metabolites, and/or cell-wall components, known as postbiotics, have undeniable beneficial effects and should be investigated as biotherapeutic approaches. This would provide a safe alternative to chemical drug treatment (Bourebaba et al., 2022).

An evolutionary conserved regulatory signal integrator that monitors the energy state of cells and systems is serine/threonine protein kinase, also known as AMP-activated protein kinase (AMPK). This definition results from recent research on both people and animals. One "fuel gauge" that has been proposed to track cellular energy levels in response to food and environmental changes is AMPK. Deviations in metabolism, potentially involving AMPK, might be one reason for the emergence of the metabolic syndrome.

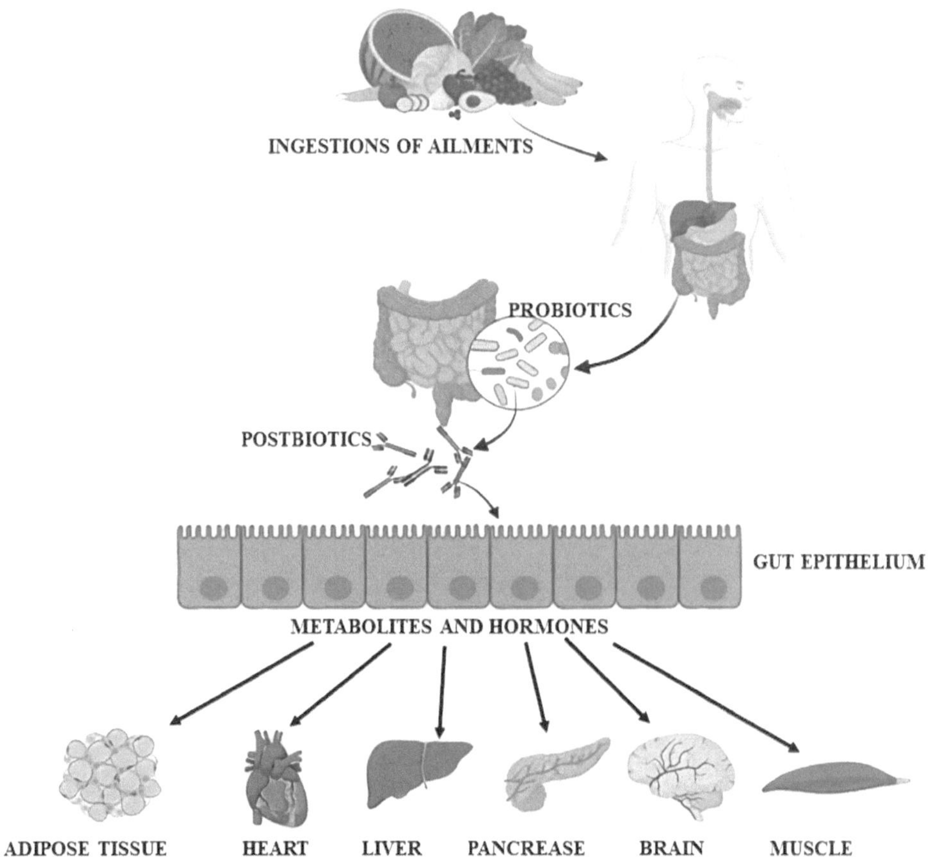

FIGURE 1.2 Probiotics have positive effects on a variety of tissues and organs.

Map all the regulatory components of the AMPK signaling pathway, pinpoint its regulatory activities, and elucidate the functional integration of this system with other intracellular pathways and cellular actions through more studies employing direct and selective AMPK activators (Viollet et al., 2007). Patients with hereditary metabolic abnormalities are becoming more common as they approach maturity as a result of improved treatments and neonatal screening programs. Treatment for many of these conditions mostly consists of dietary therapy; thus, skilled metabolic dietitians are essential components of the multidisciplinary team needed to manage these patients. A thorough monitoring of the intake of micronutrients and macronutrients throughout life is necessary for this type of therapy, which is necessary for infancy, youth, and maturity (Boyer et al., 2015).

Alginates are naturally occurring substances that are obtained from marine brown algae. They have long been widely utilized as food industry components and additives. However, because of their characteristics, which include their nontoxicity, biodegradability, biocompatibility, and functional flexibility with a range of matrices and substrates. Since products for the treatment of metabolic diseases including diabetes and obesity have been developed, the usage of alginates has increased significantly. Alginate has been thoroughly investigated as an antidiabetic and as a drug delivery mechanism in addition to its significance in regulating food intake and obesity (Gheorghita Puscaselu et al., 2020). While there is evidence that gut bacteria have a role in the pathogenesis of metabolic illnesses, including obesity and diabetes mellitus, it is important to acknowledge that this is an attractive therapeutic target. Numerous variables, such as genetics, consuming foods high in energy, and engaging in little or no physical exercise, might contribute to metabolic conditions. In light of this, if gut microbiota modification is effective, it may potentially support existing therapies for metabolic disorders (Erejuwa et al., 2014). A lot of focus has been placed on the gut microbiota's role in metabolic disorders. Many plants have phytochemicals with specific microbicidal action that can change the ratio of Bacteroidetes to Firmicutes, which has favorable impacts on health. Furthermore, beneficial prebiotic effects may be derived from nondigestible fibers and phytochemicals like polyphenols found in some plants. It is essential to address the impact of metabolic disease on healthcare delivery by focusing on the development of innovative plant-derived medications, since this has great potential for managing the disease (Nyakudya et al., 2020).

The most prevalent pathophysiologies associated with metabolic illnesses are epigenetic modifications, Nrf2 pathways, OS, and changes in miRNA expression. Growing enthusiasm for using phytotherapy as an alternative to synthetic medications for treatment. Natural products are still a good source for discovering novel drugs, as seen by the vast number of substances produced from them, including flavonoids, saponins, alkaloids, coumarins, essential oils, and resins, that are presently doing clinical studies (Tabatabaei-Malazy et al., 2015).

1.7 CONCLUSION AND FUTURE PROSPECTS

Diabetes mellitus, obesity, dyslipidemia, osteoporosis, and metabolic syndrome are the most prevalent metabolic illnesses, which result from abnormalities in normal metabolic processes. The serious adverse effects of certain synthetic drugs, their expensive price, their inability to be safe or affordable in some circumstances, and their restricted access for the general public make it challenging to prevent and cure metabolic diseases. Although there is not yet enough evidence to substantiate this claim, a rising corpus of research is beginning to indicate the possible therapeutic benefits of plants over manufactured medications. To further understand the involved signaling pathways driving the reported effects, more comprehensive study is required. Unquestionably beneficial, postbiotics and naturally occurring phytochemicals have to be researched as biotherapeutic strategies for treating conditions linked to inflammation, OS, obesity, and T2DM. These methods provide a secure substitute for chemical medication therapy.

REFERENCES

American Diabetes Association. (2010). Diagnosis and classification of diabetes mellitus. *Diabetes Care*, *33*(Supplement_1), S62–S69.

Anderson, E. L., Howe, L. D., Jones, H. E., Higgins, J. P., Lawlor, D. A., & Fraser, A. (2015). The prevalence of non-alcoholic fatty liver disease in children and adolescents: a systematic review and meta-analysis. *PloS One*, *10*(10), e0140908.

Bourebaba, Y., Marycz, K., Mularczyk, M., & Bourebaba, L. (2022). Postbiotics as potential new therapeutic agents for metabolic disorders management. *Biomedicine & Pharmacotherapy*, *153*, 113138.

Boyer, S. W., Barclay, L. J., & Burrage, L. C. (2015). Inherited metabolic disorders: aspects of chronic nutrition management. *Nutrition in Clinical Practice*, *30*(4), 502–510.

Chang, M. H., Yesupriya, A., Ned, R. M., Mueller, P. W., & Dowling, N. F. (2010). Genetic variants associated with fasting blood lipids in the US population: Third National Health and Nutrition Examination Survey. *BMC Medical Genetics*, *11*(1), 1–13.

Dallongeville, J., Cottel, D., Arveiler, D., Tauber, J. P., Bingham, A., Wagner, A., ... & Amouyel, P. (2004). The association of metabolic disorders with the metabolic syndrome is different in men and women. *Annals of Nutrition and Metabolism*, *48*(1), 43–50.

Das, U. N. (2010). Obesity: genes, brain, gut, and environment. *Nutrition*, *26*(5), 459–473.

Dongiovanni, P., Romeo, S., & Valenti, L. (2015). Genetic factors in the pathogenesis of nonalcoholic fatty liver and steatohepatitis. *BioMed Research International*, 2015, 460190.

Dongiovanni, P., & Valenti, L. (2016). Genetics of nonalcoholic fatty liver disease. *Metabolism*, *65*(8), 1026–1037.

Erejuwa, O. O., Sulaiman, S. A., & AbWahab, M. S. (2014). Modulation of gut microbiota in the management of metabolic disorders: the prospects and challenges. *International Journal of Molecular Sciences*, *15*(3), 4158–4188.

Exley, M. A., Hand, L., O'Shea, D., & Lynch, L. (2014). Interplay between the immune system and adipose tissue in obesity. *Journal of Endocrinology*, *223*(2), R41–R48.

Garuti, R., Jones, C., Li, W. P., Michaely, P., Herz, J., Gerard, R. D., ... & Hobbs, H. H. (2005). The modular adaptor protein autosomal recessive hypercholesterolemia (ARH) promotes low density lipoprotein receptor clustering into clathrin-coated pits. *Journal of Biological Chemistry*, *280*(49), 40996–41004.

Gheorghita Puscaselu, R., Lobiuc, A., Dimian, M., & Covasa, M. (2020). Alginate: from food industry to biomedical applications and management of metabolic disorders. *Polymers*, *12*(10), 2417.

Goldstone, A. P., & Beales, P. L. (2008). Genetic obesity syndromes. *Obesity and Metabolism*, *36*, 37–60.

Guerrero, R. B., Salazar, D., & Tanpaiboon, P. (2018). Laboratory diagnostic approaches in metabolic disorders. *Annals of Translational Medicine*, *6*(24), 470.

Gutiérrez-Cirlos, C., Ordóñez-Sánchez, M. L., Tusié-Luna, M. T., Patterson, B. W., Schonfeld, G., & Aguilar-Salinas, C. A. (2016). Familial hypobetalipoproteinemia in a hospital survey: genetics, metabolism and non-alcoholic fatty liver disease. *Annals of Hepatology*, *10*(2), 155–164.

Haas, J. T., & Biddinger, S. B. (2009). Dissecting the role of insulin resistance in the metabolic syndrome. *Current Opinion in Lipidology*, *20*(3), 206.

Hamada, Y., Fujii, H., & Fukagawa, M. (2009). Role of oxidative stress in diabetic bone disorder. *Bone*, *45*, S35–S38.

Hara, K., Shojima, N., Hosoe, J., & Kadowaki, T. (2014). Genetic architecture of type 2 diabetes. *Biochemical and Biophysical Research Communications*, *452*(2), 213–220.

Heindel, J. J., Blumberg, B., Cave, M., Machtinger, R., Mantovani, A., Mendez, M. A., ... & VomSaal, F. (2017). Metabolism disrupting chemicals and metabolic disorders. *Reproductive Toxicology*, *68*, 3–33.

Heller, D. A., de Faire, U., Pedersen, N. L., Dahlen, G., & McClearn, G. E. (1993). Genetic and environmental influences on serum lipid levels in twins. *New England Journal of Medicine*, *328*(16), 1150–1156.

Jager, G., & Witkamp, R. F. (2014). The endocannabinoid system and appetite: relevance for food reward. *Nutrition Research Reviews*, *27*(1), 172–185.

Klimentidis, Y. C., Beasley, T. M., Lin, H. Y., Murati, G., Glass, G. E., Guyton, M., ... & Allison, D. B. (2011). Canaries in the coal mine: a cross-species analysis of the plurality of obesity epidemics. *Proceedings of the Royal Society B: Biological Sciences*, *278*(1712), 1626–1632.

Le Barz, M., Anhê, F. F., Varin, T. V., Desjardins, Y., Levy, E., Roy, D., ... & Marette, A. (2015). Probiotics as complementary treatment for metabolic disorders. *Diabetes & Metabolism Journal*, *39*(4), 291–303.

Legler, J., Fletcher, T., Govarts, E., Porta, M., Blumberg, B., Heindel, J. J., & Trasande, L. (2015). Obesity, diabetes, and associated costs of exposure to endocrine-disrupting chemicals in the European Union. *The Journal of Clinical Endocrinology & Metabolism*, *100*(4), 1278–1288.

Locke, A. E., Kahali, B., Berndt, S. I., Justice, A. E., Pers, T. H., Day, F. R., ... & Lindström, J. (2015). Genetic studies of body mass index yield new insights for obesity biology. *Nature*, *518*(7538), 197–206.

Lyssenko, V., & Laakso, M. (2013). Genetic screening for the risk of type 2 diabetes: worthless or valuable? *Diabetes Care*, *36*(Suppl 2), S120.

Manzoor, M. F., Arif, Z., Kabir, A., Mehmood, I., Munir, D., Razzaq, A., ... & Rusu, A. (2022). Oxidative stress and metabolic diseases: relevance and therapeutic strategies. *Frontiers in Nutrition*, *9*, 994309.

Muoio, D. M., & Newgard, C. B. (2008). Molecular and metabolic mechanisms of insulin resistance and β-cell failure in type 2 diabetes. *Nature Reviews Molecular Cell Biology*, *9*(3), 193–205.

Nguyen, N. T., Nguyen, X. M. T., Lane, J., & Wang, P. (2011). Relationship between obesity and diabetes in a US adult population: findings from the National Health and Nutrition Examination Survey, 1999-2006. *Obesity Surgery*, *21*, 351–355.

Nyakudya, T. T., Tshabalala, T., Dangarembizi, R., Erlwanger, K. H., & Ndhlala, A. R. (2020). The potential therapeutic value of medicinal plants in the management of metabolic disorders. *Molecules*, *25*(11), 2669.

Ogden, C. L., Carroll, M. D., Fryar, C. D., & Flegal, K. M. (2015). Prevalence of obesity among adults and youth: United States, 2011-2014.*2015*, 1–8.

Phoswa, W. N., & Khaliq, O. P. (2021). The role of oxidative stress in hypertensive disorders of pregnancy (preeclampsia, gestational hypertension) and metabolic disorder of pregnancy (gestational diabetes mellitus). *Oxidative Medicine and Cellular Longevity*, *2021*, 1–10.

Ramasamy, I. (2016). Update on the molecular biology of dyslipidemias. *Clinicachimicaacta*, *454*, 143–185.

Rani, V., Deep, G., Singh, R. K., Palle, K., & Yadav, U. C. (2016). Oxidative stress and metabolic disorders: pathogenesis and therapeutic strategies. *Life Sciences*, *148*, 183–193.

Romeo, S., Kozlitina, J., Xing, C., Pertsemlidis, A., Cox, D., Pennacchio, L. A., ... & Hobbs, H. H. (2008). Genetic variation in PNPLA3 confers susceptibility to nonalcoholic fatty liver disease. *Nature Genetics*, *40*(12), 1461–1465.

Schellekens, H., Finger, B. C., Dinan, T. G., & Cryan, J. F. (2012). Ghrelin signalling and obesity: at the interface of stress, mood and food reward. *Pharmacology & Therapeutics*, *135*(3), 316–326.

Seuring, T., Archangelidi, O., & Suhrcke, M. (2015). The economic costs of type 2 diabetes: a global systematic review. *Pharmacoeconomics*, *33*, 811–831.

Speliotes, E. K., Willer, C. J., Berndt, S. I., Monda, K. L., Thorleifsson, G., Jackson, A. U., ... & Homuth, G. (2010). Association analyses of 249,796 individuals reveal 18 new loci associated with body mass index. *Nature Genetics*, *42*(11), 937–948.

Suzuki, K., Jayasena, C. N., & Bloom, S. R. (2011). The gut hormones in appetite regulation. *Journal of Obesity*, 2011, 528401.

Tabatabaei-Malazy, O., Larijani, B., & Abdollahi, M. (2015). Targeting metabolic disorders by natural products. *Journal of Diabetes & Metabolic Disorders*, *14*, 1–21.

Thayer, K. A., Heindel, J. J., Bucher, J. R., & Gallo, M. A. (2012). Role of environmental chemicals in diabetes and obesity: a National Toxicology Program workshop review. *Environmental Health Perspectives*, *120*(6), 779–789.

Todd, J. A., Bell, J. I., & McDevitt, H. O. (1987). HLA-DQ β gene contributes to susceptibility and resistance to insulin-dependent diabetes mellitus. *Nature*, *329*(6140), 599–604.

Trasande, L., Attina, T. M., & Blustein, J. (2012). Association between urinary bisphenol A concentration and obesity prevalence in children and adolescents. *JAMA*, *308*(11), 1113–1121.

Vehik, K., Ajami, N. J., Hadley, D., Petrosino, J. F., & Burkhardt, B. R. (2013). The changing landscape of type 1 diabetes: recent developments and future frontiers. *Current Diabetes Reports*, *13*, 642–650.

Viollet, B., Mounier, R., Leclerc, J., Yazigi, A., Foretz, M., & Andreelli, F. (2007). Targeting AMP-activated protein kinase as a novel therapeutic approach for the treatment of metabolic disorders. *Diabetes & Metabolism*, *33*(6), 395–402.

Volkow, N. D., Wang, G. J., Tomasi, D., & Baler, R. D. (2013). Obesity and addiction: neurobiological overlaps. *Obesity Reviews*, *14*(1), 2–18.

Waalen, J. (2014). The genetics of human obesity. *Translational Research*, *164*(4), 293–301.

Wild, S., Roglic, G., Green, A., Sicree, R., & King, H. (2004). Global prevalence of diabetes: estimates for the year 2000 and projections for 2030. *Diabetes Care*, *27*(5), 1047–1053.

Yadav, U., Rani, V., Deep, G., Singh, R. K., & Palle, K. (2016). Oxidative stress in metabolic disorders: pathogenesis, prevention, and therapeutics. *Oxidative Medicine and Cellular Longevity*, *148,* 183–193.

Younossi, Z. M., Koenig, A. B., Abdelatif, D., Fazel, Y., Henry, L., & Wymer, M. (2016). Global epidemiology of nonalcoholic fatty liver disease-meta-analytic assessment of prevalence, incidence, and outcomes. *Hepatology*, *64*(1), 73–84.

Zakir, F., Mohapatra, S., Farooq, U., Mirza, M. A., & Iqbal, Z. (2022). Introduction to metabolic disorders. In *Drug Delivery Systems for Metabolic Disorders* (pp. 1–20). Academic Press.

2 Targeting Signaling Pathway and Mechanism of Prebiotics, Probiotics, and Synbiotics to Manage Metabolic Disorders

Monika Kaushik, Prathap Madeswaraguptha, Murugesan Vanangamudi, Vijayaraj Surendran, Navaneetha Krishnan Subramaniyan, and Ashok Kumar

2.1 INTRODUCTION

The fast emergence of metabolic disorders (MS) in recent years can be attributed to considerable changes in our lifestyle and dietary habits brought about by improvements in quality of life (QoL) and rapid economic growth. The word "metabolic syndrome" mentions to a group of metabolic diseases that include obesity, non-alcoholic fatty liver disease (NAFLD), diabetes mellitus, insulin resistance, inflammation, dyslipidemia, hypertension, hyperglycemia, oxidative stress, and neurodegeneration. Metabolic disorders are associated with gut microbiota and pose a significant risk to public health (Larsen et al., 2022). Due to their potent ability to regulate gut microbiota, probiotics, prebiotics, synbiotics, and postbiotics may be able to prevent metabolic disorders. While their metabolites, identified as postbiotics and these microbes secrete, can be extremely important as antimicrobials against a wide range of pathogenic bacteria, probiotics are known to promote health through stimulating native gut microbiota, host immunity, cholesterol reduction, and numerous other roles. Prebiotics are substrates that host bacteria specifically use to provide health benefits. Probiotics and prebiotics are carefully chosen to form synbiotics, which work together to promote health (da Silva et al., 2021; Yadav et al., 2022). The word "probiotic" refers to "living microbes that, when directed in acceptable amounts, provide a health advantage to the host," according to a consensus statement provided by the International Scientific Association for Probiotics and Prebiotics (ISAPP). The Canadian Public Health Agency and the Italian Health Ministry recommend consuming 1×109 colony forming units (CFUs) per meal on a daily basis. One of the main benefits of probiotics, according to Canada and Italy, is their ability to sustain a healthy gut flora. However, several nations classify probiotic strains under different headings in their laws. For example, in the USA, probiotics are classified as biological agents, dietary complements, medicinal foodstuffs, pharmaceuticals, and alive biotherapeutic agents as anticipated use; in Canada, probiotics are classified as natural health products; in Belgium and Germany, they are classified as biotherapeutic/pharmaceuticals; in Finland, Denmark, and Sweden, they are classified as food supplements; and in far-flung Asian nations like Japan, China, and Malaysia, they are classified as functional foods (Xavier-Santos et al., 2020). It is currently believed that the gut microbiota affects several host processes and is involved in the regulation of numerous physiological pathways. Probiotics' actions have been explained by four major methods. The first method involves elevating SCFAs generated from bacteria, which causes L cells to express GPR-43 and secrete GLP-1 and GLP-2. These hormones have a widespread variety of effects on metabolism plus cell division. The second process involves a rise in BSH activity. The physiological processes of the host are influenced by bacterial bile salt hydrolase (BSH) enzymes in the gut, which lowers plasma cholesterol levels and prevents weight gain. Using the anti-inflammatory properties of probiotics to ameliorate steatosis, insulin sensitivity, glucose intolerance, and low-grade inflammation is the third method. Adipogenesis normalization and energy homeostasis management are affected by the fourth pathway, which is the downregulation of eCB system receptiveness. Modulation of serum lipids, plasma glucose, appetite, and pro-inflammatory cytokines by the gut microbiota has been demonstrated. Furthermore, the commonly used probiotics and prebiotics that alter the microbiota can lower low-grade gut inflammation and strengthen the reliability of the gut barrier, which lowers serum lipid and plasma glucose levels, promotes weight reduction, and lessens insulin resistance. (Halloran and Underwood, 2019; Latif et al., 2023; Li et al., 2021a) The correlation between probiotics, prebiotics, synbiotics, postbiotics, and metabolic diseases is thoroughly summarized in this book chapter. Both positive and controversial results are presented, and special attention is given to illuminating probable mechanisms and therapeutic effects that may aid in future Probiotics, prebiotics, synbiotics, and postbiotics (PPSP) research and development.

DOI: 10.1201/9781032702438-2

2.2 METABOLIC DISORDERS: AN OVERVIEW

Metabolic disorders encompass a diverse group of medical conditions that disrupt the normal processes of energy production, storage, and utilization within the human body. These disorders can manifest in various ways, from childhood onset to adulthood, and their effects can range from mild inconveniences to life-threatening complications (Yeoh et al., 2019). They are often the result of genetic mutations that interfere with enzymes, hormones, or other essential molecules responsible for maintaining metabolic balance. One of the most well-known metabolic disorders is diabetes mellitus, which affects billions of people globally. In diabetes, the body struggles to regulate blood sugar levels properly. Type 1 diabetes is an autoimmune disease in which the immune system erroneously assaults and kills insulin-producing cells in the pancreas, leading to a lifelong dependence on insulin injections for glucose regulation. Conversely, type 2 diabetes generally manifests in adulthood and is marked by insulin resistance, a condition in which the body's cells fail to respond efficiently to insulin (Rathod, 2022). Diet, physical activity, and obesity are all lifestyle variables that contribute to the development of type 2 diabetes.

Another group of metabolic disorders includes lysosomal storage diseases (LSDs) (Stephens et al., 2020), such as Gaucher disease and Tay–Sachs disease. LSDs result from the buildup of specific substances in the lysosomes, the cell's recycling centers. These substances accumulate due to genetic defects in enzymes responsible for their breakdown. Gaucher disease, for example, causes the accumulation of a fatty substance called glucocerebroside, leading to symptoms such as an enlarged spleen and liver, bone pain, and fatigue (Basilicata et al., 2023). Tay–Sachs disease, on the other hand, results in the buildup of a lipid called GM2 ganglioside, leading to severe neurological impairments in affected individuals, often starting in infancy. Phenylketonuria (Patel and Patel, 2017) is another metabolic disorder caused by a genetic defect that affects the breakdown of an amino acid called phenylalanine. Individuals with PKU lack an enzyme called phenylalanine hydroxylase, which converts phenylalanine into another amino acid, tyrosine. Without this enzyme, phenylalanine levels in the blood become elevated, leading to intellectual disabilities and other neurological problems if left untreated. Early diagnosis and dietary management, which restricts phenylalanine intake, are crucial to prevent these complications.

In contrast to PKU, porphyrias are a group of metabolic conditions considered by the abnormal accumulation of porphyrins, which are essential for the production of heme, a component of hemoglobin (Basilicata et al., 2023). Porphyrias can affect various organ systems and manifest with symptoms ranging from abdominal pain and skin sensitivity to neuropsychiatric disturbances. The types and severity of symptoms depend on the specific enzyme deficiency involved and the accumulation of different porphyrins.

Mitochondrial disorders represent a class of metabolic disorders that disrupt the function of the mitochondria. The cellular organelles are accountable for producing energy in the form of adenosine triphosphate (ATP). These disorders can affect nearly any organ system because of their widespread distribution in the body. Mitochondrial disorders may present with a wide array of symptoms, including muscle weakness, fatigue, developmental delays, and organ dysfunction. Mitochondrial diseases can be challenging to diagnose due to their heterogeneity and the complex interplay of genetic and environmental factors that contribute to their growth.

The importance of early detection and intervention cannot be overstated when it comes to metabolic disorders. Newborn screening programs have been instrumental in identifying certain conditions like PKU, allowing for early dietary interventions that can prevent the onset of severe symptoms. However, many metabolic disorders may not manifest symptoms until later in life, making early diagnosis more challenging. Genetic testing and advances in diagnostic technologies have improved our ability to identify these conditions earlier, enabling healthcare providers to implement timely interventions and treatments.

Treatment approaches for metabolic disorders vary depending on the specific condition and its underlying genetic cause. In some cases, treatment may involve dietary modifications, such as the restriction of certain nutrients or the supplementation of deficient molecules. For example, individuals with PKU must adhere to a low-phenylalanine diet and may require special medical formulas to ensure adequate nutrition. In Gaucher disease, enzyme replacement therapy has been developed to supplement the deficient enzyme and alleviate symptoms. In the case of mitochondrial disorders, treatment often focuses on symptom management and support, as there are currently limited options for directly targeting mitochondrial dysfunction (Giraldo et al., 2018). Gene therapy and other emerging therapies hold promise for the future treatment of metabolic disorders. Researchers are exploring ways to correct genetic mutations responsible for these conditions, potentially offering a cure or more effective treatments. Advances in personalized medicine and precision therapies are paving the way for more tailored approaches to managing metabolic disorders, taking into account an individual's unique genetic makeup and disease characteristics.

2.2.1 Types of Metabolic Disorders

2.2.1.1 Inborn Errors of Metabolism (IEM)

Inborn errors of metabolism, also known as congenital metabolic disorders, are genetic conditions that impact the body's capability to process specific substances. These disorders result from mutations in genes that code for enzymes involved in metabolic pathways. Examples of IEMs include:

a. ***Phenylketonuria (Patel and Patel)***: PKU is marked by the incapacity to metabolize phenylalanine, prominent to a buildup of this amino acid in the blood. If left untreated, it can lead to severe intellectual disabilities.
b. ***Maple Syrup Urine Disease (MSUD)***: MSUD prevents the breakdown of certain amino acids, resulting in a distinctive odor in urine and neurological complications.
c. ***Galactosemia***: This disorder impairs the body's capacity to metabolize galactose, a sugar present in milk and other dairy items (Lillich et al., 2020).

2.2.1.2 Diabetes Mellitus

Diabetes mellitus is a collection of metabolic disorders characterized by high blood sugar levels (hyperglycemia) as a result of inadequate insulin synthesis or poor insulin cellular responsiveness. Diabetes may be classified into two categories:

a. ***Type 1 Diabetes***: An autoimmune condition where the body's immune system attacks and destroys the insulin-producing beta cells in the pancreas.
b. ***Type 2 Diabetes***: Often linked to lifestyle factors, this form of diabetes involves insulin resistance and reduced insulin production.

2.2.1.3 Metabolic Syndrome

Metabolic syndrome comprises a group of conditions that elevate the likelihood of developing heart disease, stroke, and type 2 diabetes. The key components of metabolic syndrome include obesity, high blood pressure, elevated blood sugar, abnormal lipid profiles, and insulin resistance.

2.2.1.4 Hyperthyroidism and Hypothyroidism

Thyroid disorders, such as hyperthyroidism (overactive thyroid) and hypothyroidism (underactive thyroid), can significantly affect metabolic function (Stephens et al., 2020). Thyroid hormones, which are produced by the thyroid gland, play an important part in regulating the body's metabolism.

2.2.1.5 Lipid Metabolism Disorders

Disorders in lipid metabolism led to abnormal levels of fats (lipids) in the blood. These conditions include:

a. ***Hyperlipidemia***: Characterized by elevated intensities of cholesterol and triglycerides in the blood, increasing the risk of cardiovascular diseases.
b. ***Familial Hypercholesterolemia***: A genetic condition that results in extremely high levels of low-density lipoprotein (LDL) cholesterol.

2.2.1.6 Metabolic Bone Disorders

Metabolic bone disorders affect the bones' structure and mineral composition, leading to conditions like osteoporosis, rickets, and Paget's disease of the bone.

2.2.1.6.1 Causes of Metabolic Disorders

Metabolic disorders have various causes, often rooted in genetics, lifestyle, or a combination of both. Some key factors include:

1. ***Genetic Mutations***: Many metabolic disorders are inherited, resulting from mutations in specific genes that code for enzymes or proteins involved in metabolic pathways.
2. ***Poor Nutrition***: Diets high in sugar, unhealthy fats, and processed foods can contribute to metabolic disorders; particularly type 2 diabetes and metabolic syndrome.
3. ***Sedentary Lifestyle***: Absence of physical movement and obesity can disrupt metabolism and contribute to conditions like insulin resistance.
4. ***Hormonal Imbalances***: Conditions affecting hormone-producing organs, such as the thyroid or adrenal glands, can disrupt metabolic processes.
5. ***Medications and Environmental Factors***: Some drugs and environmental toxins can interfere with metabolism, causing disorders like drug-induced diabetes or metabolic bone disorders.

2.2.1.6.2 Management and Treatment

The management and treatment of metabolic disorders vary depending on the specific disorder and its underlying causes. However, there are common strategies and principles that apply to many of these conditions:

1. ***Dietary Modifications:*** Dietary changes can play a critical role in managing metabolic disorders. For example, individuals with diabetes must monitor their carbohydrate intake and manage blood sugar levels through diet (Kivimäki et al., 2023). In the case of lipid metabolism disorders, a diet low in saturated and Tran's fats is often recommended.
2. ***Medications***: Depending on the disorder, medications may be prescribed to help regulate metabolic processes. For instance, insulin therapy is a cornerstone of treatment for type 1 diabetes, while various medications are available for managing type 2 diabetes.
3. ***Hormone Replacement (Klein and Phillips, 2019)***: In cases of thyroid disorders, hormone replacement therapy may be necessary to restore normal thyroid function.
4. ***Enzyme Replacement Therapy (de la Fuente et al., 2021):*** Some inborn errors of metabolism can be managed with enzyme replacement therapy to supplement deficient enzymes.
5. ***Lifestyle Changes:*** Encouraging physical activity and weight management is vital in managing metabolic disorders like metabolic syndrome and obesity-related conditions.

6. ***Genetic Counseling***: For inherited metabolic disorders, genetic counseling can provide guidance to affected individuals and their families regarding inheritance patterns, risk assessment, and family planning (Bagheri et al., 2021).

2.2.2 Prevalence and Impact of Metabolic Disorders

Metabolic disorders are a growing health concern with significant global prevalence and far-reaching impacts on individuals and public health systems. These disorders encompass a range of conditions that disrupt the intricate processes governing energy production, growth, and biochemical regulation within the human body (Kivimäki et al., 2023). Understanding their prevalence and the impact they have on individuals and society is essential for addressing this emerging health crisis.

2.2.2.1 Prevalence of Metabolic Disorders

The prevalence of metabolic disorders has been progressively rising over the past few decades, largely due to changes in lifestyle, including sedentary behavior, increased consumption of processed foods, and rising rates of obesity. Here are some key metabolic disorders and their prevalence:

1. ***Diabetes Mellitus:*** Diabetes, both type 1 and type 2, has become a global epidemic. According to the International Diabetes Federation, as of my preceding knowledge update in September 2021, approximately 537 million people were living with diabetes worldwide, with projections suggesting a further increase in the coming years.
2. ***Metabolic Syndrome (Rochlani et al., 2017):*** The prevalence of metabolic syndrome has surged in parallel with obesity rates. More than one in every three persons in the United States, for example, is thought to have metabolic syndrome, which is linked to an eminent risk of heart disease, stroke, and type 2 diabetes.
3. ***Inborn Errors of Metabolism (IEM):*** IEMs are relatively rare compared to conditions like diabetes, but their impact can be severe. These conditions, collectively, affect thousands of individuals worldwide, with regional variations in prevalence.
4. ***Thyroid Disorders (Moeller, 2023):*** Disorders of the thyroid gland, including hyperthyroidism and hypothyroidism, are common. For example, an estimated 20 million Americans have some form of thyroid disease.
5. ***Lipid Metabolism Disorders (Amadi et al., 2022):*** Conditions like hyperlipidemia and familial hypercholesterolemia are prevalent, contributing to the high incidence of cardiovascular diseases globally.

2.2.2.2 Impact of Metabolic Disorders

Metabolic disorders have a profound impact on individuals, communities, and healthcare systems. Here are some of the key consequences:

1. ***Health Implications:*** Metabolic disorders often lead to severe health complications. For instance, diabetes can result in heart disease, kidney failure, blindness, and limb amputations if poorly managed. Metabolic syndrome is linked to a higher risk of cardiovascular events such as strokes and cardiac arrest (Li et al., 2021). IEMs can cause intellectual disabilities, developmental delays, and organ damage. Thyroid disorders can disrupt the body's metabolism, leading to a wide variety of symptoms and consequences.
2. ***Economic Burden:*** The economic burden of metabolic disorders is immense. These conditions require ongoing medical care, medications, and, in some cases, surgeries. The costs of healthcare and lost productivity due to these disorders strain both individuals and healthcare systems.
3. ***Quality of Life:*** Metabolic disorders can significantly diminish an individual's QoL. Managing these conditions often involves dietary restrictions, medication regimens, and lifestyle changes, which can be physically and emotionally challenging.
4. ***Public Health Challenges:*** On a societal level, metabolic disorders pose public health challenges. They increase the overall burden on healthcare systems, necessitating increased funding for prevention, treatment, and research. Moreover, the impacts on productivity and the workforce are substantial, affecting economies worldwide.
5. ***Psychosocial Impact:*** Living with a metabolic disorder can be emotionally taxing. Stigmatization and discrimination are not uncommon, especially in cases of obesity-related conditions (Stephens et al., 2020). The psychosocial impact of these disorders can lead to anxiety, depression, and reduced social participation.
6. ***Interconnectedness of Disorders:*** It's important to note that many metabolic disorders are interconnected (Stephens et al., 2020). For example, obesity often underlies conditions like type 2 diabetes, metabolic syndrome, and certain lipid metabolism disorders. This interplay complicates treatment and management.

2.2.3 Underlying Mechanisms

Metabolic disorders are a class of illnesses that impair the body's capacity to transform food into energy. This can cause an accumulation of toxic compounds in the blood, which can eventually damage organs and tissues. Genetic mutations, environmental causes, or a mix of both can cause metabolic diseases. Type 2 diabetes is one of the most common metabolic illnesses. Type 2 diabetes is characterized by insulin resistance, which implies that the cells in the body fail to respond adequately to the hormone insulin. Insulin helps the body to absorb glucose from the blood and use it for energy. When cells are insulin resistant, glucose levels in the blood rise, leading to hyperglycemia. Another common metabolic disorder is metabolic syndrome. Metabolic syndrome is a cluster of risk factors that increase the risk of developing type 2 diabetes, heart disease, and stroke. Central obesity, high blood pressure, high triglycerides, poor HDL cholesterol, and high fasting blood sugar are all risk factors.

The underlying mechanisms of metabolic disorders are complex and not fully understood. However, there are a number of factors that are thought to play a role. One important factor is inflammation. Inflammation is a normal immune response that helps the body to heal from injury or infection. However, chronic inflammation can damage cells and tissues. Chronic inflammation is thought to be a major contributor to insulin resistance and other metabolic disorders.

Oxidative stress is another major element in the development of metabolic diseases. Oxidative stress is a state that arises when free radicals and antioxidants are in equilibrium. Free radicals are unstable molecules with the potential to harm cells. Antioxidants are molecules that neutralize free radicals. When there is too much oxidative stress, cells can become damaged and dysfunctional. Oxidative stress is thought to contribute to the onset of insulin resistance, type 2 diabetes, and other metabolic disorders.

Genetic factors also contribute to the emergence of metabolic disorders. Some people are born with genes that make them more susceptible to developing these diseases. People with a family history of type 2 diabetes, for example, are more likely to get the condition themselves.

Environmental variables, such as nutrition and lifestyle, can also play a role in the emergence of metabolic diseases. A high-processed-food, sugary-drink, and unhealthy-fat diet can raise the risk of developing metabolic syndrome and type 2 diabetes. Sedentary behavior poses an additional risk for metabolic diseases.

2.2.3.1 Treatment for Metabolic Disorders

The treatment for metabolic disorders depends on the specific disorder and its severity. For some people, lifestyle changes, such as losing weight, eating a healthy diet, and exercising regularly, may be enough to manage the disorder. Others may need to take medication or insulin to control their blood sugar levels or other metabolic problems.

2.2.3.2 Prevention of Metabolic Disorders

Maintaining a healthy lifestyle is the greatest strategy to avoid metabolic problems. This involves consuming a nutritious food, exercising on a regular basis, and keeping a healthy weight. If you have a family history of metabolic disorders, it is important to talk to your doctor about ways to reduce your risk.

2.2.3.3 The Underlying Mechanisms of Metabolic Disorders

- ***Insulin resistance***: Insulin resistance is a hallmark of many metabolic disorders, including type 2 diabetes and metabolic syndrome. When cells are insulin resistant, they do not respond properly to the hormone insulin. This means that glucose cannot easily enter the cells, and glucose levels in the blood rise.
- ***Inflammation***: Inflammation is a complex process that is involved in many different diseases, including metabolic disorders. Chronic inflammation can damage cells and tissues, and it is thought could contribute to insulin resistance, type 2 diabetes, and other metabolic diseases.
- ***Oxidative stress:*** Oxidative stress is a state that arises when free radicals and antioxidants are in equilibrium. Free radicals are unstable molecules that can damage cells. Antioxidants are molecules that neutralize free radicals. Oxidative stress is thought to contribute to the emergence of insulin resistance, type 2 diabetes, and other metabolic disorders.
- ***Genetic factors***: Some people are born with genes that make them more susceptible to developing metabolic disorders. For example, people with a family history of type 2 diabetes are more likely to develop the disease themselves.
- ***Environmental factors***: Environmental factors, such as diet and lifestyle, can also contribute to the development of metabolic disorders. A high-processed-food, sugary-drink, and unhealthy-fat diet can raise the risk of developing metabolic syndrome and type 2 diabetes. Physical inactivity is another risk factor for metabolic diseases (Table 2.1).

2.3 GUT MICROBIOTA AND METABOLIC HEALTH

Microbial communities seem to mediate or modify a substantial amount of the environmental impact on human health and illness risk, according to the results of recent epidemiological, physiological, and omics-based investigations, which were supplemented by cellular studies and tests in animals (Joyce and Gahan, 2014). The wide array of interrelated archaea, bacteria, bacteriophages, eukaryotic viruses, and fungus that dwell on human surfaces and in all bodily cavities are referred to as the microbiota. The first place where nutrients are broken down and absorbed is in the small intestine, which is also where vitamins and bile acids are taken in. There is a spectrum of 103 (duodenum) to 108 (ileum) bacteria per ml has been found to exist in the small intestine's microbiota, which has received less research than that of the large intestine (Fan and Pedersen, 2021; Lynch and Pedersen, 2016). Low pH, bile acids, secretory immunoglobulin A, and antimicrobial peptides are all thought to contribute to this comparatively low biomass

TABLE 2.1
Type of Metabolic Disorder and Their Prevalence and Impact (Zhao et al., 2021)

Type of Metabolic Disorder	Prevalence	Impact	Mechanism
Type 2 Diabetes	Affects over 422 million people worldwide	Risk of heart disease, stroke, blindness, renal failure, and amputations is increased	Insulin resistance, impaired insulin secretion, and a rise in liver glucose production
Metabolic Syndrome	Affects about 25% of adults worldwide	Increases the risk of type 2 diabetes, heart disease, and stroke	Central obesity, insulin resistance, dyslipidemia, and hypertension
Obesity	Affects over 650 million adults worldwide	Rises the chance of developing type 2 diabetes, heart disease, stroke, some cancers, and arthritic conditions	Imbalance between energy intake and expenditure, genetic factors, and environmental factors
Dyslipidemia	Affects over 1 billion people worldwide	Increases the risk of heart disease and stroke	Elevated levels of LDL cholesterol, low levels of HDL cholesterol, and elevated levels of triglycerides
Hypertension	Affects over 1 billion people worldwide	Increases the risk of heart disease, stroke, kidney failure, and dementia	Genetic factors, environmental factors, and lifestyle factors
Maple syrup urine disease (MSUD)	1 in 185,000 newborns	Brain damage, seizures, and death if not treated	A genetic disorder that prevents the body from breaking down certain amino acids
Homocystinuria	1 in 332,000 newborns	Intellectual disability, eye problems, and blood clots if not treated	A genetic disorder that prevents the body from breaking down an amino acid called homocysteine
Alkaptonuria	1 in 250,000–1,000,000 people	Arthritis, heart problems, and kidney stones	A genetic disorder that prevents the body from breaking down an amino acid called tyrosine
Gaucher disease	1 in 50,000–100,000 people	Liver and spleen enlargement, anemia, and bone marrow problems	A genetic disorder that prevents the body from breaking down a fatty substance called glucocerebroside
Fabry disease	1 in 40,000–60,000 males	Kidney disease, heart disease, and skin problems	A genetic disorder that prevents the body from breaking down a fatty substance called globotriaosylceramide
Pompe disease	1 in 40,000–120,000 newborns	Muscle weakness, respiratory problems, and heart problems	A genetic disorder that prevents the body from breaking down a sugar called glycogen
Tay–Sachs disease	1 in 320,000 Ashkenazi Jewish newborns	Progressive neurological deterioration and death	A genetic disorder that prevents the body from breaking down a fatty substance called ganglioside GM2

(Fan and Pedersen, 2021). Most human-dwelling microbes live in the intestines and are impacted by the host's diet, lifestyle, medications genetic makeup, and way of birth. The host's immune system, food digestion, metabolism, detoxification, gut endocrine function, pharmacological action, neurological signaling, and production of many substances that affect the host are all influenced by the gut microbiome (Fan and Pedersen, 2021).

An examination of the small intestine microbiota has revealed the presence of enterobacteria established in the lumen, mucosa-associated Bacteroidetes, and Clostridium XIVa and IV groups (Joyce and Gahan, 2014; Zoetendal et al., 2012). Notable bacterial pathway expression levels connected to the metabolism of carbohydrates and amino acids were found in this microbial community by metagenomic analysis, with facultative anaerobes (Streptococcus species a) accounting for the majority of the activity (Joyce and Gahan, 2014; Zoetendal et al., 2012).

This section of the gastrointestinal tract (GIT)'s metabolic activities is highly active, and small intestinal enterocytes have the ability to absorb metabolites. These factors suggest that interactions between microbes and hosts in the small intestine are important, albeit little-known, for maintaining the host's metabolic fitness. The study looks at how the host's metabolic health is affected by the gastrointestinal microbiota. It specifically emphasizes the possible role that the small intestinal microbiota may have in illness as well as wellness (Joyce and Gahan, 2014) (Figure 2.1).

2.3.1 The Gut Microbiota Composition

Trillions of microbes reside in our bodies both before and after birth in the human body (Baothman et al., 2016). Before the baby is introduced to the mother's vaginal bacteria during a typical delivery, the infant's digestive tract is free of microorganisms during. The germs on the mother's skin can affect the composition of microorganisms in the infant's intestines after a Cesarean section (Makino et al., 2013). Infants who are breastfed have a distinct makeup of gut microbiota than those who are formula fed, suggesting that feeding is another source of bacteria (Baothman et al., 2016; Makino et al., 2013). Another change in the composition of newborns' flora of intestine is the introduction of solid food.

Up until old age, when the makeup changes once more, the gut microbiota then stays largely unchanged. Compared to the cells that make up the human body, adult humans have around ten times as many bacteria in them. Viral, fungal, and other microorganisms are still present in the GI tract, but bacteria make up the majority of the microbiota there. The microbiota of the intestinal tract is mostly composed of microbiome from four phyla: Actinobacteria, Bacteroidetes, Firmicutes, and Proteobacteria, although each individual

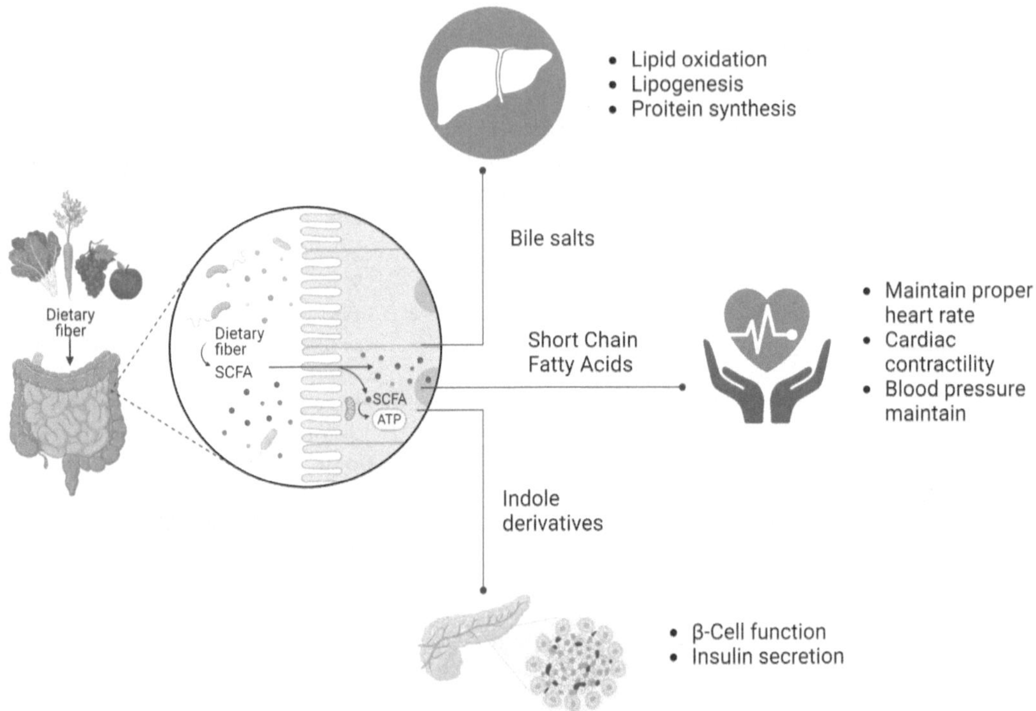

FIGURE 2.1 Gut microbiota and metabolic health.

has a different microbiota composition (Baothman et al., 2016). There are more than 1,011 bacteria per gramme of intestinal content in the large intestine, which is home to most bacteria. There are 108–109 bacteria in the ileum, compared to 1,012 in the mouth. However, the stomach has the fewest bacteria (103–104), while the jejunum harbors 105–106 (Baothman et al., 2016; Tlaskalová-Hogenová et al., 2011). The gut microbiota has greatly benefited from the invention of molecular biology techniques like next-generation sequencing, even if we are still far from fully illustrating or even recognizing all of the bacteria in our system. An excellent resource for comprehending the function of introducing defined bacterial strains and monitored bacterial cultures into animals was made possible by the use of gnotobiological techniques to grow mice in a sterile setting using a variety of proteomic and genomic methods to study their impact (Tlaskalová-Hogenová et al., 2011).

2.3.2 Gut Microbiota–Host Interactions

Long before multicellular life began to evolve, for more than 3 billion years, microbial communities were present on our planet. The emergence of organelles, cellular structure, and functional compartmentalization, and the creation of new metabolic pathways in host cells were all made possible by endosymbiosis, which was also crucial for the development of eukaryotes (Popkes and Valenzano, 2020). The complex interactions determining the structure and functionality of the gut microbiota are influenced by the host's nutrition, lifestyle, and DNA and occur codeveloping with the host from birth. Because the intestinal fauna regulates several host metabolism processes, it plays an interactive role in the metabolic processes, communication, and immune-inflammatory axes that biologically interconnect the gut, liver, muscle, and brain. To optimize treatment approaches to modify the intestinal fauna for the purpose to fight disease and promote health, a greater comprehension of these axes is necessary. Metabolites that impact the illness states of the host can be produced by the gut microbiota.

Combinatorial metabolic processes of targets by the intestinal microbiome and the genome of the host are achieved through the sequential modulation of metabolic reactions within these metabolic axes through various genomes of bacterium, as demonstrated by the production of choline, short-chain fatty acids (SCFAs), and bile acids—all of which are essential for the overall well-being of the host (Popkes and Valenzano, 2020; Zhang et al., 2007). A summary of a few of these metabolites and their most plausible microbiological link to illness is given below (Table 2.2):

2.3.2.1 Acetaldehyde Production from Ethanol

Small intestinal microbes have the ability to naturally produce ethanol, which is then metabolized by the liver and absorbed by blood (Joyce and Gahan, 2014).

Consuming ethanol, on the other hand, has the potential to change the microbiota's composition and increase the number of Proteobacteria, which in turn can encourage bacterial overgrowth in the digestive tract, damage the small intestine's barrier integrity, rise in duodenal permeability (Joyce and Gahan, 2014), which may have an impact on epithelial tight junctions (Elamin et al., 2013). Alcohol can be converted by intestinal microorganisms

TABLE 2.2
Gut Microbiota Metabolites and Host Interactions

Metabolites	Sub-Metabolites	Microorganism	Target Sites	Functions	Diseases	References
Ethanol	Acetaldehyde	Firmicutes, Bacterioides, Bifidobacterium, Atopobium, Faecalibacterium, Ruminococcus, Pseudobutyrivibrio, Subdoligranulum, and Lactobacillus	P2X and P2Y receptors are triggered by triphosadenine.	Synthesis, use, or modification of connected pathways, such as the endocannabinoid system, can be done directly or indirectly.	Bacterial overgrowth in small intestine	Joyce & Gahan (2014), Nicholson et al. (2012), Liu et al. (2022a)
Choline, Trimethylamines, Phosphatidyl-choline	Methylamine, dimethylamine, trimethylamine, dimethylglycine, betaine	Bifidobacterium, Aecalibacterium prausnitzii	Unclear direct target, although it can trigger NLRP3 inflammasome, PKC NF-κB,	Adjust glucose homeostasis and lipid metabolism	Associated with non-alcoholic fatty liver damage, diabetes, and overweight brought on by dietary habits, and cardiovascular disease	Joyce & Gahan (2014), Nicholson et al. (2012), Liu et al. (2022)
Dietary fibers, SCFAs	Isovalerate, hexanoate, valerate, butyrate, acetate, propionate, isobutyrate	Coprococcu Clostridial clusters IV, Faecalibacterium, and XIVa of Firmicutes, including species of Eubacterium, and Roseburia	Act on GPR109A, GPR91, GPR81, GPR43, GPR41, HDAC3, HDAC1	Stimulates the absorption of water and sodium, prevents the spread of infections, aids in cholesterol production, and gives colonic epithelial cells energy	Reduced colonic pH reduced human obesity, insulin resistance, type 2 diabetes, and colorectal cancer,	Joyce & Gahan (2014), Nicholson et al. (2012), Liu et al. (2022)
Bile acids	Cholate, deoxycholate, hyocholate, chenodeoxycholate, glycocholate, muricholate, taurocholate, taurochenoxycholate, glycochenodeoxycholate, taurocholate, tauro-muricholate, lithocholate	Bacteroides, Clostridium, Enterobacter, Bifidobacteria, and Lactobacillus	Directly act on PXR/SXR, CAR, VDR, TGR5, FXR, S1PR2, mAChR, FPR,	Preserve the intestinal barrier's health, increase the absorption of lipids, absorb fats from food, and absorb vitamins soluble in fat, regulate blood sugar, triglycerides, cholesterol, and energy balance. (31-31), (-30)	Alzheimer's disease, obesity, non-alcoholic fatty liver disease, non-alcoholic atherosclerosis, Parkinson's disease, ulcerative colitis, steatohepatitis, multiple sclerosis, hepatic encephalopathy, cancer	Joyce & Gahan (2014), Nicholson et al. (2012), Liu et al. (2022)
Phenol	Hippuric acid, benzoic acid, 4-Cresol, 3-Hydroxybenzoic acid, 3-Hydroxyphenyl propionate, 2-Hydroxyhippuric acid, tyrosine, & 4-Cresyl glucuronide, phenylacetate,	Subdoligranulum, F. prausnitzii, Bifidobacterium, Clostridium difficile, and Lactobacillus species.	P2X and P2Y receptors are triggered by triphosadenine.	Utilizing polyphenols, xenobiotic detoxification, and gut microbial makeup and activity are all indicated.	Obesity, severe autism, hypertension, urinary colorectal cancer.	Joyce & Gahan (2014), Nicholson et al. (2012), Liu et al. (2022)

from ethanol to acetaldehyde. Through alcohol dehydrogenase (Bandyopadhyay et al., 2019) action, microorganisms in the colon can metabolize ethanol to acetaldehyde that profoundly rearranges actin and seriously disrupts cellular junctions and E-cadherin (Joyce and Gahan, 2014).

2.3.2.2 Choline and Trimethylamines Production from Phosphatidylcholine

Phosphatidylcholine, or lecithin, is the source of choline, a semi-essential vitamin. Trimethylamine N-oxide (TMAO) and choline are examples of phosphatidylcholine metabolites that have been identified as plasma indicators linked to contributes to atherosclerosis, a higher probability of cardiovascular disease in people, and the microbiota's involvement in TMAO production (Joyce and Gahan, 2014). The human intestinal fauna holds significant importance in the metabolism of TMAO, as evidenced by the large increase in TMAO levels observed in response to phosphatidylcholine ingestion, which is followed by a dramatic suppression following antibiotic therapy (Tang et al., 2013).

2.3.2.3 SCFAs Production from Dietary Fibers

GPR41 and GPR43, GPRs expressed by enteroendocrine cells of intestine, sense dietary fibers (complex carbohydrates), are broken down by the gut bacteria into SCFA (butyrate, propionate, and acetate). Along with performing as a local source of vitamins and minerals for colonocytes and an insignificant source of nourishment for bacteria such as *Desulfotomaculum* spp. in the digestive tract, n-butyrate additionally has been observed in cell-culture designs along with mice to maintain the equilibrium of energy by triggering leptin production in adipocytes and encouraging glucagon-like peptide-1 (GLP-1) production via the GI endocrine L cells (Nicholson et al., 2012). Microbes such as eubacteria, roseburia, and clostridia are the primary producers of butyrate. n-Butyrate exhibits anti-inflammatory properties by lowering the release of cytokines and chemokines from human immune cells, but it also controls neutrophil function and migration, suppresses the inflammatory cytokines'-induced production of vascular cell adhesion molecule-1 and boosts the expression of tight junction proteins in colon epithelia. The target of the future may be n-butyrate or certain species of butyrate-producing gut bacteria in order to reestablish host immune system health, preserve membrane integrity, and regulate the breakdown of energy. Epithelial cells of colon can also directly produce carbon dioxide and ketone bodies by utilizing n-butyrate.

2.3.2.4 Bile Acids Production from Cholesterol

Bile acids production from cholesterol support cholesterol and fat-soluble nutrient absorption as well as the metabolic activity of dietary fat. Made from cholesterol in the liver and released as bile, bile acids are steroid acids. Distinct bile acid moieties, mucus, phospholipids, and biliverdin make up bile released into the duodenum through the common bile duct. Bile acids play a major physiological role in the small intestine by emulsifying fats, releasing fat-soluble vitamins, and regulating cholesterol metabolism (Begley et al., 2005). FXR, PXR, VDR, TGR5, and other host receptors are all selectively ligand-activated or -repressed by certain bile acids. Bile acids can thus change host gene-expression profiles (Joyce and Gahan, 2014) and function as systemic signaling molecules and Host–Gut Microbiota Metabolic Interaction. They affect the metabolism of xenobiotics and regulate the production and transport of bile acids (Joyce and Gahan, 2014). The liver's regulation of bile acid synthesis is significantly influenced by the powerful FXR antagonists tauro-beta and tauro alphamuricholic acid, which are particular bile acids (Joyce and Gahan, 2014). Crucially, signaling processes mediated by specific bile acids have the power to modify adipose and liver tissue's energy metabolism, which in turn affects mice's obesity (Watanabe et al., 2011).

2.3.2.5 Cresol Production from Phenol

Either 50–100 mg of volatile phenols are excreted daily by humans, mostly as phenol and 4-cresol (mostly as sulfate conjugates and glucuronide), with lesser amounts of 4-ethylphenol (Nicholson et al., 2012). Many species of *Bacteroides fragilis*, *Bifidobacterium*, and *Clostridium* have been linked to the cresol's synthesis from tyrosine in mammals. The synthesis of phenol is linked to other bacteria, including *E. coli*. A wide range of physiological and pathological disorders, including inflammatory bowel illness and weight loss, have been linked to changed amounts of metabolites from 4-cresol in human urine.

2.3.3 Gut Microbiota and Metabolic Disorders

Human propensity to inflammatory bowel disease (IBD), obesity, and type 2 diabetes appears to be influenced by abundance of microbial genes and species complexity. Decreased variation in species is linked to geriatric frailty (Joyce and Gahan, 2014), ulcerative colitis, Crohn's disease, and other IBD. Disease conditions have been associated with a deviation of butyrate-producing organism's abundance (Joyce and Gahan, 2014), according to metabolite analyses and random-access metagenomic sequences. A recent study that used massive shotgun sequencing of the fecal microbiome from volunteers with varying BMI discovered that individuals naturally partition into "low gene count" (LGC) and "high gene count" (HGC) groups. HGC represents the relative richness and variety of the microbiota. Obesity with elevated body weight and fat mass % was substantially more common in those with an LGC. Microbiomes with a lipogenic growth community (LGC) exhibit a decrease in butyrate production capacity, an increase in hydrogen sulfide production capacity, and a rise in the abundance of bacterial species linked to inflammation, according to a detailed examination of each microbiome (Joyce and Gahan, 2014). An energy-restricted diet was found to be effective in enhancing gene richness in LGC obese and overweight persons while lowering circulating cholesterol and overweight, according to a similar investigation (Le Chatelier et al., 2013).

This suggests that antibiotics might have potential to change the host's metabolism as evidenced by the reduced bacterial diversity observed in persons after antibiotic medication (Cotillard et al., 2013). Surprisingly, a study on mice given subtherapeutic antibiotic treatment (STAT) revealed that during their early growth, they were more obese (Joyce and Gahan, 2014). SCFA production by bacteria increased as a result of the impact, which was linked to a change in the microbiota's community structure (Cho et al., 2012). A human birth cohort research conducted over an extended period of time revealed a similar correlation between reduced body weight between ten and 38 months of age and early life antibiotic exposure (<6 months of age) (Joyce and Gahan, 2014). Despite the fact that antibiotics have been shown to disturb human microbial communities, there is evidence of the microbiome's ability to affect human's processes of metabolism.

2.4 PREBIOTICS: MODULATING GUT MICROBIOTA

2.4.1 Definition and Types of Prebiotics

Prebiotics are indigestible dietary elements that specifically promote the activity and/or growth of good bacteria in the stomach, enhancing the health of the host. Research indicates that prebiotics have the ability to both directly and indirectly control immune response and microbiota (Davani-Davari et al., 2019). By encouraging the development of good bacteria like *Lactobacilli* and *Bifidobacteria,* which can create SCFAs that decrease colonic pH and stop the growth of pathogens, they can interact with the gut microbiota. Prebiotics can alter the immune response by boosting the production of anti-inflammatory cytokines and reducing the production of pro-inflammatory cytokines (Khan et al., 2020).

Prebiotics operate as microbiota in the gut modulators by directly entering the intestine and exerting anti-inflammatory effects, preventing pathogen colonization by interacting with them, fermentation by intestinal microbiota, and stimulating helpful microorganisms. The most prevalent prebiotics are FOS, GOS, and TOS. SCFAs such as butyric acid, lactic acid, and propionic acid are produced by gut microbial fermentation of prebiotics. The most widely investigated prebiotics are fructooligosaccharides and inulin-type fructans (ITFs), which have been shown to considerably change the balance of the large intestine microbial population by raising the quantity of bifidobacteria and lactic acid bacteria (Guarino et al., 2020). GOS has also been demonstrated to improve the functioning of intestinal barriers and to influence gut flora (Macfarlane et al., 2008; Rauf et al., 2022).

2.4.2 Mechanism of Action of Prebiotics in Modulating Gut Microbiota

Prebiotics are non-digestible dietary components, primarily carbohydrates that play a crucial role in shaping and promoting a healthy gut microbiota (Guarino et al., 2020). Their mechanism of action involves several key steps.

2.4.2.1 Selective Nourishment

Prebiotics are not absorbed in the upper GIT but instead reach the colon largely intact. Once in the colon, they serve as a selective source of nutrition for beneficial gut bacteria, such as *Bifidobacteria* and *Lactobacilli* (Wang et al., 2020).

2.4.2.2 Fermentation

Beneficial bacteria can ferment prebiotics, breaking them down into SCFAs, such as butyrate, acetate, and propionate. SCFAs serve as an energy source for colonocytes and play a crucial role in maintaining gut health (den Besten et al., 2013).

2.4.2.3 pH Modulation

As prebiotics are fermented, they produce SCFAs, which lower the colonic pH. This acidic environment suppresses the proliferation of harmful bacteria while promoting the growth of beneficial microorganisms.

2.4.2.4 Enhanced Barrier Function

Prebiotics support the integrity of the gut barrier by promoting the production of mucin, which helps protect the gut lining. This enhanced barrier function reduces the risk of harmful bacteria crossing into the bloodstream.

2.4.2.5 Immune System Modulation

Prebiotics can influence the gut-associated immune system. They promote the development and activity of immune cells, which help maintain a balanced and regulated immune response.

2.4.2.6 Anti-Inflammatory Effects

The SCFAs produced through prebiotic fermentation have anti-inflammatory properties and can reduce inflammation in the gut, which is linked to various gastrointestinal and systemic diseases.

2.4.2.7 Nutrient Absorption

Prebiotics enhance the absorption of certain minerals, like calcium and magnesium, by promoting the growth of bacteria that are involved in mineral metabolism.

2.4.2.8 Metabolic Effects

Prebiotics have the ability to alter metabolic health by regulating the gut bacteria and their metabolic activity. They could assist in appetite regulation, insulin sensitivity, and regulating body mass (Figure 2.2).

Prebiotics work by fostering the growth of SCFAs, preserving the veracity of the gut barrier, adjusting the immune system, and affecting other facets of metabolic health in addition to specifically feeding beneficial gut bacteria. Prebiotics support a balanced and healthy gut microbiota, which has broad implications for general health by promoting the growth and activity of helpful microorganisms while preventing the formation of harmful bacteria (Megur et al., 2022).

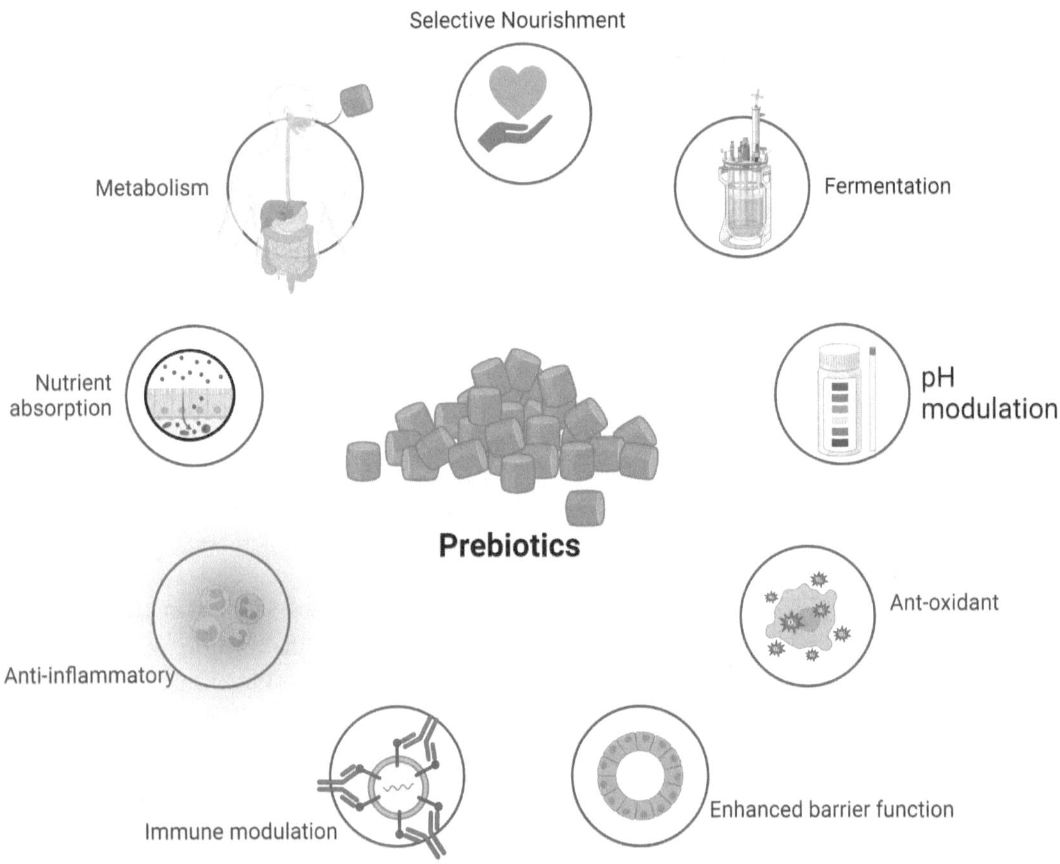

FIGURE 2.2 Mechanism of action of prebiotics.

2.4.3 Clinical Evidence in Metabolic Disorders

Clinical evidence suggests that prebiotics can have a positive impact on metabolic disorders, particularly obesity, type 2 diabetes, and metabolic syndrome.

A study by Wiciński et al. (2020) found that prebiotic supplementation led to decreased body weight and adipose tissue in overweight and obese individuals. Prebiotics may help regulate appetite and reduce calorie intake by promoting the production of satiety hormones. Research work done by Ojo et al. published in the journal *Diabetes Care* showed that prebiotic consumption improved glycemic control in individuals with type 2 diabetes. Prebiotics may enhance insulin sensitivity and reduce blood glucose levels.

Wastyk et al. (2023) demonstrated and reported a randomized controlled trial in the *Journal of Nutrition* that prebiotic intake improved several components of metabolic syndrome, including reduced waist circumference, blood pressure, and triglyceride levels.

Prebiotics have been shown to reduce systemic inflammation, which is often elevated in metabolic disorders. Lowering inflammation can help mitigate the risk and severity of metabolic conditions. Prebiotics are shown to have positive influence in liver health. Prebiotic supplementation has been associated with improved liver function and a reduction in non-NAFLD, a complaint often linked to metabolic disorders. It's crucial to highlight that the impact of prebiotics on insulin sensitivity can vary from person to person, depending on their baseline health, diet, genetics, and the specific prebiotic used. Incorporating prebiotic-rich foods or supplements, under the guidance of a healthcare professional, may be beneficial for individuals looking to improve insulin sensitivity and overall metabolic health. Studies have indicated that prebiotics can enhance insulin sensitivity, which is beneficial for managing blood glucose levels and reducing the risk of type 2 diabetes.

Incorporating prebiotic-rich foods or supplements into one's diet may help a person feel fuller for longer, reduce overeating, and ultimately support healthier eating habits and weight management. However, individual responses to prebiotics can vary, before making any modifications to one's diet, it is critical to talk with a healthcare practitioner. Prebiotics may influence the gut–brain axis, helping to regulate appetite and food intake, which can be beneficial for weight management.

Markowiak-Kopeć and Śliżewska (2020) reported that prebiotics are essential for SCFA production in the gut, and SCFAs have a crucial function in preserving gut well-being, regulating metabolism, and influencing systemic health. Consuming a diet rich in prebiotic-containing foods can support a healthy gut microbiome and the production of beneficial SCFAs. SCFAs, produced during the fermentation of prebiotics, have been linked to improved metabolic health by regulating glucose and lipid metabolism (Yadav et al., 2022).

It's noteworthy to emphasize the impacts of prebiotics, can vary based on the type of prebiotic, dosage, and individual factors. While the clinical evidence is promising, more research is needed to further understand the specific mechanisms and long-term effects of prebiotics on metabolic disorders (Bull and Plummer, 2014). Additionally, dietary changes and prebiotic supplementation should be considered as part of a comprehensive approach to managing metabolic conditions, including a balanced diet and regular physical activity.

2.5 PROBIOTICS: BENEFICIAL BACTERIA

2.5.1 Definition and Types of Probiotics

The FAO of the UNs and the WHO define probiotics as bacteria that are alive that, when fed in adequate quantities, aid in maintaining the health of the host (Bermudez-Brito et al., 2012). Lactic acid bacteria and bifido-bacteria are the kinds of bacteria that are most commonly utilized as probiotics. Although the exact processes underlying these effects are still being studied, probiotics have shown great promise as treatment possibilities for a number of disorders (Bermudez-Brito et al., 2012; Guarner and Malagelada, 2003). A few key mechanisms behind the antagonistic impacts of probiotics on various bacteria are as follows: modification of adherence to the mucosa that is competitive among the gut microbiota and epithelium, fortifying the barrier between the gut and epithelium and immune system regulation to provide the host an advantage.

Toll-like receptors and protein-like receptors with oligomerization domains that bind nucleotides are two examples of pattern recognition receptors that probiotics use to interact with the host. These receptors either boost or repress expression and influence subsequent processes by modulating key signaling processes, such as mitogen-triggered protein kinase and nuclear factor-B (Bermudez-Brito et al., 2012). The ability to comprehend is essential for causing minimal inflammatory tissue damage while evoking controlled antimicrobial responses. Probiotic strains that are suitable for a given application can be chosen with clarity thanks to these mechanisms, which may also reveal new activities for probiotics. Probiotics have demonstrated antibacterial (Bermudez-Brito et al., 2012) and anti-colorectal cancer activity (Liong, 2008), reduced irritable bowel symptoms, prevented IBD, alleviated lactose intolerance, and reduced surgical complications (Bermudez-Brito et al., 2012; Woodard et al., 2009). The benefits of probiotics differ based on the exertion, it is crucial to note, therefore generalizations about their possible health advantages should be avoided. Because of this, the health benefits associated with one strain may not apply to another, even within the same species (Bermudez-Brito et al., 2012).

2.5.2 Types of Probiotics

2.5.2.1 Bacillus and Bifdobacterium

The term "bifidobacterium" comes from the A species of specialized, classified as gramme-anaerobic microbes which usually has a branched end (Henrick et al., 2018; You et al., 2022). One of the most significant groups of probiotics for humans is this physiological bacterium, which is found in the human body. In order to maintain intestinal health, bifidobacterium can withstand anaerobic conditions, proliferate, metabolize, and secrete bifidogenic substances that have probiotic properties in the end and middle of the large and small intestine (Valdemiro Carlos, 2011). 32 species and 9 subspecies of Bifidobacterium are known to exist today; 14 of them have been isolated from human beings (Klaassens et al., 2009). These are the primary physiological roles of Bifidobacterium: (i) Like other LAB, Bifidobacterium has the ability to block pro-inflammatory cytokines and preserve the equilibrium of normal intestinal bacterial flora by limiting the growth of pathogenic bacteria (You et al., 2022). In vitro and in vivo protection against gut barrier disruption has also been shown by related investigations with Bifidobacterium. This protective impact is linked to improved intestinal tight junction integrity, reduction of vimentin release, and pro-inflammatory cytokine secretion. (ii) *Bifidobacterium bifidum* is believed to enhance bone health because it promotes calcium bioavailability and synthesizes amino acids and vitamins in the colon (Dubey & Patel, 2018; You et al., 2022). (iii) The anti-tumor properties of Bifidobacterium bifidum. Anti-tumor properties are exhibited by Bifidobacterium bifidum. A Bifidobacterium longum strain with the ability to localize and grow while secreting C-CPE-PE23 and multiply selectively in tumors was successfully generated by Shimizu et al. (Figure 2.3 and Table 2.3).

2.5.2.2 Lactobacillus

The three main categories of probiotics are bifidobacteria, lactobacilli, and other species. Probiotics are widely distributed and come in a variety of forms. Due to its status as the probiotic that best exemplifies within the LAB group, the LAB group is currently the focus of the majority of studies conducted on probiotic species. Importantly, because it inhibits the growth of pathogenic microorganisms, lactobacillus improves intestinal microecology and is a valuable prevalent probiotic in the examination of human intestinal microorganisms, closely tied to human health. It also summarizes vital vitamins and amino acids and makes intake easier of minerals (Milani et al., 2017; You et al., 2022) enhances body weight and size, and promotes host growth. Furthermore, colonic epithelial cells' normal morphology and SCFAs are a crucial metabolite of Lactobacillus that aid in the bacterium's development as well as reproduction, which in turn lowers the amount of Escherichia coli in the intestine (Ding et al., 2019; You et al., 2022). For instance, Lactobacillus plantarum ZJUFT17 (T17), also known as Lactiplanti bacillus plantarum in the updated microbial taxonomy, was isolated from traditional Chinese sour dough and shown to have anti-obesity or weight-loss properties. It also has the potential

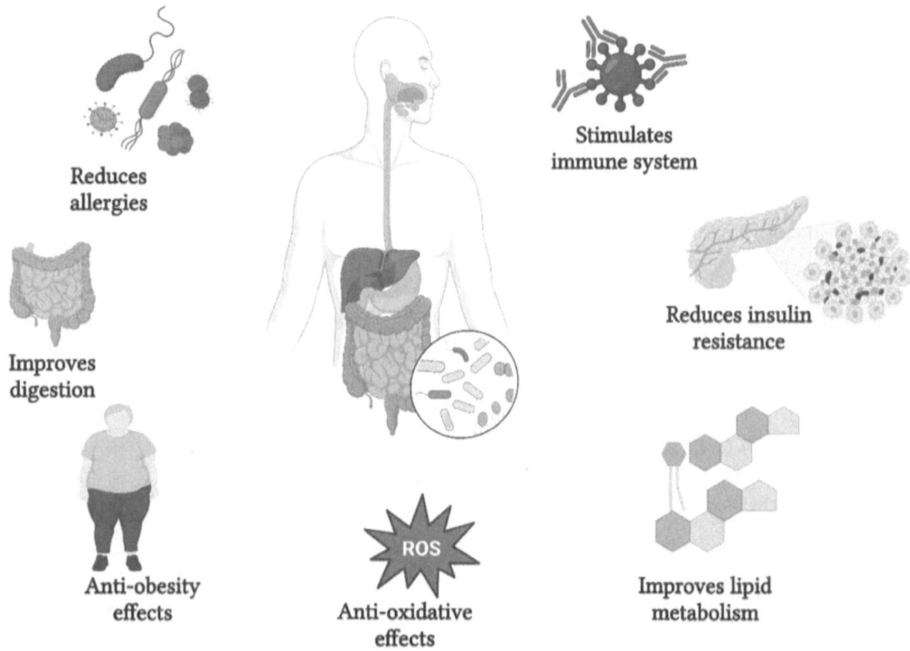

FIGURE 2.3 Health benefits of probiotics.

TABLE 2.3
Benefits and Uses for Probiotics

Microorganism	Benefits and Uses	References
Lactobacillus acidophilus	Lowers cytokines to treat diarrhea, lower cholesterol, improve cancer, and treat inflammatory bowel disease. Used in clinics and medicine.	You et al. (2022)
Lactobacillus casei	Preventive measures or management for disorders affecting the gut flora. Used in Dairy fermentation	Hill et al. (2018)
Lactobacillus rhamnosus	Possesses the capacity to combat harmful microbiome and fungus in the genitourinary tract, protecting postmenopausal women from developing recurrent UTIs used in the fermentation of milk, fruit juice, medications, and millet.	You et al. (2022)
Lactococcus lactis	Produces volatile flavor compounds by breaking down metabolic amino acids, which also helps to improve the texture and flavor profile of fermented foods. Used to ferment cheese.	You et al. (2022)
Bifidobacterium adolescentis	It modifies the microbiota of the colon and cecum and lessens inflammation in the brain and spleen. Used in clinics and medicine	You et al. (2022)
Bifidobacteria	It modifies the microbiota of the colon and cecum and lessens inflammation in the brain and spleen. Used in clinics and medicine	Xu et al. (2019)
Bacillus subtilis	Aquaculture: enhanced immunity, growth, nutrition, and disease resistance in aquatic species	You et al. (2022)
Bacillus coagulans	It has the ability to control the balance of intestinal flora, enhance immunity, support nutrient metabolism and utilization, and withstand high temperatures, acids, and bile utilized in both animal husbandry and medicine.	Mu and Cong (2019)

to function as a beneficial bacteria and can lessen resistance to insulin and inflammation in the system, both of which are regulated by the microbiota of the intestines.

2.5.2.3 Additional Species of Bacteria

Nowadays, the food sector often uses Gram-positive parthenococci such as Enterococcus in addition to Bifidobacterium and Lactobacillus. The capacity of strains belonging to Enterococcus to persist, clash, and stick to host cells in the colon is one of their most valuable probiotic characteristics. In addition, Enterococcus is highly resistant to a broad range of pH and temperature and has a notable capacity to manufacture bacteriocin, a naturally occurring antibacterial agent that can be used in the food industry (Hanchi et al., 2018).

The popular selective and probiotic non-pathogenic Saccharomyces cerevisiae is being employed in the manufacturing of probiotic meals on a commercial scale.

Saccharomyces boulardii is widely utilized in the treatment of problems with digestion, including symptoms of gastroenteritis, and has been thoroughly studied for its probiotic effect; it is especially useful when used in conjunction with antibiotic therapy. In addition, in the digestive tract, Saccharomyces boulardii is more likely to survive than other probiotics, which aids in preserving the configuration of the normal intestinal microbiota. In pathogenic infections or chronic disorders, it also exerts immunomodulatory actions that adjust immunological pathways (You et al., 2022).

Apart from the yeasts and enterococci already given, other probiotic categories that are more widely available are Streptococcus species, *E. coli*, Bacillus species. The functions and uses of a few typical probiotics were compiled in Table 2.4, based on recently published research.

2.5.3 Mechanisms of Action

Some of the primary mechanisms of action of probiotics include the improvement of the epithelial barrier, stronger attachment to intestinal mucosa and simultaneously suppression of pathogen adhesion, competitive elimination of pathogenic microbes, the generation of anti-microorganism substances, and modulation of the immune system (Figure 2.4).

2.5.3.1 Strengthening the Epithelium Barrier

The enteric flora, which is dynamic and changing, and the luminal contents are in constant touch with the intestinal epithelium. An essential defense system, the intestinal

TABLE 2.4
Investigations Detailing the Impact of Probiotics in Animal Models

Circumstances	Description & Dosage of Probiotics	Animal Models	Outcomes	References
Atherosclerosis	Probiotics delivered through water; 109 CFU/mL of Pediococcus acidilactici AS185 (1 × per day for 8 weeks)	Mature Sprague Dawley rats	Reduction: TNFα, IL-1β, IL-6, IFN-γ, TG, TC, OX-LDL-C, LDL-C, and IL-10 and HDL-C should rise	Wang et al. (2019)
Persistent inflammation	Lactobacillus plantarum LS/07 CCM7766 (109 CFU/mL), 8% BeneoSynergy1 (oligofructose-enriched inulin), 4% oil (improved with flaxseed oil), and probiotic culture were transported via skim milk. The regimen was followed for 28 weeks, with one serving each day.	Both men and women Dawley Sprague rats,	Reduction of IL-6, IL-and IL-2, 17, Elevate: IL-10, NF-κB, TNF-α,	Štofilová et al. (2015)
Heart problems	PBS-delivered probiotic culture: Lactobacillus reuteri GMNL-263 (Lr263) (1 × daily for 8 weeks) at 11 × 10^9 CFU/mL for 1 day. Two times 1010 CFU/mL	Sprague Dawley rats	Reduction of TG and TC	Liao et al. (2016)
Hypercholesterolemia	Double-coated probiotic Lactobacillus plantarum KCTC3928, a live cell with 109 CFU/mL, delivered once daily for 4 weeks. One daily for 4 weeks of Lactobacillus plantarum KCTC3928 dead cell (1010 CFU/mL).	Male C57BL/6 mice	Reduction: AST, ALT (live cell), HDL-C/TC, TG, HDL-C/LDL-C, and LDL-C Boost: dead cell HDL-C	Jeun et al. (2010)
Metabolic syndrome	Salted solution containing Lactobacillus fermentum NCIMB 5221 (2 × 1010 CFU/mL) at a dose of one microliter each day for 8 weeks.	Male ZDF (Leprfa) rats	Reduction: INS, HOMA-IR, TG, LDL-C, TG/HDL-C, and LDL-C/HDL-C	(Xavier-Santos et al. 2020)
Metabolic syndrome	Saline solution with Bifidobacterium longum BIF CGMCC NO.2107 (2 × 109 CFU/mL) probiotic (1H daily for 12 weeks)	Male Wistar rats	Reduction: BW, SBP, BG, TG, and INS	Chen et al., (2011)
Metabolic syndrome	PBS probiotic: Enterococcus faecium WEFA23-H (5 × 109 CFU/mL) 1 × daily for 5 weeks	Female BALB/c mice and male Sprague Dawley rats	Reduction: BW, TC, TG, LDL-C, BG, and HOM-IR	Zhang et al. (2017)
Obesity	Water-based probiotic: 1.5 × 1010 CFU of Streptococcus thermophilus (CNCM strain number I1630), Lactobacillus bulgaricus (CNCM strain numbers I-1632 and I1519), Lactobacillus lactis subsp. lactis (CNCM strain number I-1631); Lactobacillus acidophilus; Streptococcus thermophiles; Lactobacillus plantarum; Bifidobacterium lactis (CNCM I-2494); Lactobacillus reuteri (DSM 17938) (3 g/200 mL for each animal) (1 × daily for 4 weeks)	Male Syrian golden hamsters	Reduction: BW	Avolio et al. (2019)
Obesity	PBS Lactobacillus rhamnosus GG (1 × 107 CFU/mL) probiotic (1 × daily for 10 weeks)	Male C57BL/6J mice	Reduction: BW, IL-12p70, and Leptin Increase: AD	Ji et al. (2018)

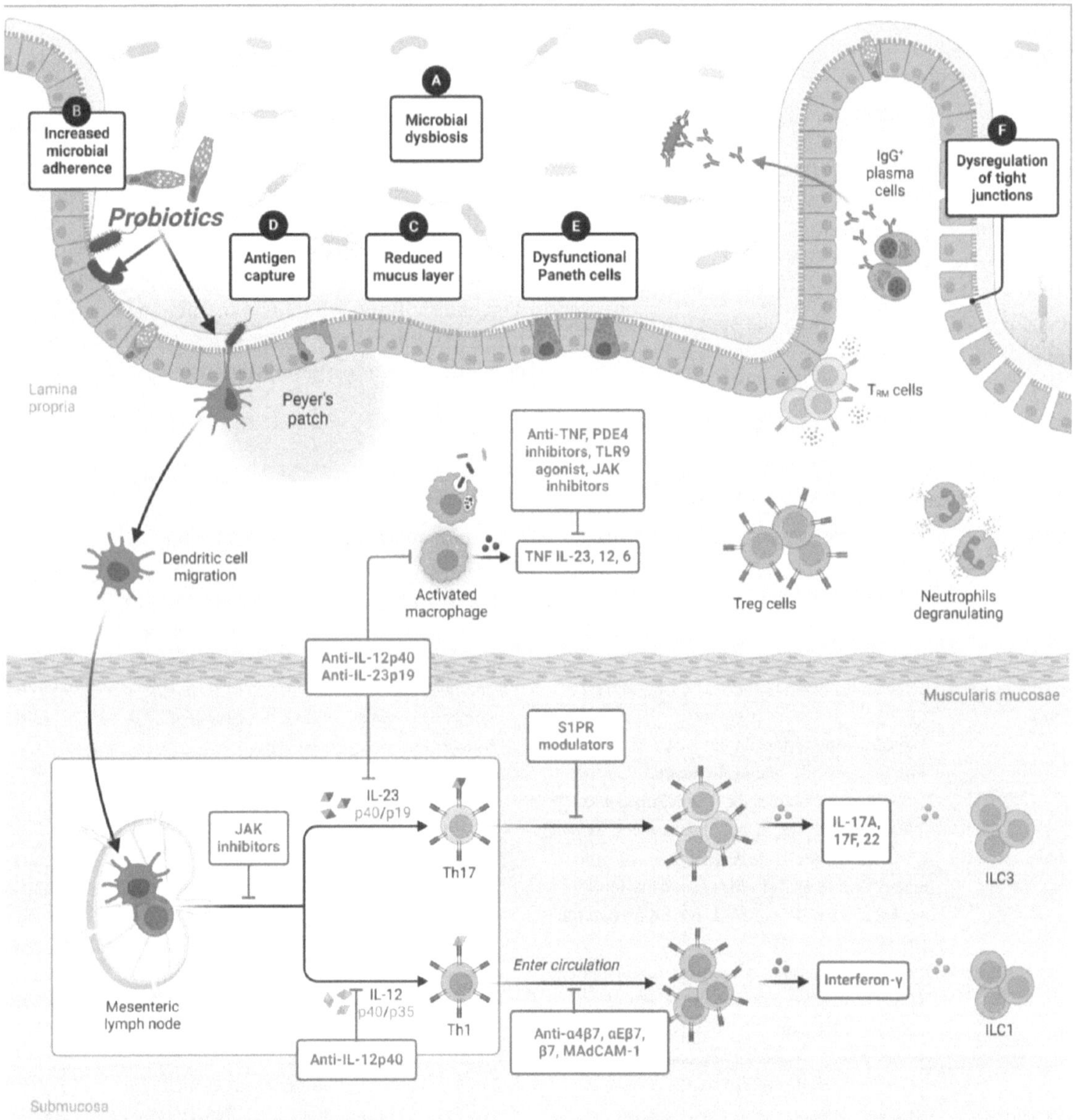

FIGURE 2.4 Mechanism of action of probiotics.

barrier, protects the organism from the environment and maintains epithelial integrity. According to Ohland and MacNaughton (2010), the intestinal barriers the defensive mechanisms include the mucous layer, secretory IgA, antimicrobial peptides, and the epithelial junction adhesion complex. Intestinal diseases like IBD may arise from the disruption of this barrier function, which allows bacteria and the submucosa to be damaged by food substances, which can then cause inflammatory responses (Bermudez-Brito et al., 2012). Consuming non-pathogenic bacteria may affect how the intestinal barrier functions, and probiotic bacteria's contribution to barrier maintenance has been well studied.

The intestinal mucosa serves as the first physical barrier to keep the intestine safe from toxins found in the intestinal lumen. Once probiotics have entered the intestine, they will interact with intestinal bacteria. Following their entry into the colon, probiotics will interact with bacteria to strengthen their mechanical, chemical, biological, and immunological barriers (Cheng et al., 2020). Probiotics enter the colon and interact with intestinal cells to preserve the strength of the mucosal membrane and the normal operation of the intestinal mechanical barrier, as well as to stimulate mucus production, promote mucosal regeneration, and restore intestinal permeability (You et al., 2022). As an illustration, certain research has revealed that antibiotics damage the intestinal barrier and disturb natural intestinal flora. Nonetheless, by boosting intestinal sIgA secretion and reducing inflammation, Fagopyrum esculentum water-soluble polysaccharide Moench bee pollen can improve intestinal barrier integrity and reduce microbial dysbiosis brought on by antibiotics.

2.5.3.2 Augmentation of the System's Immunological Reaction

Some probiotics in the gut are of the immunostimulatory type, which means they can act as immune regulators and control inflammation by directly or indirectly influencing the function of different immune cells in the body, such as B cells, macrophages, monocytes, natural killer (NK) cells, and T cells (You et al., 2022). By inhibiting the growth of cancerous cells, producing IL-12, which activates natural killer cells and promotes the development of these probiotics enhances non-specific cellular immune responses by stimulating Th1 cells and secreting a range of cytokines in a strain-specific and dose-dependent way. They also combat allergies by maintaining the proper balance between Th1 and Th2 cells (Azad et al., 2018). Yogurt is a good way to supply the necessary probiotics to boost the immunological response of the intestinal mucosal immune system, for example, by increasing the frequency of IgA+ cells and cytokine-producing cells in the intestine effector sites. The cellular immunological activity of the body can also be improved by short-term probiotic treatment. According to one study, when elderly individuals took supplements of the right doses of probiotics, their bodies' ability to perform polymorphonuclear phagocytosis and the tumor-killing activity of natural killer cells rose.

2.5.3.3 Suppression of the Adsorption and Colonization of Harmful Microorganisms

By altering the metabolism of microorganisms and enhancing human health, probiotics control the colonization and intervention of gut microbes. By creating antimicrobial factors to create colonization resistance and limit infection by intestine pathogenic microbes, or by competing for nutrition, probiotics prevent gastrointestinal disorders. The intestinal tract of rabbits can be effectively colonized by the autogenous strain Enterococcus faecalis EF2019 (CCM7420), which also has the ability to diminish coagulase-positive staphylococci, coliforms, and clostridia (You et al., 2022). Additionally, Ent7420 produces the antimicrobial enterococci. Apart from the digestive tract, probiotics can also reproduce and produce antimicrobial metabolites on the epithelial surface that can regulate and preserve the vaginal microbiome. As well as adhering to mucus and epithelial cells to provide them a competitive advantage over harmful bacteria, probiotics can attach themselves to the host to strengthen bonds and enhance the immune response (Zhang et al., 2019). As foreign bacteria colonize the human intestine, probiotics can be absorbed by competing with pathogenic bacteria for nutrients (Figures 2.5 and 2.6).

2.5.3.4 Impact of Probiotics on the Gut–Brain Axis

It is believed that the relationship between the gut and the brain is a mechanism inside the central nervous system (CNS) that regulates the brain's and the gut's reciprocal interactions at the neuronal, endocrine, and immune levels. Its significance in preserving equilibrium in the body has long been recognized (You et al., 2022; Zhang et al., 2019). Understanding the significance of the gut–brain axis has been of significant interest to microbiota, since they are one of the key regulators of this system. The gut microbiota and the brain communicate through a variety of pathways, including the immune system, tryptophan

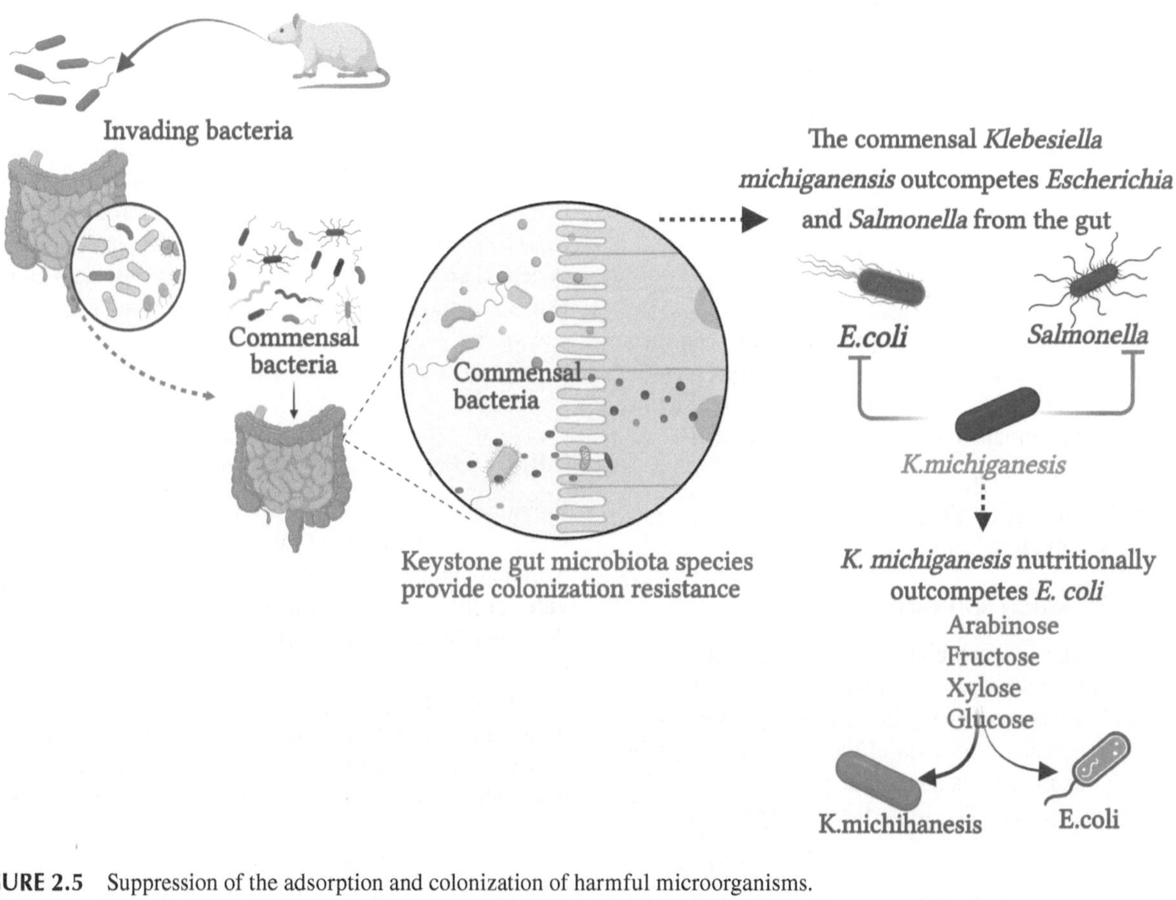

FIGURE 2.5 Suppression of the adsorption and colonization of harmful microorganisms.

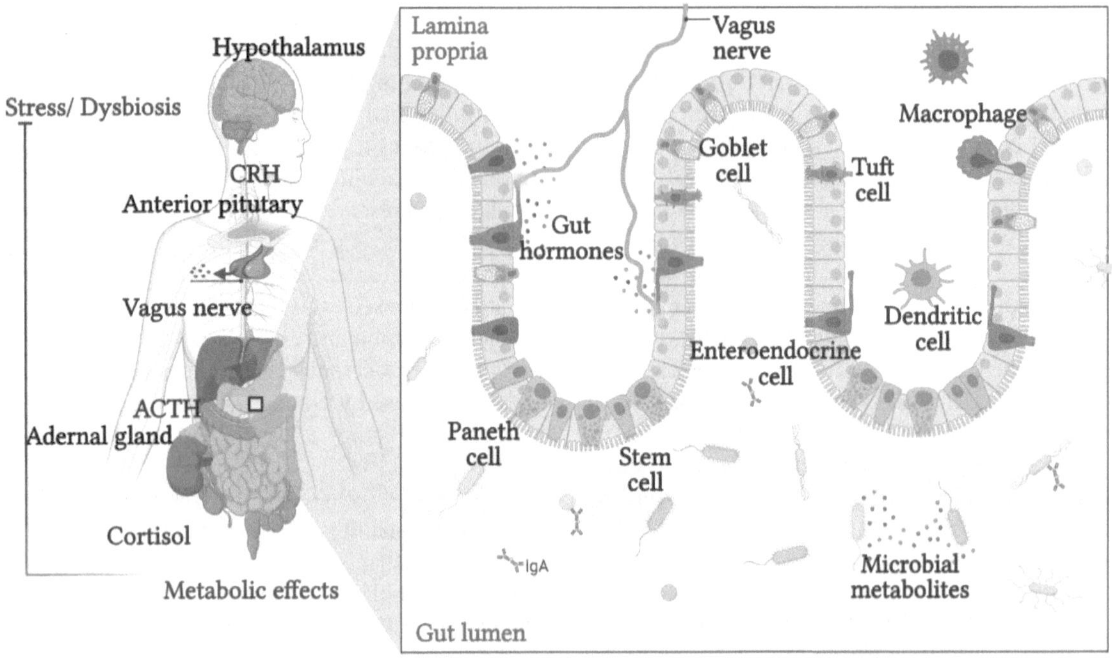

FIGURE 2.6 Impact of probiotics on the gut–brain axis.

metabolism, the vagus and enteric nervous systems, and other mechanisms that may be involved in gut microbial signaling to the brain involving microbial metabolites like SCFAs, branched-chain amino acids, and peptidoglycans. By means of the autonomic nervous system, microbes' composition and behavior can be altered by the brain.

2.5.4 Clinical Evidence in Metabolic Disorders

Consuming products containing probiotics has been recommended by several studies as a dietary therapy to prevent MetS. The research demonstrating the probiotic effects on MetS risk variables using animal models is included in Table 2.4.

2.6 SYNBIOTICS: THE SYNERGY OF PREBIOTICS AND PROBIOTICS

2.6.1 Definition and Importance

Synbiotics refer to a combination of prebiotics and probiotics in a single product or dietary supplement. Prebiotics are indigestible substances that stimulate the development and function of beneficial bacteria in the gut, whereas probiotics are living microorganisms that provide health advantages when ingested. The importance of synbiotics lies in their synergistic effect on the gut microbiota. By providing both prebiotics and probiotics together, synbiotics create an optimal environment for beneficial bacteria to thrive and establish themselves in the gut. This can result in enhanced gut health, improved digestion, strengthened immune function, and potentially, positive impacts on various aspects of overall health, including metabolic health and the immune system (Pandey et al., 2015). Synbiotics provide a comprehensive method for promoting and preserving a harmonious and varied gut microbiota, which is increasingly acknowledged as a crucial factor in our general health.

2.6.2 Complementary Mechanisms

Prebiotics and probiotics work in concert to support a better gut microbiota and, in turn, general well-being through complementary processes of synbiotics. Prebiotics provide probiotics with nutrition, which promotes their development and activity. In exchange, prebiotics are broken down by probiotics into advantageous substances like SCFAs, which support gut health and inhibit the growth of pathogenic microbes. The gut microbiota becomes more varied and balanced as a result of this reciprocal support, which increases the effectiveness of probiotics and prebiotics. Probiotics add to a healthy gut environment by introducing and sustaining beneficial living bacteria in the ecosystem, while prebiotics provide the groundwork for one. When combined, they form a potent alliance that can improve immunological response, inflammation, metabolism, and digestion. The complementary mechanisms of synbiotics underscore their potential as a comprehensive approach to gut health and offer a promising strategy for maintaining a balanced and resilient microbial community.

2.6.3 Clinical Applications of Synbiotics

Prebiotics and probiotics work synergistically to form synbiotics, which are becoming more and more well-known for their possible medicinal uses. This all-encompassing approach tackles the complex connection between general health and gut bacteria (Murphy et al., 2021). The clinical uses of synbiotics in a range of medical disorders as well as their potential for treatment are discussed below.

2.6.3.1 Gastrointestinal Disorders

Synbiotics have demonstrated clinical efficacy in managing various gastrointestinal disorders. Synbiotics can be beneficial in restoring gut microbial equilibrium, mitigating inflammation, and alleviating symptoms such as stomach discomfort and diarrhea in disorders including IBD and irritable bowel syndrome (IBS). Clinical trials have shown improvements in both disease activity and QoL for individuals with these conditions.

2.6.3.2 Immune Health

The gut microbiota exerts a substantial influence on the regulation of the immune system. Research has been conducted on the potential of synbiotics to enhance immune function. Clinical studies have indicated that synbiotic supplementation may enhance immune responses, reducing the risk of infections and improving vaccine effectiveness. This is especially relevant in populations with weakened immune systems, such as the elderly or those with chronic illnesses.

2.6.3.3 Metabolic Health

Synbiotics have shown promise in the context of metabolic health, particularly in addressing obesity and type 2 diabetes. Synbiotics can impact glucose metabolism and enhance insulin sensitivity by regulating the gut microbiota and stimulating the formation of SCFAs. Clinical evidence suggests that synbiotics can aid in weight management and metabolic control.

2.6.3.4 Allergies and Atopic Diseases

The gut microbiome is intricately linked to the development and regulation of allergic responses. Synbiotics may have a role in preventing and managing allergies and atopic diseases, such as eczema and asthma. Clinical studies have explored their potential to modulate immune responses and reduce the risk of allergic sensitization.

2.6.3.5 Mental Health and Neurological Disorders

Recent studies indicate that the connection between the gastrointestinal system and the brain is of utmost importance in the field of mental health and neurological illnesses. Synbiotics may have a therapeutic role in conditions like depression, anxiety, and neurodegenerative diseases. Clinical studies are ongoing to understand the impact of synbiotics on these complex conditions (Salminen et al., 2020).

2.6.3.6 Antimicrobial Properties

Synbiotics can exhibit antimicrobial effects by creating an environment unfavorable for pathogenic bacteria. This may have applications in preventing or treating bacterial infections, particularly in healthcare settings.

2.6.3.7 Pediatrics

Researchers are now investigating the use of synbiotics in pediatric healthcare, namely, for preventing necrotizing enterocolitis (NEC) in preterm newborns and managing pediatric allergy illnesses.

2.6.3.8 Women's Health

In gynecological health, synbiotics are being studied for their potential in managing conditions like bacterial vaginosis and urinary tract infections. They may help maintain a healthy vaginal microbiome.

A flexible and promising method for enhancing patient outcomes in a range of healthcare settings is the use of synbiotics. Their capacity to impact the gut microbiota and its multifarious relationships with many bodily systems renders them a subject of ongoing investigation and a promising adjunctive treatment for an extensive array of medical ailments. Synbiotics may become an increasingly more useful tool in the care and prevention of complicated health difficulties, from gastrointestinal illnesses to mental health conditions, as our understanding of the gut–brain–immune axis expands. However, it is crucial to bear in mind that the therapeutic use of synbiotics must be customized to suit the individual requirements of each patient and guided by evidence-based protocols (Deshmukh & Patole, 2021).

2.7 SIGNALING PATHWAYS IMPACTED BY PREBIOTICS, PROBIOTICS, AND SYNBIOTICS

2.7.1 AMP-Activated Protein Kinase (AMPK) Pathway

A proposal has been made to replace the term "non-alcoholic fatty liver disease" (NAFLD) with "metabolic-associated fatty liver disease" (MAFLD) in order to more accurately represent the diverse nature and underlying mechanisms of the illness (Méndez-Sánchez et al., 2022). The onset and course of MAFLD may be impacted by a variety of risk factors, including obesity (Baboota et al.,

2022). Investigating the functions of mitophagy and mitochondrial ROS in MAFLD could be significant.

In general, damaged mitochondria can be specifically destroyed by mitophagy to lower the amount of ROS generated by damaged mitochondria which might damage healthy mitochondria and result in mitochondrial malfunction. Consequently, to maintain mitochondrial integrity in MAFLD, defective mitochondria may also be broken down via mitophagy, a crucial mechanism of mitochondrial quality control (Cai et al., 2022). As a result, active mitophagy would finally reduce oxidative stressors and/or inflammatory reactions that cause ROS (Vachliotis et al., 2022).

The alterations in hepatic inflammation may support the need to assess the efficacy of the synbiotic treatment for MAFLD (Scorletti et al., 2020). Prebiotics have been shown to be effective in treating MAFLD, specifically through modulating the PI3K/AKT/mTOR/AMPK pathway. Furthermore, a number of ingestible phytochemicals may stimulate mitophagy to ameliorate mitochondrial damage, which represents a potentially effective treatment approach for MAFLD by protecting the liver. The modulation of Th17/Treg balance has been proposed as a potential role for the PI3K/AKT/mTOR signaling pathway, which could potentially contribute to the pathogenesis of MAFLD (Figure 2.1).

Additionally, it has been proposed that the Th17/Treg balance is crucial to the pathophysiology of major depressive illnesses (Yoshikawa et al., 2023). The research articles cited above suggest that the molecular etiology for MAFLD may involve neurodegenerative illnesses and/or disorders associated to aging.

2.7.1.1 AMPK Activation by Probiotics

Probiotics fortified with selenium (SP) exhibit an anti-inflammatory impact in the NAFLD model caused by a western diet. To generate an animal model resembling NAFLD, male Sprague Dawley rats weighing between 160 and 180 grams were administered a high-fat diet consisting of 58% of their caloric intake from fat. Additionally, their meal was supplemented with a fructose solution at a concentration of 30% by weight/volume. This dietary regimen was maintained for a duration of 12 weeks. The expression of AMPK, SIRT-1, and autophagy proteins such as LC-3 A/B and Beclin was dramatically downregulated in NAFLD control rats, suggesting downregulation of autophagy. On the other hand, supplementing with SP reduces hepatic steatosis as seen by better biochemical indicators and autophagic activation through increased SIRT-1 and AMPK pathway expression, highlighting the significance of autophagy in the pathogenesis of the disease (Pant et al., 2023).

2.7.1.2 AMPK Activation by Synbiotics

A year of a synbiotic supplementation changed the fecal microbiome in a randomized study of NAFLD patients, but it had no effect on liver fat content or liver fibrosis signs (Scorletti et al., 2020).

2.7.2 Insulin Signaling Pathway: Probiotics on Insulin Sensitivity and Glucose Metabolism in Human Trials

Administering a probiotic capsule containing three freeze-dried strains of Lactobacillus acidophilus (2109 CFU/g), Bifidobacterium bifidum (2109 CFU/g), and Lactobacillus casei (2109 CFU/g) on a daily basis for 6 weeks resulted in enhanced insulin sensitivity, as determined by the homeostasis model assessment for insulin resistance and the quantitative insulin sensitivity check index. This enhancement was noted in comparison to a placebo pill containing cellulose. The treatment of probiotics resulted in a reduction in TAG and VLDL levels. However, this study did not evaluate HbA1c levels. The source cited is Karamali et al. (2016). In addition, a 4-week oral treatment of L. acidophilus NCFM improved insulin sensitivity, as assessed by hyperinsulinemic-euglycemic clamp, compared to a placebo group. However, there were no changes observed in inflammatory markers such as IL-Ira, TNF-α, IL-6, and high-sensitivity C-reactive protein (Andreasen et al., 2010).

2.7.2.1 Prebiotics on Insulin Sensitivity and Glucose Metabolism in Human Trials

a. ***Fructooligosaccharides:*** A double-blind crossover study was conducted with twelve healthy participants. During the study, the participants were given a daily supplementation of 20 g of fructose syrup (FOS) for 4 weeks. The results showed that this supplementation reduced the production of glucose in the liver, without affecting the uptake of glucose stimulated by insulin or the production of glucose suppressed by insulin during a hyperinsulinemic clamp. The reference is Luo et al. (1996).
b. ***Resistant starch:*** The application of resistant starch enhanced insulin sensitivity in persons without health issues (Robertson et al., 2005) and decreased the levels of glucose or insulin after a meal in individuals with type 2 diabetes (Johnston et al., 2010).

2.7.2.2 Synbiotics on Insulin Sensitivity and Glucose Metabolism in Human Trials

The synbiotic bread, including 1 × 108 CFU of the probiotic Lactobacillus sporogeneses and 007 g of inulin per gram as a prebiotic, was taken by participants with type 2 diabetes for 8 weeks. The purpose was to enhance lipid profiles, insulin metabolism, NO levels, plasma, and the amount of malondialdehyde. The experiment was done using a randomized, double-blind, placebo-controlled approach (Bahmani, et al., 2016; Tajadadi-Ebrahimi et al., 2014).

2.7.3 Prebiotics on Inflammation and NF-κB Pathway

One potential approach for managing diabetes is to preserve beta cells by controlling NF-κB. Considering the association found between NF-kB and gut microbiota, probiotic-mediated NF-kB targeted therapy may be explored as a potential treatment for diabetes and other illnesses with inflammatory and metabolic disorders. Numerous Lactobacillus strains have demonstrated the ability to control NF-κB expression both in vivo and in vitro. Promising biotherapeutic targets for diabetes include NF-κB, which can be regulated through dietary intervention incorporating probiotics, according to emerging leads from existing data. It may be possible to use specific probiotic strains to control NF-κB in order to preserve health and prevent diabetes. Signaling pathways activate NF-κB and are probably regulated by probiotics. Probiotics can control NF-κB by several mechanisms, including inactivating IKK, phosphorylating IkBα, inhibiting ubiquitination, blocking the degradation of IkBα by proteasomes, preventing the translocation of NF-κB dimers to the nucleus, and inhibiting transcription.

2.7.3.1 Prebiotics on Inflammation and NF-kB Pathway

Probiotics constitute beneficial bacteria that help with IBD by modifying inflammatory signaling pathways. When compared to cells treated with Sonicat, the probiotic cocktail caused the NF-κB pathway's RIP, NEMO, IRAK4, and TIRAP, genes to be downregulated. The administration of probiotics has been found to cause a significant reduction in IL-1βand IL-6 production. The probiotic cocktail being studied, namely, Bifidobacterium spp., demonstrated anti-inflammatory effects on HT-29 cells via altering the JAK/STAT and NF-κB signaling pathways. Patients with IBD may find that using probiotics with the fewest adverse effects is an effective treatment, even in the early stages of inflammation (Aghamohammad et al., 2022).

2.7.3.2 Synbiotics on Inflammation and NF-kB Pathway

Research on synbiotic in IBD-affected animals is promising, and clinical outcomes for IBD patients are positive, but there are still few placebo-controlled trials and a lack of data. Before recommendations for the routine use of synbiotic to treat IBD can be made, more double-blind, placebo-controlled studies are needed. Probiotic use appears to be generally safe, effective, and potentially well-tolerated in IBD patients. Scientific data suggests that they can help patients with mild to moderately active ulcerative colitis with their clinical symptoms (Fujimori et al., 2009).

On intestinal epithelial cells (IECs) and monocytes, Streptococcus salivarius showed anti-inflammatory properties. These microorganisms generate a symbiotic relationship well with their host. HT-29/kB-luc-E, a reporter clone stimulated by tumour necrosis factor alpha (TNF-α), was used to screen strains. Each strain's supernatant decreased the activation of NF-κB. Two strains that were the most productive generated an active metabolite, which was able to inhibit the proinflammatory chemokine interleukin-8 (IL-8) release (Kaci et al., 2011).

2.7.4 Probiotic, Prebiotic, and Synbiotic Hormone Signaling and the Gut–Brain Axis

Multiple studies have shown evidence of the influence of gut microbiota on the connection between the gut and the brain, known as the gut–brain axis, and its capacity to potentially prevent and manage many brain illnesses, such as depression, insomnia, and Alzheimer's disease (Alli et al., 2022; Pluta et al., 2020). Probiotics enhance the gut–brain axis and enhance the management of some brain disorders by directly modulating the composition of gut bacteria toward beneficial functioning. Furthermore, the therapeutic effects of prebiotics on mental illnesses are achieved through both direct and indirect mechanisms, including the modification of the composition of intestinal microbiota and the promotion and augmentation of probiotics in the colon. Probiotics have the ability to directly modify the biochemistry of the CNS, leading to changes in the levels of serotonin, g-aminobutyric acid (GABA), brain-derived neurotrophic factor (BDNF), dopamine (DA), and c-Fos. These changes subsequently impact behavior and cognition. Specific probiotic strains exert an influence on the vagus and enteric nerves, which play a crucial role in the communication between the gut and the brain. In addition, probiotic bacteria regulate the composition of beneficial bacteria and indirectly enhance the diversity of the gut microbiota. Subsequently, the gut microbiota might indirectly enhance CNS function by modifying metabolites such as tryptophan, exopolysaccharides, and SCFAs. In addition, there is a synbiotic relationship between the gut microbiota and the immune, endocrine, and CNSs. Probiotics and prebiotics enhance the vagus nerve and enteric nervous system (ENS), thereby impacting brain function through the modification and augmentation of metabolites such as tryptophan and SCFAs. The secretion levels of specific brain factors, such as dopamine, brain-derived neurotrophic factor, serotonin/5 hydroxy tryptamine, gamma-aminobutyric (GABA), and brain-derived neurotrophic factor, have a significant impact on mental illnesses. Probiotics and prebiotics activate the immune system, leading to the release of pro-inflammatory cytokines. These cytokines modify the hormone system and neurons, hence decreasing inflammation in the specific brain region (Ansari et al., 2020; Ojeda et al., 2021; Tabrizi et al., 2019). Research has shown that the utilization of synbiotic products, comprising prebiotics such as resistant starch and inulin, and probiotics like Lactobacillus, Enterococcus, and Bifidobacterium, results in an elevated production of neurotransmitters and neuropeptides such as brain-derived-neurotrophic factor and GABA. This leads to enhanced CNS function and improved cognitive abilities, including the management of psychiatric conditions like anxiety, stress, depression, and memory impairment (Li et al., 2021; Swanson et al., 2020; Tan et al., 2021).

2.8 CLINICAL STUDIES AND TRIALS

2.8.1 Human Trial on Probiotics

The clinical research has shifted its attention toward probiotics and postbiotics due to their unique therapeutic advantages and prospective benefits. This is supported by a growing body of preclinical studies that have shown their effectiveness in treating different diseases. The amount of clinical trial registrations in the ClinicalTrials.gov database has shown a considerable growth in probiotic-related clinical research since 2001.

Moreover, an analysis of clinical research data spanning from 2001 to 2023 indicates that the predominant focus of studies on probiotics has been on infections, diarrhea, IBD, and IBS. This may be linked to the well-established primary therapeutic mechanisms of probiotics, which encompass the management of gut microbiota, modification of immunological response, and enhancement of gastrointestinal function.

Hyperuricemia is a frequently occurring metabolic disorder. The probiotics Limosilactobacillus fermentum GR-3 have been proven to enhance the elimination of uric acid and improve hyperuricemia in humans. This was demonstrated by a significant decrease in serum uric acid levels (26.2%±2.3%) in a randomized, controlled, double-blind study involving 120 patients with hyperuricemia. The study is registered in the Chinese Clinical Trial Registry under the identifier ChiCTR2100053287 (Zhao et al., 2022). A recent clinical study conducted by Spencer et al. in 2021 has substantiated the beneficial effects of probiotic supplements in the context of melanoma immunotherapy. Probiotics have demonstrated their efficacy as a novel approach to address malnutrition in neonates (Table 2.5).

2.8.1.1 New concerns regarding the safety of probiotics in vulnerable target populations

There are few long-term trials aimed at proving the safety of probiotics in populations at risk (older adults, premature infants, and those with compromised or weakened immune systems). Immunocompromised hosts may be more susceptible to adverse events (AEs) despite the good effects of probiotics being documented in these populations. This is because of their weakened defenses against microbial challenges (Sanders et al., 2010).

Short-term observations provide evidence that in elderly, stressed, or immunocompromised people, certain probiotic strains may act as opportunistic infections or neonatal populations (Kothari et al., 2019). Probiotic risks for mothers who are pregnant or nursing have been investigated. Just 28 out of the 100 pertinent research on the use of probiotics during pregnancy revealed AEs. Of these, only 11 reported AEs—such as headaches, nausea, and gastrointestinal issues—that might be causally linked to the medication were made; neither the mother nor the child had any significant health difficulties. AEs were not reported in the 72 remaining investigations (Elias et al., 2011; Jarde et al., 2018; Sheyholislami & Connor, 2021).

TABLE 2.5
Evidence of Probiotics in Clinical Trials (2018–2023)

S. No.	NCT Number	Probiotic	Target Disease	Aim	Clinical Phase
1	NCT05570942	*L. rhamnosus* TCELL-1	Colorectal cancer (CRC)	Evaluation the Effectiveness of *L. rhamnosus* TCELL-1 Upon CRC	Phase 2
2	NCT01667627	Probiotic combination (BIO-25)	Irritable bowel syndrome (IBS)	Analyze the medical results of the multispecies probiotic combination "BIO-25" in persons diagnosed with irritable bowel syndrome with diarrhea (IBS-D).	Phase 4
3	NCT04223479	Probiotic formula capsule	Inflammatory bowel syndrome (IBD)	Probiotic adjuvant therapy's positive effects on people with ulcerative colitis	Phase 2
4	NCT03047291	*L. reuteri* Prodentis (PerioBalance©R)	Mucositis	An assessment of L. reuteri Prodentis's efficacy in the management of periimplantitis and mucositis	Phase 4
5	NCT03047291	*L. helveticus* Rosell ©R –52	Metabolic syndrome	Evaluating the impact of probiotics on metabolic syndrome	Phase 3
6	NCT03261466	*B. breve* BR03 and B632	Obesity	Assessing the effectiveness of probiotics in promoting weight reduction	Phase 4
7	NCT05629468	Probiotic formula (Hi- Flora)	Acne vulgaris	Evaluate the effectiveness of probiotics in treating Acne vulgaris.	Phase 3
8	NCT03568812	*Thermophiles, B. L. plantarum, S. bifidum, "Rillus©R"*	HIV Infections	Explore the potential of Rillus©R in alleviating gastrointestinal inflammation in individuals with HIV.	Phase 2
9	NCT03695432	*L. acidophilus* Rossel-52, *L. rhamnosus* Rosell-11	Influenza-like illness	Assessing the effectiveness of probiotics to lower H. pylori bacterial load and alter gut microbiota	Phase 2
10	NCT04567147	Formula probiotic	Depression	Investigated the effect of formula probiotic on depression	Phase 1

Every data of information in Table 2.5 was obtained from https://clinicaltrials.gov.

2.8.2 Human Trials on Prebiotics

Prebiotics, mostly consisting of dietary fibers, promote the growth and function of gut bacteria that are advantageous to the human body (Gibson et al., 2017). Postbiotics refer to the advantageous substances generated by probiotics. Each component significantly contributes to the overall balance of the body's internal stability and plays a distinct function in the mutually beneficial relationship with the human host (Chaluvadi et al., 2016).

Manage a variety of conditions, from mental health to gastrointestinal illnesses, by utilizing the benefits of probiotics and prebiotics to support gut microbiota health and immune system strength (Varsha et al., 2021). Gum Arabic (GA) has been used to treat a number of medical ailments, including rheumatoid arthritis, kidney illness, metabolic disorders, periodontitis, gastrointestinal disorders, and sickle cell anemia. GA also showed anti-inflammatory, prebiotic, and antibacterial qualities (Al-Jubori et al., 2023).

Worldwide, colorectal cancer (CRC) stands among the most dangerous cancer types and is the third most prevalent appearance. While over 90% of occurrences of colorectal cancer are sporadic, lifestyle choices such as heavy alcohol use, smoking, eating processed meat, and taking antibiotics often may contribute to the development of CRC. The progression of colorectal cancer (CRC) is heavily impacted by several variables, such as the diversity of an individual's intestinal microbiota, the integrity of the intestinal barrier, and the existence of helpful and harmful compounds that might cause mutations or cancer. As a result, probiotics and prebiotics have drawn emphasis due to their potential as microbiome-modulating agents and their effectiveness in CRC prevention and treatment. In addition to reviewing the current mechanisms that support the efficacy of prebiotic and probiotic supplements for CRC prevention and therapy, this report summarized the benefits of this approach. Apoptosis and the inhibition of cancer cell growth may be brought about by mechanisms that include creating helpful metabolites, strengthening the intestinal barrier, lowering intestinal inflammation, and balancing the composition of the gut microbiota (Wang et al., 2023).

2.8.3 Human Trials in Synbiotics

Patients with metabolic illnesses have been shown to benefit from the use of synbiotic. A symbiosis is a synergistic blend of probiotics and prebiotics that enhances the viability and stimulates the proliferation of advantageous and health-enhancing bacterial species in the GIT, hence benefitting the host (Gibson and Roberfroid, 1995). Recent clinical trials have shown that a 10-week synbiotic treatment is beneficial in improving blood pressure and QoL in people with hypothyroidism, although it may not improve depression or serum TSH levels (Ramezani et al., 2023).

2.9 CHALLENGES AND FUTURE DIRECTIONS

2.9.1 Regulatory Challenges

Despite the promising evidence for the use of prebiotics, probiotics, and synbiotics in managing metabolic disorders, there are several regulatory challenges that need to be addressed. One challenge is that there is no clear definition of what constitutes a prebiotic, probiotic, or synbiotics. This makes it difficult for regulators to develop clear and consistent regulations for these products.

Another challenge is that the mechanisms by which prebiotics, probiotics, and synbiotics exert their health effects are not fully understood (Cunningham et al., 2021). This makes it difficult for regulators to assess the safety and efficacy of these products. Regulatory bodies face challenges in standardizing definitions for prebiotics, probiotics, and synbiotics. A consensus on criteria for product classification and quality control is essential for ensuring consistency and reliability in research and development. Determining optimal doses and specific strains for therapeutic efficacy poses a significant challenge. The heterogeneity of gut microbiota among individuals adds complexity, making it difficult to establish universal guidelines for product formulations. Regulatory agencies require robust scientific evidence to support health claims associated with prebiotics, probiotics, and synbiotics. Establishing a causal relationship between microbial interventions and specific metabolic outcomes necessitates rigorous clinical trials and long-term observational studies. Ensuring the safety of microbial interventions is paramount. Regulatory bodies must assess the potential risks, including adverse reactions and unintended consequences. Standardized safety assessments and reporting mechanisms are crucial for consumer protection (Markowiak and Śliżewska, 2017).

The exploration of prebiotics, probiotics, and synbiotics as therapeutic tools for managing metabolic disorders offers a promising avenue for research and innovation. However, addressing regulatory challenges is imperative to translate these findings into safe and effective interventions. A collaborative effort among researchers, industry stakeholders, and regulatory bodies is essential to navigate the intricate landscape of signaling pathways, ensuring that these microbial interventions contribute positively to the management of metabolic disorders while upholding rigorous standards of safety and efficacy.

There is currently a dearth of standardized clinical trials to assess the impact of prebiotics, probiotics, and synbiotics on metabolic health. This poses a challenge for regulators in making well-informed choices about the regulation of these items.

2.9.2 Personalized Approaches

Personalized approaches start with understanding an individual's gut microbial profile. Advances in metagenomics allow for comprehensive analysis, identifying specific bacterial strains and their functional capacities. This microbial profiling forms the basis for tailoring prebiotics, probiotics, and synbiotics to an individual's unique microbiota composition. Personalized nutrition examines the complex interaction between an individual's genetic composition and their reaction to nutritional treatments (Yadav et al., 2022). Tailoring prebiotics to stimulate the growth of beneficial microbes and selecting probiotic strains based on an individual's microbial deficiencies enables precision nutrition that targets specific signaling pathways associated with metabolic health. Integrating genomic and metabolomic data provides a holistic understanding of the host-microbiota interaction. This approach allows for the identification of genetic factors influencing response to microbial interventions and enables the development of personalized strategies to modulate signaling pathways associated with metabolic disorders. Advancements in wearable technology and biomarker monitoring enable the real-time monitoring of metabolic parameters. Continuous monitoring enables the adjustment of prebiotic, probiotic, and synbiotic interventions based on an individual's dynamic metabolic responses, ensuring personalized precision over time. Personalized approaches extend beyond microbial interventions to include lifestyle modifications. Tailoring recommendations for physical activity, sleep, and stress management complements the targeted modulation of signaling pathways, creating a comprehensive and individualized approach to metabolic disorder management.

This can be achieved through a combination of:

Gut microbiota analysis: This involves sequencing the DNA of the gut microbiota to identify the specific bacteria that are present and their relative abundance (Chen et al., 2019).

Metabolomics analysis: This involves measuring the levels of different metabolites in the blood or urine to identify markers of metabolic dysregulation.

Genetic testing: This can be used to identify genetic variants that are associated with metabolic disorders.

Once the individual's gut microbiota composition, metabolic profile, and genetic risk factors are known, a personalized prebiotic, probiotic, or synbiotic intervention can be designed.

This intervention may involve:

Selecting specific prebiotics, probiotics, or synbiotic strains: Different strains of bacteria have different effects on the gut microbiota and metabolism. By selecting specific strains, it is possible to target specific signaling pathways and mechanisms.

Determining the optimal dose: The appropriate dosage of prebiotics, probiotics, and synbiotics will differ based on the specific requirements of each individual. Commencing with a minimal dosage and progressively augmenting it till the desired outcomes are attained is of utmost significance (Markowiak and Śliżewska, 2017).

Monitoring and adjusting the intervention: It is important to monitor the individual's response to the intervention and adjust it as needed. This may need doing iterative gut microbiota study and metabolomics analysis to evaluate the influence of the intervention on the gut microbiota and metabolism. In conclusion, the era of personalized medicine has ushered in a new frontier for the management of metabolic disorders. Precision targeting of signaling pathways through personalized prebiotics, probiotics, and synbiotics holds the potential to revolutionize therapeutic strategies. As technology continues to advance, integrating diverse data sources and refining personalized interventions, the journey toward truly personalized and effective management of metabolic disorders is well underway.

2.9.3 Emerging Therapies and Technologies

2.9.3.1 Emerging Therapies

Targeted probiotic delivery: This involves developing delivery systems that can deliver specific probiotic strains to specific locations in the gut. This can be achieved using a variety of methods, such as encapsulation, microgels, and nanoparticles.

Microbial engineering: This involves using genetic engineering techniques to modify probiotic strains to enhance their beneficial effects. For example, probiotics could be engineered to produce more SCFAs or to target specific signaling pathways (Arun et al., 2023).

Fecal microbiota transplantation (FMT): This involves transplanting the gut microbiota from a healthy person to a person with a metabolic disorder. FMT has been shown to be effective in treating certain metabolic disorders, such as Clostridioides difficile infection and IBD. Nevertheless, further investigation is required to assess the safety and effectiveness of this medication for additional metabolic illnesses (Kim and Gluck, 2019).

Precision Prebiotics: Advances in microbiome research have led to the identification of specific prebiotics that selectively nourish beneficial microbial strains associated with improved metabolic outcomes. Precision prebiotics target individualized microbial profiles, fostering the growth of key bacteria involved in signaling pathways related to insulin sensitivity, inflammation modulation, and lipid metabolism (Fan et al., 2023).

Designer Probiotics: The concept of designer probiotics involves the engineering of microbial strains with enhanced functionalities. These genetically modified probiotics can be tailored to express specific enzymes or metabolites that actively participate in signaling pathways critical for metabolic health. Designer probiotics offer a bespoke approach to address individual variations in gut microbiota composition (Chua et al., 2017).

2.9.3.2 Emerging Technologies

Artificial intelligence (AI): AI is being used to develop personalized prebiotic, probiotic, and synbiotic interventions based on individual gut microbiota data and metabolic profiles. AI can also be used to screen and identify new prebiotic and probiotic strains with potential beneficial effects on metabolism.

Omics technologies: Omics technologies, including genomics, metagenomics, and metabolomics, are now employed to investigate the gut microbiota and its impact on metabolic health. This research is leading to a better understanding of how prebiotics, probiotics, and synbiotics work to improve metabolic health.

Microfluidic devices: Microfluidic devices are being used to develop new methods for culturing and studying the gut microbiota. These devices may be utilized to generate intricate gut-like habitats for the purpose of examining the impact of prebiotics, probiotics, and synbiotics on the gut microbiota and metabolism. Emerging therapies and technologies are being developed to target signaling pathways and mechanisms of prebiotics, probiotics, and synbiotics in more precise ways. This has the potential to improve the efficacy and safety of these interventions for the management of metabolic disorders (Yu et al., 2022). As the scientific community continues to push the boundaries of innovation, the integration of these emerging approaches holds tremendous potential for transforming the landscape of metabolic disorder management. From precision prebiotics to designer probiotics and synthetic synbiotics, coupled with advancements in nanotechnology and machine learning, the journey toward more effective, personalized, and futuristic interventions is underway.

2.10 CONCLUSION

We have progressively established a new function for bacteria in health and illness after decades of research. Dysbiosis of the gut microbiota is intimately linked to metabolic disorders. PPSP's emphasis on gut flora yields beneficial effects in managing metabolic disorders, including type 2 diabetes mellitus and obesity. Since PPSP has been shown to be advantageous in reducing metabolic illnesses, researchers have been experimenting with various workable methods to find the most effective treatment. It has been shown that co-intervention with numerous live bacterial strains may be a viable approach. To maximize the positive benefits, new food processing techniques have also been developed, such as probiotic-fermented natural foods and enzyme-modified prebiotics. Furthermore, the findings from both in vitro and in vivo assays indicate that one of the most effective ways for PPSP to mitigate metabolic illness is through the modulation of the arrangement of the gut microbiota. This is demonstrated by the regulation of the abundance of various microorganisms, including Lactobacillus, Proteobacteria, Rikenellaceae, Ruminococcaceae, Yersinia, Clostridiaceae, Collinsella, Christensenellaceae, Firmicutes, Desulfovibrionaceae, Lactobacillus, Lachnospiraceae, Bacteroidetes, Blautia, Bifidobacteria, and Bifidobacterium. Probiotics may improve intestinal barrier function, competitive exclusion of pathogens, host-body immunomodulation, and neurotransmitter production, among other important pathways. By competing with pathogens for resources and receptor-binding positions, probiotics hinder their ability to thrive in the GIT. Probiotics also produce chemicals such as hydrogen peroxide, bacteriocins, SCFA, and organic acids which have antimicrobial qualities that lessen pathogenic bacteria in the digestive system. By stimulating the production of mucin proteins, regulating the manifestation of snug connection proteins like claudin 1 and occluding, and regulating the immune response inside the gut, probiotics also improve the function of the gut barrier. Additionally, probiotics affect B and T lymphocytes, dendritic cells (DC), and macrophages, which regulate the inherent and adaptive immune response. Probiotics have the capacity to connect with intestinal epithelial cells, attract macrophages and mononuclear cells, and increase the release of cytokines that reduce inflammation. Probiotics can also stimulate the synthesis of neurotransmitters in the stomach by means of the gut–brain axis. Dopamine, gamma-aminobutyric acid (GABA), and serotonin levels may be changed by certain probiotic strains, and these changes can affect gut motility, mood, behavior, and stress-related pathways (Latif et al., 2023). In addition, PPSP indirectly enhances metabolic problems by regulating gut microbial metabolites such as butyrate, acetate, propionate, lactic acid, isovalerate, and palmitoylethanolamide. It also inhibits the creation of LPS and TMAO, while reducing bile acid accumulation. Furthermore, the increase in the levels of occludin 1, GLP1, IL-10, claudin 1, and ZO-1 leads to a notable improvement in the function of the intestinal barrier, which plays a crucial role in reducing metabolic diseases. By targeting multiple key signaling pathways, such as GPR43, NLCR3, NOD2, Akt, AMPK, CPR1α, ERK, PPARα, SIRT1, TLR2, GLUT2/4, IRF4, p38 MAPK, and TRAF6-mediated pathways, and inhibiting TLR4, ACE, NF-κB, TNF-α, and NOD1-related pathways, these mechanisms collectively improve the overall metabolic system. Additionally, PPSP has been shown to have an impact on metabolic illnesses in a total of clinical trials. However, further study is required to determine how the treatment works in pregnant patients. Clinical studies are yet required to examine the effectiveness and efficiency of existing or proposed therapies with regard to therapeutic applications in metabolic syndrome. More research should be done on the synbiotics' ideal recipe and the particular benefits of postbiotics for people. Furthermore, the majority of recent studies have concentrated on the mechanisms and effects of PPSP on type 2 diabetes and obesity. Considering these recent developments, treating MS may include targeting the gut microbiota.

REFERENCES

Aghamohammad, S., Sepehr, A., Miri, S. T., Najafi, S., Rohani, M., & Pourshafiea, M. R. (2022). The effects of the probiotic cocktail on modulation of the NF-kB and JAK/STAT signaling pathways involved in the inflammatory response in bowel disease model. *BMC Immunology, 23*(1), 8. https://doi.org/10.1186/s12865-022-00484-6

Al-Jubori, Y., Ahmed, N. T. B., Albusaidi, R., Madden, J., Das, S., & Sirasanagandla, S. R. (2023). The efficacy of gum arabic in managing diseases: A systematic review of evidence-based clinical trials. *Biomolecules, 13*(1), 138. https://doi.org/10.3390/biom13010138

Alli, S. R., Gorbovskaya, I., Liu, J. C. W., Kolla, N. J., Brown, L., & Müller, D. J. (2022). The gut microbiome in depression and potential benefit of prebiotics, probiotics and Synbiotics: A systematic review of clinical trials and observational studies. *International Journal of Molecular Sciences, 23*(9), 4494. https://doi.org/10.3390/ijms23094494

Amadi, P. U., Gu, H.-M., Yin, K., Jiang, X.-C., & Zhang, D.-w. (2022). Lipid metabolism and human diseases, 13, 1072903

Andreasen, A. S., Larsen, N., Pedersen-Sko lease provide source details such as volume and issue numbers and page range and journal title for the journal article in reference 'Amadi et al. 2022'.vsgaard, T., Berg, R. M., Møller, K., Svendsen, K. D., Jakobsen, M., & Pedersen, B. K. (2010). Effects of Lactobacillus acidophilus NCFM on insulin sensitivity and the systemic inflammatory response in human subjects. *British Journal of Nutrition*, *104*(12), 1831–1838. https://doi.org/10.1017/S0007114510002874

Ansari, F., Pourjafar, H., Tabrizi, A., & Homayouni, A. (2020). The effects of probiotics and prebiotics on mental disorders: A review on depression, anxiety, Alzheimer, and autism Spectrum disorders. *Current Pharmaceutical Biotechnology*, *21*(7), 555–565. https://doi.org/10.2174/1389201021666200107113812

Arun, K. B., Nisha, P., & Finamore, A. (2023) Editorial. Emerging perspectives on probiotics, prebiotics, and synbiotics for prevention and management of chronic disease, *10*, 309140.

Ashraf, R., & Shah, N. P. (2014, January 1). Immune system stimulation by probiotic microorganisms. *Critical Reviews in Food Science and Nutrition*, *54*(7), 938–956. https://doi.org/10.1080/10408398.2011.619671

Avolio, E., Fazzari, G., Zizza, M., De Lorenzo, A., Di Renzo, L., Alò, R., Facciolo, R. M., & Canonaco, M. (2019, January 1). Probiotics modify body weight together with anxiety states via pro-inflammatory factors in HFD-treated Syrian golden hamster. *Behavioural Brain Research*, *356*, 390–399. https://doi.org/10.1016/j.bbr.2018.09.010

Azad, M. A. K., Sarker, M., & Wan, D. (2018, October 23). Immunomodulatory effects of probiotics on cytokine profiles. *BioMed Research International*, *2018*, 8063647. https://doi.org/10.1155/2018/8063647

Baboota, R. K., Spinelli, R., Erlandsson, M. C., Brandao, B. B., Lino, M., Yang, H., Mardinoglu, A., Bokarewa, M. I., Boucher, J., Kahn, C. R., & Smith, U. (2022). Chronic hyperinsulinemia promotes human hepatocyte senescence. *Molecular Metabolism*, *64*, 101558. https://doi.org/10.1016/j.molmet.2022.101558

Bagheri, P., Khalili, D., Seif, M., & Rezaianzadeh, A. (2021). Dynamic behavior of metabolic syndrome progression: A comprehensive systematic review on recent discoveries. *BMC Endocrine Disorders*, *21*(1), 54. https://doi.org/10.1186/s12902-021-00716-7

Bahmani, F., Tajadadi-Ebrahimi, M., Kolahdooz, F., Mazouchi, M., Hadaegh, H., Jamal, A. S., Mazroii, N., Asemi, S., & Asemi, Z. (2016). The consumption of synbiotic bread containing Lactobacillus sporogenes and inulin affects nitric oxide and malondialdehyde in patients with type 2 diabetes mellitus: Randomized, double-blind, placebo-controlled trial. *Journal of the American College of Nutrition*, *35*(6), 506–513. https://doi.org/10.1080/07315724.2015.1032443

Bandyopadhyay, A., Chowdhury, S. K., Dey, S., Moses, J. C., & Mandal, B. B. (2019). Silk: A promising biomaterial opening new vistas towards affordable healthcare solutions. *Journal of the Indian Institute of Science*, *99*(3), 445–487. https://doi.org/10.1007/s41745-019-00114-y

Baothman, O. A., Zamzami, M. A., Taher, I., Abubaker, J., & Abu-Farha, M. (2016, December). The role of gut microbiota in the development of obesity and diabetes. *Lipids in Health and Disease*, *15*(1), 108. https://doi.org/10.1186/s12944-016-0278-4

Basilicata, M., Marrone, G., Di Lauro, M., Sargentini, E., Paolino, V., Hassan, R., D'Amato, G., Bollero, P., & Noce, A. (2023). Gaucher disease in internal medicine and dentistry. *Applied Sciences*, *13*(6), 4062. https://doi.org/10.3390/app13064062

Begley, M., Gahan, C. G., & Hill, C. (2005, September 1). The interaction between bacteria and bile. *FEMS Microbiology Reviews*, *29*(4), 625–651. https://doi.org/10.1016/j.femsre.2004.09.003

Bermudez-Brito, M., Plaza-Díaz, J., Muñoz-Quezada, S., Gómez-Llorente, C., & Gil, A. (2012, October 2). Probiotic mechanisms of action. *Annals of Nutrition and Metabolism*, *61*(2), 160–174. https://doi.org/10.1159/000342079

Bull, M. J., & Plummer, N. T. (2014, December). Part 1: The human gut microbiome in health and disease. *Integrative Medicine*, *13*(6), 17–22.

Cai, J., Huang, J., Yang, J., Chen, X., Zhang, H., Zhu, Y., Liu, Q., & Zhang, Z. (2022). The protective effect of selenoprotein M on non-alcoholic fatty liver disease: The role of the AMPKα1-MFN2 pathway and Parkin mitophagy. *Cellular and Molecular Life Sciences*, *79*(7), 354. https://doi.org/10.1007/s00018-022-04385-0

Chaluvadi, S., Hotchkiss, A. T., & Yam, K. L. (2016). Chapter 36. Gut micro-biota: Impact of probiotics, prebiotics, Synbiotics, pharmabi-otics, and postbiotics on human health. In R. R. Watson & V. R. Preedy (Eds.), *Probiotics, Prebiotics, and Synbiotics* (pp. 515–523). Academic Press.

Chen, M. X., Wang, S. Y., Kuo, C. H., & Tsai, I. L. (2019). Metabolome analysis for investigating host-gut microbiota interactions. *Journal of the Formosan Medical Association*, *118*(Suppl. 1), S10–S22. https://doi.org/10.1016/j.jfma.2018.09.007

Chen, J. J., Wang, R., Li, X. F., & Wang, R. L. (2011). Bifidobacterium longum supplementation improved high-fat-fed-induced metabolic syndrome and promoted intestinal Reg I gene expression. *Experimental Biology and Medicine (Maywood, N.J.)*, *236*(7), 823–831. https://doi.org/10.1258/ebm.2011.010399

Cheng, F. S., Pan, D., Chang, B., Jiang, M., & Sang, L. X. (2020, April 4). Probiotic mixture VSL # 3: An overview of basic and clinical studies in chronic diseases. *World Journal of Clinical Cases*, *8*(8), 1361–1384. https://doi.org/10.12998/wjcc.v8.i8.1361

Cho, I., Yamanishi, S., Cox, L., Methé, B. A., Zavadil, J., Li, K., Gao, Z., Mahana, D., Raju, K., Teitler, I., Li, H., Alekseyenko, A. V., & Blaser, M. J. (2012, August 30). Antibiotics in early life alter the murine colonic microbiome and adiposity. *Nature*, *488*(7413), 621–626. https://doi.org/10.1038/nature11400

Chua, K. J., Kwok, W. C., Aggarwal, N., Sun, T., & Chang, M. W. (2017). Designer probiotics for the prevention and treatment of human diseases. *Current Opinion in Chemical Biology*, *40*, 8–16. https://doi.org/10.1016/j.cbpa.2017.04.011

Cotillard, A., Kennedy, S. P., Kong, L. C., Prifti, E., Pons, N., Le Chatelier, E., Almeida, M., Quinquis, B., Levenez, F., Galleron, N., Gougis, S., Rizkalla, S., Batto, J. M., Renault, P., ANR MicroObes consortium, Doré, J., Zucker, J. D., Clément, K., & Ehrlich, S. D. (2013, August 29). Dietary intervention impact on gut microbial gene richness. *Nature*, *500*(7464), 585–588. https://doi.org/10.1038/nature12480

Cunningham, M., Azcarate-Peril, M. A., Barnard, A., Benoit, V., Grimaldi, R., Guyonnet, D., Holscher, H. D., Hunter, K., Manurung, S., Obis, D., Petrova, M. I., Steinert, R. E., Swanson, K. S., van Sinderen, D., Vulevic, J., & Gibson, G. R. (2021). Shaping the future of probiotics and prebiotics. *Trends in Microbiology*, *29*(8), 667–685. https://doi.org/10.1016/j.tim.2021.01.003

daSilva, T. F., Casarotti, S. N., de Oliveira, G. L. V., & Penna, A. L. B. (2021). The impact of probiotics, prebiotics, and Synbiotics on the biochemical, clinical, and immunological markers, as well as on the gut microbiota of obese hosts. *Critical Reviews in Food Science and Nutrition*, *61*(2), 337–355. https://doi.org/10.1080/10408398.2020.1733483

Davani-Davari, D., Negahdaripour, M., Karimzadeh, I., Seifan, M., Mohkam, M., Masoumi, S. J., Berenjian, A., & Ghasemi, Y. (2019). Prebiotics: Definition, types, sources, mechanisms, and clinical applications. *Foods*, *8*(3), 92. https://doi.org/10.3390/foods8030092

de la Fuente, M., Lombardero, L., Gómez-González, A., Solari, C., Angulo-Barturen, I., Acera, A., Vecino, E., Astigarraga, E., & Barreda-Gómez, G. (2021). Enzyme therapy: Current challenges and future. *Perspectives*, *22*(17), 9181.

denBesten, G., van Eunen, K., Groen, A. K., Venema, K., Reijngoud, D. J., & Bakker, B. M. (2013, September). The role of short-chain fatty acids in the interplay between diet, gut microbiota, and host energy metabolism. *Journal of Lipid Research*, *54*(9), 2325–2340. https://doi.org/10.1194/jlr.R036012

Deshmukh, M., & Patole, S. (2021). Current status of probiotics for preterm infants. *Indian Journal of Pediatrics*, *88*(7), 703–708. https://doi.org/10.1007/s12098-021-03736-2

Ding, S., Wang, Y., Yan, W., Li, A., Jiang, H., & Fang, J. (2019, June 13). Effects of *Lactobacillus plantarum* 15-1 and fructooligosaccharides on the response of broilers to pathogenic *Escherichia coli* O78 challenge. *PLOS One*, *14*(6), e0212079. https://doi.org/10.1371/journal.pone.0212079

Dubey, M. R., & Patel, V. P. (2018, August 31). Probiotics: A promising tool for calcium absorption. *Open Nutrition Journal*, *12*(1), 59–69. https://doi.org/10.2174/1874288201812010059

Elamin, E. E., Masclee, A. A., Dekker, J., & Jonkers, D. M. (2013, July 1). Ethanol metabolism and its effects on the intestinal epithelial barrier. *Nutrition Reviews*, *71*(7), 483–499. https://doi.org/10.1111/nure.12027

Elias, J., Bozzo, P., & Einarson, A. (2011). Are probiotics safe for use during pregnancy and lactation? *Canadian Family Physician Medecin de Famille Canadien*, *57*(3), 299–301.

Fan, S., Zhang, Z., Zhao, Y., Daglia, M., Zhang, J., Zhu, Y., Bai, J., Zhu, L., & Xiao, X. (2023). Recent advances in targeted manipulation of the gut microbiome by prebiotics: From taxonomic composition to metabolic function. *Current Opinion in Food Science*, *49*, 100959. https://doi.org/10.1016/j.cofs.2022.100959

Fan, Y., & Pedersen, O. (2021, January). Gut microbiota in human metabolic health and disease. *Nature Reviews. Microbiology*, *19*(1), 55–71. https://doi.org/10.1038/s41579-020-0433-9

Fujimori, S., Gudis, K., Mitsui, K., Seo, T., Yonezawa, M., Tanaka, S., Tatsuguchi, A., & Sakamoto, C. (2009). A randomized controlled trial on the efficacy of synbiotic versus probiotic or prebiotic treatment to improve the quality of life in patients with ulcerative colitis. *Nutrition*, *25*(5), 520–525. https://doi.org/10.1016/j.nut.2008.11.017

Gibson, G. R., Hutkins, R., Sanders, M. E., Prescott, S. L., Reimer, R. A., Salminen, S. J., Scott, K., Stanton, C., Swanson, K. S., Cani, P. D., Verbeke, K., & Reid, G. (2017). Expert consen-sus document: The International Scientific Association for Probiotics and Prebiotics (ISAPP) consensus statement onthe definition and scope of prebiotics. *Nature Reviews Gastroenterology and Hepatology*, *14*(8), 491–502. https://doi.org/10.1038/nrgastro.2017.75

Gibson, G. R., & Roberfroid, M. B. (1995). Dietary modulation of the human colonic microbiota: Introducing the concept of prebiotics. *Journal of Nutrition*, *125*(6), 1401–1412. https://doi.org/10.1093/jn/125.6.1401

Giraldo, P., López De Frutos, L., & Cebolla, J. J. (2018). Biomarker combination is necessary for the assessment of Gaucher disease? *Annals of Translational Medicine*, *6*(Suppl. 1), S81. https://doi.org/10.21037/atm.2018.10.69

Guarino, M. P. L., Altomare, A., Emerenziani, S., Di Rosa, C., Ribolsi, M., Balestrieri, P., Iovino, P., Rocchi, G., & Cicala, M. (2020, April 9). Mechanisms of action of prebiotics and their effects on gastro-intestinal disorders in adults. *Nutrients*, *12*(4), 1037. https://doi.org/10.3390/nu12041037

Guarner, F., & Malagelada, J. R. (2003, February 8). Gut flora in health and disease. *Lancet*, *361*(9356), 512–519. https://doi.org/10.1016/S0140-6736(03)12489-0

Halloran, K., & Underwood, M. A. (2019). Probiotic mechanisms of action. *Early Human Development*, *135*, 58–65. https://doi.org/10.1016/j.earlhumdev.2019.05.010

Hanchi,H.,Mottawea,W.,Sebei,K.,&Hammami,R.(2018,August3). The genus Enterococcus: Between probiotic potential and safety concerns-An update. *Frontiers in Microbiology*, *9*, 1791. https://doi.org/10.3389/fmicb.2018.01791

Henrick, B. M., Hutton, A. A., Palumbo, M. C., Casaburi, G., Mitchell, R. D., Underwood, M. A., Smilowitz, J. T., & Frese, S. A. (2018, April 25). Elevated fecal pH indicates a profound change in the breastfed infant gut microbiome due to reduction of Bifidobacterium over the past century. *mSphere*, *3*(2), e00041–e00018. https://doi.org/10.1128/mSphere.00041-18

Hill, D., Sugrue, I., Tobin, C., Hill, C., Stanton, C., & Ross, R. P. (2018). The *Lactobacillus casei* group: History and health related applications. *Frontiers in Microbiology*, *9*, 2107. https://doi.org/10.3389/fmicb.2018.02107

Jarde, A., Lewis-Mikhael, A. M., Moayyedi, P., Stearns, J. C., Collins, S. M., Beyene, J., & McDonald, S. D. (2018). Pregnancy outcomes in women taking probiotics or prebiotics: A systematic review and meta-analysis. *BMC Pregnancy and Childbirth*, *18*(1), 14. https://doi.org/10.1186/s12884-017-1629-5

Jeun, J., Kim, S., Cho, S. Y., Jun, H. J., Park, H. J., Seo, J. G., Chung, M. J., & Lee, S. J. (2010, March 1). Hypocholesterolemic effects of *Lactobacillus plantarum* KCTC3928 by increased bile acid excretion in C57BL/6 mice. *Nutrition*, *26*(3), 321–330. https://doi.org/10.1016/j.nut.2009.04.011

Ji, Y., Park, S., Park, H., Hwang, E., Shin, H., Pot, B., & Holzapfel, W. H. (2018). Modulation of active gut microbiota by Lactobacillus rhamnosus GG in a diet induced obesity murine model. *Frontiers in Microbiology*, *9*, 710. https://doi.org/10.3389/fmicb.2018.00710

Johnston, K. L., Thomas, E. L., Bell, J. D., Frost, G. S., & Robertson, M. D. (2010). Resistant starch improves insulin sensitivity in metabolic syndrome. *Diabetic Medicine*, *27*(4), 391–397. https://doi.org/10.1111/j.1464-5491.2010.02923.x

Joyce, S. A., & Gahan, C. G. (2014, March 1). The gut microbiota and the metabolic health of the host. *Current Opinion in Gastroenterology*, *30*(2), 120–127. https://doi.org/10.1097/MOG.0000000000000039

Kaci, G., Lakhdari, O., Doré, J., Ehrlich, S. D., Renault, P., Blottière, H. M., & Delorme, C. (2011, July). Inhibition of the NF-kappaB pathway in human intestinal epithelial cells by commensal *Streptococcus salivarius*. *Applied and Environmental Microbiology*, *77*(13), 4681–4684. https://doi.org/10.1128/AEM.03021-10.

Karamali, M., Dadkhah, F., Sadrkhanlou, M., Jamilian, M., Ahmadi, S., Tajabadi-Ebrahimi, M., Jafari, P., & Asemi, Z. (2016). Effects of probiotic supplementation on glycaemic control and lipid profiles in gestational diabetes: A randomized, double-blind, placebo-controlled trial. *Diabetes and Metabolism*, *42*(4), 234–241. https://doi.org/10.1016/j.diabet.2016.04.009.

Khan, S., Moore, R. J., Stanley, D., & Chousalkar, K. K. (2020, June 17). The gut microbiota of laying hens and its manipulation with prebiotics and probiotics to enhance gut health and food safety. *Applied and Environmental Microbiology*, *86*(13), e00600–e00620. https://doi.org/10.1128/AEM.00600-20

Kim, K. O., & Gluck, M. (2019). Fecal microbiota transplantation: An update on clinical practice. *Clinical Endoscopy*, *52*(2), 137–143. https://doi.org/10.5946/ce.2019.009

Kivimäki, M., Bartolomucci, A., & Kawachi, I. (2023). The multiple roles of life stress in metabolic disorders. *Nature Reviews. Endocrinology*, *19*(1), 10–27. https://doi.org/10.1038/s41574-022-00746-8

Klaassens, E. S., Boesten, R. J., Haarman, M., Knol, J., Schuren, F. H., Vaughan, E. E., & De Vos, W. M. (2009, May 1). Mixed-species genomic microarray analysis of fecal samples reveals differential transcriptional responses of bifidobacteria in breast- and formula-fed infants. *Applied and Environmental Microbiology*, *75*(9), 2668–2676. https://doi.org/10.1128/AEM.02492-08

Klein, K. O., & Phillips, S. A. (2019). Review of hormone replacement therapy in girls and adolescents with hypogonadism. *Journal of Pediatric and Adolescent Gynecology*, *32*(5), 460–468. https://doi.org/10.1016/j.jpag.2019.04.010

Kothari, D., Patel, S., & Kim, S. K. (2019). Probiotic supplements might not be universally-effective and safe: A review. *Biomedicine and Pharmacotherapy*, *111*, 537–547. https://doi.org/10.1016/j.biopha.2018.12.104

Larsen, O. F. A., van der Grint, M., Wiegers, C., & van de Burgwal, L. H. M. (2022). The gut microbiota: Master of puppets connecting the epidemiology of infectious, autoimmune, and metabolic disease. *Frontiers in Microbiology*, *13*, 902106. https://doi.org/10.3389/fmicb.2022.902106

Latif, A., Shehzad, A., Niazi, S., Zahid, A., Ashraf, W., Iqbal, M. W., Rehman, A., Riaz, T., Aadil, R. M., Khan, I. M., Özogul, F., Rocha, J. M., Esatbeyoglu, T., & Korma, S. A. (2023). Probiotics: Mechanism of action, health benefits and their application in food industries. *Frontiers in Microbiology*, *14*, 1216674. https://doi.org/10.3389/fmicb.2023.1216674

LeChatelier, E., Nielsen, T., Qin, J., Prifti, E., Hildebrand, F., Falony, G., Almeida, M., Arumugam, M., Batto, J. M., Kennedy, S., Leonard, P., Li, J., Burgdorf, K., Grarup, N., Jørgensen, T., Brandslund, I., Nielsen, H. B., Juncker, A. S., Bertalan, M.,. . . & Pedersen, O. (2013, August 29). Richness of human gut microbiome correlates with metabolic markers. *Nature*, *500*(7464), 541–546. https://doi.org/10.1038/nature12506

Li, H. Y., Zhou, D. D., Gan, R. Y., Huang, S. Y., Zhao, C. N., Shang, A., Xu, X. Y., & Li, H. B. (2021a). Effects and mechanisms of probiotics, prebiotics, Synbiotics, and postbiotics on metabolic diseases targeting gut microbiota: A narrative review. *Nutrients*, *13*(9). https://doi.org/10.3390/nu13093211

Li, X., Zhai, Y., Zhao, J., He, H., Li, Y., Liu, Y., Feng, A., Li, L., Huang, T., Xu, A., & Lyu, J. (2021b). Impact of metabolic syndrome and it's components on prognosis in patients with cardiovascular diseases: A meta-analysis. *Frontiers in Cardiovascular Medicine*, *8*, 704145. https://doi.org/10.3389/fcvm.2021.704145.

Liao, P. H., Liao, P., Kuo, W., Kuo, C., Yeh, Y., Shen, C., Chen, Y., Chen, R., Padma, V. V., Chen, Y., & Huang, C. (2016, January 1). *Lactobacillus reuteri* GMNL-263 reduces hyperlipidaemia and the heart failure process in high-calorie diet-fed induced heart dysfunction in rats. *Journal of Functional Foods*, *20*, 226–235. https://doi.org/10.1016/j.jff.2015.11.009

Lillich, F. F., Imig, J. D., & Proschak, E. (2020). Multi-target approaches in metabolic syndrome. *Frontiers in Pharmacology*, *11*, 554961. https://doi.org/10.3389/fphar.2020.554961

Liong, M. T. (2008, April 1). Safety of probiotics: Translocation and infection. *Nutrition Reviews*, *66*(4), 192–202. https://doi.org/10.1111/j.1753-4887.2008.00024.x

Liu, J., Tan, Y., Cheng, H., Zhang, D., Feng, W., & Peng, C. (2022a, July 7). Functions of gut microbiota metabolites, current status and future perspectives. *Aging and Disease*, *13*(4), 1106–1126. https://doi.org/10.14336/AD.2022.0104

Liu, N., Wang, H., Yang, Z., Zhao, K., Li, S., & He, N. (2022b, July 4). The role of functional oligosaccharides as prebiotics in ulcerative colitis. *Food and Function*, *13*(13), 6875–6893. https://doi.org/10.1039/d2fo00546h

Luo, J., Rizkalla, S. W., Alamowitch, C., Boussairi, A., Blayo, A., Barry, J. L., Laffitte, A., Guyon, F., Bornet, F. R., & Slama, G. (1996). Chronic consumption of short-chain fructooligosaccharides by healthy subjects decreased basal hepatic glucose production but had no effect on insulin-stimulated glucose metabolism. *American Journal of Clinical Nutrition*, *63*(6), 939–945. https://doi.org/10.1093/ajcn/63.6.939

Lynch, S. V., & Pedersen, O. (2016, December 15). The human intestinal microbiome in health and disease. *New England Journal of Medicine*, *375*(24), 2369–2379. https://doi.org/10.1056/NEJMra1600266

Macfarlane, G. T., Steed, H., & Macfarlane, S. (2008). Bacterial metabolism and health-related effects of galacto-oligosaccharides and other prebiotics. *Journal of Applied Microbiology*, *104*(2), 305–344. https://doi.org/10.1111/j.1365-2672.2007.03520.x

Markowiak, P., & Śliżewska, K. (2017, September 15). Effects of probiotics, prebiotics, and Synbiotics on human health. *Nutrients*, *9*(9), 1021. https://doi.org/10.3390/nu9091021

Markowiak-Kopeć, P., & Śliżewska, K. (2020, April 16). The effect of probiotics on the production of short-chain fatty acids by human intestinal microbiome. *Nutrients*, *12*(4), 1107. https://doi.org/10.3390/nu12041107

Megur, A., Daliri, E. B., Baltriukienė, D., & Burokas, A. (2022, May 29). Prebiotics as a tool for the prevention and treatment of obesity and diabetes: Classification and ability to modulate the gut microbiota. *International Journal of Molecular Sciences*, *23*(11), 6097. https://doi.org/10.3390/ijms23116097

Méndez-Sánchez, N., Bugianesi, E., Gish, R. G., Lammert, F., Tilg, H., Nguyen, M. H., Sarin, S. K., Fabrellas, N., Zelber-Sagi, S., Fan, J. G., Shiha, G., Targher, G., Zheng, M. H., Chan, W. K., Vinker, S., Kawaguchi, T., Castera, L., Yilmaz, Y., Korenjak, M.,. . . & Global Multi-stakeholder Consensus on the Redefinition of Fatty Liver Disease. (2022). Global multi-stakeholder endorsement of the MAFLD definition. *Lancet. Gastroenterology and Hepatology*, *7*(5), 388–390. https://doi.org/10.1016/S2468-1253(22)00062-0

Milani, C., Duranti, S., Bottacini, F., Casey, E., Turroni, F., Mahony, J., Belzer, C., Delgado Palacio, S., Arboleya Montes, S., Mancabelli, L., Lugli, G. A., Rodriguez, J. M., Bode, L., de Vos, W., Gueimonde, M., Margolles, A., van Sinderen, D., & Ventura, M. (2017). The first microbial colonizers of the human gut: Composition, activities, and health implications of the infant gut microbiota. *Microbiology and Molecular Biology Reviews*, *81*(4), e00036–e00017. https://doi. https://doi.org/10.1128/MMBR.00036-17

Moeller, L. C. (2023). Translational perspectives from TSHR, MCT8 and TRα research. *Nature Reviews. Endocrinology*, *19*(2), 74–75. https://doi.org/10.1038/s41574-022-00785-1

Mu, Y., & Cong, Y. (2019). Bacillus coagulans and its applications in medicine. *Beneficial Microbes*, *10*(6), 679–688. https://doi.org/10.3920/BM2019.0016

Murphy, K., Ross, R. P., Ryan, C. A., Dempsey, E. M., & Stanton, C. (2021, September 7). Probiotics, prebiotics, and Synbiotics for the prevention of necrotizing enterocolitis. *Frontiers in Nutrition*, *8*, 667188. https://doi.org/10.3389/fnut.2021.667188

Nicholson, J. K., Holmes, E., Kinross, J., Burcelin, R., Gibson, G., Jia, W., & Pettersson, S. (2012). Host-gut microbiota metabolic interactions. *Science*, *336*(6086), 1262–1267. https://doi.org/10.1126/science.1223813

Ohland, C. L., & MacNaughton, W. K. (2010, June). Probiotic bacteria and intestinal epithelial barrier function. *American Journal of Physiology. Gastrointestinal and Liver Physiology*, *298*(6), G807–G819. https://doi.org/10.1152/ajpgi.00243.2009

Ojeda, J., Ávila, A., & Vidal, P. M. (2021). Gut microbiota interaction with the central nervous system throughout life. *Journal of Clinical Medicine*, *10*(6), 1299. https://doi.org/10.3390/jcm10061299

Pandey, K. R., Naik, S. R., & Vakil, B. V. (2015, December). Probiotics, prebiotics and Synbiotics- a review. *Journal of Food Science and Technology*, *52*(12), 7577–7587. https://doi.org/10.1007/s13197-015-1921-1

Pant, R., Sharma, N., Kabeer, S. W., Sharma, S., & Tikoo, K. (2023, March). Selenium-enriched probiotic alleviates western diet-induced non-alcoholic fatty liver disease in rats via modulation of autophagy through AMPK/SIRT-1 pathway. *Biological Trace Element Research*, *201*(3), 1344–1357. https://doi.org/10.1007/s12011-022-03247-x.

Patel, S., & Patel, N. (2017). How to use QbD to select packaging components. https://www.pda.org/pda-letter-portal/home/full-article/how-to-use-qbd-to-select-packaging-components. Last Accessed on 07/05/2024.

Pluta, R., Ułamek-Kozioł, M., Januszewski, S., & Czuczwar, S. J. (2020). Gut microbiota and pro/prebiotics in Alzheimer's disease. *Aging*, *12*(6), 5539–5550. https://doi.org/10.18632/aging.102930

Popkes, M., & Valenzano, D. R. (2020, September 28). Microbiota-host interactions shape ageing dynamics. *Philosophical Transactions of the Royal Society of London Series B*, *375*(1808), 20190596.

Ramezani, M., Reisian, M., & Sajadi Hezaveh, Z. (2023, February 6). The effect of synbiotic supplementation on hypothyroidism: A randomized double-blind placebo controlled clinical trial. *PLOS One*, *18*(2), e0277213. https://doi.org/10.1371/journal.pone.0277213.

Rathod, S. (2022). Novel insights into the immunotherapy-based treatment strategy for autoimmune Type 1 diabetes. *Diabetology*, *3*(1), 79–96. https://doi.org/10.3390/diabetology3010007

Rauf, A., Khalil, A. A., Rahman, U. U., Khalid, A., Naz, S., Shariati, M. A., Rebezov, M., Urtecho, E. Z., de Albuquerque, R. D. D. G., Anwar, S., Alamri, A., Saini, R. K., & Rengasamy, K. R. R. (2022). Recent advances in the therapeutic application of short-chain fatty acids (SCFAs): An updated review. *Critical Reviews in Food Science and Nutrition*, *62*(22), 6034–6054. https://doi.org/10.1080/10408398.2021.1895064

Robertson, M. D., Bickerton, A. S., Dennis, A. L., Vidal, H., & Frayn, K. N. (2005). Insulin-sensitizing effects of dietary resistant starch and effects on skeletal muscle and adipose tissue metabolism. *American Journal of Clinical Nutrition*, *82*(3), 559–567. https://doi.org/10.1093/ajcn.82.3.559

Rochlani, Y., Pothineni, N. V., Kovelamudi, S., & Mehta, J. L. (2017). Metabolic syndrome: Pathophysiology, management, and modulation by natural compounds. *Therapeutic Advances in Cardiovascular Disease*, *11*(8), 215–225. https://doi.org/10.1177/1753944717711379

Salminen, S., Stahl, B., Vinderola, G., & Szajewska, H. (2020). Infant formula supplemented with biotics: Current knowledge and future perspectives. *Nutrients*, *12*(7), 1952. https://doi.org/10.3390/nu12071952

Sanders, M. E., Akkermans, L. M., Haller, D., Hammerman, C., Heimbach, J., Hörmannsperger, G., Huys, G., Levy, D. D., Lutgendorff, F., Mack, D., Phothirath, P., Solano-Aguilar, G., & Vaughan, E. (2010). Safety assessment of probiotics for human use. *Gut Microbes*, *1*(3), 164–185. https://doi.org/10.4161/gmic.1.3.12127

Scorletti, E., Afolabi, P. R., Miles, E. A., Smith, D. E., Almehmadi, A., Alshathry, A., Childs, C. E., Del Fabbro, S., Bilson, J., Moyses, H. E., Clough, G. F., Sethi, J. K., Patel, J., Wright, M., Breen, D. J., Peebles, C., Darekar, A., Aspinall, R., Fowell, A. J., . . . & Byrne, C. D. (2020). Synbiotics alter fecal microbiomes, but not liver fat or fibrosis, in a randomized trial of patients with nonalcoholic fatty liver disease. *Gastroenterology*, *158*(6), 1597–1610.e7. https://doi.org/10.1053/j.gastro.2020.01.031

Sheyholislami, H., & Connor, K. L. (2021). Are probiotics and prebiotics safe for use during pregnancy and lactation? A systematic review and meta-analysis. *Nutrients*, *13*(7), 2382. https://doi.org/10.3390/nu13072382

Stephens, C. R., Easton, J. F., Robles-Cabrera, A., Fossion, R., de la Cruz, L., Martínez-Tapia, R., Barajas-Martínez, A., Hernández-Chávez, A., López-Rivera, J. A., & Rivera, A. L. (2020). The impact of education and age on metabolic disorders. *Frontiers in Public Health*, *8*, 180. https://doi.org/10.3389/fpubh.2020.00180

ofilová, J., Szabadosová, V., Hrčková, G., Salaj, R., Bertková, I., Hijová, E., Strojný, L., & Bomba, A. (2015, February 1). Co-administration of a probiotic strain *Lactobacillus plantarum* LS/07 CCM7766 with prebiotic inulin alleviates the intestinal inflammation in rats exposed to N,N-dimethylhydrazine. *International Immunopharmacology*, *24*(2), 361–368. https://doi.org/10.1016/j.intimp.2014.12.022

Swanson, K. S., Gibson, G. R., Hutkins, R., Reimer, R. A., Reid, G., Verbeke, K., Scott, K. P., Holscher, H. D., Azad, M. B., Delzenne, N. M., & Sanders, M. E. (2020). The international scientific Association for Probiotics and Prebiotics (Isapp) consensus statement on the definition and scope of Synbiotics. *Nature Reviews. Gastroenterology and Hepatology*, *17*(11), 687–701. https://doi.org/10.1038/s41575-020-0344-2

Tabrizi, A., Khalili, L., Homayouni-Rad, A., Pourjafar, H., Dehghan, P., & Ansari, F. (2019). Prebiotics, as promising functional food to patients with psychological disorders: A review on mood disorders, sleep, and cognition. *NeuroQuantology*, *17*, 2189. doi: 10.14704/nq.2019.17.06.2189.].

Tajadadi-Ebrahimi, M., Bahmani, F., Shakeri, H., Hadaegh, H., Hijijafari, M., Abedi, F., & Asemi, Z. (2014). Effects of daily consumption of synbiotic bread on insulin metabolism and serum high-sensitivity C-reactive protein among diabetic patients: A double-blind, randomized, controlled clinical trial. *Annals of Nutrition and Metabolism*, *65*(1), 34–41. https://doi.org/10.1159/000365153

Tan, Q., Orsso, C. E., Deehan, E. C., Kung, J. Y., Tun, H. M., Wine, E., Madsen, K. L., Zwaigenbaum, L., & Haqq, A. M. (2021). Probiotics, prebiotics, synbiotics, and fecal microbiota transplantation in the treatment of behavioral symptoms of autism spectrum disorder: A systematic review. *Autism Research*, *14*(9), 1820–1836. https://doi.org/10.1002/aur.2560

Tang, W. H., Wang, Z., Levison, B. S., Koeth, R. A., Britt, E. B., Fu, X., Wu, Y., & Hazen, S. L. (2013, April 25). Intestinal microbial metabolism of phosphatidylcholine and cardiovascular risk. *New England Journal of Medicine*, *368*(17), 1575–1584. https://doi.org/10.1056/NEJMoa1109400

Vachliotis, I., Goulas, A., Papaioannidou, P., & Polyzos, S. A. (2022). Nonalcoholic fatty liver disease: Lifestyle and quality of life. *Hormones*, *21*(1), 41–49. https://doi.org/10.1007/s42000-021-00339-6

ValdemiroCarlos, S. (2011). The importance of prebiotics in functional foods and clinical practice. *Food and Nutrition Sciences*, *2*(2), 133–144.

Varsha, K. K., Maheshwari, A. P., & Nampoothiri, K. M. (2021). Accom-plishment of probiotics in human health pertaining to immunoregulation and disease control. *Clinical Nutrition ESPEN*, *44*, 26–37. https://doi.org/10.1016/j.clnesp.2021.06.020

Wang, B., Kong, Q., Li, X., Zhao, J., Zhang, H., Chen, W., & Wang, G. (2020, October 20). A high-fat diet increases gut microbiota biodiversity and energy expenditure due to nutrient difference. *Nutrients*, *12*(10), 3197. https://doi.org/10.3390/nu12103197

Wang, C., Wang, H., Zhao, Z., Xiao, S., Zhao, Y., Duan, C., Gao, L., Li, S., & Wang, J. (2019, September 1). Pediococcus acidilactici AS185 attenuates early atherosclerosis development through inhibition of lipid regulation and inflammation in rats. *Journal of Functional Foods*, *60*, 103424. https://doi.org/10.1016/j.jff.2019.103424

Wang, H., Chen, K., Ning, M., Wang, X., Wang, Z., Yue, Y., Yuan, Y., & Yue, T. (2023). Intake of Pro- and/or prebiotics as a promising approach for prevention and treatment of colorectal cancer. *Molecular Nutrition and Food Research*, *67*(3), e2200474. https://doi.org/10.1002/mnfr.202200474

Wastyk, H. C., Perelman, D., Topf, M., Fragiadakis, G. K., Robinson, J. L., Sonnenburg, J. L., Gardner, C. D., & Sonnenburg, E. D. (2023, January–December). Randomized controlled trial demonstrates response to a probiotic intervention for metabolic syndrome that may correspond to diet. *Gut Microbes*, *15*(1), 2178794. https://doi.org/10.1080/19490976.2023.2178794

Watanabe, M., Horai, Y., Houten, S. M., Morimoto, K., Sugizaki, T., Arita, E., Mataki, C., Sato, H., Tanigawara, Y., Schoonjans, K., Itoh, H., & Auwerx, J. (2011, July 29). Lowering bile acid pool size with a synthetic farnesoid X receptor (FXR) agonist induces obesity and diabetes through reduced energy expenditure. *Journal of Biological Chemistry*, *286*(30), 26913–26920. https://doi.org/10.1074/jbc.M111.248203

Wiciński, M., Gębalski, J., Gołębiewski, J., & Malinowski, B. (2020, July 29). Probiotics for the treatment of overweight and obesity in humans-A review of clinical trials. *Microorganisms*, *8*(8), 1148. https://doi.org/10.3390/microorganisms8081148

Woodard, G. A., Encarnacion, B., Downey, J. R., Peraza, J., Chong, K., Hernandez-Boussard, T., & Morton, J. M. (2009, July). Probiotics improve outcomes after Roux-en-Y gastric bypass surgery: A prospective randomized trial. *Journal of Gastrointestinal Surgery*, *13*(7), 1198–1204. https://doi.org/10.1007/s11605-009-0891-x

Xavier-Santos, D., Bedani, R., Lima, E. D., & Saad, S. M. I. (2020, January 1). Impact of probiotics and prebiotics targeting metabolic syndrome. *Journal of Functional Foods*, *64*, 103666. https://doi.org/10.1016/j.jff.2019.103666

Xu, Y., Cui, Y., Yue, F., Liu, L., Shan, Y., Liu, B., Zhou, Y., & Lü, X. (2019, September 1). Exopolysaccharides produced by lactic acid bacteria and bifidobacteria: Structures, physiochemical functions and applications in the food industry. *Food Hydrocolloids*, *94*, 475–499. https://doi.org/10.1016/j.foodhyd.2019.03.032

Yadav, M. K., Kumari, I., Singh, B., Sharma, K. K., & Tiwari, S. K. (2022). Probiotics, prebiotics and synbiotics: Safe options for next-generation therapeutics. *Applied Microbiology and Biotechnology*, *106*(2), 505–521. https://doi.org/10.1007/s00253-021-11646-8

Yeoh, C., Teng, H., Jackson, J., Hingula, L., Irie, T., Legler, A., Levine, C., Chu, I., Chai, C., & Tollinche, L. (2019). Metabolic disorders and anesthesia. *Current Anesthesiology Reports*, *9*(3), 340–359. https://doi.org/10.1007/s40140-019-00345-w

Yoshikawa, S., Taniguchi, K., Sawamura, H., Ikeda, Y., Asai, T., Tsuji, A., & Matsuda, S. (2023). Metabolic associated fatty liver disease as a risk factor for the development of central nervous system disorders. *Livers*, *3*(1), 21–32. https://doi.org/10.3390/livers3010002

You, S., Ma, Y., Yan, B., Pei, W., Wu, Q., Ding, C., & Huang, C. (2022, October 5). The promotion mechanism of prebiotics for probiotics: A review. *Frontiers in Nutrition*, *9*, 1000517. https://doi.org/10.3389/fnut.2022.1000517

Yu, Y., Wen, H., Li, S., Cao, H., Li, X., Ma, Z., She, X., Zhou, L., & Huang, S. (2022). Emerging microfluidic technologies for microbiome research. *Frontiers in Microbiology*, *13*, 906979. https://doi.org/10.3389/fmicb.2022.906979

Zhang, C. X., Wang, H. Y., & Chen, T. X. (2019, November 20). Interactions between intestinal microflora/probiotics and the immune system. *BioMed Research International*, *2019*, 6764919. https://doi.org/10.1155/2019/6764919

Zhang, M. M., Poulsen, M., & Currie, C. R. (2007, August). Symbiont recognition of mutualistic bacteria by acromyrmex leaf-cutting ants. *ISME Journal*, *1*(4), 313–320. https://doi.org/10.1038/ismej.2007.41

Zhang, F., Qiu, L., Xu, X., Liu, Z., Zhan, H., Tao, X., Shah, N. P., & Wei, H. (2017). Beneficial effects of probiotic cholesterol-lowering strain of Enterococcus faecium WEFA23 from infants on diet-induced metabolic syndrome in rats. *Journal of Dairy Science*, *100*(3), 1618–1628. https://doi.org/10.3168/jds.2016-11870

Zhao, S., Feng, P., Hu, X., Cao, W., Liu, P., Han, H., Jin, W., & Li, X. (2022). Probiotic *Limosilactobacillus fermentum* GR-3 ameliorates human hyperuricemia via degrading and promoting excretion of uric acid. *iScience*, *25*(10), 105198. https://doi.org/10.1016/j.isci.2022.105198

Zhao, Y., Zhang, P., Lee, J. T., Oldenburg, B., van Heusden, A. v., Haregu, T. N., & Wang, H. (2021). The prevalence of metabolic disease multimorbidity and its associations with spending and health outcomes in middle-aged and elderly Chinese adults. *Frontiers in Public Health*, *9*, 658706. https://doi.org/10.3389/fpubh.2021.658706

Zoetendal, E. G., Raes, J., Van Den Bogert, B., Arumugam, M., Booijink, C. C., Troost, F. J., Bork, P., Wels, M., De Vos, W. M., & Kleerebezem, M. (2012, July). The human small intestinal microbiota is driven by rapid uptake and conversion of simple carbohydrates. *ISME Journal*, *6*(7), 1415–1426. https://doi.org/10.1038/ismej.2011.212

3 Potential Role of Probiotics, Prebiotics, and Synbiotics in Management of Metabolic Syndrome and Chronic Metabolic Disease

Md. Khokon Miah Akanda and Sanzia Mehjabin

3.1 INTRODUCTION

A number of metabolism-related illnesses are called metabolic syndrome. In addition to excessive triglycerides, obesity, impaired fasting glucose, poor HDL cholesterol, high blood pressure, and metabolic factors that contribute to the illness. Diabetes, cardiovascular disease, stroke, or all three are all more likely to occur in those who have metabolic syndrome. About 25% of Americans have metabolic syndrome, the number develops with age, especially among persons of color and ethnic minorities (Brown et al., 2012; Falkner and Cossrow, 2014). The digestive system is composed of many organs associated with one another. It digests nutrients and delivers food-derived energy. With a well-known anatomical architecture, this complex system has a surface area of around 300 square meters in adults and measures approximately 7 m in length. An estimated 10,000 cells, over a kilogram, and a thousand species make up the bacterial flora of the human large intestine (Diamant et al., 2011). A diverse array of microbiota can be found in the mouth and intestines. The microbiota includes both aerobic and anaerobic species, including yeasts, lactobacilli, bacteroides, and streptococci. More than double size of the human genome, the microbiome is thought to include more than two million genes. High-throughput techniques and powerful analytical tools allow for more accurate gut microbial characterization than ever previously. This has enabled comparisons between various disease states and healthy states to be performed (Quigley, 2013).

Now, metabolic syndrome is linked to this dynamic yet stable environment. The gut microbiome of persons without diabetes and those with type 2 diabetes differs, as evidenced by the research, and it may have an impact on metabolism and energy storage in both lean and obese people (Alonso and Guarner, 2013; Larsen et al., 2010). The bacteria that live in the gut are primarily responsible for three different functions: metabolic, protective, and trophic. Alterations to one's eating routine are, without a question, the most essential non-pharmacological component in the treatment of risk factors for metabolic syndrome, a number of dietary therapies have been investigated (Guarner and Malagelada, 2003; Simão et al., 2013). The scientific literature has referred to the use of probiotic, prebiotic, and synbiotic products as one of the dietary therapies to prevent metabolic syndrome risk factors.

3.2 METABOLIC SYNDROME ASSOCIATE DISEASE

Obesity, dyslipidemia, insulin resistance, and hypertension are all symptoms of metabolic syndrome. It is linked to a number of serious disorders, each with its own set of issues and health risks. The syndrome greatly raises the risk of cardiovascular complications due to accelerated atherosclerosis. This leads to conditions including coronary artery disease, heart attacks, and stroke, which are exacerbated by the metabolic syndrome's role in vascular inflammation and atherosclerosis. People with metabolic syndrome are more prone to cardiac issues as a result of this (Haque et al., 2016; McCracken et al., 2018). The syndrome greatly raises the risk of insulin resistance which leads to type 2 diabetes and cardiovascular complications due to accelerated atherosclerosis. Blood sugar control should be the patient's top priority in the prevention of diabetes (Bonomini et al., 2015). There is a link between metabolic syndrome and non-alcoholic fatty liver disease, both of which cause the liver to store fat. Non-alcoholic steatohepatitis may lead to fibrosis, cirrhosis, failure, and inflammation of the liver. This trend focuses on keeping an eye on and controlling metabolic risk factors to avoid getting chronic liver disease (Marceau et al., 1999). Diabetes and high blood pressure often lead to chronic kidney disease. According to Peralta et al. (2006), treatment and early intervention of metabolic syndrome may be advantageous in the prevention or postponement of renal illness. Individuals with metabolic syndrome often have obstructive sleep apnea, which causes breathing interruptions during sleep. This syndrome may cause daytime fatigue, cardiovascular problems, and other health issues. The link between sleep apnea and obesity,

DOI: 10.1201/9781032702438-3

a component of metabolic syndrome, emphasizes the necessity of weight control (McCracken et al., 2018). Osteoarthritis and metabolic syndrome are linked, in part because obesity puts more stress on joints and because metabolic syndrome is linked to systemic inflammation. This may lower movement and cause joint pain, which would lower quality of life (Courties et al., 2017; Parvez and Akanda, 2019). Gout is frequently brought on by elevated blood uric acid levels, which are frequently linked to metabolic syndrome. Gout is a painful inflammation of the joints, especially the big toes. It can be controlled by eating a well-balanced diet and preserving kidney function, both of which are impacted by metabolic syndrome (McCracken et al., 2018). Many eye conditions, such as retinopathy, glaucoma, and cataracts, are associated with metabolic syndrome. It is crucial for people with metabolic syndrome to get routine eye exams since these disorders can cause vision loss or impairment if they are not appropriately treated (Chopra et al., 2012). The connection between hypothyroidism and metabolic syndrome highlights the intricate interactions between hormonal and metabolic processes in the body. Fatigue, weight gain, and other health problems can result from hypothyroidism, which makes managing metabolic syndrome more difficult. The metabolic syndrome substantially raises the risk of colon, breast, and prostate cancers, among other malignancies. It has a stronger correlation with several cancers in women, such as rectal and pancreatic cancer. The syndrome's constituents—obesity, hypertension, and excessive cholesterol levels—contribute to this elevated risk and also result in less favorable outcomes for cancer patients (Esposito et al., 2012). Metabolic syndrome is a multidimensional disorder that necessitates a comprehensive approach to care due to its impact on numerous physiological systems and the possibility of major health problems, as seen in Figure 3.1.

3.3 PATHOPHYSIOLOGY OF METABOLIC SYNDROME

The metabolic syndrome pathophysiology includes multiple complex pathways that have yet to be fully understood. It is still contested whether the various components of metabolic syndrome constitute separate illnesses or are part of a larger pathogenic process (Dizaji, 2018; Uzzaman et al., 2018). Many variables contribute to metabolic syndrome. These factors include excessive eating and a lack of physical activity. Other factors, including genetic and epigenetic factors, have also been identified as contributors. Caloric consumption may cause metabolic syndrome because visceral obesity activates most metabolic syndrome pathways (Matsuzawa et al., 2011; Pekgor et al., 2019). Figure 3.2 depicts the theorized causes of metabolic syndrome.

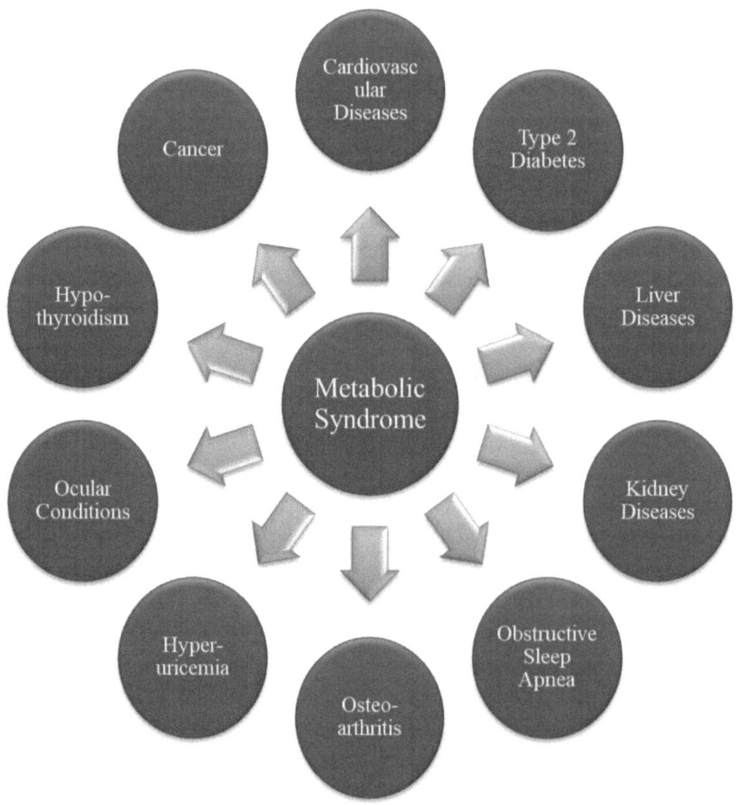

FIGURE 3.1 Metabolic syndrome-associated disease.

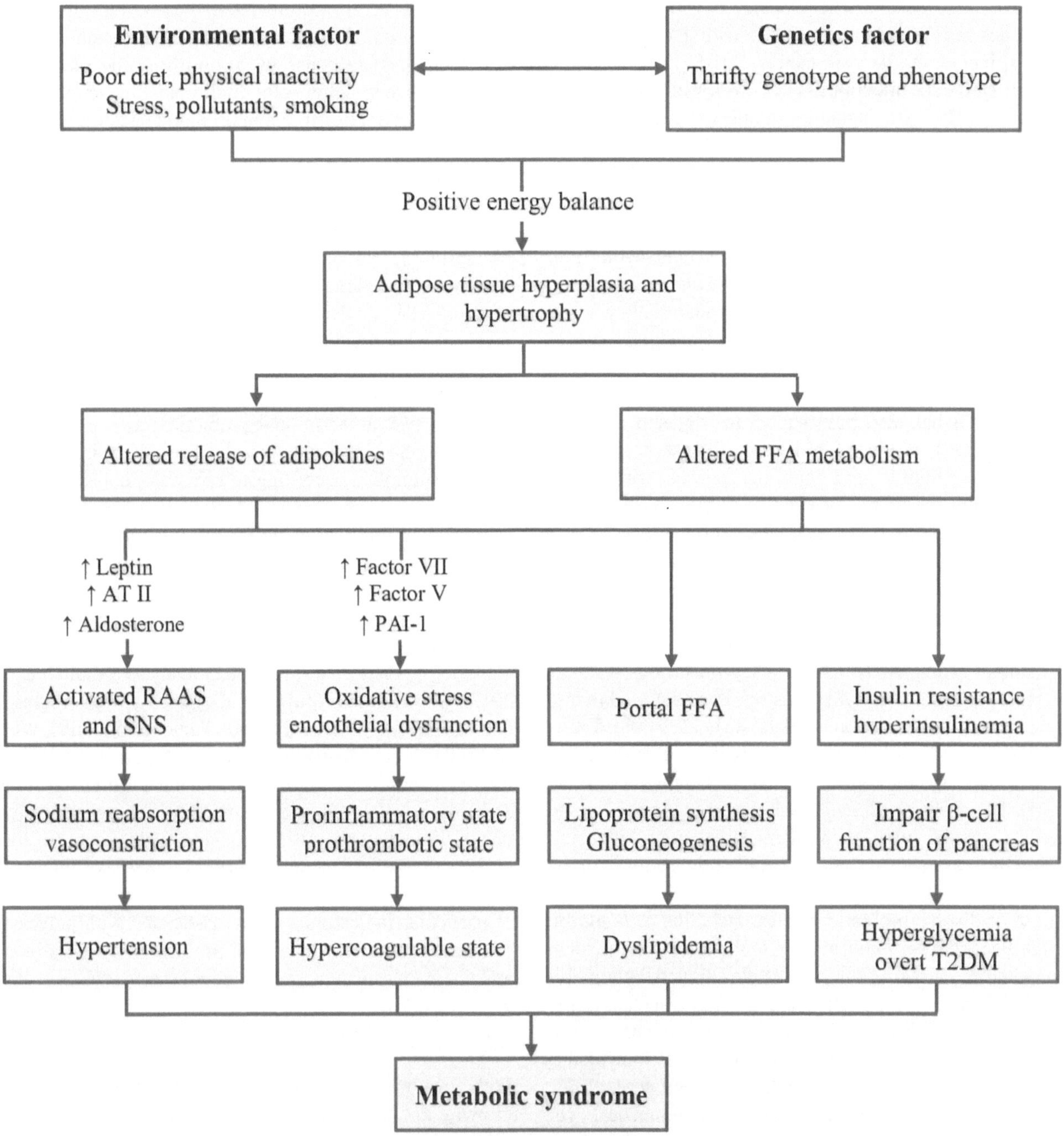

FIGURE 3.2 Metabolic syndrome: a schematic representation. Abbreviations: FFA: free fatty acid, ATII: angiotensin II, PAI-1: plasminogen activator inhibitor-1, RAAS: renin angiotensin aldosterone system, SNS: sympathetic nervous system.

3.4 PROBIOTICS

"Probiotic" is a term that originates from the Greek for "life." Still, its definition has changed over time as the popularity of live bacterial supplements has grown and probiotic mechanisms of action have been better understood. Animal feed additives that balanced intestinal flora and tissue extracts stimulated microbial development (Fuller, 1989). The contemporary definition of probiotics is "live microorganisms that, when administered in adequate amounts, confer a health benefit on the host." It is feasible that the definition might be altered in the context of food by highlighting the fact that the positive impact is exerted by microorganisms "when consumed in adequate amounts as part of food" (FAO/WHO, 2001).

3.5 POTENTIAL ROLE OF PROBIOTICS

Multiple meta-analyses showed that point to the potential efficacy of probiotic supplements in improving established markers of lipid profiles, inflammation, and oxidative stress, in people who have chronic kidney disease. Both of these conditions are widely recognized as risk factors for cardiovascular disease (Zheng et al., 2021). It is shown that probiotics relieve symptoms linked with a variety of conditions, including allergies, cancer, AIDS, lung infections, and urinary tract infections. They work well for treating a variety of illnesses, including aging, exhaustion, autism, osteoporosis, type 2 diabetes, and obesity according to a number of studies (Harish and Varghese, 2006). It has been established that probiotics are a beneficial adjunct to rehydration therapy (Szymański et al., 2006). Recent findings from a major clinical trial that included patients with *C. difficile*-associated colitis indicate that *S. boulardii* only protected against the return of disease in individuals who had a history of several *C. difficile* infections in a quick succession. Proteases generated by *S. boulardii* will break down toxins produced by *C. difficile* and will block gut receptors for toxins. It has also been shown to trigger a particular antitoxin that is produced in the digestive tract. An immunoglobulin manufactured with the purpose of combating the agent that is responsible for diarrhea (Hord, 2008; Parvez et al., 2016). Probiotics, which are made up of yeast *S. boulardii* and many different types of bacteria, can help lower the number of cases of diarrhea caused by antibiotics (Macfarlane et al., 2006). Eight types of probiotics, such as *Lactobacillus plantarum*, reduce gas and stomach pain (Chapman et al., 2011). The efficacy of various probiotic mixtures in mitigating symptoms was demonstrated in multiple studies involving adults (Hatakka et al., 2008). Taking *B. bifidum* MIMBb75 supplements for 28 days helped people with irritable bowel syndrome (Guglielmetti et al., 2011). The probiotic *E. coli* Nissle 1917 can cure IBS, especially in people with changed intestinal microbiota (e.g., following gastroenterocolitis or antibiotic administration) (Akanda and Hasan, 2021; Kruis et al., 2012). The application of diverse probiotic species, including *S. boulardii*, *Bifidobacterium bifidum*, and *Lactobacillus casei*, has demonstrated encouraging outcomes (Kelesidis and Pothoulakis, 2012). Fermented milk that contains bacteria such as *L. acidophilus, B. bifidum,* and *B. breve* has the potential to promote a moderation of remission in patients, as indicated by preliminary studies (Afroja et al., 2017; Sheil et al., 2007). Working probiotic strains can induce unique mucosal cytokines including IL-10, IL-4. By modifying the phosphorylation of cytoskeletal, tight junction proteins, probiotics have the potential to improve the function of the intestinal barrier (Howarth, 2008). The antioxidant enzymes found in probiotics, such as catalase and superoxide dismutase, have an effect on the stability and interactions between cells in the mucosa, which in turn reduces the symptoms of inflammatory bowel disease. Bacteria that function as probiotics possess adjuvant-like characteristics, induce anti-inflammatory activity, and modulate both humoral and cell-mediated immunity. It is well-established that probiotic bacteria secrete factors that regulate immune responses. As an illustration, *L. reuteri* secretes substances that lower cell proliferation and raise mitogen-activated protein kinase levels by blocking the production of NF-κB-dependent genes. This process is crucial for the initiation of apoptosis (Delcenserie et al., 2008). Nevertheless, the administration of the probiotic culture impeded the modulation of the aforementioned response by diminishing the secretion of IL-8, even when Salmonella dublin, a pathogen, was present (Hardy et al., 2013). Some probiotic bacteria, including *Bacillus bulgaricus*, *Bacillus reuteri*, and *Bacillus coagulans*, may exhibit hypocholeremic effects. Humans who consumed *L. acidophilus* L1 milk had significantly lower serum cholesterol levels, according to research. As a result of consuming low-fat yogurt that included *B. longum* BL1, a substantial reduction in triglycerides, total blood cholesterol, LDL cholesterol was observed in research that involved 32 individuals who were diagnosed with hypercholesterolemia. According to Lee et al. (2012), there was an extra 14.5% increase in HDL cholesterol concentrations. *L. bulgaricus*, an additional probiotic, has been shown to have anticancer activities in solid Ehrlich ascites and sarcoma-180 tumors, according to research published by Lee et al. (2012). There was a reduction in colon carcinogenesis in mice that were caused by 1, 2-dimethylhydrazine when FOS was mixed with Bifidobacteria probiotics. Additionally, the production of breast and liver tumors in rats was suppressed and decreased. Adult hypercholesterolemic patients who take probiotics have lower total and LDL cholesterol based on a recent meta-analysis (Niamah et al., 2017). According to Nguyen et al. (2007), cholesterol might decrease by *L. plantarum* PH40 (Yadav et al., 2019). When administered to a hypercholesterolemic rat model, probiotic treatment results in a reduction in total serum cholesterol. According to Parnell and Reimer (2010), rats were given one of three diets that were enhanced with either 0%, 10%, or 20% prebiotic fiber for a period of 10 weeks. The utilization of probiotics may have resulted in an improvement of particular indicators that are associated with polycystic ovarian syndrome include lipid profiles, body mass index, and fasting plasma glucose (Angoorani et al., 2023).

3.6 PREBIOTICS

Prebiotics, introduced in 1995, enhance human health by growing and activating a few microorganisms outside the colon (Davani-Davari et al., 2019). By this definition, a few substances that fall under the carbohydrate group are categorized as prebiotics. These include galactooligosaccharides, lactulose, and short- and long-chain fructans. Gibson et al. (2017) define dietary prebiotics as fermented compounds that affect the microbiota's composition and/or activity in the intestines, enhancing host health, according to the "International Scientific Association of Probiotics and Prebiotics (ISAPP)." This definition was presented at the sixth meeting of the ISAPP in 2008. A multitude of prebiotic definitions have been utilized in the scientific literature. In general, prebiotics lack a universally agreed-upon definition; nevertheless, the association between prebiotic intake and human health continues to be the central theme in all initial and subsequent definitions (Davani-Davari et al., 2019). According to a study by Bindels et al. (2015), the initial definition of "selectivity," which refers to the effectiveness of prebiotics in stimulating the development of specific microflora in the gastrointestinal tract, included a provision that has since generated controversy.

3.7 POTENTIAL ROLE OF PREBIOTICS

Prebiotics have also been demonstrated to help treat inflammatory bowel disease. Patients with chronic pouchitis who received 24 g of inulin daily had fewer bacteriodetes in their feces (Langen and Dieleman, 2009). According to the investigations, prebiotics also appear to increase hypercholesterolemic activity. In hamsters, Nguyen et al. (2007) found that inulin lowered total cholesterol and triglycerides by 29% and 63%. Chicory inulin decreased hydroxy-corticosteroids in hypercholesterolemic individuals, XOS prebiotic therapy decreased triglyceride levels by 27% in male Sprague-Dawley rats (Parnell and Reimer, 2010). By modulating the composition of gut flora, prebiotics like polyphenols have been shown in multiple studies to impede the progression of obesity (Luo et al., 2020). Prebiotics may treat metabolic diseases; hence food processing methods are being studied to improve them. Altering resistant starch with *Deinococcus geothermalis* amylosucrase is one possible approach (Vo et al., 2019). Fermented *Momordica charantia* juice with *L. plantarum* was found to be more beneficial in avoiding diabetes than local diets, according to Gao et al. (2019). Prebiotics like *Cyclocarya paliurus* polysaccharides can improve the body's metabolism, lower chronic inflammation by boosting Bacteroidetes, and stop the TLR4-MAPK signaling pathway from working (Wu et al., 2020). Prebiotics alter gut microbial metabolites, which may affect metabolism. Acetic and butyric acid concentrations in glucometabolic illness patients are affected by maltodextrin. In mice, rye and oat bran fiber lowers inflammation, glucose metabolism, body weight SCFA production, tryptophan-serotonin, and bile acid metabolism (Lee et al., 2018). In overweight or obese youngsters, maize starch prebiotic dextrin and lentil-based diets increase Actinobacteria and Bacteroidetes and decrease Firmicutes (Barczynska et al., 2016). Prebiotics play a crucial role in regulating gut microbial metabolites which can potentially impact metabolism (Liu et al., 2020). Prebiotics like maltodextrin can improve insulin resistance by restoring the intestinal barrier and lowering blood endotoxin levels (Hann et al., 2019).

3.8 SYNBIOTICS

Synbiotic diet supplements restore normal bacterial flora by combining probiotics, prebiotics, usually oligosaccharides, or inulin (Pandey et al., 2015). The phrase "synbiotic" was first employed to explain mixtures of probiotics and prebiotics that beneficially affect the host by improving the survival and implantation of live microbial dietary supplements in the gastrointestinal tract, by selectively stimulating the growth and/or by activating the metabolism of one or a limited number of health-promoting bacteria, thus improving host welfare (Gibson and Roberfroid, 1995).

The study on this notion is preliminary, with no high-quality clinical proof that such benefits exist. Synbiotics can be complementary, in which each component is chosen independently for its potential influence on host health, or synergistic. Selecting a prebiotic component boosts probiotic function. Synbiotics, which are said to boost the growth and health advantages of existing probiotics, are being studied to see whether they can be optimized. Probiotics are living bacteria that are designed to colonize the large intestine, although no proof is present that adding dietary bacteria to healthy people offers any further benefit. Prebiotics are supplements that boost healthy bacteria. A fiber can be a prebiotic, but it is not invariably one. Given the vast variety of conceivable synbiotic combinations, using synbiotics to alter microbiota in the human digestive tract looks to hold considerable promise (De Vrese and Schrezenmeir, 2008; Gourbeyre et al., 2011; Scavuzzi et al., 2014).

3.9 POTENTIAL ROLE OF SYNBIOTIC

For the purpose of enhancing immune function, synbiotics appear to be an incredibly intriguing remedy. By using *B. coagulans* and inulin as dietary supplements for a period of 6 weeks, C-reactive protein dropped substantially, while the levels of glutathione were simultaneously increased (Panda et al., 2006). The administration of synbiotic supplementation consisting of 10% FOS, *Lactobacillus*, and *Bifidobacterium*, effectively reduced intestinal and systemic inflammation in rodents that were administered low-fiber diet, a high-fat. These comparable effects to those observed with FOS supplementation alone (Delcenserie et al., 2008). Another study proved that synbiotics have potential in regulating lipid profiles, as evidenced by a study in which rice bran fermented with *L. acidophilus* was fed to hypercholesterolemic male rodents (Oberreuther-Moschner et al., 2004). It was shown that the injection of a synbiotic reduced the inhibition of the activity of NK cells in Peyer's patches that were produced by azoxymethane. Treatments with probiotics and prebiotics alone did not have this effect (Saulnier et al., 2009). It has also suggested that synbiotics could modify the colonic microbiota composition, decrease inflammation in the gut mucosa, and elicit remission in inflammatory bowel disease, in addition to preventing travelers' diarrhea and enhancing patients' quality of life as a whole (Pokusaeva et al., 2011; Romeo et al., 2010). It has been established in a number of studies that including synbiotics into one's diet can enhance glucose homeostasis and lipid metabolism in those who have type 2 diabetes (Mahboobi et al., 2018). Studies show that synbiotics like yogurts may lessen cardiovascular disease risk in high-cholesterol patients (Mofid et al., 2020). Patients on hemodialysis may see a reduction in intracellular adhesion molecule type 1 (ICAM-1) levels after 12 weeks of taking synbiotic supplements (Haghighat et al., 2019). Synbiotics may enhance energy metabolism biomarkers in non-alcoholic fatty liver disease patients, given that ICAM-1 is a major contributor to the development of cardiovascular disease

(Li et al., 2022). Redesigning the metabolic profile using synbiotic components may help obese people, since they give the right target for changing the gut flora. Functional meals that incorporate synbiotic components may help reduce obesity, a significant chronic illness risk factor (Hijová, 2022). Studies show that synbiotic supplements can alter hormone, neurotransmitter, and inflammatory secretion, potentially reducing food triggers causing weight gain (Aoun et al., 2020). Table 3.1 shows a summary of the impacts and processes that probiotics, prebiotics, and synbiotics have on the digestive system's metabolic disorders based on the experiments' results.

The clinical outcomes that are linked with the utilization of synbiotics, probiotics, and prebiotics in the therapy of metabolic illnesses are summarized in Table 3.2, which offers an overview of these relationships.

3.10 SAFETY AND EFFICACY

The increased requirement for temperature and moisture-stable probiotics and prebiotics in new food supplements has made difficult quality assurance methods (Luo et al., 2019). To increase consumer and stakeholder trust, studies have questioned the quality, purity of commercial probiotic, synbiotic products, recommending standardized prebiotic assessment, and certification. Valid identification determines probiotic strain genus, species, subspecies, and strain. Most commercial quality control labs use phenotypic approaches, which have poor resolution to the genus level (Huys et al., 2013). Whole-genome sequencing, next-generation sequencing has revolutionized microbiological community studies, enabling the establishment of quality, safety standards for food. However, despite their ability to detect probiotics in multistrain combinations and potential contaminants, they are rarely used in quality control labs (Quigley, 2013). According to Courtin et al. (2009), one of the most important goals for the future is to enhance the stability of living cells in goods throughout their shelf life across a variety of product shapes. Utilizing big data and machine learning to comprehend strain phenomics and fluxomics could potentially facilitate the mastery of product efficacy and stability across a multitude of applications. It is widely recognized that food processing techniques, such as heat and pH changes, can lead to the degradation of prebiotics. Thus, standardized prebiotic product quality assurance is essential for maintaining various prebiotic product availability, effective, and dependable products in the future. Molecular integrity maintenance and dosage determination can be accomplished through chemical and structural analyses pertaining to prebiotic quality assurance. Alternatively, functional assays can be employed to gauge the prebiotic's activity retention, specifically in terms of microbial metabolism and the resulting health benefits transmitted to final products (Lebeer et al., 2018). In-depth information regarding novel candidate prebiotics can be obtained through the utilization of environmental scanning electron microscopy for microstructural morphological examination and spectroscopic techniques for detailed structural analysis (Zeng et al., 2018).

TABLE 3.1
Experimental Studies Show How Probiotics, Prebiotics, Synbiotics Affect Metabolic Illnesses

Supplements	Target Disease	Doses	Mechanisms and Main Effects	Refs.
Probiotics				
Bifidobacterium lactis LMG P-28149 and *Lactobacillus rhamnosus LMG S-28148*	Obesity and insulin resistance	10^8 CFU	*Rikenellaceae* and *Akkermansia* muciniphila restoration. Lipoprotein lipase and PPARγ expression are upregulated. TG clearance and insulin sensitivity enhancement A reduction in *Lactobacillaceae*.	Alard et al. (2016)
Ligilactobacillus salivarius PI2 and *Bifidobacterium longum PI10*	Obesity	5×10^8 CFU	Expression of GLP1 and IL-10 is upregulated.	Alard et al. (2021)
Bifidobacterium longum NK49 and Lactobacillus plantarum NK3 worked together	Obesity and osteoporosis	1×10^9 CFU	Enhancing the intestinal barrier. Inhibiting the production of LPS. The downregulation of TNF-α expression linked to NF-κB.	Kim et al. (2019)
Lactobacillus fermentum MCC2760	Type 2 diabetes mellitus	10^9 CFU	Improving the intestinal barrier. The expression of GLUT4, GLP1, and ZO-1 is enhanced.	Archer et al. (2021)
Lactobacillus casei	Hypertension	2×10^8 CFU	*Akkermansia* and *Lactobacillus* are proliferating. Reduced Firmicutes to Bacteroidetes Ratio and Expression of Aces.	Hsu et al. (2019)
Lactobacillus fermentum CECT5716 and Bifidobacterium breve CECT7263	Hypertension	10^9 CFU	An increase in bacteria associated to butyrate. Raising the butyrate concentration in the plasma. Lower the production of LPS.	Vera et al. (2020)

(*Continued*)

TABLE 3.1 (*Continued*)
Experimental Studies Show How Probiotics, Prebiotics, Synbiotics Affect Metabolic Illnesses

Supplements	Target Disease	Doses	Mechanisms and Main Effects	Refs.
Lactobacillus reuteri and *Lactobacillus johnsonii*	Inflammatory bowel disease and Osteoporosis	10^{10} CFU	Enhancing the metabolism of tetrathionate. Yersinia enterocolitica reduction.	Kamdar et al. (2016)
Lactobacillus paracasei	Colitis with metabolic disorder	0.8–1.2 × 10^9 CFU	Palmitoylethanolamide production for intestinal function maintenance.	Esposito et al. (2021)
Lactobacillus reuteri LR6	Protein-energy malnutrition	1 × 10^9 CFU	Proliferation of Bifidobacteria, Firmicutes, and Lactobacilli.	Garg et al. (2020)
Prebiotics				
Maize starch dextrin and Lentil	Obesity	70.8% red lentil diet	A reduction in Firmicutes. Bacteroidetes and Actinobacteria proliferate.	Barczynska et al. (2016), Siva et al. (2018)
Inulin oligofructose	Obesity	5% in diet, 0.6 g/day	Proliferation of *Bifidobacterium*. A reduction in the ratio of *Firmicutes* to *Bacteroidetes*.	Kumar et al. (2016), de Cossío et al. (2017)
Chicory oligofructose	Obesity	10% in diet	*Collinsella* and *Bifidobacterium* are proliferating.	Klancic et al. (2020)
Amylosucrase-modified chestnut starch	Obesity	1500 mg/kg	SCFA upregulation via the GPR43-mediated pathway.	Lee et al. (2018)
Fuji FF	Obesity	10% in diet	Increasing production of propionic, butyric, and acetic acids.	Igarashi et al. (2020)
Oligosaccharides of unsaturated alginate	Obesity	400 mg/kg	Expression of ZO-1 and ccluding is increased.	Li et al. (2020a)
Polysaccharides from acorns and sago	Obesity and type 2 diabetes mellitus	1% *v/v*, 5% in diet	Mitigating mucosal inflammation and gastrointestinal hyperpermeability biomarkers.	Ahmadi et al. (2019)
Galactooligosaccharides	Obesity and Insulin resistance	7% *w/w*	Elevating the expression of GLP1. Decreased excretion of bile acid in the feces.	Mistry et al. (2020)
Dextrin derived from resistant wheat and maize starch	Type 2 diabetes mellitus	5 g/kg	The populations of Akkermansia and Prevotella are growing. The pathways IRS1-Akt-GLUT2 and SIRT1-AMPK-PPAR-CPR1 are becoming increasingly active.	Hu et al. (2020)
Isomaltodextrin	Insulin resistance	1%, 2.5%, 5% in drinking water	Increasing the production of acetic and butyric acids. Enhancing the intestinal barrier. Reduce the level of endotoxins in circulation.	Hann et al. (2019)
Whole garlic	Dyslipidemia	5% in diet	The expansion of *Lachnospiraceae*. Reduced *Prevotella* dosage.	Chen et al. (2019)
Fucoidan and galactooligosaccharides	Dyslipidemia	100, 800 mg/kg	Bacteroidetes have grown in number, as has *Lactobacillus casei* DM8121's bile salt hydrolase activity and proteobacteria. Actinobacteria and Firmicutes are declining.	Ahmadi et al. (2019)
Brans of oats and rye dietary fiber.	Metabolic disorder	10% in diet	Bile acid and tryptophan-serotonin metabolic pathways are regulated.	Kundi et al. (2021)
Agave salmiana fructan	Metabolic disorder	10% in diet	Increasing lactic acid production.	Regalado-Rentería et al. (2020)
Glycolipids from tilapia heads	Colitis with metabolic disorder	30 mg/kg	The occurrence of Ackermansia, Allobaculum, Bifidobacterium, Coprococcus, Oscillospira, and Prevotellaceae is increasing.	Gu et al. (2020)
Long-chain inulin	Hypertension	5% in diet	Lowering plasma TMAO and feces acetate and propionate.	Scheithauer et al. (2020)
Synbiotics				
Omega-3 Fatty Acids, Lactobacillus, Lactococcus, Bifidobacterium, and *Propionibacterium*	Obesity	2.5 mL/kg	The combination of probiotics and lipid buildup significantly reduced hepatic steatosis and lipid accumulation when compared to probiotics alone.	Kobyliak et al. (2017), Kobyliak et al. (2018)

(*Continued*)

TABLE 3.1 (*Continued*)
Experimental Studies Show How Probiotics, Prebiotics, Synbiotics Affect Metabolic Illnesses

Supplements	Target Disease	Doses	Mechanisms and Main Effects	Refs.
Bacillus licheniformis, xylosaccharides	Obesity	7.5×10^8 CFU/mL and 2 g/mL	Working synergistically to promote weight and lipid metabolism. Ruminococcaceae and Desulfovibrionaceae are declining.	Li et al. (2020b)
Chia seeds, L. plantarum PMO 08	Obesity	1×10^9 CFU/mL and 4% in diet	Positively synergistic obesity improvement. Boosting L. plantarum	Oh et al. (2019)
Xylo-oligosaccharides with L. paracasei HII01	Obesity	1×10^8 CFU and 10% in PBS	Inhibiting metabolic endotoxemia. Enterobacteriaceae and Firmicutes-Bacteroidetes ratio reduction.	Thiennimitr et al. (2018)
Salvia miltiorrhiza polysaccharide, Bifidobacterium bifidum V, and Lactobacillus plantarum X	NAFLD	1–2 $\times 10^8$ CFU and 50 mg/kg	Reduced hepatic steatosis and insulin resistance. Lowering LPS.	Wang et al. (2019)
Corn bran with Clostridium butyricum	Metabolic intestinal disability	1×10^8 CFU/g and 5% in diet	Boosting acetate-producing bacteria and isovalerate synthesis. Pathogens are declining.	Zhang et al. (2018)

Abbreviations: ACE, angiotensin-converting enzyme; Akt, protein kinase B; AMPK, adenosine monophosphate kinase; CPR1α, carnitine palmitoyl transferase 1α; ERK, extracellular regulated protein kinases; GLP1, glucagon-like peptide 1; GLUT2/4, glucose transporter 2; GPR43, G-protein coupled receptor; IL-10, interleukin-10; IRF4, interferon regulatory factor 4; IRS1, insulin receptor substrate 1; LPS, lipopolysaccharide; NF-κB, nuclear factor kappa B; NLCR3, nucleotide-binding oligomerization domain-like receptors 3; NOD2, nucleotide-binding oligomerization domain-containing protein 2; p38 MAPK, p38 mitogen-activated protein kinase; PPARα/γ, peroxisome proliferators activated receptor α/γ; SCFAs, short-chain fatty acids; SIRT1, sirtuin 1; TLR2/4, TG, triglycerides; Toll-like receptor 2/4; TMAO, trimethylamine-n-oxide; TNF-α, tumor necrosis factor α; TRAF6, TNF receptor-associated factor 6; ZO-1, zonula occludens-1

TABLE 3.2
Probiotics, Prebiotics, and Synbiotics' Clinical Effects on Metabolic Disorders

Supplements	Target Disease	Doses	Duration	Sample Size	Main Effects	Refs.
Probiotics						
Streptococcus thermophiles and *Lactobacillus acidophilus SGL11, delbrueckii DSM 20081, lactis SGLc01, plantarum SGL07, reuteri SGL01*	Obesity	1.5×10^{10} CFU	3 weeks	60	Improving body composition, bacterial composition, and psychopathological status.	De Lorenzo et al. (2017)
Bifidobacterium lactis	Obesity	2.72×10^{10} CFU	45 days	45	Improved obesity, blood lipids, and TNF- and IL-6 indicators.	Bernini et al. (2016)
Lactobacillus plantarum CBT LP3 and *Bifidobacterium breve CBT BR3*	Obesity	15×10^{10} CFU	12 weeks	50	Obesity biomarkers are improved more successfully in patients with Prevotella-rich enterotypes than in those with Bacteroides-rich enterotypes.	Song et al. (2020)
Lactobacillus acidophilus La-5 and *Bifidobacterium lactis BB-12*	Type 2 diabetes mellitus	10^9 CFU	6 weeks	50	Improving fructosamine, HbA1c and IL-10 levels.	Tonucci et al. (2017)
Lactobacillus reuteri strain ADR-1 and ADR-3	Type 2 diabetes mellitus	4×10^9 CFU for ADR-1 2×10^{10} CFU for ADR-3	12 weeks	68	Decreasing HbA1c and cholesterol levels.	Hsieh et al. (2018)
Lactobacillus casei strain Shirota fermentation milk	Type 2 diabetes mellitus	80 mL	16 weeks	70	Increase the concentrations *of C. coccoides, C. leptum*, and Lactobacillus. Translocated intestinal microorganisms are decreasing.	Sato et al. (2017)

(*Continued*)

TABLE 3.2 (*Continued*)
Probiotics, Prebiotics, and Synbiotics' Clinical Effects on Metabolic Disorders

Supplements	Target Disease	Doses	Duration	Sample Size	Main Effects	Refs.
Lactobacillus rhamnosus HN001	Gestational diabetes mellitus	6 × 10^9 CFU	14–16 weeks' gestation	423	Decreasing the relapse prevalence of diabetes mellitus.	Wickens et al. (2017)
Lactobacillus rhamnosus with Bifidobacterium lactis	Gestational diabetes mellitus	1 × 10^9 CFU	16–28 weeks' gestation	411	Not preventing gestational diabetes mellitus.	Callaway et al. (2019)
Lactobacillus rhamnosus GG with Bifidobacterium lactis BB12	Gestational diabetes mellitus	6.5 × 10^9 CFU	17–36 weeks' gestation	230	Not improving depression, anxiety, and physical well-being status.	Dawe et al. (2020)
Lactobacillus acidophilus, Lactobacillus casei, and *Bifidobacterium bifidum*	Major depressive with metabolic disorder	2 × 10^9 CFU/g	8 weeks	40	Insulin resistance, C-reactive protein, and total glutathione levels are all improving.	Akkasheh et al. (2016)
Prebiotics						
Yacon	Obesity	25 g	6 weeks	26–40	Increasing the antioxidant capability of the plasma. Reducing oxidative stress and fecal SCFAs.	Machado et al. (2021), Adriano et al. (2020)
Inulin oligofructose	Obesity	8 g/day	16 weeks	42	Modifying appetite to reduce energy intake.	Hume et al. (2017)
Oligofructose	Obesity	21 g	12 weeks	37	Enhanced metabolic endotoxemia. PAI1 level is decreasing.	Parnell et al. (2017)
Whey protein and Inulin-type fructan	Obesity	5–8 g	12 weeks	125	Appetite control. Increase the amount of Bifidobacterium.	Reimer et al. (2017)
Inulin oligofructose	Type 2 diabetes mellitus	10 g/day	2 months	46	Increasing glycemic control, lipid profiles, and immunological markers	Dehghan et al. (2016)
Inulin	Obesity-related major depressive	10 g/day	8 weeks	45	Increasing the positive effects of calorie restriction on fat mass and TC level.	Vaghef-Mehrabany et al. (2021)
Inulin	NAFLD	10 g/day	3 months	75	Fatty liver and serum aminotransferase enzyme quality improvement.	Javadi et al. (2017)
Synbiotics						
Growing up milk	Obesity	300 mL	12 months	160	Improving body fat gain.	Wall et al. (2019)
Bifidobacterium bifidum, Lactobacillus acidophilus, Lactobacillus casei, plus inulin	Obesity	2 × 10^9 CFU/g and 0.8 g	8 weeks	59	Improving lipid profiles and mental health. BMI, blood pressure, glucose metabolism, and waist circumference are not improved.	Hadi et al. (2019)
The mixture includes Lactobacillus acidophilus, Lactobacillus plantarum, and *Lactobacillus reuteri, together with inulin and fructo-oligosaccharides.*	Metabolic disorder	1 × 10^9 CFU and 12.97% in liquid	2 months	60	Decreasing metabolic syndrome prevalence	Cicero et al. (2021)
Probiotic yogurt plus Coix lacryma-jobi	Type 2 diabetes mellitus	100 mL and 25 g	12 weeks	60	Reducing body weight and fasting blood glucose	Djaja et al. (2019)
Bifidobacterium bifidum W23, W51, and W52. Also found were galacto-oligosaccharides P11 and fructo-oligosaccharides P6	Type 2 diabetes mellitus	1.5 × 10^{10} CFU and 8 g	6 months	26	Improving hip circumference, zonulin and lipoprotein. Not affecting glucose metabolism.	Horvath et al. (2020)
Bifidobacterium, Lactobacillus, and *Streptococus thermophilus* plus fructo-oligosaccharide	Type 2 diabetes mellitus	500 mg/day	9 weeks	70	HbA1c, BMI, and microalbuminuria are all improving. Fasting blood glucose, lipid profiles, and creatinine levels are unaffected.	Ebrahimi et al. (2017)

(*Continued*)

TABLE 3.2 (*Continued*)
Probiotics, Prebiotics, and Synbiotics' Clinical Effects on Metabolic Disorders

Supplements	Target Disease	Doses	Duration	Sample Size	Main Effects	Refs.
Lactobacillus acidophilus, Bifidobacterium bifidum, Bifidobacterium lactis, Bifidobacterium longum, and inulin	Prediabetes mellitus	1.5 × 10⁹ CFU and 6 g	6 months	120	Not restoring the balance of gut microbiota.	Kassaian et al. (2020)
Bifidobacterium lactis plus fructo-oligosaccharides	Digestive disorder	5 × 10⁹ CFU/ bag and 4.95 g/bag	30 days	27	Improving intestinal function. Decreasing IL-6, IL-8, IL-17α, and IFN-γ levels.	Neyrinck et al. (2021)
Chicory inulin, Bifidobacterium lactis, Lactobacillus acidophilus, and *Lactobacillus casei*	NAFLD	7 × 10⁹ CFU and 100 mg	4 months	28	Improving fatty liver grade, and inflammatory and antioxidative status.	Çakır et al. (2017)
Selenium, Bifidobacterium bifidum, Bifidobacterium longum, and Lactobacillus acidophilus	Alzheimer's disease with metabolic disorder	2 × 10⁹ CFU and 200 mg	12 weeks	79	Improving the cognitive function and metabolic function.	Tamtaji et al. (2019)

Abbreviations: BMI, body mass index; HbA1c, hemoglobin A1c; IL-6/8/10/17α, interleukin-6/8/10/17α; IFN-γ, interferon-γ; PAI1, plasminogen activator inhibitor 1; SCFAs, short-chain fatty acids; TC, total cholesterol; TNF-α, tumor necrosis factor α

3.11 FUTURE PERSPECTIVE TO CONTROL METABOLIC DISORDERS

Recent advancements in prebiotic and probiotic fields have significantly impacted the field, this trend is expected to continue eventually. These developments have been made possible by significant advancements in technology and associated approaches. To synthesize novel oligosaccharides, recent developments in enzyme technology are being implemented. The production of small quantities of novel oligosaccharides allows for in vitro fermentations to examine their prebiotic potential. This research enhances understanding of enzyme accessibility and activities by examining changes in bacterial populations and fermentation products. Probiotics that possess observable health benefits should be identified and recommended for use, notwithstanding the presence of certain detrimental effects such as gastric acidity, bile secretions, pancreatic effluent, and (likely the most significant) competition for colonization sites, nutrients with highly active resident flora. Strategies for surmounting this issue may be contemplated. The probiotic could be enhanced by protective coatings or increased resistance to certain factors, such as acid, and could be further enhanced through genetic engineering by incorporating genes encoding proteins involved in mammalian cell adhesion, potentially enhancing its survivability (Crittenden and Playne, 1996). In order to establish the safety of probiotic, prebiotic, and including substances, additional corroborating evidence linking alterations in intestinal bacterial communities to physiological aspects in humans is required. Additionally, a greater comprehension of how probiotics and prebiotics alter the structure of microbial communities is necessary (Fuller and Gibson, 1997). By applying molecular techniques to the study of intestinal microbial ecology, these research objectives can be more effectively attained. Utilizing oligonucleotide probes that target 16S ribosomal RNA, human large intestine, and rumen microbial ecology have been studied (Robinson et al., 2010).

3.12 CONCLUSION

In summary, the significance of prebiotics, probiotics, and synbiotics in mitigating metabolic disorders highlights complicated interaction between gastrointestinal health and metabolic wellness as a whole. Probiotics, prebiotics, and numerous interventions that are affiliated with microbiome-targeted nutrition and therapeutics have been significantly broadened by the abundance of research in these areas. In order to target an expanding array of compositional, functional niches within the microbiome, numerous substances will be discovered to fulfill economic and environmental requirements. Industry developments and customer preferences will drive the use of probiotic, prebiotic, and other bioactive compounds in several forms. Delivery and quality assurance innovations will boost demand. Prolonged progressions in biotechnology and bioinformatics are poised to yield comprehensive mechanistic understandings of pathways of prebiotic and probiotic actions, in addition to facilitating the discovery of novel candidate organisms and substrates. The ongoing improvement of validation and discovery methods will enhance the dependability and replicable nature of research outcomes. This will facilitate the comparison of data sets and the generation of broader aggregated insights across various research streams. Further investment in large intervention and population-based studies, coupled with these insights, will reveal novel approaches to enhance the clinical relevance and effectiveness of dietary interventions while also customizing them to the biology and microbiome of individual subjects.

REFERENCES

Adriano, L. S., Dionísio, A. P., Pinto de Abreu, F. A., Wurlitzer, N. J., Cordeiro de Melo, B. R., Ferreira Carioca, A. A., & de Carvalho Sampaio, H. A. (2020). Acute postprandial effect of yacon syrup ingestion on appetite: A double blind randomized crossover clinical trial. *Food Research International*, *137*, 109648. https://doi.org/10.1016/j.foodres.2020.109648

Afroja, S., Falgunee, F. N., Jahan, M. M., Akanda, K. M., Mehjabin, S., & Parvez, G. M. M. (2017). Antibacterial activity of different citrus fruits. *Specialty Journal of Medical Research and Health Science*, *2*(1), 25–32.

Ahmadi, S., Nagpal, R., Wang, S., Gagliano, J., Kitzman, D. W., Soleimanian-Zad, S., Sheikh-Zeinoddin, M., Read, R., & Yadav, H. (2019). Prebiotics from acorn and sago prevent high-fat-diet-induced insulin resistance via microbiome-gut-brain axis modulation. *The Journal of Nutritional Biochemistry*, *67*, 1–13. https://doi.org/10.1016/j.jnutbio.2019.01.011

Akanda, Md. K. M., & Hasan, A. H. M. N. (2021). Characterization of pharmacological properties of methanolic seed and stem bark extracts of *Ziziphus mauritiana* (BAU Kul) using in-vitro and in-vivo animal (*Swiss albino* male mice) model. *Clinical Phytoscience*, *7*(1), 8. https://doi.org/10.1186/s40816-020-00246-0

Akkasheh, G., Kashani-Poor, Z., Tajabadi-Ebrahimi, M., Jafari, P., Akbari, H., Taghizadeh, M., Memarzadeh, M. R., Asemi, Z., & Esmaillzadeh, A. (2016). Clinical and metabolic response to probiotic administration in patients with major depressive disorder: A randomized, double-blind, placebo-controlled trial. *Nutrition*, *32*(3), 315–320. https://doi.org/10.1016/j.nut.2015.09.003

Alard, J., Cudennec, B., Boutillier, D., Peucelle, V., Descat, A., Decoin, R., Kuylle, S., Jablaoui, A., Rhimi, M., Wolowczuk, I., Pot, B., Tailleux, A., Maguin, E., Holowacz, S., & Grangette, C. (2021). Multiple selection criteria for probiotic strains with high potential for obesity management. *Nutrients*, *13*(3), Article 3. https://doi.org/10.3390/nu13030713

Alard, J., Lehrter, V., Rhimi, M., Mangin, I., Peucelle, V., Abraham, A.-L., Mariadassou, M., Maguin, E., Waligora-Dupriet, A.-J., Pot, B., Wolowczuk, I., & Grangette, C. (2016). Beneficial metabolic effects of selected probiotics on diet-induced obesity and insulin resistance in mice are associated with improvement of dysbiotic gut microbiota. *Environmental Microbiology*, *18*(5), 1484–1497. https://doi.org/10.1111/1462-2920.13181

Alonso, V., & Guarner, F. (2013). Linking the gut microbiota to human health. *The British Journal of Nutrition*, *109*(Suppl 2), S21–S26. https://doi.org/10.1017/S0007114512005235

Angoorani, P., Ejtahed, H.-S., Ettehad Marvasti, F., Taghavi, M., Mohammadpour Ahranjani, B., Hasani-Ranjbar, S., & Larijani, B. (2023). The effects of probiotics, prebiotics, and synbiotics on polycystic ovarian syndrome: An overview of systematic reviews. *Frontiers in Medicine*, *10*. https://www.frontiersin.org/articles/10.3389/fmed.2023.1141355

Aoun, A., Darwish, F., & Hamod, N. (2020). The influence of the gut microbiome on obesity in adults and the role of probiotics, prebiotics, and synbiotics for weight loss. *Preventive Nutrition and Food Science*, *25*(2), 113–123. https://doi.org/10.3746/pnf.2020.25.2.113

Archer, A. C., Muthukumar, S. P., & Halami, P. M. (2021). Lactobacillus fermentum MCC2759 and MCC2760 alleviate inflammation and intestinal function in high-fat diet-fed and streptozotocin-induced diabetic rats. *Probiotics and Antimicrobial Proteins*, *13*(4), 1068–1080. https://doi.org/10.1007/s12602-021-09744-0

Barczynska, R., Kapusniak, J., Litwin, M., Slizewska, K., & Szalecki, M. (2016). Dextrins from maize starch as substances activating the growth of bacteroidetes and actinobacteria simultaneously inhibiting the growth of firmicutes, responsible for the occurrence of obesity. *Plant Foods for Human Nutrition*, *71*(2), 190–196. https://doi.org/10.1007/s11130-016-0542-9

Bernini, L. J., Simão, A. N. C., Alfieri, D. F., Lozovoy, M. A. B., Mari, N. L., de Souza, C. H. B., Dichi, I., & Costa, G. N. (2016). Beneficial effects of *Bifidobacterium lactis* on lipid profile and cytokines in patients with metabolic syndrome: A randomized trial. Effects of probiotics on metabolic syndrome. *Nutrition*, *32*(6), 716–719. https://doi.org/10.1016/j.nut.2015.11.001

Bindels, L. B., Delzenne, N. M., Cani, P. D., & Walter, J. (2015). Towards a more comprehensive concept for prebiotics. *Nature Reviews. Gastroenterology & Hepatology*, *12*(5), 303–310. https://doi.org/10.1038/nrgastro.2015.47

Bonomini, F., Rodella, L. F., & Rezzani, R. (2015). Metabolic syndrome, aging and involvement of oxidative stress. *Aging and Disease*, *6*(2), Article 2. https://doi.org/10.14336/AD.2014.0305

Brown, K., DeCoffe, D., Molcan, E., & Gibson, D. L. (2012). Diet-induced dysbiosis of the intestinal microbiota and the effects on immunity and disease. *Nutrients*, *4*(8), 1095–1119. https://doi.org/10.3390/nu4081095

Çakır, M., İşbilen, A. A., Eyüpoğlu, İ., Sağ, E., Örem, A., Şen, T. M., Kaklıkkaya, N., & Kaya, G. (2017). Effects of long-term synbiotic supplementation in addition to lifestyle changes in children with obesity-related non-alcoholic fatty liver disease. *Turkish Journal of Gastroenterology*, *28*, 377–383. https://doi.org/10.5152/tjg.2017.17084. https://doi.org/10.5152/tjg.2017.17084

Callaway, L. K., McIntyre, H. D., Barrett, H. L., Foxcroft, K., Tremellen, A., Lingwood, B. E., Tobin, J. M., Wilkinson, S., Kothari, A., Morrison, M., O'Rourke, P., Pelecanos, A., & Dekker Nitert, M. (2019). Probiotics for the prevention of gestational diabetes mellitus in overweight and obese women: Findings from the SPRING double-blind randomized controlled trial. *Diabetes Care*, *42*(3), 364–371. https://doi.org/10.2337/dc18-2248

Chapman, C. M. C., Gibson, G. R., & Rowland, I. (2011). Health benefits of probiotics: Are mixtures more effective than single strains? *European Journal of Nutrition*, *50*(1), 1–17. https://doi.org/10.1007/s00394-010-0166-z

Chen, K., Xie, K., Liu, Z., Nakasone, Y., Sakao, K., Hossain, M. A., & Hou, D.-X. (2019). Preventive effects and mechanisms of garlic on dyslipidemia and gut microbiome dysbiosis. *Nutrients*, *11*(6), Article 6. https://doi.org/10.3390/nu11061225

Chopra, R., Chander, A., & Jacob, J. J. (2012). Ocular associations of metabolic syndrome. *Indian Journal of Endocrinology and Metabolism*, *16*(Suppl1), S6. https://doi.org/10.4103/2230-8210.94244

Cicero, A. F. G., Fogacci, F., Bove, M., Giovannini, M., & Borghi, C. (2021). Impact of a short-term synbiotic supplementation on metabolic syndrome and systemic inflammation in elderly patients: A randomized placebo-controlled clinical trial. *European Journal of Nutrition*, *60*(2), 655–663. https://doi.org/10.1007/s00394-020-02271-8

Courties, A., Sellam, J., & Berenbaum, F. (2017). Metabolic syndrome-associated osteoarthritis. *Current Opinion in Rheumatology*, *29*(2), 214. https://doi.org/10.1097/BOR.0000000000000373

Courtin, C. M., Swennen, K., Verjans, P., & Delcour, J. A. (2009). Heat and pH stability of prebiotic arabinoxylooligosaccharides, xylooligosaccharides and fructooligosaccharides. *Food Chemistry*, *112*(4), 831–837. https://doi.org/10.1016/j.foodchem.2008.06.039

Crittenden, R. G., & Playne, M. J. (1996). Production, properties and applications of food-grade oligosaccharides. *Trends in Food Science & Technology*, *7*(11), 353–361. https://doi.org/10.1016/S0924-2244(96)10038-8

Davani-Davari, D., Negahdaripour, M., Karimzadeh, I., Seifan, M., Mohkam, M., Masoumi, S. J., Berenjian, A., & Ghasemi, Y. (2019). Prebiotics: Definition, types, sources, mechanisms, and clinical applications. *Foods*, *8*(3), 92. https://doi.org/10.3390/foods8030092

Dawe, J. P., McCowan, L. M. E., Wilson, J., Okesene-Gafa, K. A. M., & Serlachius, A. S. (2020). Probiotics and maternal mental health: A randomised controlled trial among pregnant women with obesity. *Scientific Reports*, *10*(1), Article 1. https://doi.org/10.1038/s41598-020-58129-w

de Cossío, L. F., Fourrier, C., Sauvant, J., Everard, A., Capuron, L., Cani, P. D., Layé, S., & Castanon, N. (2017). Impact of prebiotics on metabolic and behavioral alterations in a mouse model of metabolic syndrome. *Brain, Behavior, and Immunity*, *64*, 33–49. https://doi.org/10.1016/j.bbi.2016.12.022

De Lorenzo, A., Costacurta, M., Merra, G., Gualtieri, P., Cioccoloni, G., Marchetti, M., Varvaras, D., Docimo, R., & Di Renzo, L. (2017). Can psychobiotics intake modulate psychological profile and body composition of women affected by normal weight obese syndrome and obesity? A double blind randomized clinical trial. *Journal of Translational Medicine*, *15*(1), 135. https://doi.org/10.1186/s12967-017-1236-2

de Vrese, M., & Schrezenmeir, J. (2008). Probiotics, prebiotics, and synbiotics. *Advances in Biochemical Engineering/Biotechnology*, *111*, 1–66. https://doi.org/10.1007/10_2008_097

Dehghan, P., Farhangi, M. A., Tavakoli, F., Aliasgarzadeh, A., & Akbari, A. M. (2016). Impact of prebiotic supplementation on T-cell subsets and their related cytokines, anthropometric features and blood pressure in patients with type 2 diabetes mellitus: A randomized placebo-controlled trial. *Complementary Therapies in Medicine*, *24*, 96–102. https://doi.org/10.1016/j.ctim.2015.12.010

Delcenserie, V., Martel, D., Lamoureux, M., Amiot, J., Boutin, Y., & Roy, D. (2008). Immunomodulatory effects of probiotics in the intestinal tract. *Current Issues in Molecular Biology*, *10*(1–2), 37–54.

Diamant, M., Blaak, E. E., & de Vos, W. M. (2011). Do nutrient-gut-microbiota interactions play a role in human obesity, insulin resistance and type 2 diabetes? *Obesity Reviews: An Official Journal of the International Association for the Study of Obesity*, *12*(4), 272–281. https://doi.org/10.1111/j.1467-789X.2010.00797.x

Djaja, N., Permadi, I., Witjaksono, F., Soewondo, P., Abdullah, M., Agustina, R., & Ali, S. (2019). The effect of job's tears-enriched yoghurt on GLP-1, calprotectin, blood glucose levels and weight of patients with type 2 diabetes mellitus. *Mediterranean Journal of Nutrition and Metabolism*, *12*(2), 163–171. https://doi.org/10.3233/MNM-180258

Ebrahimi, Z. sadat, Nasli-Esfahani, E., Nadjarzade, A., & Mozaffari-khosravi, H. (2017). Effect of symbiotic supplementation on glycemic control, lipid profiles and microalbuminuria in patients with non-obese type 2 diabetes: A randomized, double-blind, clinical trial. *Journal of Diabetes & Metabolic Disorders*, *16*(1), 23. https://doi.org/10.1186/s40200-017-0304-8

Esposito, G., Pesce, M., Seguella, L., Lu, J., Corpetti, C., Del Re, A., De Palma, F. D. E., Esposito, G., Sanseverino, W., & Sarnelli, G. (2021). Engineered *Lactobacillus paracasei* producing palmitoylethanolamide (PEA) prevents colitis in mice. *International Journal of Molecular Sciences*, *22*(6), Article 6. https://doi.org/10.3390/ijms22062945

Esposito, K., Chiodini, P., Colao, A., Lenzi, A., & Giugliano, D. (2012). Metabolic syndrome and risk of cancer: A systematic review and meta-analysis. *Diabetes Care*, *35*(11), 2402–2411. https://doi.org/10.2337/dc12-0336

Falkner, B., & Cossrow, N. D. F. H. (2014). Prevalence of metabolic syndrome and obesity-associated hypertension in the racial ethnic minorities of the United States. *Current Hypertension Reports*, *16*(7), 449. https://doi.org/10.1007/s11906-014-0449-5

Fathi Dizaji, B. (2018). The investigations of genetic determinants of the metabolic syndrome. *Diabetes & Metabolic Syndrome*, *12*(5), 783–789. https://doi.org/10.1016/j.dsx.2018.04.009

Fuller, R. (1989). Probiotics in man and animals. *The Journal of Applied Bacteriology*, *66*(5), 365–378.

Gao, H., Wen, J.-J., Hu, J.-L., Nie, Q.-X., Chen, H.-H., Xiong, T., Nie, S.-P., & Xie, M.-Y. (2019). Fermented *Momordica charantia* L. juice modulates hyperglycemia, lipid profile, and gut microbiota in type 2 diabetic rats. *Food Research International*, *121*, 367–378. https://doi.org/10.1016/j.foodres.2019.03.055

Garg, S., Singh, T. P., & Malik, R. K. (2020). *In vivo* implications of potential probiotic *Lactobacillus reuteri* LR6 on the gut and immunological parameters as an adjuvant against protein energy malnutrition. *Probiotics and Antimicrobial Proteins*, *12*(2), 517–534. https://doi.org/10.1007/s12602-019-09563-4

Gibson, G. R., Hutkins, R., Sanders, M. E., Prescott, S. L., Reimer, R. A., Salminen, S. J., Scott, K., Stanton, C., Swanson, K. S., Cani, P. D., Verbeke, K., & Reid, G. (2017). Expert consensus document: The International Scientific Association for Probiotics and Prebiotics (ISAPP) consensus statement on the definition and scope of prebiotics. *Nature Reviews. Gastroenterology & Hepatology*, *14*(8), 491–502. https://doi.org/10.1038/nrgastro.2017.75

Gibson, G. R., & Roberfroid, M. B. (1995). Dietary modulation of the human colonic microbiota: Introducing the concept of prebiotics. *The Journal of Nutrition*, *125*(6), 1401–1412. https://doi.org/10.1093/jn/125.6.1401

Gourbeyre, P., Denery, S., & Bodinier, M. (2011). Probiotics, prebiotics, and synbiotics: Impact on the gut immune system and allergic reactions. *Journal of Leukocyte Biology*, *89*(5), 685–695. https://doi.org/10.1189/jlb.1109753

Gu, Z., Zhu, Y., Jiang, S., Xia, G., Li, C., Zhang, X., Zhang, J., & Shen, X. (2020). Tilapia head glycolipids reduce inflammation by regulating the gut microbiota in dextran sulphate sodium-induced colitis mice. *Food & Function*, *11*(4), 3245–3255. https://doi.org/10.1039/D0FO00116C

Guarner, F., & Malagelada, J.-R. (2003). Gut flora in health and disease. *Lancet (London, England)*, *361*(9356), 512–519. https://doi.org/10.1016/S0140-6736(03)12489-0

Guglielmetti, S., Mora, D., Gschwender, M., & Popp, K. (2011). Randomised clinical trial: *Bifidobacterium bifidum* MIMBb75 significantly alleviates irritable bowel syndrome and improves quality of life – a double-blind, placebo-controlled study. *Alimentary Pharmacology & Therapeutics*, *33*(10), 1123–1132. https://doi.org/10.1111/j.1365-2036.2011.04633.x

Hadi, A., Sepandi, M., Marx, W., Moradi, S., & Parastouei, K. (2019). Clinical and psychological responses to synbiotic supplementation in obese or overweight adults: A randomized clinical trial. *Complementary Therapies in Medicine*, *47*, 102216. https://doi.org/10.1016/j.ctim.2019.102216

Haghighat, N., Mohammadshahi, M., Shayanpour, S., & Haghighizadeh, M. H. (2019). Effect of synbiotic and probiotic supplementation on serum levels of endothelial cell adhesion molecules in hemodialysis patients: A randomized control study. *Probiotics and Antimicrobial Proteins*, *11*(4), 1210–1218. https://doi.org/10.1007/s12602-018-9477-9

Hann, M., Zeng, Y., Zong, L., Sakurai, T., Taniguchi, Y., Takagaki, R., Watanabe, H., Mitsuzumi, H., & Mine, Y. (2019). Anti-inflammatory activity of isomaltodextrin in a C57BL/6NCrl mouse model with lipopolysaccharide-induced low-grade chronic inflammation. *Nutrients*, *11*(11), Article 11. https://doi.org/10.3390/nu11112791

Haque, M. U., Ahmmed, S. B., Akanda, M. K. M., Hasan, M. T., Mou, S. A., Sajon, S. R., & Islam, M. A. U. (2016). Prevalence and risk factors of obesity and hypertension among university students in Rajshahi City, Bangladesh. *Bangladesh Pharmaceutical Journal*, *19*(2), Article 2. https://doi.org/10.3329/bpj.v19i2.29277

Hardy, H., Harris, J., Lyon, E., Beal, J., & Foey, A. D. (2013). Probiotics, prebiotics and immunomodulation of gut mucosal defences: Homeostasis and immunopathology. *Nutrients*, *5*(6), 1869–1912. https://doi.org/10.3390/nu5061869

Harish, K., & Varghese, T. (2006). Probiotics in humans - evidence based review. *Calicut Medical Journal*, *4*(4), e3.

Hatakka, K., Holma, R., El-Nezami, H., Suomalainen, T., Kuisma, M., Saxelin, M., Poussa, T., Mykkänen, H., & Korpela, R. (2008). The influence of *Lactobacillus rhamnosus* LC705 together with *Propionibacterium freudenreichii* ssp. shermanii JS on potentially carcinogenic bacterial activity in human colon. *International Journal of Food Microbiology*, *128*(2), 406–410. https://doi.org/10.1016/j.ijfoodmicro.2008.09.010

Hijová, E. (2022). Synbiotic supplements in the prevention of obesity and obesity-related diseases. *Metabolites*, *12*(4), Article 4. https://doi.org/10.3390/metabo12040313

Hord, N. (2008). Eukaryotic-microbiota crosstalk: Potential mechanisms for health benefits of prebiotics and probiotics. *Annual Review of Nutrition*, *28*, 2015–2231. https://doi.org/10.1146/annurev.nutr.28.061807.155402

Horvath, A., Leber, B., Feldbacher, N., Tripolt, N., Rainer, F., Blesl, A., Trieb, M., Marsche, G., Sourij, H., & Stadlbauer, V. (2020). Effects of a multispecies synbiotic on glucose metabolism, lipid marker, gut microbiome composition, gut permeability, and quality of life in diabesity: A randomized, double-blind, placebo-controlled pilot study. *European Journal of Nutrition*, *59*(7), 2969–2983. https://doi.org/10.1007/s00394-019-02135-w

Howarth, G. S. (2008). Inflammatory bowel disease, a dysregulated host-microbiota interaction: Are probiotics a new therapeutic option? *Journal of Gastroenterology and Hepatology*, *23*(12), 1777–1779. https://doi.org/10.1111/j.1440-1746.2008.05685.x

Hsieh, M.-C., Tsai, W.-H., Jheng, Y.-P., Su, S.-L., Wang, S.-Y., Lin, C.-C., Chen, Y.-H., & Chang, W.-W. (2018). The beneficial effects of *Lactobacillus reuteri* ADR-1 or ADR-3 consumption on type 2 diabetes mellitus: A randomized, double-blinded, placebo-controlled trial. *Scientific Reports*, *8*(1), Article 1. https://doi.org/10.1038/s41598-018-35014-1

Hsu, C.-N., Hou, C.-Y., Chan, J. Y. H., Lee, C.-T., & Tain, Y.-L. (2019). Hypertension programmed by perinatal high-fat diet: Effect of maternal gut microbiota-targeted therapy. *Nutrients*, *11*(12), Article 12. https://doi.org/10.3390/nu11122908

Hu, F., Niu, Y., Xu, X., Hu, Q., Su, Q., & Zhang, H. (2020). Resistant dextrin improves high-fat-high-fructose diet induced insulin resistance. *Nutrition & Metabolism*, *17*(1), 36. https://doi.org/10.1186/s12986-020-00450-2

Hume, M. P., Nicolucci, A. C., & Reimer, R. A. (2017). Prebiotic supplementation improves appetite control in children with overweight and obesity: A randomized controlled trial1, 2, 3. *The American Journal of Clinical Nutrition*, *105*(4), 790–799. https://doi.org/10.3945/ajcn.116.140947

Huys, G., Botteldoorn, N., Delvigne, F., De Vuyst, L., Heyndrickx, M., Pot, B., Dubois, J.-J., & Daube, G. (2013). Microbial characterization of probiotics-advisory report of the working group "8651 probiotics" of the Belgian Superior Health Council (SHC). *Molecular Nutrition & Food Research*, *57*(8), 1479–1504. https://doi.org/10.1002/mnfr.201300065

Igarashi, M., Morimoto, M., Suto, A., Nakatani, A., Hayakawa, T., Hara, K., & Kimura, I. (2020). Synthetic dietary inulin, Fuji FF, delays development of diet-induced obesity by improving gut microbiota profiles and increasing short-chain fatty acid production. *PeerJ*, *8*, e8893. https://doi.org/10.7717/peerj.8893

Javadi, L., Ghavami, M., Khoshbaten, M., Safaiyan, A., Barzegari, A., & Pourghassem Gargari, B. (2017). The effect of probiotic and/or prebiotic on liver function tests in patients with nonalcoholic fatty liver disease: A double blind randomized clinical trial. *Iranian Red Crescent Medical Journal*, *19*(4). https://doi.org/10.5812/ircmj.46017

Joint FAO/WHO Expert Consultation on Risk Assessment of Microbiological Hazards in Foods : hazard identification, exposure assessment and hazard characterization of Campylobacter spp. in broiler chickens and Vibrio spp. in seafood, WHO headquarters, Geneva, Switzerland, 23–27 July 2001. World Health Organization. https://iris.who.int/handle/10665/67090

Kamdar, K., Khakpour, S., Chen, J., Leone, V., Brulc, J., Mangatu, T., Antonopoulos, D. A., Chang, E. B., Kahn, S. A., Kirschner, B. S., Young, G., & DePaolo, R. W. (2016). Genetic and metabolic signals during acute enteric bacterial infection alter the microbiota and drive progression to chronic inflammatory disease. *Cell Host & Microbe*, *19*(1), 21–31. https://doi.org/10.1016/j.chom.2015.12.006

Kassaian, N., Feizi, A., Rostami, S., Aminorroaya, A., Yaran, M., & Amini, M. (2020). The effects of 6 mo of supplementation with probiotics and synbiotics on gut microbiota in the adults with prediabetes: A double blind randomized clinical trial. *Nutrition*, *79–80*, 110854. https://doi.org/10.1016/j.nut.2020.110854

Kelesidis, T., & Pothoulakis, C. (2012). Efficacy and safety of the probiotic *Saccharomyces boulardii* for the prevention and therapy of gastrointestinal disorders. *Therapeutic Advances in Gastroenterology*, *5*(2), 111–125. https://doi.org/10.1177/1756283X11428502

Kim, D.-E., Kim, J.-K., Han, S.-K., Jang, S.-E., Han, M. J., & Kim, D.-H. (2019). *Lactobacillus plantarum* NK3 and *Bifidobacterium longum* NK49 alleviate bacterial vaginosis and osteoporosis in mice by suppressing NF-κB-linked TNF-α expression. *Journal of Medicinal Food*, *22*(10), 1022–1031. https://doi.org/10.1089/jmf.2019.4419

Klancic, T., Laforest-Lapointe, I., Choo, A., Nettleton, J. E., Chleilat, F., Noye Tuplin, E. W., Alukic, E., Cho, N. A., Nicolucci, A. C., Arrieta, M.-C., & Reimer, R. A. (2020). Prebiotic oligofructose prevents antibiotic-induced obesity risk and improves metabolic and gut microbiota profiles in rat dams and offspring. *Molecular Nutrition & Food Research*, *64*(16), 2000288. https://doi.org/10.1002/mnfr.202000288

Kobyliak, N., Falalyeyeva, T., Bodnar, P., & Beregova, T. (2017). Probiotics supplemented with omega-3 fatty acids are more effective for hepatic steatosis reduction in an animal model of obesity. *Probiotics and Antimicrobial Proteins*, *9*(2), 123–130. https://doi.org/10.1007/s12602-016-9230-1

Kobyliak, N., Falalyeyeva, T., Boyko, N., Tsyryuk, O., Beregova, T., & Ostapchenko, L. (2018). Probiotics and nutraceuticals as a new frontier in obesity prevention and management. *Diabetes Research and Clinical Practice*, *141*, 190–199. https://doi.org/10.1016/j.diabres.2018.05.005

Kruis, W., Chrubasik, S., Boehm, S., Stange, C., & Schulze, J. (2012). A double-blind placebo-controlled trial to study therapeutic effects of probiotic *Escherichia coli* Nissle 1917 in subgroups of patients with irritable bowel syndrome. *International Journal of Colorectal Disease*, *27*(4), 467–474. https://doi.org/10.1007/s00384-011-1363-9

Kumar, S. A., Ward, L. C., & Brown, L. (2016). Inulin oligofructose attenuates metabolic syndrome in high-carbohydrate, high-fat diet-fed rats. *British Journal of Nutrition*, *116*(9), 1502–1511. https://doi.org/10.1017/S0007114516003627

Kundi, Z. M., Lee, J. C.-Y., Pihlajamäki, J., Chan, C. B., Leung, K. S., So, S. S. Y., Nordlund, E., Kolehmainen, M., & El-Nezami, H. (2021). Dietary fiber from oat and rye brans ameliorate western diet-induced body weight gain and hepatic inflammation by the modulation of short-chain fatty acids, bile acids, and tryptophan metabolism. *Molecular Nutrition & Food Research*, *65*(1), 1900580. https://doi.org/10.1002/mnfr.201900580

Langen, M. A. C., & Dieleman, L. A. (2009). Prebiotics in chronic intestinal inflammation. *Inflammatory Bowel Diseases*, *15*(3), 454–462. https://doi.org/10.1002/ibd.20737

Larsen, N., Vogensen, F. K., Berg, F. W. J. van den, Nielsen, D. S., Andreasen, A. S., Pedersen, B. K., Al-Soud, W. A., Sørensen, S. J., Hansen, L. H., & Jakobsen, M. (2010). Gut microbiota in human adults with type 2 diabetes differs from non-diabetic adults. *PLOS ONE*, *5*(2), e9085. https://doi.org/10.1371/journal.pone.0009085

Lebeer, S., Bron, P. A., Marco, M. L., Van Pijkeren, J.-P., O'Connell Motherway, M., Hill, C., Pot, B., Roos, S., & Klaenhammer, T. (2018). Identification of probiotic effector molecules: Present state and future perspectives. *Current Opinion in Biotechnology*, *49*, 217–223. https://doi.org/10.1016/j.copbio.2017.10.007

Lee, E.-S., Lee, B.-H., Shin, D. U., Lim, M.-Y., Chung, W.-H., Park, C.-S., Baik, M.-Y., Nam, Y.-D., & Seo, D.-H. (2018). Amelioration of obesity in high-fat diet-fed mice by chestnut starch modified by amylosucrase from *Deinococcus geothermalis*. *Food Hydrocolloids*, *75*, 22–32. https://doi.org/10.1016/j.foodhyd.2017.09.019

Lee, J. H., Nam, S. H., Seo, W. T., Yun, H. D., Hong, S. Y., Kim, M. K., & Cho, K. M. (2012). The production of surfactin during the fermentation of *cheonggukjang* by potential probiotic *Bacillus subtilis* CSY191 and the resultant growth suppression of MCF-7 human breast cancer cell. *Food Chemistry*, *131*(4), 1347–1354. https://doi.org/10.1016/j.foodchem.2011.09.133

Li, S., Liu, J., Wang, Z., Duan, F., Jia, Z., Chen, X., & Li, S. (2022). The promising role of probiotics/prebiotics/synbiotics in energy metabolism biomarkers in patients with NAFLD: A systematic review and meta-analysis. *Frontiers in Public Health*, *10*. https://www.frontiersin.org/articles/10.3389/fpubh.2022.862266

Li, S., Wang, L., Liu, B., & He, N. (2020a). Unsaturated alginate oligosaccharides attenuated obesity-related metabolic abnormalities by modulating gut microbiota in high-fat-diet mice. *Food & Function*, *11*(5), 4773–4784. https://doi.org/10.1039/C9FO02857A

Li, Y., Liu, M., Liu, H., Wei, X., Su, X., Li, M., & Yuan, J. (2020b). Oral supplements of combined Bacillus licheniformis zhengchangsheng® and xylooligosaccharides improve high-fat diet-induced obesity and modulate the gut microbiota in rats. *BioMed Research International*, *2020*, e9067821. https://doi.org/10.1155/2020/9067821

Liu, Z., Li, L., Ma, S., Ye, J., Zhang, H., Li, Y., Sair, A. T., Pan, J., Liu, X., Li, X., Yan, S., & Liu, X. (2020). High-dietary fiber intake alleviates antenatal obesity-induced postpartum depression: Roles of gut microbiota and microbial metabolite short-chain fatty acid involved. *Journal of Agricultural and Food Chemistry*, *68*(47), 13697–13710. https://doi.org/10.1021/acs.jafc.0c04290

Luo, G., Li, B., Yang, C., Wang, Y., Bian, X., Li, W., Liu, F., & Huo, G. (2019). Major traditional probiotics: Comparative genomic analyses and roles in gut microbiome of eight cohorts. *Frontiers in Microbiology*, *10*. https://www.frontiersin.org/articles/10.3389/fmicb.2019.00712

Luo, Q., Zhang, J.-R., Li, H.-B., Wu, D.-T., Geng, F., Corke, H., Wei, X.-L., & Gan, R.-Y. (2020). Green extraction of antioxidant polyphenols from green tea (*Camellia sinensis*). *Antioxidants*, *9*(9), Article 9. https://doi.org/10.3390/antiox9090785

Macfarlane, S., Macfarlane, G. T., & Cummings, J. H. (2006). Review article: Prebiotics in the gastrointestinal tract. *Alimentary Pharmacology & Therapeutics*, *24*(5), 701–714. https://doi.org/10.1111/j.1365-2036.2006.03042.x

Machado, A. M., da Silva, N. B. M., de Freitas, R. M. P., de Freitas, M. B. D., Chaves, J. B. P., Oliveira, L. L., Martino, H. S. D., & de Cássia Gonçalves Alfenas, R. (2021). Effects of yacon flour associated with an energy restricted diet on intestinal permeability, fecal short chain fatty acids, oxidative stress and inflammation markers levels in adults with obesity or overweight: A randomized, double blind, placebo controlled clinical trial. *Archives of Endocrinology and Metabolism*, *64*(5), 597–607. https://doi.org/10.20945/2359-3997000000225

Mahboobi, S., Rahimi, F., & Jafarnejad, S. (2018). Effects of prebiotic and synbiotic supplementation on glycaemia and lipid profile in type 2 diabetes: A meta-analysis of randomized controlled trials. *Advanced Pharmaceutical Bulletin*, *8*(4), Article 4. https://doi.org/10.15171/apb.2018.065

Marceau, P., Biron, S., Hould, F.-S., Marceau, S., Simard, S., Thung, S. N., & Kral, J. G. (1999). Liver pathology and the metabolic syndrome X in severe obesity. *The Journal of Clinical Endocrinology & Metabolism*, *84*(5), 1513–1517. https://doi.org/10.1210/jcem.84.5.5661

Matsuzawa, Y., Funahashi, T., & Nakamura, T. (2011). The concept of metabolic syndrome: Contribution of visceral fat accumulation and its molecular mechanism. *Journal of Atherosclerosis and Thrombosis*, *18*(8), 629–639. https://doi.org/10.5551/jat.7922

McCracken, E., Monaghan, M., & Sreenivasan, S. (2018). Pathophysiology of the metabolic syndrome. *Clinics in Dermatology*, *36*(1), 14–20. https://doi.org/10.1016/j.clindermatol.2017.09.004

Mistry, R. H., Liu, F., Borewicz, K., Lohuis, M. A. M., Smidt, H., Verkade, H. J., & Tietge, U. J. F. (2020). Long-term β-galacto-oligosaccharides supplementation decreases the development of obesity and insulin resistance in mice fed a western-type diet. *Molecular Nutrition & Food Research*, *64*(12), 1900922. https://doi.org/10.1002/mnfr.201900922

Mofid, V., Izadi, A., Mojtahedi, S. Y., & Khedmat, L. (2020). Therapeutic and nutritional effects of synbiotic yogurts in children and adults: A clinical review. *Probiotics and Antimicrobial Proteins*, *12*(3), 851–859. https://doi.org/10.1007/s12602-019-09594-x

Neyrinck, A. M., Rodriguez, J., Taminiau, B., Amadieu, C., Herpin, F., Allaert, F.-A., Cani, P. D., Daube, G., Bindels, L. B., & Delzenne, N. M. (2021). Improvement of gastrointestinal discomfort and inflammatory status by a synbiotic in middle-aged adults: A double-blind randomized placebo-controlled trial. *Scientific Reports*, *11*(1), Article 1. https://doi.org/10.1038/s41598-020-80947-1

Nguyen, T. D. T., Kang, J. H., & Lee, M. S. (2007). Characterization of *Lactobacillus plantarum* PH04, a potential probiotic bacterium with cholesterol-lowering effects. *International Journal of Food Microbiology*, *113*(3), 358–361. https://doi.org/10.1016/j.ijfoodmicro.2006.08.015

Niamah, A. K., Sahi, A. A., & Al-Sharifi, A. S. N. (2017). Effect of feeding soy milk fermented by probiotic bacteria on some blood criteria and weight of experimental animals. *Probiotics and Antimicrobial Proteins*, *9*(3), 284–291. https://doi.org/10.1007/s12602-017-9265-y

Oberreuther-Moschner, D. L., Jahreis, G., Rechkemmer, G., & Pool-Zobel, B. L. (2004). Dietary intervention with the probiotics *Lactobacillus acidophilus* 145 and *Bifidobacterium longum* 913 modulates the potential of human faecal water to induce damage in HT29clone19A cells. *British Journal of Nutrition*, *91*(6), 925–932. https://doi.org/10.1079/BJN20041108

Oh, Y. J., Kim, H. J., Kim, T. S., Yeo, I. H., & Ji, G. E. (2019). Effects of *Lactobacillus plantarum* PMO 08 alone and combined with chia seeds on metabolic syndrome and parameters related to gut health in high-fat diet-induced obese mice. *Journal of Medicinal Food*, *22*(12), 1199–1207. https://doi.org/10.1089/jmf.2018.4349

Panda, A. K., Rao, S. V. R., Raju, M. V. L. N., & Sharma, S. R. (2006). Dietary supplementation of *Lactobacillus sporogenes* on performance and serum biochemico-lipid profile of broiler chickens. *The Journal of Poultry Science*, *43*(3), 235–240. https://doi.org/10.2141/jpsa.43.235

Pandey, Kavita R., Naik, Suresh R., & Vakil, Babu V. (2015). Probiotics, prebiotics and synbiotics- a review. *Journal of Food Science and Technology*, *52*(12), 7577–7587. https://doi.org/10.1007/s13197-015-1921-1

Parnell, J. A., Klancic, T., & Reimer, R. A. (2017). Oligofructose decreases serum lipopolysaccharide and plasminogen activator inhibitor-1 in adults with overweight/obesity. *Obesity*, *25*(3), 510–513. https://doi.org/10.1002/oby.21763

Parnell, J. A., & Reimer, R. A. (2010). Effect of prebiotic fibre supplementation on hepatic gene expression and serum lipids: A dose-response study in JCR:LA-cp rats. *The British Journal of Nutrition*, *103*(11), 1577–1584. https://doi.org/10.1017/S0007114509993539

Parvez, G. M. M., & Akanda, K. M. (2019). Chapter 1- Foods and arthritis: An overview. In R. R. Watson & V. R. Preedy (Eds.), *Bioactive Food as Dietary Interventions for Arthritis and Related Inflammatory Diseases* (Second Edition) (pp. 3–22). Academic Press. https://doi.org/10.1016/B978-0-12-813820-5.00001-5

Parvez, G. M. M., Akanda, K. M., Karim, R., Mou, S. M., Zahan, P., Mosaddik, A. (2016). Comparative phytochemical screening and antimicrobial evaluation of different varieties of banana (Musa sapientum). *International Journal of Innovative Pharmaceutical Sciences and Research*, *4*(4), 372–383.

Pekgor, S., Duran, C., Berberoglu, U., & Eryilmaz, M. A. (2019). The role of visceral adiposity index levels in predicting the presence of metabolic syndrome and insulin resistance in overweight and obese patients. *Metabolic Syndrome and Related Disorders*, *17*(5), 296–302. https://doi.org/10.1089/met.2019.0005

Peralta, C. A., Kurella, M., Lo, J. C., & Chertow, G. M. (2006). The metabolic syndrome and chronic kidney disease. *Current Opinion in Nephrology and Hypertension*, *15*(4), 361. https://doi.org/10.1097/01.mnh.0000232875.27846.7e

Pokusaeva, K., Fitzgerald, G. F., & van Sinderen, D. (2011). Carbohydrate metabolism in bifidobacteria. *Genes & Nutrition*, *6*(3), 285–306. https://doi.org/10.1007/s12263-010-0206-6

Quigley, E. M. M. (2013). Gut bacteria in health and disease. *Gastroenterology & Hepatology*, *9*(9), 560–569.

Regalado-Rentería, E., Aguirre-Rivera, J. R., Godínez-Hernández, C. I., García-López, J. C., Oros-Ovalle, A. C., Martínez-Gutiérrez, F., Martinez-Martinez, M., Ratering, S., Schnell, S., Ruíz-Cabrera, M. Á., & Juárez-Flores, B. I. (2020). Effects of agave fructans, inulin, and starch on metabolic syndrome aspects in healthy wistar rats. *ACS Omega*, *5*(19), 10740–10749. https://doi.org/10.1021/acsomega.0c00272

Reimer, R. A., Willis, H. J., Tunnicliffe, J. M., Park, H., Madsen, K. L., & Soto-Vaca, A. (2017). Inulin-type fructans and whey protein both modulate appetite but only fructans alter gut microbiota in adults with overweight/obesity: A randomized controlled trial. *Molecular Nutrition & Food Research*, *61*(11), 1700484. https://doi.org/10.1002/mnfr.201700484

Robinson, C. J., Bohannan, B. J. M., & Young, V. B. (2010). From structure to function: The ecology of host-associated microbial communities. *Microbiology and Molecular Biology Reviews: MMBR*, *74*(3), 453–476. https://doi.org/10.1128/MMBR.00014-10

Romeo, J., Nova, E., Wärnberg, J., Gómez-Martínez, S., Díaz Ligia, L. E., & Marcos, A. (2010). Immunomodulatory effect of fibres, probiotics and synbiotics in different life-stages. *Nutricion Hospitalaria*, *25*(3), 341–349.

Sato, J., Kanazawa, A., Azuma, K., Ikeda, F., Goto, H., Komiya, K., Kanno, R., Tamura, Y., Asahara, T., Takahashi, T., Nomoto, K., Yamashiro, Y., & Watada, H. (2017). Probiotic reduces bacterial translocation in type 2 diabetes mellitus: A randomised controlled study. *Scientific Reports*, *7*(1), Article 1. https://doi.org/10.1038/s41598-017-12535-9

Saulnier, D. M., Spinler, J. K., Gibson, G. R., & Versalovic, J. (2009). Mechanisms of probiosis and prebiosis: Considerations for enhanced functional foods. *Current Opinion in Biotechnology*, *20*(2), 135–141. https://doi.org/10.1016/j.copbio.2009.01.002

Scavuzzi, B., Henrique, F., Miglioranza, L., Simão, A., & Dichi, I. (2014). Impact of prebiotics, probiotics and synbiotics on components of the metabolic syndrome. *Annals of Nutritional Disorders & Therapy*, *1*, 1009.

Scheithauer, T. P. M., Rampanelli, E., Nieuwdorp, M., Vallance, B. A., Verchere, C. B., van Raalte, D. H., & Herrema, H. (2020). Gut microbiota as a trigger for metabolic inflammation in obesity and type 2 diabetes. *Frontiers in Immunology*, *11*, 571731. https://doi.org/10.3389/fimmu.2020.571731

Sheil, B., Shanahan, F., & O'Mahony, L. (2007). Probiotic effects on inflammatory bowel disease 1, 2. *The Journal of Nutrition*, *137*(3), 819S–824S. https://doi.org/10.1093/jn/137.3.819S

Simão, T. N. C., Lozovoy, M. A. B., Simão, A. N. C., Oliveira, S. R., Venturini, D., Morimoto, H. K., Miglioranza, L. H. S., & Dichi, I. (2013). Reduced-energy cranberry juice increases folic acid and adiponectin and reduces homocysteine and oxidative stress in patients with the metabolic syndrome. *The British Journal of Nutrition*, *110*(10), 1885–1894. https://doi.org/10.1017/S0007114513001207

Siva, N., Johnson, C. R., Richard, V., Jesch, E. D., Whiteside, W., Abood, A. A., Thavarajah, P., Duckett, S., & Thavarajah, D. (2018). Lentil (*Lens culinaris* Medikus) diet affects the gut microbiome and obesity markers in rat. *Journal of Agricultural and Food Chemistry*, *66*(33), 8805–8813. https://doi.org/10.1021/acs.jafc.8b03254

Song, E.-J., Han, K., Lim, T.-J., Lim, S., Chung, M.-J., Nam, M. H., Kim, H., & Nam, Y.-D. (2020). Effect of probiotics on obesity-related markers per enterotype: A double-blind, placebo-controlled, randomized clinical trial. *EPMA Journal*, *11*(1), 31–51. https://doi.org/10.1007/s13167-020-00198-y

Szymański, H., Pejcz, J., Jawień, M., Chmielarczyk, A., Strus, M., & Heczko, P. B. (2006). Treatment of acute infectious diarrhoea in infants and children with a mixture of three *Lactobacillus rhamnosus* strains - a randomized, double-blind, placebo-controlled trial. *Alimentary Pharmacology & Therapeutics*, *23*(2), 247–253. https://doi.org/10.1111/j.1365-2036.2006.02740.x

Tamtaji, O. R., Heidari-soureshjani, R., Mirhosseini, N., Kouchaki, E., Bahmani, F., Aghadavod, E., Tajabadi-Ebrahimi, M., & Asemi, Z. (2019). Probiotic and selenium co-supplementation, and the effects on clinical, metabolic and genetic status in Alzheimer's disease: A randomized, double-blind, controlled trial. *Clinical Nutrition*, *38*(6), 2569–2575. https://doi.org/10.1016/j.clnu.2018.11.034

Thiennimitr, P., Yasom, S., Tunapong, W., Chunchai, T., Wanchai, K., Pongchaidecha, A., Lungkaphin, A., Sirilun, S., Chaiyasut, C., Chattipakorn, N., & Chattipakorn, S. C. (2018). *Lactobacillus paracasei* HII01, xylooligosaccharides, and synbiotics reduce gut disturbance in obese rats. *Nutrition*, *54*, 40–47. https://doi.org/10.1016/j.nut.2018.03.005

Tonucci, L. B., Santos, K. M. O. dos, Oliveira, L. L. de, Ribeiro, S. M. R., & Martino, H. S. D. (2017). Clinical application of probiotics in type 2 diabetes mellitus: A randomized, double-blind, placebo-controlled study. *Clinical Nutrition*, *36*(1), 85–92. https://doi.org/10.1016/j.clnu.2015.11.011

Uzzaman, S., Akanda, K. M., Mehjabin, S., Parvez, M. A. (2018) Short review on a nutritional fruit: Guava. *Open Access: Toxicology & Research*, *1*(1), 1–8.

Vaghef-Mehrabany, E., Ranjbar, F., Asghari-Jafarabadi, M., Hosseinpour-Arjmand, S., & Ebrahimi-Mameghani, M. (2021). Calorie restriction in combination with prebiotic supplementation in obese women with depression: Effects on metabolic and clinical response. *Nutritional Neuroscience*, *24*(5), 339–353. https://doi.org/10.1080/1028415X.2019.1630985

Vera, I., Toral, M., de la Visitación, N., Sánchez, M., Gómez-Guzmán, M., Romero, M., Yang, T., Izquierdo-Garcia, J. L., Jiménez, R., Ruiz-Cabello, J., Guerra-Hernández, E., Raizada, M. K., Pérez-Vizcaíno, F., & Duarte, J. (2020). Probiotics prevent dysbiosis and the rise in blood pressure in genetic hypertension: Role of short-chain fatty acids. *Molecular Nutrition & Food Research*, *64*(6), 1900616. https://doi.org/10.1002/mnfr.201900616

Vo, T. D., Lynch, B. S., & Roberts, A. (2019). Dietary exposures to common emulsifiers and their impact on the gut microbiota: Is there a cause for concern? *Comprehensive Reviews in Food Science and Food Safety*, *18*(1), 31–47. https://doi.org/10.1111/1541-4337.12410

Wall, C. R., Hill, R. J., Lovell, A. L., Matsuyama, M., Milne, T., Grant, C. C., Jiang, Y., Chen, R. X., Wouldes, T. A., & Davies, P. S. W. (2019). A multicenter, double-blind, randomized, placebo-controlled trial to evaluate the effect of consuming growing up milk "Lite" on body composition in children aged 12-23 mo. *The American Journal of Clinical Nutrition*, *109*(3), 576–585. https://doi.org/10.1093/ajcn/nqy302

Wang, W., Xu, A.-L., Li, Z.-C., Li, Y., Xu, S.-F., Sang, H.-C., & Zhi, F. (2019). Combination of probiotics and *Salvia miltiorrhiza* polysaccharide alleviates hepatic steatosis via gut microbiota modulation and insulin resistance improvement in high fat-induced NAFLD mice. *Diabetes & Metabolism Journal*, *44*(2), 336–348. https://doi.org/10.4093/dmj.2019.0042

Wickens, K. L., Barthow, C. A., Murphy, R., Abels, P. R., Maude, R. M., Stone, P. R., Mitchell, E. A., Stanley, T. V., Purdie, G. L., Kang, J. M., Hood, F. E., Rowden, J. L., Barnes, P. K., Fitzharris, P. F., & Crane, J. (2017). Early pregnancy probiotic supplementation with *Lactobacillus rhamnosus* HN001 may reduce the prevalence of gestational diabetes mellitus: A randomised controlled trial. *British Journal of Nutrition*, *117*(6), 804–813. https://doi.org/10.1017/S0007114517000289

Wu, T., Shen, M., Guo, X., Huang, L., Yang, J., Yu, Q., Chen, Y., & Xie, J. (2020). *Cyclocarya paliurus* polysaccharide alleviates liver inflammation in mice via beneficial regulation of gut microbiota and TLR4/MAPK signaling pathways. *International Journal of Biological Macromolecules*, *160*, 164–174. https://doi.org/10.1016/j.ijbiomac.2020.05.187

Yadav, R., Khan, S. H., Mada, S. B., Meena, S., Kapila, R., & Kapila, S. (2019). Consumption of probiotic *Lactobacillus fermentum* MTCC: 5898-fermented milk attenuates dyslipidemia, oxidative stress, and inflammation in male rats fed on cholesterol-enriched diet. *Probiotics and Antimicrobial Proteins*, *11*(2), 509–518. https://doi.org/10.1007/s12602-018-9429-4

Zeng, H., Chen, P., Chen, C., Huang, C., Lin, S., Zheng, B., & Zhang, Y. (2018). Structural properties and prebiotic activities of fractionated lotus seed resistant starches. *Food Chemistry*, *251*, 33–40. https://doi.org/10.1016/j.foodchem.2018.01.057

Zhang, J., Sun, J., Chen, X., Nie, C., Zhao, J., Guan, W., Lei, L., He, T., Chen, Y., Johnston, L. J., Zhao, J., & Ma, X. (2018). Combination of *Clostridium butyricum* and corn bran optimized intestinal microbial fermentation using a weaned pig model. *Frontiers in Microbiology*, *9*. https://www.frontiersin.org/articles/10.3389/fmicb.2018.03091

Zheng, H. J., Guo, J., Wang, Q., Wang, L., Wang, Y., Zhang, F., Huang, W.-J., Zhang, W., Liu, W. J., & Wang, Y. (2021). Probiotics, prebiotics, and synbiotics for the improvement of metabolic profiles in patients with chronic kidney disease: A systematic review and meta-analysis of randomized controlled trials. *Critical Reviews in Food Science and Nutrition*, *61*(4), 577–598. https://doi.org/10.1080/10408398.2020.1740645

4 Synbiotics and Gut Microflora
Mechanisms and Therapeutic Rationality and Clinical Applications for Management of Type 2 Diabetes

Nisha Sharma, Prakash Chandra Gupta, Swarnakshi Upadhyay, and Kamla Pathak

4.1 INTRODUCTION

Based on data provided by the International Diabetes Federation (IDF), it is anticipated a rise to 783 million diabetic individuals by the year 2045 (Sun et al., 2021). Diabetes has been linked to various notable health effects arteriosclerosis, hypertension, dyslipidemia, and kidney issues along with key risks like blindness, cardiac problems, lower limb amputation, etc. Historically, type 2 diabetes mellitus (T2DM) was primarily observed in older individuals. However, emerging evidence indicates a rising incidence of T2DM in young individuals and research suggests that around 16% of the global adult population with T2DM develop it during adolescence (Temneanu et al., 2016).

The prevalence of T2DM has experienced a significant surge in recent decades, resulting in its widespread manifestation as a metabolic illness. Insulin and a range of oral hypoglycemic medications are presently employed as pharmacological interventions for the management of T2DM. Nonetheless, it is worthwhile to note that T2DM poses challenges in terms of achieving a complete cure (Galicia-Garcia et al., 2020). The efficacy of previous therapeutic approaches for T2DM has been constrained by the presence of insulin resistance and insulin insufficiency.

In recent years, the bond between the body's microbiota and obesity-related T2DM has opened up a novel avenue for mitigating the risk of T2DM. The gut microbiome owns genetic makeup about 150 times more than that identified in other parts of the body (Hou et al., 2022). Lipid and glucose metabolism are straightly altered by intestinal activities, namely, digestion, absorption, metabolism, and neuromodulation, which are tremendously improved by the act of microbes of gut (Jandhyala et al., 2015). The gut microbiota is a complicated ecological mesh of a varying cluster of microorganisms, enveloping an enormous populace of bacteria that embodies at least 1,000 evident species (Rajilić-Stojanović et al., 2014; Mirjana & Willem, 2014). The gut microbiota on the whole consists of bacteria, apart from other commensal organisms, together with archea, viruses, fungi, and protists (Hou et al., 2022).

The clinical potency of T2DM is linked to peculiar alteration in the gut microbiota amid impacted individuals. The dominance of synbiotics, on the potency of T2DM, can be seen by the managing the balance of intestinal microbiota in persons with T2DM (Jiang et al., 2022). This chapter's goal is to provide a concise summation of synbiotics and gut microbiota, its mechanisms, therapeutic rationale, and clinical strategies in controlling T2DM.

4.2 TYPE 2 DIABETES MELLITUS T2DM

T2DM, a chronic metabolic disease, is evident by deviations in the metabolism of fats and carbohydrates, resulting in cardiovascular disease, retinopathy, nephropathy, neuropathy, leg ulcers, and gangrene. The susceptible nature linked with T2DM covers obesity, advanced age, genetic predisposition, tobacco use, a sedentary lifestyle, and hypertension. As per the recent research progressive T2DM may result due to modifications to the gut microbiota's makeup, caused by obesity (Kim et al., 2014).

Minor fatigue and thirst are the starting in the persons with T2DM and finally a glucose tolerance test is the only method to verify inflated blood sugar (Drivsholm et al., 2005). Insulin and oral hypoglycemics were used for the treatment of diabetes during the 1920s, with over 40 anti-diabetic medications (Guo, 2015). Additionally, drugs like glinide insulin secretagogues, insulin sensitizers, and α-glucosidase inhibitors were used to treat T2DM, which had invariable drawbacks (Raptis & Dimitriadis, 2001), like glinides are difficult for patients to be taken again and again, glucosease inhibitors causes distension in the abdomen, and insulin sensitizers may upraise the threat of myocardial infarction (Juan, 2014).

According to the studies, the amelioration of T2DM is correlated to gut microbiota. In T2DM patients, the prebiotics and synbiotic supplements may enhance antioxidant enzyme activity, promote glucose homeostasis, and lipid metabolism (Mahboobi et al., 2018; Mirmiranpour et al., 2020). Synbiotics

DOI: 10.1201/9781032702438-4

have been increasingly used by researchers to ameliorate the gut microbe environment of T2DM patients so as to increase the potency of T2DM treatment making it a promising area that demands in-depth research. It offers a peerless merit in controlling blood sugar in T2DM persons as compared to standard chemical medications.

4.3 SYNBIOTICS

"Synbiotics", initially coined in 1995, is a synergistic blend of probiotics and prebiotics. They have a positive impact on the gastrointestinal tract by fostering and buildup of live microorganism as health supplements and improve the growth or rejuvenate the metabolism of particular groups of favorable bacteria (Gibson & Roberfroid, 1995). This concept is fundamentally consistent with the characterization of probiotics and prebiotics, which possess complementary and synergistic roles (Kolida & Gibson, 2011). There exist two distinct categories of synbiotics, specifically complementary and synergistic synbiotics.

Complementary synbiotics refer to the fusion of a probiotic and a prebiotic, which might involve several instances of each component. These components function autonomously to attain one or more advantageous effects on health. The necessity to demonstrate selective use in the study is not necessary, as it has already been established by earlier research on prebiotics. A synergistic synbiotic is comprised of a viable microbe and a particularly utilized substrate, with the intention of these constituents functioning in tandem (Abdullah, 2022).

4.3.1 Synbiotics: Components and Function

Synbiotics refer to fusion of probiotics and prebiotics, benefiting the host by boosting the gastrointestinal tract's beneficial bacteria' viability and functionality. It consists of live microbes and certain substrates that are concisely consumed by microbes residing in the host, resulting in a constructive influence on the health of the host organism. Examples include combinations of Bifidobacteria or lactobacilli with fructo-oligosaccharides, inulin, or galacto-oligosaccharides (Abdullah, 2022).

Probiotics are live microbes that can help a host's health if appropriately eaten. Probiotics have become popular worldwide for health and wellness. Many probiotic strains and combinations have mixed clinical results (Suez et al., 2019). By interacting with their metabolites, probiotics can preserve the ideal composition of intestinal flora. Probiotics have been shown to reduce blood lipids and cholesterol in animal research and clinical trials (Ooi & Liong, 2010).

In order to retain the gut microbiota of the host in a healthy condition, prebiotics encourages the proliferation and enzymatic activation of colonic microbials (Terpou et al., 2019).

The microecological balance and homeostasis are improved inside the gut by strengthening the growth and multiplication of useful bacteria in the gut (Sarao & Arora, 2017). Synbiotics are beneficial to the host either by triggering bacterial metabolic pathways contributing the human vigor or enhance the proliferation of probiotic microorganisms, thereby enhancing the viability rate of probiotics within the gastrointestinal tract and promoting a more beneficent climate in the gut (Rao, 2002). The most important role of synbiotics is to foster intestinal hydration and govern the composition of the microbes of intestine (Maftei, 2019).

4.3.2 Synbiotics in the Treatment of T2DM

The effect of synbiotics on the intestinal environment and T2DM have been extensively studied demonstrating the utility of synbiotics in the management of T2DM although the basic etiology behind it still is under the scope of research. Insulin resistance and glucose metabolism in the host may be improved by using synbiotics to alter the gut microbiome (Han & Lin, 2014). The intestinal microbe composition is precisely linked to T2DM, and it has been observed that individuals with T2DM have larger proportions of Proteus and Basilides and relatively lower of firmicutes (Hulston et al., 2015).

Currently, medication-assisted blood glucose management and insulin therapy are the two main therapeutic treatments for T2DM. The therapeutic benefits of controlling the gut microbiota balance on patients, however, are not well supported by research. The intestine's ability to absorb and digest food is precisely linked to the metabolism of fats and carbohydrates, and the metabolic processes of gut bacteria are essential to this process. The therapeutic effectiveness of T2DM patients may be impacted by modifications in the gut microecological balance. Commercial oral liquids (syrups, solutions, drinks, etc.) for diabetics are primarily made of one type of dietary fiber or a dietary fiber derivative such as lactulose and arabinose (Xiao et al., 2019). In individuals with diabetes, pre-prandial medication can effectively manage constipation, regulate weight, and moderate postprandial blood glucose. But this type of dietary fiber is hard to absorb and digest. In order to regulate blood glucose and cholesterol levels, it is crucial to counteract the adverse effects of the dietary fiber. A formulation consisting of 40% *Lactobacillus plantarum* and 60% carbohydrate prebiotics, such as lactulose and arabinose, making the total weight of the synbiotics was reported in a study (Jiang et al., 2022).

Lactulose a naturally prevailing disaccharide, in syrup form, is built up of galactose and fructose (Aït-Aissa & Aïder, 2014). It had prebiotic properties, which showed effective mitigation in fasting and postprandial glucose levels, besides inflammation markers, enhances insulin sensitivity, and benefits the lipid profile in persons with prediabetes (Barengolts, 2016).

L-arabinose a natural component of plant polysaccharides and an inhibitor of α-glucosidase demonstrated selectively to hinder the activity of intestinal sucrase in a noncompetitive manner, leading to the suppression of the enhanced postprandial glucose levels usually occurring after the ingestion of sucrose. L-arabinose given with sucrose to mice and rats led to the suppression of blood glucose and insulin responses.

The levels of postprandial glucose, insulin, and C-peptide in humans decreased by including 4% L-arabinose in sucrose-based beverages and it boosted the response of glucagon-like peptide-1 irrespective of causing any harmful effects on the gastrointestinal system. L-arabinose helps in managing diabetes and weight loss as it prevents metabolic conversion of sucrose (Hu, 2018), suggesting L-arabinose imparts advantageous properties in relation to hyperglycemia, glycemic index, and fat storage. In one of the studies, administration of a low dose of L-arabinose resulted in a prominent augmentation of glucose intolerance and restoration of gut microbiota dysbiosis in T2DM induced by an elevated fat diet and streptozotocin (Shen et al., 2021).

L. plantarum and inulin potentially alleviated the cognitive impairment in diabetic rats (Li et al., 2014), confirming the ability of *L. plantarum* to modulate insulin and glucagon secretion, besides improving insulin sensitivity in rats with diabetes. The bacterium *L. plantarum* has an impact on the metabolic processes of blood glucose by augmenting the release of insulin and glucose tolerance (Hosseinifard et al., 2020). A probiotic combination including *L. plantarum*, lactulose, and arabinose can effectively control blood glucose, cholesterol levels, and body weight in patients of T2DM. The body's immune system, growth of harmful germs, and equilibrium of gut flora can be controlled by lactulose. Therefore, synbiotics help in detoxification, hypoglycemia, and lipid reduction, maintain stable blood sugar and lipid levels, and prevent obesity in patients with T2DM (de Vries et al., 2006) (Figure 4.1).

4.3.3 Animal Model

Researchers looked into the effectiveness of the aforementioned synbiotic combination in treating T2DM in a model of diseased mice in order to confirm its effectiveness. In T2DM animal model, with a high-fat diet for one month, tested for the effective synbiotic combination on T2DM using various dosages. A study revealed that the synbiotic blend of lactulose, arabinose, and *L. plantarum* exhibited a substantial enhancement in the fat and sugar metabolism of mice with T2DM and notably diminished the levels of fat and glucose in the bloodstream, leading to substantial reduction in body weight among while contrasting the mice in the control group with those in the experimental treatment group. By enhancing probiotics and suppressing pathogenic bacteria, this synbiotic combination can ameliorate the health of the intestinal microenvironment (Jiang et al., 2022).

The impact of administering yogurt to rats induced with T2DM induced by streptozotocin and a high-fat diet, exhibited enhanced regulation of blood glucose levels, with a notable decline in insulin resistance and glycosylated hemoglobin levels, in comparison to the rats that were given yogurt sweetened with sucrose. Additionally, the rats fed with synbiotic yogurt demonstrated a remarkable improvement in the levels of short-chain fatty acids (SCFAs) and the overall status of their gut microbiota (Ban et al., 2020). *L. rhamnosus* given orally in an animal model of T2DM showed significant efficacy in ameliorating glucose intolerance, hyperglycemia, and pancreatic damage in a mice model of diabetes (Chen et al., 2014).

4.3.4 Clinical Studies

During the last 10 years, more clinical research has been conducted on the use of synbiotics to treat T2DM. It has been demonstrated that certain synbiotics improve insulin receptor substrates, lower levels of cell adhesion molecule-1, and lower levels of fat and insulin resistance. Furthermore, several probiotics enhanced insulin sensitivity, fasting glucose, antioxidant status, and metabolic stress reduction in T2DM participants (Sáez-Lara et al., 2016).

Twenty T2DM patients were given *B. bifidum*, *L. acidophilus*, and oligofructose for 2 weeks, during which in the patients on fasting, glycemia was lowered and their HDL-C level (Moroti et al., 2012). A three-month experiment on the combined effects of powdered cinnamon and *L. acidophilus* in 136 patients with T2DM revealed a slight improvement in antioxidant enzyme activity (Soleimani et al., 2019). *L. acidophilus*, *L. casei*, *Bifidobacterium bifidum*, and inulin showed decreased blood glucose, insulin levels, and insulin

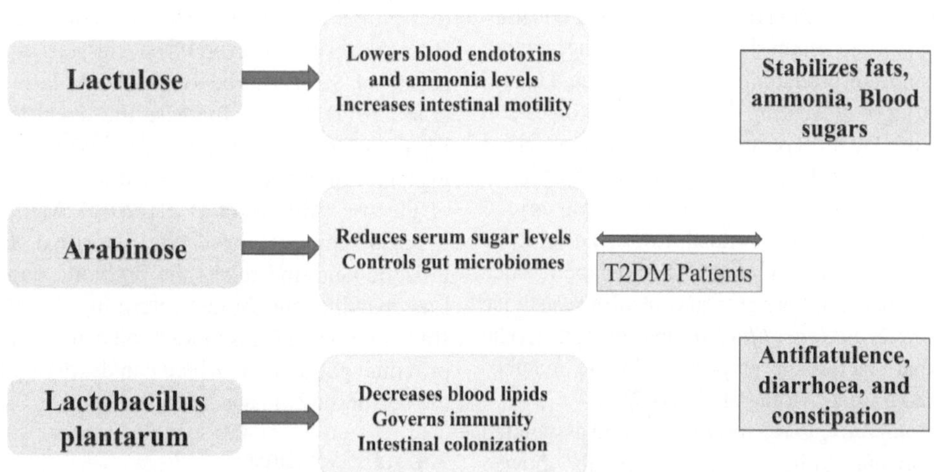

FIGURE 4.1 Influence of lactulose, arabinose, and Lactobacillus plantarum in the treatment of T2DM.

resistance (Velayati et al., 2021). As evidenced by the aforementioned clinical trials, various synbiotic combinations have the potential to positively impact T2DM treatment and efficiently manage a patient's condition. Synbiotics therapy offers a new opportunity for the benefit of T2DM patients as compared to typical medication therapy because it is suited for the majority of patients and has noticeable results.

4.4 GUT MICROFLORA

More than 1,000 different types of bacteria make up the gut microbiota. These bacteria are mostly distributed throughout nine phyla, with the majority of them being attribute of the Actinobacteria, Firmicutes, Bacteroidetes, and Proteobacteria (Schloissnig et al., 2013). The digestion and absorption of food, improved host immunity, biological antagonist, heightened anticancer responses, and the synthesis of advantageous chemicals are among the primary physiological roles of gut microbiota (Jandhyala et al., 2015). A disbalance in the gut microbiota can induce cancer, autoimmune diseases, metabolic diseases, and cardiovascular disorders (Valdes et al., 2018). The gut microbiome is significant in T2DM, as insulin sensitivity and glucose levels are regulated by the gut flora. Modifying gut microbiota can help individuals with diabetes feel better since it reverses the effects of prediabetes' decreased glucose tolerance and elevated fasting glucose.

4.4.1 Gut Microflora of T2DM

There were 42 human research investigations that looked at T2D and the bacterial microbiota. Most of them found links between certain groups and the disease or its symptoms. The first research on T2DM gut microbiota was published in 2010 (Larsen et al., 2010). In T2DM individuals, the amount of class Betaproteobacteria was significantly elevated and firmly correlated with plasma glucose (Qin et al., 2012). According to a study, individuals with diabetes had greater amounts of four intestinal Lactobacillus species and diminished levels of five Clostridium species (Karlsson et al., 2013). Diabetes and a decrease in butyrate are positively associated (Sanna et al., 2019). Thus, boosting gut bacteria's capacity to synthesize butyrate or augmenting the quantity of butyrate-producing bacteria may be a useful strategy for treating or preventing diabetes. Bacteroides and Bifidobacterium are the most prevalent advantageous genera in T2D investigations. Most studies support Bifidobacterium as a genus with defensive microorganisms. Most animal research on Bifidobacterium revealed improved glucose tolerance against T2D (Kikuchi et al., 2018). Diabetic mice showed reduced glucose intolerance and insulin resistance after receiving *Bacteroides acidifaciens* and uniformis. The findings show that Bacteroides improves glucose metabolism in people and animals (Yang et al., 2017).

Akkermansia muciniphila is a newly identified associated microbiota component. Animal models originally showed its glucose metabolism benefits (Plovier et al., 2017). The bacterium *L. plantarum*, commonly present in fermented food products, has been intensely studied in animal models. Numerous explorations have demonstrated that *L. plantarum* has a positive impact on glucose metabolism in transgenic and diet-induced T2DM models (Martinic et al., 2018).

4.4.2 Relationship between Gut Microflora and Prediabetes

Research on gut microbiota in sizable cohorts has shown the complex link between T2DM and gut flora. Research conducted on sterile mice has revealed that disease development is significantly impacted by the gut microbiota (Backhed et al., 2004). In comparison to typical mice, the sterile mice exhibit reduced insulin resistance and a decreased body fat percentage (Turnbaugh et al., 2006). The genuine proof that gut microbiota and T2DM are causally related was eventually found in a human trial including 952 volunteers in the Netherlands. Clinical parameters, quantities of fecal SCFA, whole genomes, and intestinal metagenomes have been evaluated in clinical trials. Mendelian Randomization analyses conducted in both directions were used to assess the causal relationship between blood glucose parameters and microbiological features *Roseburia intestinalis* and *Eubacterium abundances* rose, and the increased risk of T2DM was linked to aberrant propionate absorption or synthesis. Thus, butyrate may increase the production of propionate in stools and postprandial insulin release, elevating the risk of T2DM (Sanna et al., 2019).

4.4.3 Gut Microflora and Anti-diabetic Drugs

4.4.3.1 Metformin

Since the middle of the 20th century, metformin—which can reduce hepatic gluconeogenesis and increase insulin sensitivity—has been the drug of choice for treating T2DM. Metformin targets the gut microbiota to influence glucose metabolism in different ways like restoring the balance of intestinal microbiota in T2DM patients in order to move them toward a more healthy condition and maintaining the ecology of gut microbes. It increases bacterial count that produces SCFAs, such as Shewanella, Lactobacillus, Bifidobacterium, Prevotella species, etc., and improving the ability of SCFAs to be synthesized (de la Cuesta-Zuluaga et al., 2017). SCFAs increase the liberation of GLP-1 and PYY, can enhance insulin sensitivity, and have a hypoglycemic impact bile acid route to control the metabolism of glucose (Mccreight et al., 2016). Metformin induces a hypoglycemic response via intestinal Bacteroides fragilisbile acid and raises the probiotic population (such as Lactobacillus and Bifidobacterium). According to a recent study on mice, glucose induction can activate SGLT1 in the proximal gut of mice, which can decrease glucose synthesis (de la Cuesta-Zuluaga et al., 2017).

4.4.3.2 Acarbose

As an inhibitor of α-glucosidase, acarbose lowers the quantity of carbohydrates absorbed and digested in the small intestine, which declines blood glucose levels after meals. Since acarbose operates exclusively in the intestinal framework of the distal gut microbiota may be somewhat impacted. An earlier study revealed that taking acarbose caused a considerable alteration in the gut microbiota of prediabetes, with an enrichment of Lactobacillus, Faecalibacterium, and Dialister (Zhang et al., 2017). Dialister was found to have a negative correlation with HbA1c in people with prediabetes, suggesting that it may play a function in regulating glucose metabolism. In T2DM patients, acarbose can also lead to a rise in the quantity of *Bifidobacterium longum* and *Enterococcus faecalis*. The concentration of LPS and *B. longum* had a contrary correlation, but the concentration of HDL cholesterol and *E. faecalis* had a positive correlation (Su et al., 2015). Data from patients recently diagnosed with T2DM revealed that acarbose drastically decreased the amount of Bacteroides while augmenting the amount of probiotics Lactobacillus and Bifidobacterium (Gu et al., 2017).

4.4.3.3 Traditional Chinese Medicine (TCM)

Insulin resistance is one way that TCM has been shown to help T2DM patients live better life (Wang et al., 2020). TCM has a distinct effect even if many of its ingredients do not enter the bloodstream. Gut bacteria may have a mediating role in its effectiveness (Nie et al., 2019). Individuals diagnosed with T2DM saw an appreciable decline in high blood sugar levels (hyperglycemia) and high lipid levels (hyperlipidemia) by utilizing AMC, a combination of eight traditional Chinese medications. Additionally, the use of AMC resulted in alterations to the gut flora (Tong et al., 2018). They augment the synbiotic bacteria that Blautia spp. need to maintain glucose and lipid balance considerably. The efficacy of berberine in reducing individuals' HbA1c levels has been established and has been found to exhibit inhibitory effects on the biotransformation of dicarboxylic acid in T2DM, mostly through its interaction with *Ruminococcus bromii* (Zhang et al., 2020).

4.4.3.4 Traditional Indian Medicine

The efficacy of traditional Indian medicine in improving the quality of life for individuals with T2DM has been substantiated by its ability to mitigate insulin resistance. An *in vivo* investigation utilizing rats proved the effectiveness of the methanol extract of *Barringtonia racemosa* in preventing the increase in blood glucose levels following maltose delivery (Gowri et al., 2007). *Syzygium cumini* (L.) has been shown in studies utilizing diabetic rats to reduce cholesterol, free fatty acids, blood sugar, and postprandial glucose (Prince et al., 1998). *S. cumini* extracts have demonstrated α-glucosidase inhibitory effects in pharmacological studies. The anti-diabetic potency of *Tinospora cordifolia* was reported in mice with diabetes mellitus (DM). The administration of the plant's aqueous and alcoholic extract has been found to augment the glucose tolerance of rats with DM (Grover et al., 2000). It has been discovered that the water-soluble extract of *O. basilicum* inhibits the activities of maltase, pig pancreatic α-amylase, and rat intestinal sucrase suggesting that the extract may hold potent therapeutic benefits in managing DM (Agrawal et al., 2012). The findings of research suggested that *O. basilicum* possibly be prescribed dietary therapy for moderate T2DM (El-Beshbishy & Bahashwan, 2012).

4.4.4 Role of Gut Microflora in Pathophysiology of T2DM

The progression of different ailments is mainly controlled by diverse signaling pathways that are modulated by metabolite composition and gut microbiota components. SCFAs, bile acids, branched-chain amino acids (BCAAs), imidazole propionate, and lipopolysaccharide offer important roles as regulators in T2DM.

SCFAs a metabolite, synthesized in the intestines by the bacteria, control the metabolism and utilization of dietary fiber, including the generation of acetate, propionate acid, and butyrate (Gurung et al., 2020). SCFAs trigger intestinal hormone and exert an impact on sensitivity to insulin and glucose metabolism through different pathways impacting the progression of diabetes. SCFAs are energy-regulated signaling molecules that bind directly to the intestinal L cells' free fatty acid receptors. It delayed gastric emptying, appetite suppression, increased insulin secretion, and decreased glucagon levels (Cummings et al., 1987). SCFAs, particularly butyrate, make roughly 5%–10% of the total energy used in a typical colon (Psichas et al., 2015). Butyrate stimulates the expression of genes linked to intestinal gluconeogenesis. Among these genes is FFAR3, which controls the metabolism of fats and blood sugar (Koh et al., 2016).

Primary bile acids excreted into the gastrointestinal tract are commonly transformed by gut bacteria into secondary bile acids. This process influences insulin sensitivity and glucose metabolism via many signaling pathways (Fiorucci & Distrutti, 2015). FGF19/15 ligands act to increase glucose tolerance and insulin sensitivity. Moreover, secondary bile acid can increase muscle energy expenditure and intestinal L cells' production of GLP-1, turn on the TGR-5 (thiol guanosine receptor) receptor, and treat insulin resistance and aberrant glucose metabolism (Shapiro et al., 2018). When enterochromaffin cells are stimulated to secrete 5-hydroxytryptamine by bile acid, the outcome is a diminished insulin release and rise in glucagon production (Martin et al., 2019).

The high levels of lipopolysaccharide (LPS) in the peripheral distribution, patients with T2DM have low levels of inflammation (Pussinen et al., 2011). Gram-negative bacteria are primarily responsible for producing high levels of serum LPS, thereby raise intestinal permeability and elevate LPS in the peripheral circulation. With the aid of CD14, LPS binds to the receptor TLR4, activating the NF-κB inflammatory signaling cascade and the generation of inflammatory proteins like TNF-γ, IL-1β, IL-6, and TNF-α, as well as causing macrophage aggregation. Following then, insulin resistance and aberrant phosphorylation of the insulin receptor substrate happen (Creely et al., 2007).

Leucine, isoleucine, and valine are the three primary amino acids that make up BCAAs and are necessary for human health. They must be received through nutrition, are unable to be produced by the host, and are mostly created by gut microbial metabolism (Rodes et al., 2013). Insulin resistance and T2DM are encouraged by diets high in BCAAs (Zheng et al., 2016). *Bacteroides vulgatus* and *Prevotella copri* are the primary bacteria that drive the production of BCAAs. Insulin resistance, decreased glucose tolerance, and elevated plasma BCAAs can result from *P. copri* feces microbiota transplantation in a mouse model.

Imidazole propionate directly affects mitogen-activated protein kinase (MAPK) and consequently stimulates the phosphorylation of the p62 protein, triggering the phosphorylation of mTORC1S2448. Insulin resistance, aberrant serine phosphorylation of the insulin receptor substrate, and IRS breakdown result from the additional activation of the downstream S6K1 protein phosphorylation. In individuals with T2DM and prediabetes who had low microbial gene abundance and the Bacteroides 2 enterotype, imidazole propionate was more common. *Ruminococcus gnavus*, *Clostridium baumannii*, and *C. parasymbiotics* are all favorably correlated with it, while anti-inflammatory bacteria are negatively correlated with it (The Meta Cardis Consortium, 2020).

4.5 MECHANISM OF GUT MICROFLORA BY SYNBIOTIC

Numerous genes found in bacteria are essential for preserving the gut flora's ability to operate (Guinane & Cotter, 2013). Research has shown that the presence of several illnesses is attributed with disturbance of the intestinal microbiota (Rao, 2002). Disbalance in the framework of the gut microbiota can impact metabolic processes, resulting into obesity and metabolic illnesses including diabetes, dyslipidemia, and metabolic syndrome (Safari & Gérard, 2019). However, the administration of synbiotics has shown promise in enhancing the intestinal microenvironment and consequently managing T2DM.

4.5.1 Molecular Mechanisms of Microflora on Metabolism in T2DM

The therapeutic management of T2DM by the processes that synbiotics utilize is of great interest. Regulation of the processes of nutrient absorption and energy utilization is greatly done by gut microbiota. The carbohydrates present in dietary sources, indigestible by the host organism, are fermented by the gut microbiota which is obtained by generation of various glycoside hydrolases, facilitating the conversion of these carbohydrates into monosaccharides and SCFAs. Due to the synthesis of SCFAs, persons with obesity and type T2DM experience alteration in their gut microbiota influencing the expression of receptors for SCFAs and impacting the host's cycle of starvation and repletion (Remely et al., 2014). The presence of intestinal flora-derived products, including methane and SCFAs, has been seen to have an inhibitory effect on intestinal peristalsis. This inhibition leads to a prolonged transit time of intestinal contents and an increased absorption of enteral nutrition, including glucose. Furthermore, these products have a direct impact on postprandial blood glucose levels.

The intestinal microbiota has a noteworthy function in the processes of lipogenesis and storage. T2DM is characterized by notable pathophysiological attributes, namely, insulin resistance coupled with a shortfall in insulin production, which can be either absolute or relative in nature. This deficiency arises from impaired pancreatic beta-cell activity. Additionally, noteworthy that there exists a strong affinity between obesity and insulin resistance. The gut microflora have the ability to trigger the pathway of host lipogenesis and deposition through many mechanisms. Low-grade persistent inflammatory responses can be attributed to disruptions in the composition of gut flora.

T2DM exhibits a range of chronic low-grade inflammatory reactions that are depicted by endocannabinoid system dysfunction and metabolic endotoxemia (Bessac et al., 2018). In animals, the gut microbiota may impact lipid metabolism and initiate long-term, low-grade inflammatory reactions. Such processes can eventually lead to the initiation of obesity and insulin resistance. The impact of the gut microbiota on pathogenesis may surpass the contribution of inherent genetic defects in animals (Tumminia et al., 2018).

4.5.2 Microbiota on Metabolism in the T2DM

The microbiota exerts an influence on inflammation, engages in interactions with food elements, impacts intestinal permeability, influences metabolism of fats and glucose, affects insulin susceptibility, and contributes to the general regulation of energy balance in the mammalian host. The influence of microbiota on metabolism in T2DM takes place in the following steps.

4.5.2.1 Modulation of Inflammation

In general, T2DM is correlated with high levels of inflammatory proteins, chemokines, and pro-inflammatory cytokines. Certain gut microorganisms and their metabolites, particularly lipopolysaccharides, have been found to contribute to minimally inflammatory response and metabolic endotoxemia. Conversely, there are also gut microbes that elicit the generation of anti-inflammatory cytokines and chemokines.

Increased glucose metabolism may result from the stimulation of IL-10 by a number of species, including *L. plantarum*, *B. fragilis*, *R. intestinalis*, and *A. muciniphila* (Shen et al., 2018). This is manifested by increased expression of IL-10 in muscle tissue providing protection against insulin resistance associated with aging (Hoffmann et al., 2016).

Beneficial microorganisms employ the strategy of inhibiting pro-inflammatory cytokines and chemokines as a means to mitigate inflammation. Lactobacillus, namely,

L. plantarum, *L. paracasei*, and *L. casei*, have been found to diminish the levels of IL-1b, Monocyte Chemoattractant Protein-1, IL-8, and C-reactive protein (Liu et al., 2018). *L. paracasei* and *B. fragilis* inhibits IL-6 expression (Sun et al., 2017). Generation of IL-22, an anti-inflammatory cytokine is enhanced by *R. intestinalis* (Hoffmann et al., 2016). The role of IL-22 in restoring insulin sensitivity and providing relief from diabetes is well recognized (Wang et al., 2014).

4.5.2.2 Gut Permeability

The intestines become more susceptible in T2DM patients. There is a transfer of microbial products from gut into the bloodstream, which leads to metabolic endotoxemia.

The beneficial effects *B. vulgatus* and *B. dorei* on T2DM to increase the colon's tight junction gene expression were demonstrated on a mice model. This upregulation in expression reduced gut permeability, lessened lipopolysaccharide production, and improved endotoxemia, suggesting a positive impact of these species on T2DM. Butyrate, synthesized by *Faecali bacterium* and Roseburia, decreases intestinal permeability by acting on serotonin transporters and PPAR-g pathways (Kinoshita et al., 2002).

4.5.2.3 Glucose Metabolism

T2DM is manipulated by gut microbiota and balance between glucose and insulin resistance in important metabolic organs. The digestion of carbohydrates and the synthesis of gut hormones regulating the physiological process is affected by the gut microbiota (Kim et al., 2014). *Bifidobacterium lactis* enhances glycogen production by reducing the expression of genes connected to hepatic gluconeogenesis. The expression of GLUT-4 in muscle tissue is enhanced by *L. gasseri* providing an effective diabetes management (Kang et al., 2013). Insulin resistance by upregulation of mRNA expression of key molecules involved in insulin signaling pathways, including phosphatidylinositol-3-kinase (PI3K), insulin receptor substrate 2 (IRS2), AMP-activated protein kinase (AMPK), and glycogen production in the liver improved by giving *L. casei*. Decrease in hyperglycemia with exchange of bile acids and chloride, leading to the upregulation of many genes was seen with *L. casei* (Neyazi et al., 2017).

Gut hormones and enzymes are highly influenced by microbiota and its byproducts leading to enhanced insulin resistance and glucose tolerance. Butyrate a ligand for G-protein coupled receptors located in the gastrointestinal tract enabled entero-endocrine L cells, resulting in the release of gut hormones such as GLP-1, PYY, and GLP-2 (Arora & Bäckhed, 2016).

4.5.2.4 Fatty Acid Oxidation, Synthesis, and Energy Expenditure

Augmenting fatty acid oxidation and energy use while concurrently decreasing fatty acid production can help mitigate obesity and therefore ameliorate T2DM. Adipose tissue can be made more conducive to fatty acid oxidation by *L. gasseri*, *B. acidifaciens*, *A. muciniphila*, and SCFA's by reducing the expression of PPAR-g by butyrate, propionate, and acetate, three SCFAs. This reduction subsequently leads to an increase in fatty acid oxidation. By upregulating genes linked to fatty acid oxidation and downregulating those linked to fatty acid synthesis, *L. gasseri* has shown promise in reducing obesity (Kang et al., 2013). The serum concentration of malondialdehyde, a biomarker indicating lipid oxidative damage, was observed to decrease in diabetic rodents following administration of *A. muciniphila* and *L. casei* (Li et al., 2016). Therefore, the microbiota members that have a positive consequence on T2DM regulate the metabolism of fatty acids and the subsequent energy expenditure in the host, leading to the reduction of obesity and the alleviation of T2D.

4.5.2.5 Combined Effects of Microflora

Apart from the aforementioned mechanisms, certain microorganisms have the ability to determine the physiological state of the host by encouraging the proliferation of other potentially advantageous microbiota or by engaging in cross-feeding interactions. Cross-feeding interactions between various species of Bifodobacterium and other bacteria, including Faecalibacterium and Roseburia, have been shown (Moens et al., 2016). The presence of *L. rhamnosus* in the cecum of rats enhanced Bifidobacterium population. The population of butyrate-producing bacteria was greatly enhanced by *L. casei* (Wang et al., 2017).

4.6 THERAPIES FOR T2DM BASED ON GUT MICROFLORA

Manipulation of intestinal flora in regulating T2DM to prevent and treat diabetes is an area of intense investigation. As per the available literature, the effects of conventional treatment can be influenced by the unique qualities gut flora in an individual.

4.6.1 Fecal Microflora Transplantation

Fecal microbiota transplantation (FMT), with antibiotic therapy, is a purposeful therapeutic strategy for gastrointestinal disorders like irritable bowel syndrome, *Clostridium difficile* infection, and ulcerative colitis that do not respond well (Antushevich, 2020). In total, 60% of patients showed recovery within a month without severe side effects in the treatment of *C. difficile* infections proving its effectiveness (Cui et al., 2015).

In a first-ever clinical trial in 2012 making use of FMT, the metabolic syndrome patients received FMT of healthy, thin donors for 6 weeks and there was a drastic change in insulin sensitivity and butyrate-producing bacteria (Vrieze et al., 2012). Patients significantly showed decreased peripheral resistance to insulin, as demonstrated by a fall in HbA1c and a rise in plasma γ-aminobutyric acid (GABA). The patients who had lower levels of intestinal flora diversity showed better results which ensured influence of gut microbiota of patient in the treatment. Transplanting MTS-D intestinal flora for 2 weeks, insulin of patients with metabolic syndrome lowered, with an increase in isolithocholic acid, deoxycholic acid, and lithocholic acid (Kootte, 2017).

4.6.2 Dietary Fibers

Dietary fibers have been shown to improve T2DM, confirming that altering the food composition can help in managing diabetes (Velázquez-López et al., 2016). In T2DM, 25–30 g of fiber, with whole grains and legumes up 1/3rd of the main diet carbohydrates is recommended to prevent T2DM (Hu et al., 2020). The Ma-pi diet is high in sea salt, beans, fermented foods, complex carbohydrates, and green tea, enhance the range of microbiome in gut, enrich bacteria that produce mucus and SCFA's, including Faecalibacterium, Akkermansia, Bacteroides, and Roseburia, and inhibit pro-inflammatory bacteria like Streptococcus and Collinsella. It can also reduce inflammation in people with T2DM (Fallucca et al., 2014). Dietary fiber can boost intestinal SCFA levels, enhance number of SCFA-generating bacteria, inhibit the proliferation of pathogenic bacteria, and raise patient HbA1c and insulin levels. With lower HbA1c, more SCFA-producing bacteria are present. The gut microbiota after the consumption of barley bread indicated a higher abundance of Prevotella in individuals who exhibited a positive response to the dietary intervention compared to those who did not respond. It is thought that a high-fiber diet has a direct impact on Prevotella (Zhao et al., 2018).

4.6.3 Probiotics

Probiotics are described as live microorganisms that provide sufficient health advantages to humans, typically in the form of gram-positive bacteria. Probiotics for diabetes primarily come in three varieties, according to recent research:

4.6.3.1 Common Probiotics

These bacteria, which primarily come from the Lactobacillus and Bifidobacterium genera, are highly safe to use and are frequently employed in food fermentation. Numerous clinical trials have tried probiotic intervention in T2DM patients; however, the outcomes have been mixed. In many clinical trials, probiotics have been shown to lower fasting insulin, HbA1c, and FBG while enhancing the effectiveness of HOMA-IR (Singh et al., 2013), lowering oxidative stress indicators (TAS, TAS, and MDA), suggesting that probiotics improve antioxidant strain rather than glucose metabolism to treat diabetes (Tao et al., 2020). Ardeshirlarijani et al. in a meta-analysis reported that probiotic capsules and multistrains together significantly lowered HbA1c and FBG in individuals with T2DM, only in those without additional risk factors (Ardeshirlarijani et al., 2019).

4.6.3.2 Novel Probiotics

A. muciniphila is an effective probiotic treatment for various ailments (Sun & Buys, 2016). Mice administered *A. muciniphila* given through oral route showed decreased inflammation, enhanced glucose tolerance, repaired intestinal barrier, and increased GLP-1 release in colon cells (Ansaldo et al., 2019). The presence of *F. prausnitzii* plays a critical role in T2DM management by fecal transplantation, medication, diet, and other methods (Plovier et al., 2017).

4.6.3.3 Genetically Engineered Bacteria

Strains are genetically modified for developing biological components for treating any disease. To treat T2DM, the use of *L. lactis* as a transporter to generate GLP-1 is a good example. *L. lactis* given orally to rats increased insulin concentrations and decreased blood glucose (Agarwal et al., 2014).

4.6.3.4 Exercise

Exercise is crucial for lowering blood sugar, decreasing inflammation, and increasing insulin sensitivity. A fresh viewpoint on how exercise controls diabetes is offered by research on gut bacteria. Exercise boosts the diverse gut microbiota related with a negative correlation to obesity and T2DM because it increases the *A. muciniphila* in the intestinal microbiota of athletes (Clarke et al., 2014). Following exercise training, the abundance of Bacteroides increased although that of the Clostridium species and Blautia dropped (Motiani et al., 2020). Exercise may lower blood glucose levels in diabetic patients by influencing their gut microbiota, as changes in the gut flora are positively correlated with glucose absorption. Exercise-induced improvements in insulin resistance due to gut microbiota have been proven in mice using FMT (Hamasaki, 2018).

4.7 CLINICAL APPLICATIONS FOR THE MANAGEMENT OF T2DM

The interaction between medications and gut bacteria is currently attracting significant attention (Whang et al., 2019). The modulation of microbiota and the potential improvement of diabetes have been observed through the administration of antibiotics, non-antibiotic medicines (Maier et al., 2018), and anti-diabetic medications. The microbiota at baseline has the potential to have both positive and negative influences on the pharmacokinetics and pharmacodynamics of medicines and other substances through a range of pathways, as discussed in a previous review (Klaassen & Cui, 2015). There is less research on influence of modifying gut microbiota, specifically through the utilization of pre- and/or probiotics, on the efficacy of anti-diabetic medications. The results of a study to investigate chicory inulin improved with oligofructose on liver enzyme levels in diabetic patients conducted showed an appreciable decline in liver enzyme levels when the prebiotic was administered alone, however, with synbiotic formulation containing *B. coagulans* and beta carotene, no significant variation in hepatic biomarkers were observed (Al-Najjar et al., 2022). Previous investigations have proven the advantageous effects of probiotics that include *L. acidophilus* and *L. casei*, *L. plantarum*, *L. plantarum*, *L. gasseri*, *L. reuteri*, and *L. rhamnosus*. However, the benefits have not been observed with *L. bulgaricus* (Zhao et al., 2021). Experimental research on diabetes has indicated additional metabolic effects associated with the utilization of probiotics. The presence of *B. lactis* was related with decreased lipid levels and insulinaemia (Kim et al., 2014). *L. casei* CCFM0412 was observed to enhance glucose tolerance, reduce lipid levels, improve immune regulation, and mitigate oxidative stress (Chen et al., 2014). Additionally, administering *L. johnsonii* caused increased expression of proteins intricated in the maintenance of intercellular tight junctions in the gastrointestinal tract.

Research on the intake of probiotics or synbiotics among persons diagnosed with diabetes has yielded inconsistent findings. Some studies have indicated enhanced metabolic control, while others have not observed such improvements.

Strategy of administering probiotics and synbiotics for reducing fasting blood glucose levels in individuals with elevated fasting blood glucose levels was very effective (Markowiak & Śliżewska, 2017).

4.8 FUTURE PERSPECTIVES AND CONCLUSION

Managing T2DM with synbiotics is gaining importance. The potential mechanism behind the regulation of gut microbiota and synbiotics has been investigated. Theoretically, it is viable to opt for variety of suitable blends of synbiotics to manipulate the balance of intestinal microbiota of T2DM patients which has been substantiated by many research works.

In the coming years, manipulating the gut microbiota could be a very beneficial strategy for the prophylaxis of diabetes, apart from investigating the relation between gut microbiota, obesity, and T2DM (Mahboobi et al., 2018).

The various technological advancements like 16S rRNA, gradient gel electrophoresis making use of PCR denaturation, metagenomics, metatranscriptomics, and microarrays, have potent role in the research of diverse gut microbiota. The beneficial association between gut microbiota and T2DM needs to be explored (Jiang et al., 2022). An extensive understanding of the underlying mechanism between different components will open up new possibilities for developing innovative treatment strategies that specifically target the intestinal flora. These strategies will help regulate the gut microbiota environment and hence intervene in the progression of type 2 diabetes mellitus (T2DM) by maintaining its homeostasis.

Making use of synbiotics will effectively improve the framework of intestinal microbiota. It will promote the maintenance of homeostasis and offer a newer therapeutic strategy for the management of T2DM. Synbiotics have the potential to emerge as an efficacious strategy for the treatment of T2DM.

It is important to explore the specific microbial species playing a role in the pathophysiology of diabetes, along with the underlying molecular pathways involved in this process.

REFERENCES

Abdullah, Z. (2022). A commentary on mechanism of action and types of synbiotics. *Journal of Probiotics & Health*, *10*(9), 1000290.

Agarwal, P., Khatri, P., Billack, B., et al. (2014). Oral delivery of glucagon like peptide-1 by a recombinant *Lactococcus lactis*. *Pharmaceutical Research*, 31, 3404–3414.

Agrawal, S.S., Naqvi, S., Gupta, S.K., et al. (2012). Prevention and management of diabetic retinopathy in STZ diabetic rats by *Tinospora cordifolia* and its molecular mechanisms. *Food and Chemical Toxicology*, 50, 3126–3132.

Aït-Aissa, A., & Aïder, M. (2014). Lactulose: Production and use in functional food, medical and pharmaceutical applications. Practical and critical review. *International Journal of Food Science & Technology*, 49, 1245–1253.

Al-Najjar, Y., Arabi, M., Paul, P., et al. (2022). Can probiotic, prebiotic, and synbiotic supplementation modulate the gut-liver axis in type 2 diabetes? A narrative and systematic review of clinical trials. *Frontiers in Nutrition*, 9, 1052619. doi.org/10.3389/fnut.2022.1052619.

Ansaldo, E., Slayden, L.C., Ching, K.L., et al. (2019). Akkermansia muciniphilainduces intestinal adaptive immune responses during homeostasis. *Science*, 364, 1179–1184.

Antushevich, H. (2020). Fecal microbiota transplantation in disease therapy. *Clinica Chimica Acta*, 503, 90–98.

Ardeshirlarijani, E., Tabatabaei-Malazy, O., Mohseni, S., et al. (2019). Effect of probiotics supplementation on glucose and oxidative stress in type 2 diabetes mellitus: A meta-analysis of randomized trials. *DARU-Journal of Pharmaceutical Sciences*, 27, 827–837.

Arora, T., & Bäckhed, F. (2016). The gut microbiota and metabolic disease: Current understanding and future perspectives. *Journal of Internal Medicine*, 280(4), 339–349. doi.org/10.1111/joim.12508

Backhed, F., Ding, H., Wang, T., et al. (2004). The gut microbiota as an environmental factor that regulates fat storage. *Proceedings of the National Academy of Sciences of the United States of America*, 101, 15718–15723.

Ban, Q., Cheng, J., Sun, X., et al. (2020). Effects of a synbiotic yogurt using monk fruit extract as sweetener on glucose regulation and gut microbiota in rats with type 2 diabetes mellitus. *Journal of Dairy Science*, 103, 2956–2968. doi.org/10.3168/jds.2019-17700

Barengolts, E. (2016). Gut microbiota, prebiotics, probiotics, and synbiotics in management of obesity and prediabetes: Review of randomized controlled trials. *Endocrine Practice*, 22(10), 1224–1234. doi.org/10.4158/EP151157.RA

Bessac, A., Cani, P.D., Meunier, E., et al. (2018). Inflammation and gut-brain axis during type 2 diabetes: Focus on the crosstalk between intestinal immune cells and enteric nervous system. *Frontiers in Neuroscience*, 12, 725.

Chen, P., Zhang, Q., Dang, H., et al. (2014). Oral administration of *Lactobacillus rhamnosus* CCFM0528 improves glucose tolerance and cytokine secretion in high-fat-fed, streptozotocin-induced type 2 diabetic mice. *Journal of Functional Foods*, 10, 318–326. doi.org/10.1016/j.jff.2014.06.014.

Clarke, S.F., Murphy, E.F., O'Sullivan, O., et al. (2014). Exercise and associated dietary extremes impact on gut microbial diversity. *Gut*, 63, 1913–1920.

Creely, S.J., McTernan, P.G., Kusminski, C.M., et al. (2007). Lipopolysaccharide activates an innate immune system response in human adipose tissue in obesity and type 2 diabetes. *American Journal of Physiology. Endocrinology and Metabolism*, 292, E740–E747.

Cui, B., Feng, Q., Wang, H., et al. (2015). Fecal microbiota transplantation through mid-gut for refractory Crohn's disease: Safety, feasibility, and efficacy trial results. *Journal of Gastroenterology and Hepatology*, 30, 51–58.

Cummings, J.H., Pomare, E.W., Branch, W.J., et al. (1987). Short chain fatty acids in human large intestine, portal, hepatic and venous blood. *Gut*, 28, 1221–1227.

de la Cuesta-Zuluaga, J., Mueller, N.T., Corrales-Agudelo, V., et al. (2017). Metformin is associated with higher relative abundance of mucin-degrading *Akkermansia muciniphila* and several short-chain fatty acid-producing microbiota in the gut. *Diabetes Care*, 40, 54–62.

de Vries, M.C., Vaughan, E.E., Kleerebezem, M., et al. (2006). *Lactobacillus plantarum*-survival, functional and potential probiotic properties in the human intestinal tract. *The International Dairy Journal*, 16, 1018–1028.

Drivsholm, T., Olivarius, N.D.F., Nielsen, A.B.S., et al. (2005). Symptoms, signs and complications in newly diagnosed type 2 diabetic patients, and their relationship to glycaemia, blood pressure and weight. *Diabetologia*, 48, 210–214.

El-Beshbishy, H., & Bahashwan, S. (2012). Hypoglycemic effect of basil (*Ocimum basilicum*) aqueous extract is mediated through inhibition of alpha-glucosidase and alpha-amylase activities: An in vitro study. *Toxicology and Industrial Health*, 28, 42–50.

Fallucca, F., Porrata, C., Fallucca, S., et al. (2014). Influence of diet on gut microbiota, inflammation and type 2 diabetes mellitus. First experience with macrobiotic Ma-Pi 2 diet. *Diabetes/metabolism Research and Reviews*, 30, 48–54.

Fiorucci, S., & Distrutti, E. (2015). Bile acid-activated receptors, intestinal microbiota, and the treatment of metabolic disorders. *Trends in Molecular Medicine*, 21(11), 702–714.

Galicia-Garcia, U., Benito-Vicente, A., Jebari, S., et al. (2020). Pathophysiology of type 2 diabetes mellitus. *The International Journal of Molecular Sciences*, 21(17), 6275. doi.org/10.3390/ijms21176275.

Gibson, G.R., & Roberfroid, M.B. (1995). Dietary modulation of the human colonic microbiota: Introducing the concept of prebiotics. *The Journal of Nutrition*, 125, 1401–1412.

Gowri, P.M., Tiwari, A.K., Ali, A.Z., et al. (2007). Inhibition of α-glucosidase and amylase by bartogenic acid isolated from *Barringtonia racemosa* Roxb. seeds. *Phytotherapy Research*, 21, 796–799.

Grover, J.K., Vats, V., & Rathi, S.S. (2000). Anti-hyperglycemic effect of *Eugenia jambolana* and *Tinospora cordifolia* in experimental diabetes and their effects on keymetabolic enzymes involved in carbohydrate metabolism. *Journal of Ethnopharmacology*, 73, 461–470.

Gu, Y., Wang, X., Li, J., et al. (2017). Analyses of gut microbiota and plasma bile acids enable stratification of patients for antidiabetic treatment. *Nature Communications*, 8, 1785.

Guinane, C.M., & Cotter, P.D. (2013). Role of the gut microbiota in health and chronic gastrointestinal disease: Understanding a hidden metabolic organ. *Therapeutic Advances in Gastroenterology*, 6, 295–308.

Guo, L. (2015). Medication treatment of type 2 diabetes. *Clinical Medication Journal*, 13, 18–22.

Gurung, M., Li, Z., You, H., et al. (2020). Role of gut microbiota in type 2 diabetes pathophysiology. *EBioMedicine*, 51, 102590. doi.org/10.1016/j.ebiom.2019.11.051.

Hamasaki, H. (2018). Exercise and glucagon-like peptide-1: Does exercise potentiate the effect of treatment? *World Journal of Diabetes*, 9, 138–140.

Han, J.L., & Lin, H.L. (2014). Intestinal microbiota and type 2 diabetes: From mechanism insights to therapeutic perspective. *World Journal of Gastroenterology*, 20, 17737.

Hoffmann, T., Pham, H.P., Bridonneau, C., et al. (2016). Microorganisms linked to inflammatory bowel disease-associated dysbiosis differentially impact host physiology in genotobiotic mice. *The ISME Journal*, 10, 460–477. doi.org/10.1038/ismej.2015.127

Hosseinifard, E.S., Bavafa-Valenlia, K., Saghafi-Asl, M., et al. (2020). Antioxidative and metabolic effects of *Lactobacillus plantarum*, inulin, and their synbiotic on the hypothalamus and serum of healthy rats. *Nutrition and Metabolic Insights*, 13. doi.org/10.1177/1178638820925092

Hou, K., Wu, Z.X., Chen, X.Y., et al. (2022). Microbiota in health and diseases. *Signal Transduction and Targeted Therapy*, 7, 135. doi.org/10.1038/s41392-022-00974-4

Hu, B. (2018). Production and utilization of L-arabinose in China. *World Journal of Engineering and Technology*, 6, 24–36.

Hu, Y., Ding, M., Sampson, L., et al. (2020). Intake of whole grain foods and risk of type 2 diabetes: Results from three prospective cohort studies. *BMJ*, 370, m2206.

Hulston, C.J., Churnside, A.A., & Venables, M. (2015). Probiotic supplementation prevents high-fat, overfeeding-induced insulin resistance in human subjects. *British Journal of Nutrition*, 113, 596–602.

Jandhyala, S.M., Talukdar, R., Subramanyam, C., et al. (2015). Role of the normal gut microbiota. *World Journal of Gastroenterology*, 21(29), 8787–8803.

Jiang, H., Cai, M., Shen, B., et al. (2022). Synbiotics and gut microbiota: New perspectives in the treatment of type 2 diabetes mellitus. *Foods*, 11, 2438.

Juan, L.N.T. (2014). Clinical understanding of glinides secretagogues. *Chinese Journal of Practice International Medicine*, 34, 959–961.

Kang, J.H., Yun, S.I., Park, M.H., et al. (2013). Anti-obesity effect of *Lactobacillus gasseri* BNR17 in high-sucrose diet-induced obese mice. *PLoS ONE*, 8(1), e54617. doi.org/10.1371/journal.pone.0054617

Karlsson, F.H., Tremaroli, V., Nookaew, I., et al. (2013). Gut metagenome in European women with normal, impaired and diabetic glucose control. *Nature*, 498, 99–103.

Kikuchi, K., Othman, M.B., & Sakamoto, K. (2018). Sterilized bifidobacteria suppressed fat accumulation and blood glucose level. *Biochemical and Biophysical Research Communications*, 501, 1041–1047. doi.org/10.1016/j.bbrc.2018.05.105.

Kim, S.H., Huh, C.S., Choi, I.D., et al. (2014). The anti-diabetic activity of *Bifidobacterium lactis* HY8101 in vitro and in vivo. *Journal of Applied Microbiology*, 117(3), 834–845. doi.org/10.1111/jam.12573

Kinoshita, M., Suzuki, Y., & Saito, Y. (2002). Butyrate reduces colonic paracellular permeability by enhancing PPARγ activation. *Biochemical and Biophysical Research Communications*, 293(2), 827–831. doi.org/10.1016/S0006-291X(02)00294-2.

Klaassen, C.D., & Cui, J.Y. (2015). Review: Mechanisms of how the intestinal microbiota alters the effects of drugs and bile acids. *Drug Metabolism and Disposition*, 43(10), 1505–1521.

Koh, A., De Vadder, F., Kovatcheva-Datchary, P., et al. (2016). From dietary fiber to host physiology: Short chain fatty acids as key bacterial metabolites. *Cell*, 165, 1332–1345.

Kolida, S., & Gibson, G.R. (2011). Synbiotics in health and disease. *Annual Review of Food Science & Technology*, 2, 373–393.

Kootte, R.S. (2017). The treatment of insulin sensitivity after lean donor feces in metabolic syndrome is driven by baseline intestinal microbiota composition. *Cell Metabolism*, 26, 611–619.

Larsen, N., Vogensen, F.K., van den Berg, F.W., et al. (2010). Gut microbiota in human adults with type 2 diabetes differs from non-diabetic adults. *PLOS One*, 5, e9085.

Li, C., Ding, Q., Nie, S.P., et al. (2014). Carrot juice fermented with *Lactobacillus plantarum* NCU116 ameliorates type 2 diabetes in rats. *Journal of Agriculture & Food Chemistry*, 62, 11884–11891.

Li, H., Ding, R., Shan, Y., et al. (2021). L-arabinose alleviates diabetes-aggravated cerebral ischemic injury by repairing the blood-brain barrier via downregulating NF-κB signals. *Journal of Functional Foods*, 87, 104839. doi.org/10.1016/j.jff.2021.104839.

Li, X., Wang, N., Yin, B., et al. (2016). Effects of *Lactobacillus plantarum* CCFM0236 on hyperglycaemia and insulin resistance in high-fat and streptozotocin-induced type 2 diabetic mice. *Journal of Applied Microbiology*, 121(6), 1727–1736. doi.org/10.1111/jam.13276

Liu, W.C., Yang, M.C., Wu, Y.Y., et al. (2018). *Lactobacillus plantarum* reverse diabetes-induced Fmo3 and ICAM expression in mice through enteric dysbiosis-related c-Jun NH2-terminal kinase pathways. *PLOS One*, 13(5), e0196511. doi.org/10.1371/journal.pone.0196511

Maftei, N.M. (2019). Probiotic, prebiotic and synbiotic products in human health. In *Frontiers and New Trends in the Science of Fermented Food and Beverages*. IntechOpen: London, UK.

Mahboobi, S., Rahimi, F., & Jafarnejad, S. (2018). Effects of prebiotic and synbiotic supplementation on glycaemia and lipid profile in type 2 diabetes: A meta-analysis of randomized controlled trials. *Advanced Pharmaceutical Bulletin*, 8, 565–574.

Maier, L., Pruteanu, M., Kuhn, M. et al. (2018). Extensive impact of non-antibiotic drugs on human gut bacteria. *Nature*, 555, 623–628. doi.org/10.1038/nature25979

Markowiak, P., & Śliżewska, K. (2017). Effects of probiotics, prebiotics, and synbiotics on human health. *Nutrients*, 9(9), 1021. doi.org/10.3390/nu9091021

Martin, A.M., Yabut, J.M., Choo, J.M., et al. (2019). The gut microbiome regulates host glucose homeostasis via peripheral serotonin. *Proceedings of the National Academy of Sciences of the United States of America*, 116, 19802–19804.

Martinic, A., Barouei, J., Bendiks, Z., et al. (2018). Supplementation of *Lactobacillus plantarum* improves markers of metabolic dysfunction induced by a high fat diet. *Journal of Proteome Research*, 17(8), 2790–2802.

Mccreigh, L.J., Bailey, C.J., & Pearson, E.R. (2016). Metformin and the gastrointestinal tract. *Diabetologia*, 59, 426–435.

Mirmiranpour, H., Huseini, H.F., Derakhshanian, H., et al. (2020). Effects of probiotic, cinnamon, and symbiotic supplementation on glycemic control and antioxidant status in people with type 2 diabetes; a randomized, double-blind, placebo-controlled study. *Journal of Diabetes Metabolic Disorders*, 19, 53–60.

Moens, F., Weckx, S., & Vuyst, L.D. (2016). Bifidobacterial inulin-type fructan degradation capacity determines cross-feeding interactions between bifidobacteria and *Faecalibacterium prausnitzii*. *International Journal of Food Microbiology*, 231, 76–85. doi.org/10.1016/j.ijfoodmicro.2016.05.015.

Moroti, C., Souza Magri, L.F.S., de Rezende Costa, M.D.R., et al. (2012). Effect of the consumption of a new symbiotic shake on glycemia and cholesterol levels in elderly people with type 2 diabetes mellitus. *Lipids in Health Disease*, 11, 29.

Motiani, K.K., Collado, M.C., Eskelinen, J.J., et al. (2020). Exercise training modulates gut microbiota profile and improves endotoxemia. *Medicine and Science in Sports and Exercise*, 52, 94–104.

Neyazi, N., Mohammadi, F., Nouri, Z., et al. (2017). Potential efficacy of *Lactobacillus casei* IBRC_M10711 on expression and activity of insulin degrading enzyme but not insulin degradation. *Vitro Cellular & Developmental Biology-Animal*, 53, 12–19. doi.org/10.1007/s11626-016-0083-4

Nie, Q., Chen, H., Hu, J., et al. (2019). Dietary compounds and traditional Chinese medicine ameliorate type 2 diabetes by modulating gut microbiota. *Critical Reviews in Food Science and Nutrition*, 59, 848–863.

Ooi, L.G., & Liong, M.T. (2010). Cholesterol-lowering effects of probiotics and prebiotics: A review of in vivo and in vitro findings. *International Journal Molecular Science*, 11, 2499–2522.

Plovier, H., Everard, A., Druart, C., et al. (2017). A purified membrane protein from *Akkermansia muciniphila* or the pasteurized bacterium improves metabolism in obese and diabetic mice. *Nature Medicine*, 23, 107–113.

Prince, P.S.M., Menon, V.P., & Pari, L. (1998). Hypoglycaemic activity of *Syzigium cumini* seeds: Effect on lipid peroxidation in alloxan diabetic rats. *Journal of Ethnopharmacology*, 61, 1–7.

Psichas, A., Sleeth, M.L., Murphy, K.G., et al. (2015). The short chain fatty acid propionate stimulates GLP-1 and PYY secretion via free fatty acid receptor 2 in rodents. *International Journal of Obesity*, 39, 424–429.

Pussinen, P.J., Havulinna, A.S., Lehto, M., et al. (2011). Endotoxemia is associated with an increased risk of incident diabetes. *Diabetes Care*, 34, 392–397.

Qin, J., Li, Y., Cai, Z., et al. (2012). A metagenome-wide association study of gut microbiota in type 2 diabetes. *Nature*, 490, 55–60.

Rajilić-Stojanović, M., & de Vos, W.M. (2014). The first 1000 cultured species of the human gastrointestinal microbiota. *FEMS Microbiology Reviews*, 38(5), 996–1047. doi.org/10.1111/1574-6976.12075

Rao, A.V. (2002). Prebiotics and probiotics: New concepts in nutrition and health. *Heinz Infant Nutrition Institute*, 19, 1–4.

Raptis, S.A., & Dimitriadis, G.D. (2001). Oral hypoglycemic agents: Insulin secretagogues, _-glucosidase inhibitors and insulin sensitizers. *Experimental & Clinical Endocrinology & Diabetes*, 109(Suppl. S2), S265–S287.

Remely, M., Aumueller, E., Merold, C., et al. (2014). Effects of short chain fatty acid producing bacteria on epigenetic regulation of FFAR3 in type 2 diabetes and obesity. *Gene*, 537, 85–92.

Rodes, L., Khan, A., Paul, A., et al. (2013). Effect of probiotics *Lactobacillus* and *Bifidobacterium* on gut-derived lipopolysaccharides and inflammatory cytokines: An in vitro study using a human colonic microbiota model. *Journal of Microbiology and Biotechnology*, 23, 518–526.

Sáez-Lara, M.J., Robles-Sanchez, C., Ruiz-Ojeda, F.J., et al. (2016). Effects of probiotics and synbiotics on obesity, insulin resistance syndrome, type 2 diabetes and non-alcoholic fatty liver disease: A review of human clinical trials. *International Journal of Molecular Science*, 17, 928.

Safari, Z., & Gérard, P. (2019). The links between the gut microbiome and non-alcoholic fatty liver disease (NAFLD). *Cellular & Molecular Life Science*, 76(8), 1541–1558. doi.org/10.1007/s00018-019-03011

Sanna, S., van Zuydam, N.R., Mahajan, A., et al. (2019). Causal relationships among the gut microbiome, short-chain fatty acids and metabolic diseases. *Nature Genetics*, 51, 600–605.

Sarao, L.K., & Arora, M. (2017). Probiotics, prebiotics, and microencapsulation: A review. *Critical Review in Food Science & Nutrition*, 57, 344–371.

Schloissnig, S., Arumugam, M., Sunagawa, S., et al. (2013). Genomic variation landscape of the human gut microbiome. *Nature*, 493, 45–50.

Shapiro, H., Kolodziejczyk, A.A., Halstuch, D., et al. (2018). Bile acids in glucose metabolism in health and disease. *Journal of Experimental Medicine*, 215(2), 383–396.

Shen, D., Lu, Y., Tian, S., et al. (2021). Effects of L-arabinose by hypoglycemic and modulating gut microbiome in a high-fat diet- and streptozotocin-induced mouse model of type 2 diabetes mellitus. *Journal of Food Biochemistry*, 45(12), e13991. doi.org/10.1111/jfbc.13991.

Shen, Z., Zhu, C., Quan, Y., et al. (2018). Insights into Roseburia intestinalis which alleviates experimental colitis pathology by inducing anti-inflammatory responses. *Journal of Gastroenterology and Hepatology*, 33(10), 1751–1760. doi.org/10.1111/jgh.14144Ci

Singh, V.P., Sharma, J., Babu, S., et al. (2013). Role of probiotics in health and disease: A review. *Journal of the Pakistan Medical Association*, 63, 253–257.

Soleimani, A., Motamedzadeh, A., Zarrati Mojarrad, M., et al. (2019). The effects of synbiotic supplementation on metabolic status in diabetic patients undergoing hemodialysis: A randomized, double-blinded, placebo-controlled trial. *Probiotics & Antimicrobial Proteins*, 11, 1248–1256.

Su, B., Liu, H., Li, J., et al. (2015). Acarbose treatment affects the serum levels of inflammatory cytokines and the gut content of bifidobacteria in Chinese patients with type 2 diabetes mellitus. *Journal of Diabetes*, 7, 729–739.

Suez, J., Zmora, N., Segal, E., et al. (2019). The pros, cons, and many unknowns of probiotics. *Nature Medicine*, 25, 716–729.

Sun, H.S., Pouya, K., Suvi, P., et al. (2021). IDF diabetes Atlas: Global, regional and country-level diabetes prevalence estimates for 2021 and projections for 2045. *Diabetes Research and Clinical Practice*, 183, 109119. doi.org/10.1016/j.diabres.2021.109119.

Sun, J., & Buys, N.J. (2016). Glucose- and glycaemic factor lowering effects of probiotics on diabetes: A meta-analysis of randomised placebo-controlled trials. *The British Journal of Nutrition*, 115, 1167–1177.

Sun, K.Y., Xu, D.H, Xie, C., et al. (2017). Lactobacillus paracasei modulates LPS-induced inflammatory cytokine release by monocyte-macrophages via the up-regulation of negative regulators of NF-kappaB signaling in a TLR2-dependent manner. *Cytokine*, 92, 1–11. doi.org/10.1016/j.cyto.2017.01.003.

Tao, Y.W., Gu, Y.L., Mao, X.Q., et al. (2020). Effects of probiotics on type II diabetes mellitus: A metaanalysis. *Journal of Translational Medicine*, 18, 30.

Temneanu, O.R., Trandafir, L.M., & Purcarea, M.R. (2016). Type 2 diabetes mellitus in children and adolescents: A relatively new clinical problem within pediatric practice. *Journal of Medicine & Life*, 9(3), 235–239.

Terpou, A., Papadaki, A., Lappa, I., et al. (2019). Probiotics in food systems: Significance and emerging strategies towards improved viability and delivery of enhanced beneficial value. *Nutrients*, 11, 1591.

Molinaro, A., Bel Lassen, P., et al. (2020). Imidazole propionate is increased in diabetes and associated with dietary patterns and altered microbial ecology. *Nature Communications*, 11 (1), 5881.

Tong, X., Xu, J., Lian, F., et al. (2018). Structural alteration of gut microbiota during the amelioration of human type 2 diabetes with hyperlipidemia by metformin and a traditional Chinese herbal formula: A multicenter, randomized, open label clinical trial. *mBio*, 9(3), e02392-17.

Tumminia, A., Vinciguerra, F., Parisi, M., et al. (2018). Type 2 diabetes mellitus and Alzheimer's disease: Role of insulin signalling and therapeutic implications. *International Journal of Molecular Science*, 19, 3306.

Turnbaugh, P.J., Ley, R.E., Mahowald, M.A., et al. (2006). An obesity-associated gut microbiome with increased capacity for energy harvest. *Nature*, 444, 1027–1031.

Valdes, A.M., Walter, J., Segal, E., et al. (2018). Role of the gut microbiota in nutrition and health. *BMJ*, 361, k2179.

Velayati, A., Kareem, I., Sedaghat, M., et al. (2021). Does symbiotic supplementation which contains *Bacillus Coagulans Lactobacillus rhamnosus*, *Lactobacillus acidophilus* and fructooligosaccharide has favourite effects in patients with type-2 diabetes? A randomised, double-blind, placebo-controlled trial. *Archieves of Physiology & Biochemistry*, 2, 1–8.

Velázquez-López, L., Muñoz-Torres, A.V., García-Peña, C., et al. (2016). Fiber in diet is associated with improvement of glycated hemoglobin and lipid profile in Mexican patients with type 2 diabetes. *Journal of Diabetes Research*. 2016, 2980406

Vrieze, A., van Nood, E., Holleman, F., et al. (2012). Transfer of intestinal microbiota from lean donors increases insulin sensitivity in individuals with metabolic syndrome. *Gastroenterology*, 143, 913–916.

Wang, G., Li, X., Zhao, J., et al. (2017). *Lactobacillus casei* CCFM419 attenuates type 2 diabetes via a gut microbiota dependent mechanism. *Food and Function*, 9(8), 3155–3164. doi.org/10.1039/C7FO00593H

Wang, J., Ma, Q., Li, Y., et al. (2020). Research progress on traditional Chinese medicine syndromes of diabetes mellitus. *Biomedicine & Pharmacotherapy*, 121, 109565.

Wang, X., Ota, N., Manzanillo, P., et al. (2014). Interleukin-22 alleviates metabolic disorders and restores mucosal immunity in diabetes. *Nature*, 9, 514(7521), 237–241.

Whang, A., Nagpal, R., & Yadav, H. (2019). Bi-directional drug-microbiome interactions of anti-diabetics. *EBioMedicine*, 39, 591–602.

Xiao, Y., Chen, Q., Guang, C., et al. (2019). An overview on biological production of functional lactose derivatives. *Applied Microbiology & Biotechnology*, 103, 3683–3691.

Yang, J.Y., Lee, Y.S., Kim, Y., et al. (2017). Gut commensal *Bacteroides acidifaciens* prevents obesity and improves insulin sensitivity in mice. *Mucosal Immunology*, 10, 104–116. doi.org/10.1038/mi.2016.42.

Zhang, X., Fang, Z., Zhang, C., et al. (2017). Effects of acarbose on the gut microbiota of prediabetic patients: A randomized, doubleblind, controlled crossover trial. *Diabetes Therapy*, 8, 293–307.

Zhang, Y., Gu, Y., Ren, H., et al. (2020). Gut microbiome-related effects of berberine and probiotics on type 2 diabetes (the PREMOTE study). *Nature Communications*, 11, 5015.

Zhao, L., Zhang, F., Ding, X., et al. (2018). Gut bacteria selectively promoted by dietary fibers alleviate type 2 diabetes. *Science*, 359, 1151–1156.

Zhao, X., Zhong, X., Liu, X., et al. (2021). Therapeutic and improving function of Lactobacilli in the prevention and treatment of cardiovascular-related diseases: A novel perspective from gut microbiota. *Frontiers in Nutrition*, 8, 693412. doi.org/10.3389/fnut.2021.693412

Zheng, Y., Li, Y., Qi, Q., et al. (2016). Cumulative consumption of branched-chain amino acids and incidence of type 2 diabetes. *International Journal of Epidemiology*, 45, 1482–1492.

5 Exploring Gut Microbiota as Therapeutic Target to Maintain Metabolic Health

Anas Islam, Aditya Singh, Asad Ahmad, Badruddeen, Juber Akhtar, Usama Ahmad, Mohammad Irfan Khan, Mohammad Ahmad, and Yusuf Asad

5.1 INTRODUCTION

Metabolic disorders include diseases characterized by abnormal metabolic processes in the body, resulting in many health complications (Liu et al., 2020). These diseases undermine the breakdown and processing of nutrients and cause imbalances affecting energy production, hormone regulation, and various metabolic functions (Raposo et al., 2017). The symptoms encompass a variety of common conditions including obesity, type 2 diabetes (T2D), and cardiovascular disease (Pasdar et al., 2017). Metabolic diseases are a major global health concern that affect millions of people globally. The complicated bacteria that live in our intestines and may have an impact on the development and treatment of certain diseases have received special attention in recent studies (Zhu et al., 2022).

Gut microbiota may be influenced by a number of variables, but nutrition is one important element that has the potential to drastically modify the configuration of gut microbiota (Marco et al., 2020). Additionally, research has shown how the gut bacteria plays a function in the metabolic digestion of food, namely, in the conversion of carnitine and choline to trimethylamine. This process has a significant impact on metabolic diseases (Li et al., 2022). Empirical data connects alterations in gut microbiota composition to many health conditions, such as metabolic disorders and obesity. We still don't completely understand the exact processes at play in the development of many diseases, nor the extent of causation. Even though the body of research on this subject is growing, more investigation is required to establish a clear link between metabolic illnesses and disordered gut flora.

Changing the diet and adjusting the microbiota are two ways to investigate the possible therapeutic benefits of the gut microbiota for metabolic diseases. The extant research indicates that some dietary modifications and the utilization of probiotics have exhibited efficacy in modifying the makeup of gut microbiota and influencing metabolic consequences. These methods are intended to promote the synthesis of advantageous metabolites like short-chain fatty acids (SCFAs) and restore equilibrium to the gut flora. By focusing on interventions like dietary modifications, prebiotics, probiotics, and possibly pharmaceutical treatments targeted at the gut microbiota, there is a possibility for preventing and easing metabolic diseases (Zhang et al., 2015). Current investigations on the connection among the microbiota of the gut and metabolic disorders might lead to novel treatments and prophylactic measures (Han et al., 2023).

5.1.1 Significance of Gut Microbiota in Metabolic Health

The bacteria in the gut have a big impact on the metabolism's health. It does this by a number of processes, one of which is the synthesis of SCFA, which is crucial for controlling insulin sensitivity, glucose metabolism, and host energy balance (Longo et al., 2023). The metabolic effects are caused by the complicated relationships involving intestinal hormones like GLP-1 and gut microorganisms. Together with affecting hunger, this hormonal interaction also controls the glucose balance (Longo et al., 2023).

According to research, dysbiosis, which is brought on by disparity in the microbiota of gut, is connected to metabolic illnesses (Longo et al., 2023). Dysbiosis, in particular, can compromise gut permeability and elevate circulating levels of LPS, fostering low-grade inflammation that ultimately contributes to metabolic disorders (Abidi and Rtibi, 2023).

However, there is hope for improving metabolic health through dietary interventions and physical activity. Research indicates that interventions like intermittent fasting can enhance gut microbiota diversity and reduce the presence of pathogenic bacteria, resulting in reduced inflammation and improved metabolic health (Zhang et al., 2023). Likewise, it has been discovered that physical exercise, especially moderate-intensity and prolonged duration, modifies the gut microbiota's composition. This means that the beneficial bacteria that create butyrate will proliferate while the bacteria linked to metabolic disorders will decline (Zhang et al., 2023). These verdicts highlight the potential for lifestyle modifications to positively impact metabolic health.

This chapter aims to provide an in-depth analysis of the important role the gut microbiota plays in maintaining metabolic health. It seeks to clarify the ways in which the gut microbiota affects insulin sensitivity, glucose metabolism, host energy homeostasis, and gut hormones including GLP-1. This chapter tries to highlight how important it is to comprehend the function of gut microbiota in common illnesses like obesity and type 2 diabetes mellitus (T2DM) by looking at dysbiosis and its relationship to metabolic

DOI: 10.1201/9781032702438-5

disorders such as these. Furthermore, it explores therapeutic strategies, including dietary interventions and lifestyle modifications, highlighting their potential in improving metabolic health. By presenting compelling case studies and clinical evidence, this chapter bridges theory and practical application, offering insights and solutions to one of the most pressing health challenges of our era.

5.2 GUT MICROBIOTA: THE BASICS

The term "microbiome" or "gut microbiota" refers to the trillions of bacteria that live in the stomach, small intestine, and colon (Van Best et al., 2020). Numerous factors can explain individual variances in the gut microbiota's diversity and composition. The early microbial colonization is influenced by genetic predisposition, and microbial profiles vary throughout family members. Our nutrition has a major impact on the makeup of our gut bacteria. Our dietary intake provides the necessary minerals and chemicals needed for microbial development. A diet high in whole grains, fruits, and vegetables encourages the establishment of beneficial gut flora. In the process of breaking down complex carbohydrates, these microbes produce SCFAs, which are essential for preserving gut health. The gut microbiota is shaped in part by age (Iadanza et al., 2020). The microbiota of the gut is typically made up of a wide variety of microorganisms, most of which are bacteria, but there are also a few viruses, fungi, and archaea. The primary bacterial taxa found in the human gastrointestinal system are Actinobacteria, Proteobacteria, Verrucomicrobia, and Bacteroidetes. Genetics, nutrition, age, geography, and environmental exposures all affect an individual's gut microbiota diversity. Factors contributing to these variations include genetics, diet, antibiotic use, and other lifestyle choices (Brüssow, 2020). Genetic predisposition can influence the initial colonization of gut microbiota in humans. Some individuals may have genetic variations that affect their ability to metabolize certain components of the diet, which can in turn influence the composition of their gut microbiota. Increased microbial variety and substrates for the development of beneficial bacteria are provided by a diet high in plant-based fiber. The gut microbiota changes with age, with variations in microbial composition and diversity (Gomaa, 2020).

These changes can have implications for digestive health, nutrient absorption, and overall well-being, particularly in the elderly. The gut microbiota greatly influences the immune system by aiding in protection against harmful microorganisms through competition and the creation of substances that fight microbes. Breast milk is essential for promoting a healthy gut microbial community in babies, as it provides important nutrients and compounds that encourage the growth of helpful bacteria, ultimately contributing to the regulation of the host's immune reactions. Exclusive breastfeeding in term infants born vaginally appears to result in the most "beneficial" gut microbiome. This transition introduces solid foods and leads to an increased prevalence of bacteria such as Bacteroides, Bilophila, Roseburia, Clostridium, and Anaerostipes, gradually transforming the microbiome into an adult-like configuration. Solid foods prompt a shift from a Bifidobacterium-dominant microbiome to one dominated by Bacteroidetes and Firmicutes, including groups like Clostridium coccoides and Clostridium leptum. This change in diet also causes the expression of genes linked to essential metabolic processes in the adult microbiome and long-term increases in the amounts of SCFAs in feces. The gut microbiota seems to be essential for immune system education and gut tolerance modulation, especially in newborns and infants. This mutualistic relationship between host and microbiome has been well-described in germ-free animal experiments, with increasing evidence supporting its relevance in humans. According to research, compared to healthy children, babies who subsequently acquired allergy problems showed reduced IgG responses to certain clusters of microbial antigens (West et al., 2020). Additional research has shown that throughout the initial phases of infancy, babies at high menace of emerging atopic disorders had lower levels of Proteobacteria, which was associated with higher natural inflammatory responses activated by Toll-like receptor-4 (TLR-4). Additionally, a decrease in Ruminococcaceae was linked to heightened innate inflammatory responses induced by TLR-2 (Agus et al., 2021).

Infants who had a greater chance of having asthma displayed a certain pattern of gut microorganisms, such as reduced concentrations of certain bacterial species including Bifidobacterium and Faecalibacterium. Peripheral blood mononuclear cells treated with sterilized fecal water from these babies produced more CD4+ IL-4 generating cells and less regulatory Foxp3 cells (Sjödin et al., 2023). Researchers found a link between the gut bacteria Faecalibacterium and the amounts of regulatory cytokines in children with different allergies. This indicates that increasing the presence of these microorganisms could encourage a tolerogenic immune response with regulatory properties. Several key metabolites and their roles in metabolic disorders have been identified, providing insights into potential therapeutic avenues for these conditions. The gut microbiota's conversion of dietary phosphatidylcholine (L-carnitine) into trimethylamine (TMA) is one significant metabolite route. Trimethylamine N-oxide (TMAO), which is produced when liver enzymes further break down TMA, starts the inflammatory process that leads to cardiovascular disease. Leucine, isoleucine, and valine are examples of branched-chain amino acids that have been connected to insulin resistance and are found in high amounts in obese and insulin-resistant people. Bacteroides vulgatus and Prevotella copri are two examples of bacteria that have been connected to elevated blood levels of BCAAs and insulin resistance. The mechanistic links between BCAAs, insulin resistance, and gut microbiota are complex and not fully understood, but these metabolites are considered harmful. Human health is greatly impacted by the bile acids that are generated when the gut bacteria breaks down host cholesterol. Previously thought to help just in fat absorption, they are now known to be communication molecules that affect the host's metabolism through interactions with specific receptors like TGR5 and FXR. This bile acid signaling route can be modulated by altered gut microbiota, which can alter host metabolism. An inherent FXR antagonist, tauro-β-muricholic acid, contributes to the development of steatosis, insulin resistance, and obesity (Zou et al., 2020)

5.2.1 Factors Influencing Gut Microbiota

The connection among our gut flora and the meals we eat has received a lot of attention lately (Vandenplas et al., 2020). Numerous studies show that the composition of our gut microbiota is largely influenced by our food, and that this might have a substantial impact on our overall health. Let's examine the different elements that affect gut microbiota and their implications for well-being.

5.2.1.1 Dietary Fiber

There is a substantial correlation between dietary fiber and several health advantages. For example, it can reduce insulin resistance in individuals with type 2 diabetes and trigger the manufacture of beneficial metabolites like butyrate. A fiber-rich diet is crucial for preserving the variety of microorganisms in the gut.

5.2.1.2 High-Fat Diet

Diets high in fat can harm the gut by changing the makeup of microbes and how they operate metabolically. High-fat diets are frequently linked to decreased Bacteroidetes abundance and increased Firmicutes abundance. This change can lead to an overproduction of LPS and an increase in inflammation (Tanes et al., 2021).

5.2.1.3 Vegan Diet

The debate over whether a vegan diet is healthier for gut microbiota compared to a non-vegan diet is ongoing. Some studies have found that the gut bacterial community composition remains relatively consistent regardless of diet, challenging the notion that a vegan diet is definitively superior for gut health (Bakaloudi et al., 2021).

5.2.1.4 Gluten

Studies on gluten-free diets have shown mixed results. Some individuals without celiac disease or gluten intolerance choose to avoid gluten (Leonard et al., 2021).

5.2.1.5 Oxidative Stress

Oxidative stress can negatively impact gut microbial diversity and contribute to inflammation and other health problems (Pisoschi et al., 2021).

5.2.1.6 Socioeconomic Status

The economic status of a region can impact dietary choices and, subsequently, the gut microbiota. Malnourished individuals, especially undernourished infants, tend to have an unsteady gut microbiota with an abundance of enteropathogens. Restoring gut microbial diversity can be key to addressing various health conditions. Dietary interventions, such as the inclusion of microbiota-accessible carbohydrates (MACs), supplementation of missing microbial taxa, and other dietary modifications, offer potential avenues for improving gut health. To improve our understanding of how dietary decisions affect our health, it is imperative that we comprehend the complex link between nutrition and gut flora. Ongoing research and clinical trials continue to shed light on these interactions and may offer new avenues for preventing and treating autoimmune and inflammatory diseases through dietary interventions (Peverill et al., 2021).

5.2.1.7 Neurological Control

Often referred to as the "second brain," the enteric nervous system plays a vital role in regulating gut motility. It regulates the digestive tract's smooth muscle contractions, which are rhythmic.

5.2.1.8 Physical Activity

Regular physical activity can promote healthy gut motility. Exercise helps keep the muscles of the gastrointestinal tract in good shape and can prevent issues like constipation. Emotional factors, including stress and anxiety, can influence gut motility. Some individuals experience changes in motility during stressful situations, leading to symptoms like diarrhea or constipation. Certain medications, such as laxatives or antispasmodic drugs, can directly impact gut motility. They are often used to manage conditions like irritable bowel syndrome (IBS). Certain medical procedures, such as abdominal surgeries, can impact gut motility. Post-operative ileus is a temporary slowing of gut motility after surgery (Reque and Brandelli, 2021).

5.2.1.9 Gastrointestinal Disorders

Conditions like IBS, inflammatory bowel disease (IBD), and gastroparesis can disrupt normal gut motility. In IBS, for example, motility can be either increased or decreased, leading to symptoms like diarrhea or constipation.

5.2.1.10 Antibiotics and Drugs

The use of some drugs and antibiotics can significantly change the composition of the gut microbiota. The impact may differ based on factors like the specific antibiotic used, dosage, method of administration, and the individual's pre-existing microbiota (Silva et al., 2021).

5.2.1.11 Prebiotics

Prebiotics, like dietary fibers and other bioactive substances, can positively impact microbiota of the gut by encouraging the growth of good bacteria and the synthesis of SCFAs (Marco et al., 2021).

5.2.1.12 Bacterial Balance

An imbalance in the gut microbiota, such as enterobacteriaceae, may be the source of digestive complaints and problems with movement (Kim et al., 2021).

5.2.1.13 Age

Gut motility can change with age. In older individuals, it may slow down, leading to constipation. This is partly due to changes in muscle tone and nerve function (Safarimosavi et al., 2021).

5.2.1.14 Hormonal Changes

Hormones such as gastrin, cholecystokinin (CCK), and motilin can stimulate or inhibit gut motility. For example, gastrin promotes stomach motility, while CCK regulates the release of bile from the gallbladder. Hormonal fluctuations, such as those that occur during the menstrual cycle, can affect gut motility in some individuals, leading to changes in bowel habits (Gungor et al., 2021).

5.3 GUT MICROBIOTA AND METABOLISM

The complex link among gut microbiota and human metabolism is characterized by an especially fascinating aspect. This complex interaction between our gut microbiota and metabolic functions has extensive implications for our general well-being. The breakdown of food components, especially complex carbohydrates that the body finds difficult to process, is actively aided by the gut bacteria (Kim et al., 2020). After being absorbed by the bloodstream, SCFAs provide the host with a significant energy source. They are involved in lipid metabolism and energy harvesting. Via a number of pathways, gut bacteria can affect hunger and body weight. For instance, by influencing the brain's appetite centers, the synthesis of certain metabolites, such as SCFAs, may have an impact on the control of hunger. Dysbiosis can lead to increased energy extraction from food and enhanced fat storage, which can contribute to weight gain. Gut microbiota can metabolize dietary components, converting them into bioactive compounds that affect metabolism. For example, the breakdown of polyphenols in plant-based foods can yield metabolites with antioxidant properties. The transformation of dietary proteins can result in the production of bioactive peptides that may influence metabolic processes and have health-promoting effects. The gut microbiome is essential for preserving glucose homeostasis. Enhancement in insulin sensitivity has been associated with SCFAs, namely, butyrate (Jia et al., 2020).

Dysbiosis may disrupt glucose metabolism, raising the risk of type 2 diabetes and insulin resistance, among other illnesses. An unbalanced makeup of the gut microbiota might be a factor in dyslipidemia, a disorder with aberrant lipid profiles that increases the risk of cardiovascular illnesses. Chronic inflammation plays a significant role in metabolic disorders' development, which can be regulated by gut microbiota through anti-inflammatory compound production and maintenance of gut barrier integrity. Dysbiosis may lead to increased inflammation, which can contribute to metabolic syndrome and related conditions. The metabolism of bile acids, which are necessary for the breakdown and absorption of dietary lipids, can be influenced by gut bacteria. Additionally, bile acids have signaling properties. Dysbiosis can alter lipid absorption and metabolism as well as upset the bile acid balance. The makeup and function of the intestinal lining can be altered by gut bacteria, which can affect how well nutrients are absorbed. This may have an impact on how vitamins and minerals, among other nutrients, are absorbed. Entire metabolic health and effective food absorption depend on a healthy gut microbiome (Xie et al., 2020).

5.3.1 Gut Microbiota's Role in Nutrient Metabolism

Within the complex areas of nutritional metabolism, the gut microbiota emerges as a pivotal player as shown in Figure 5.2, profoundly influencing how the human body processes and utilizes essential nutrients. One of the key contributions of our microbial inhabitants is their involvement in the fermentation of dietary components that our own enzymes cannot break down. Complex carbohydrates, such as certain types of dietary fiber and resistant starches, form a substantial part of our diet but remain indigestible by human enzymes. However, our gut microbiota, composed mainly of bacteria residing in the large intestine, possess the necessary tools to ferment these complex carbohydrates (Vernocchi et al., 2020). Additionally, the metabolism of dietary proteins is influenced by the gut bacteria. When we consume proteins, they are initially broken down into peptides and amino acids during digestion. These smaller protein components can serve as substrates for the gut microbiota's metabolic activities. Specific bacteria in our intestines can metabolize amino acids into various bioactive compounds, including biogenic amines and short peptides. Certain metabolites have the ability to affect our systems systemically, affecting things like immune system modulation, blood pressure regulation, and neurotransmitter balance. Consequently, the reputation of the gut microbiota in protein metabolism goes beyond basic digestion and encompasses metabolic control and overall health (Bianchetti et al., 2023).

Moreover, the gut microbiota is closely intertwined with lipid metabolism. Dietary fats, including triglycerides, are subject to microbial modification in the gut. Certain microorganisms are proficient in degrading complex lipids into simpler forms, releasing fatty acids and glycerol. These microbial-derived fatty acids can be absorbed and utilized by our bodies for energy or stored in adipose tissue. Additionally, the gut microbiota's influence on bile acid metabolism is vital for lipid absorption and cholesterol homeostasis. Our gut bacteria influence the absorption and digestion of dietary lipids and cholesterol indirectly through the metabolism of bile acids. Dysregulation of this intricate interplay can lead to metabolic disturbances, including obesity and dyslipidemia. Gut microbiota's involvement in nutrient metabolism extends to carbohydrates, proteins, and lipids, with profound implications for overall metabolic health (Figure 5.1). Nutrient metabolism is crucial for developing strategies to promote metabolic well-being and prevent metabolic disorders, making it an important focus in the field of nutrition and health research (Litvak et al., 2018).

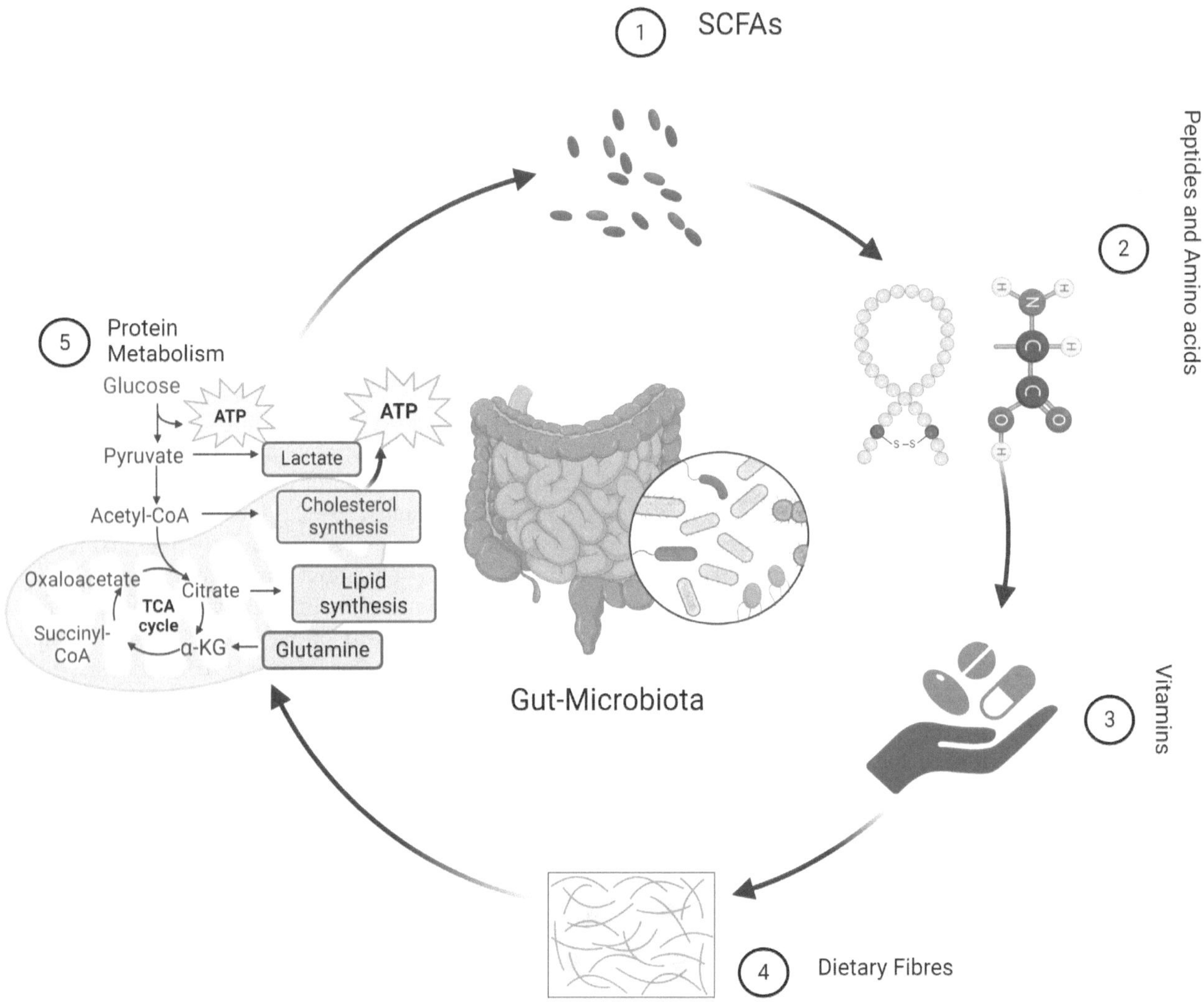

FIGURE 5.1 Gut microbiota's metabolism.

5.3.2 Influence on Energy Regulation

The human body's energy metabolism is significantly regulated by the gut flora. The complex interplay between energy management and gut microbiota has gained a lot of interest in the areas of metabolism, nutrition, and health (Xiao and Kang, 2020).

5.3.3 Caloric Extraction from Diet

The amount of calories that are extracted from the food we eat is greatly influenced by our gut bacteria. When we ingest complex carbohydrates that our own digestive enzymes cannot break down, our gut bacteria step in. They metabolize these complex carbohydrates into simpler, absorbable molecules. This microbial fermentation process releases additional calories from our food, contributing to our overall caloric intake. This caloric extraction can be a double-edged sword. Although it might provide the host more energy, if the balance between calorie intake and expenditure is thrown off, it can also lead to weight gain and obesity (Ma et al., 2020).

5.3.4 Regulation of Appetite

Through a variety of processes, the gut flora affects our hunger and feelings of fullness. Bioactive substances like SCFAs, which have an impact on the gut–brain axis, are produced by gut bacteria. These substances modulate our experience of hunger and fullness by sending messages to the brain. Furthermore, the microbial ecology in the gut can generate signaling molecules that influence the release of hunger-controlling hormones like leptin and ghrelin. These signaling pathways may be disrupted by changes in the gut flora, which might result in binge eating and weight gain (Pizarroso et al., 2021).

5.3.5 Energy Storage and Fat Accumulation

Extra energy is stored in the form of fat by the gut flora. Triglycerides accumulate in adipose tissue as a result of certain bacteria that are connected to obtaining more energy from the food. Furthermore, the gut microbiota's impact on absorbing dietary fats and controlling lipogenesis (the generation of fats) can contribute to fat accumulation. When energy intake consistently surpasses energy expenditure, additional calories are stored in adipocytes, leading to an increase in weight and obesity (Schoeler and Caesar, 2019).

5.3.6 Mitochondrial Function and Energy Expenditure

The gut microbiota can affect not only caloric intake and storage but also energy expenditure. Mitochondria play a crucial role as the energy producers in our cells, responsible for producing adenosine triphosphate, which serves as the primary source of energy in the human body. Disruptions in mitochondrial function can affect overall energy expenditure. Some gut microbes produce metabolites that support mitochondrial function, while others can hinder it. As such, the makeup of our gut microbiota can affect our resting metabolic rate as well as how much energy we use when exercising (Rath et al., 2018).

5.4 DYSBIOSIS AND METABOLIC DISORDERS

The complex and delicate balance between humans and their gut microbiota represents a complex relationship that significantly affects various aspects of health. Growing evidence is pointing to the role of dysbiosis, or an alteration in the typical makeup of the gut microbial community, in the development of metabolic diseases (Aron-Wisnewsky et al., 2021). An interesting finding regarding obesity is the disrupted ratio between two major bacterial groups: Firmicutes and Bacteroidetes. Obese people frequently have a higher ratio of Firmicutes to Bacteroidetes, which has been associated with better calorie absorption from diet because of enhanced energy extraction capacities. On the contrary, a more even balance between these groups is associated with better metabolic outcomes.

Moreover, the gut microbiota's role in metabolic conditions goes beyond just obesity. Type 2 diabetes, a common metabolic disorder distinguished by high blood sugar levels and resistance to insulin, has also been associated with imbalances in gut microorganisms. This association underscores the systemic influence of gut microbes on host metabolism, and it challenges the traditional understanding of metabolic diseases primarily as genetic or lifestyle-driven conditions. As researchers delve deeper into this relationship, various mechanisms through which dysbiosis impacts metabolic health have come to light. Dysbiotic gut microbiota can result in microbial translocation, which is the passage of bacterial fragments or even whole germs across the intestinal barrier and into the bloodstream. This disorder causes pro-inflammatory reactions, which worsen metabolic illnesses. LPS found in bacterial cell walls are crucial to this process because they bind to host cell receptors such TLR-4, which exacerbates insulin resistance and inflammation (Montanari et al., 2021).

Dysbiosis-induced intestinal barrier weakness might compromise its strength of the intestinal epithelial layer and allow more germs to enter the body. This compromised intestinal barrier is linked to inflammation in metabolic regions such as the pancreas, liver, and adipose tissue. Moreover, dysbiotic conditions can disturb the equilibrium of T helper 17 cells, an essential type of immune cell for preserving intestinal defense and stability. A decreased population of Th17 cells in the gut due to altered microbiota interactions with antigen-presenting cells has been observed. This immune dysregulation further compromises mucosal barrier integrity, exacerbating inflammation and metabolic disorders (Régnier et al., 2021).

In addition to dietary modifications, postbiotics, which are bioactive compounds produced by gut bacteria, offer potential therapeutic value. Harnessing the metabolic products of beneficial bacteria could provide a novel approach to mitigating inflammation and insulin resistance associated with metabolic disorders. Targeting bacterial recognition and translocation processes represents another avenue for intervention. Strategies that focus on preventing microbial translocation and its subsequent pro-inflammatory effects could hold promise as therapeutic interventions for metabolic disorders. The modulation of host immune responses to bacterial fragments, such as LPS, may be explored to mitigate inflammation and insulin resistance (Genua et al., 2021).

Additionally, the host's nutrient-sensing receptors are essential for modulating reactions to microbial changes (Braunsdorf et al., 2016). When dietary fibers ferment, microbiological byproducts known as SCFAs are created. These fatty acids have interactions with GPR41 and GPR43, two host receptors. The releasing of gut hormones is impacted by this interaction. Insulin secretion, stomach emptying, and calorie intake are all regulated by these hormones. Targeting these receptors with agonists could have a profound impact on metabolic health. The modulation of other nutrient-sensing receptors, including GPR119 and nuclear farnesoid X receptor (FXR), also holds potential for therapeutic interventions. For example, GPR119 is known to mediate glucose-induced insulin secretion and the release of gut hormones that influence metabolic regulation. Manipulating these receptors to enhance insulin signaling and improve metabolic outcomes represents a promising direction in metabolic disorder research. Research in the dynamic field of the relationship between imbalance in gut bacteria and metabolic conditions presents promising opportunities for novel therapeutic approaches. The future of metabolic disorder therapies may well be shaped by dietary modifications, microbiota-targeted interventions, and the development of new pharmaceutical agents aimed at modulating nutrient-sensing receptors and immune responses. As research in this area continues to advance, it brings hope for improved outcomes and enhanced well-being for individuals living with metabolic disorders (Karl, 2021).

5.4.1 Understanding Dysbiosis

The intricate and fragile equilibrium between humans and their gut microbiota is a mutually beneficial relationship that influences different aspects of health. Recent discoveries have brought this complex relationship to light, especially when it comes to the impact, dysbiosis plays in metabolic diseases (Choi et al., 2021).

The large community of microbes termed as the "gut microbiota" that inhabit the human digestive tract is made up primarily of bacteria, but it also contains viruses, fungi, archaea, and other microbes. Their variety and structure are crucial to maintaining health because these bacteria influence the host's physiological processes and metabolism, control the immune system, and facilitate food absorption. An intriguing observation related to obesity is the imbalanced proportion between two major bacterial groups: Firmicutes and Bacteroidetes. Individuals with obesity often exhibit an elevated ratio of Firmicutes to Bacteroidetes. This alteration has been associated with an increased ability to extract energy from food intake leading to heightened calorie absorption and contributing to weight gain. In contrast, a more balanced ratio of these phyla is associated with healthier metabolic outcomes (Hrncir, 2022).

Metabolic issues are related to the gut microbiota in addition to obesity. This relationship calls into question the prevalent wisdom that metabolic illnesses are predominantly caused by hereditary or lifestyle factors and emphasizes the wider influence of gut bacteria on host metabolism (Stolfi et al., 2022). Various methods via which dysbiosis affects metabolic health have emerged as researchers continue to explore this link. An imbalanced gut microbiota can result in microbial translocation, where fragments of bacteria and sometimes entire microorganisms breach the intestinal barrier and move into the bloodstream. This event initiates inflammatory reactions and worsens metabolic disorders. Bacterial cell walls include LPS, which are essential because they bind to host cell receptors such as TLR-4 and cause inflammation and resistance to insulin (Clerbaux et al., 2022).

Gut barrier dysfunction, caused by an unbalanced gut microbiota, can result from dysbiosis and impair the barrier that protects the intestinal epithelial cells. This makes it simpler for bacterial components to get through the barrier. The intestinal barrier's weakened state aggravates a number of inflammatory processes within metabolic organs, including the pancreas, liver, and adipose tissue (Stolfi et al., 2022). Dysbiotic circumstances can also upset the equilibrium of T helper 17 (Th17) cells, a group of immune cells involved in intestine defense and integrity. A decreased population of Th17 cells in the gut due to altered microbiota interactions with antigen-presenting cells has been observed. This immune dysregulation further compromises mucosal barrier integrity, exacerbating inflammation and metabolic disorders (Schreurs et al., 2021).

It's interesting to note that the gut microbiota has an impact on the synthesis of interleukin-22. Decreases in IL-22 levels associated with dysbiosis may affect the host's defenses against pathogenic microbes and integrity of the gut barrier (Schreiber et al., 2015). These complex relationships between metabolic diseases and dysbiosis of the gut microbiota provide opportunities for various treatment approaches. One possible strategy is dietary therapy, which includes the consumption of prebiotics and probiotics in order to restore microbial equilibrium. Prebiotics and probiotics can both help change the composition of the gut microbiota and improve metabolic outcomes. In addition to dietary modifications, postbiotics, which are bioactive compounds produced by gut bacteria, offer potential therapeutic value. Harnessing the metabolic products of beneficial bacteria could provide a novel approach to mitigating inflammation and insulin resistance associated with metabolic disorders.

Targeting bacterial recognition and translocation processes represents another avenue for intervention. Strategies that focus on preventing microbial translocation and its subsequent pro-inflammatory effects could hold promise as therapeutic interventions for metabolic disorders. The modulation of host immune responses to bacterial fragments, such as LPS, may be explored to mitigate inflammation and insulin resistance (Boutriq et al., 2021).

Receptors for host nutrients are also essential for reacting to alterations brought on by microbes. Dietary fibers include SCFAs, which interact with certain host receptors like GPR41 and GPR43 to influence the manufacture of gut hormones including peptide YY and glucagon-like peptide-1. Insulin secretion, stomach emptying, and calorie intake are all regulated by these hormones. The health of the metabolism may be significantly affected by using agonists that target these receptors (Shimizu et al., 2019).

The modulation of other nutrient-sensing receptors, including GPR119 and nuclear FXR, also holds potential for therapeutic interventions. For example, GPR119 is known to mediate glucose-induced insulin secretion and the release of gut hormones that influence metabolic regulation. Manipulating these receptors to enhance insulin signaling and improve metabolic outcomes represents a promising direction in metabolic disorder research (Tanes et al., 2021).

Despite being in its early stages of investigation, the complicated connection between metabolic diseases and gut microbial dysbiosis has great potential for innovative treatment methods. The future of metabolic disorder therapies may well be shaped by dietary modifications, microbiota-targeted interventions, and the development of new pharmaceutical agents aimed at modulating nutrient-sensing receptors and immune responses. As research in this area continues to advance, it brings hope for improved outcomes and enhanced well-being for individuals living with metabolic disorders (Giovannini et al., 2021).

5.4.2 Linking Dysbiosis to Metabolic Disorders

The connection between dysbiosis and metabolic disorders is shedding light on potential therapeutic interventions and dietary strategies to mitigate these health issues (Scannapieco et al., 2021).

- Obesity: One of the main metabolic disorders, obesity, has been linked to dysbiosis. When a person is obese, their body produces more potentially dangerous bacteria (like Firmicutes) than good bacteria (like Bifidobacterium and Lactobacillus). The changed microbiota in the gut may have an impact on fat accumulation and energy metabolism. Dysbiosis can cause the body to absorb more energy from food and encourage the buildup of fat, both of which are factors in obesity.

- Dietary Factors: Food selections may either promote a healthy balance in the gut microbiota or cause an imbalance. Diet has a significant influence on this composition. A diet rich in vegetables, fruits, fiber, and whole grains is linked with a more beneficial and diverse gut flora. These dietary factors can either protect against or increase the risk of metabolic disorders.
- Therapeutic Potential: The link between dysbiosis and metabolic disorders has opened up potential therapeutic strategies. The potential of probiotics—beneficial living bacteria—to help restore a balanced gut microbiota has been studied. Probiotics have the potential to help with weight management and glucose regulation, as well as to balance the composition of gut flora and decrease inflammation. Additionally, dietary interventions, such as prebiotics (food for beneficial bacteria) and a high-fiber diet, can support a healthier gut microbiota.
- Personalized Medicine: Acknowledging the unique characteristics of gut microbiota and its link to metabolic well-being, personalized medical strategies are under investigation. Evaluating the makeup and functioning of a person's gut microbiota may help tailor nutritional plans and probiotic regimens to address certain metabolic issues.

5.5 MECHANISMS OF GUT MICROBIOTA IN METABOLIC REGULATION

It is well known that the microbiota of the human gut is made up of a wide variety of bacteria and plays a critical role in regulating metabolism. These microbes engage in interactions with the host and contribute to several facets of the equilibrium of metabolism (Li et al., 2022).

5.5.1 Energy Metabolism

Gut microbiota facilitates the breakdown of complex carbohydrates and plant polysaccharides that are otherwise indigestible by human enzymes. The absorbed SCFAs can influence appetite and energy expenditure. A dysfunction in the gut flora known as dysbiosis is linked to an increased ability to get energy from meals. This may result in greater accumulation of energy stores in the form of fat tissue, contributing to obesity. Dysbiosis can also interfere with hormonal signals that regulate hunger and fullness. Metabolites and components derived from microbes, such as LPS, have the potential to trigger inflammation and disrupt insulin signaling pathways. Furthermore, the production of SCFAs by gut bacteria is important in controlling blood glucose levels. These SCFAs act as messengers by binding to specific receptors and are able to improve sensitivity to insulin in peripheral tissues (Li et al., 2022).

5.5.2 Microbiota-Host Crosstalk

The gut microbiota generates various bioactive molecules, including neurotransmitters, secondary bile acids, and endocannabinoids. These metabolites can have systemic effects on host metabolism (Fan et al., 2022).

5.5.3 Dietary and Lifestyle Influences

Consuming dietary fiber, which is fermented by gut bacteria into SCFAs, can promote a healthy gut microbiota and support metabolic regulation. Probiotics, or good live bacteria, and prebiotics, or substances that promote the growth of healthy microorganisms, can shift the gut microbiota and perhaps improve metabolic health (Zhang et al., 2021).

5.5.4 Gut Microbiota's Impact on Metabolism

Dysbiosis can disrupt the hormonal signaling related to hunger and satiety. Dysbiosis is linked to insulin resistance, a trait that characterizes type 2 diabetes. LPS, a metabolite and component generated by microbes, can cause inflammation and interfere with insulin signaling pathways. The gut bacteria's production of SCFAs is essential for maintaining glucose homeostasis. Some gut bacteria can influence hepatic gluconeogenesis, the process of glucose production in the liver. Dysbiosis can lead to elevated glucose production, contributing to hyperglycemia (Tomasova et al., 2021).

5.5.5 Lipid Metabolism

Bile acids are required for fat breakdown and absorption. Dysbiosis can disrupt bile acid metabolism, potentially affecting fat absorption (Brown et al., 2023). Specific gut bacteria are involved in cholesterol metabolism, impacting host cholesterol levels. Reducing the absorption of cholesterol is possible by some microorganisms that encourage the transformation of cholesterol to coprostanol, which is expelled in feces. Low-grade inflammation brought on by dysbiosis has been linked to changed lipid profiles. Triglycerides, high-density lipoprotein (HDL), and low-density lipoprotein (LDL) levels are all impacted by inflammatory pathways that are regulated by gut microbes.

Inflammation and metabolic issues can arise from bacteria like LPS entering the bloodstream due to a breached barrier. Systemic inflammation is influenced by the way gut bacteria interact with the immune system of the host. An ongoing, low-grade inflammatory response is a typical sign of metabolic diseases (Brown et al., 2023). The gut microbiota generates various bioactive molecules, including neurotransmitters, secondary bile acids, and endocannabinoids. These metabolites can have systemic effects on host metabolism. Consuming dietary fiber, which is fermented by gut bacteria into SCFAs, can promote a healthy gut microbiota and support metabolic regulation (Litvak et al., 2018).

Probiotic and prebiotic compounds may be able to modify the gut flora, perhaps improving metabolic health. Hormones that control hunger and energy balance, including ghrelin, leptin, and peptide YY, are secreted in different amounts depending on the gut flora. Changes in hunger and satiety can result from dysbiosis, which can interfere with these hormonal cues. LPS, a molecule and component generated by microbes, can cause inflammation and disrupt insulin signaling pathways.

When SCFAs bind to G-protein-coupled receptors (GPCRs), they function as signaling molecules generated by gut bacteria. They can enhance insulin sensitivity in peripheral tissues, contributing to improved glucose homeostasis. Certain gut bacteria influence hepatic gluconeogenesis, the production of glucose in the liver. Dysbiosis can lead to increased glucose production, resulting in elevated blood sugar levels.

5.5.6 Role of Gut-Derived Metabolites

The fermentation and metabolism of dietary ingredients that have not yet been fully digested, producing a variety of bioactive substances known as "gut-derived metabolites." Among the gut-derived metabolites that have been studied the most are SCFAs. SCFAs have a variety of effects on metabolic regulation. They give the colon's cells energy and have been connected to better glucose and insulin balance. Specifically, butyrate has demonstrated potential in improving the intestinal barrier's performance, lowering inflammation, and affecting the control of hunger. SCFAs can influence host metabolism through interactions with many host cell receptors, such as GPCRs and epigenetic modifications (Gesper et al., 2021).

Bile acids—metabolites produced in the liver and broken down by the gut microbiota—are the building blocks of secondary bile acid production. These secondary bile acids activate important receptors such as the FXR and the Takeda GPCR, which in turn influence lipid and glucose balance in metabolism, according to research. Cardiovascular health can be impacted by the makeup of bile acids in the stomach, which can alter triglyceride and cholesterol levels and disturb homeostasis (Kim et al., 2021). The gut flora affects the production of various neuromodulators and neurotransmitters. The gut–brain axis, which promotes interaction between the CNS and the digestive system, depends on these chemicals. Changes in production of these have been connected to mental health issues and mood disorders (Kim et al., 2021). Furthermore, gut-derived metabolites like LPS and endocannabinoids have gained attention for their impact on inflammation and metabolic health. Endocannabinoids produced by gut microbes may influence appetite, energy balance, and lipid metabolism (Zheng et al., 2022).

Comprehending the ways in which these molecules impact energy balance, glucose control, lipid metabolism, and even mental health, among other elements of metabolism, has great significance for the creation of innovative treatments for metabolic illnesses. Targeted interventions, such as dietary modifications, probiotics, and prebiotics, aim to modulate the production of specific gut-derived metabolites, offering potential avenues for preventing and managing conditions like obesity, type 2 diabetes, and cardiovascular disease (Glorieux et al., 2020).

Metabolites produced in the digestive system also contribute to immune regulation. The intestines are a crucial location for immune system interaction, and the metabolites that gut bacteria create greatly influence the regulation of immunological responses. Butyrate, for instance, exhibits anti-inflammatory characteristics and aids in preserving the equilibrium of immune cells within the gut, thereby decreasing susceptibility to IBD. The capacity of gut bacteria to transform food ingredients into bioactive metabolites offers several health advantages. For example, flavonoids, which are present in fruits and vegetables, can be changed into smaller phenolic compounds with improved bioavailability and possible health benefits by certain gut flora. The stomach is also necessary for metabolism and the absorption of nutrients. Metabolites originating from the gut may impact the body's capacity to absorb essential nutrients, such as minerals and vitamins (Glorieux et al., 2020).

5.6 THERAPEUTIC STRATEGIES

5.6.1 Modulating Gut Microbiota for Metabolic Health

There are various methods for modifying gut microorganisms to improve metabolic health. These strategies include lifestyle and medical interventions. Healthy diets such as intermittent fasting and regular exercise have become effective means of positively impacting the gut microorganisms and, in turn, improving metabolic health (Longo et al., 2023). There are a few more techniques in addition to these lifestyle adjustments:

1. **Probiotics**: Live bacteria known as probiotics have health advantages when ingested in appropriate amounts. Studies have identified particular strains of probiotics that can augment the microbial community and variety in the gastrointestinal tract while diminishing inflammation, ultimately resulting in enhanced metabolic well-being.
2. **Prebiotics**: Prebiotics are dietary fibers that are not digested and aid in the growth of beneficial gut flora. Consuming prebiotics has been shown to have a positive impact on the diversity and makeup of the gut microbiota, as well as to lessen inflammation and support metabolic health.
3. **Fecal Microbiota Transplantation (FMT)**: Fecal microbiota transplantation is a process that involves moving fecal matter from a donor to a recipient in order to balance the gut microbiota. Originally intended for addressing specific gastrointestinal conditions, FMT is now under investigation for its possible role in improving metabolic well-being.

4. **Antibiotics**: Antibiotics can be selectively used to target and eliminate pathogenic bacteria within the gut microbiota. However, it is crucial to exercise caution in their use, as overuse can lead to dysbiosis, potentially having adverse effects on metabolic health (Zhang et al., 2023).

These techniques provide a variety of ways to influence gut microbiota with the ultimate aim of enhancing metabolic health. It's interesting to note that bariatric surgery can change the makeup of the gut microbiota and improve metabolic health. Dietary therapies like the Mediterranean-style diet have shown promise in fostering a more diversified and favorable gut flora. To ascertain the long-term safety and efficacy of these treatments, further research is needed, underscoring the ongoing progress of our understanding in this complex field (Longo et al., 2023).

5.6.2 Dietary Interventions

The interaction between diet interventions and the microbiote of the intestine is an increasingly important topic in metabolic health. An abundant ecology of bacteria resides in the digestive tract's intestinal microbes. This complex network of organisms plays a crucial part in the breakdown of nutrients, generating various chemical compounds that impact human metabolism and triggering host responses that regulate essential bodily functions. One important finding from 2004 that emphasized the significance of the intestinal microbe in influencing host energy capture and energy storage is the fundamental knowledge of its mechanical participation in maintaining metabolic balance (Bäckhed et al., 2004). Intestinal bacteria have a significant potential to influence metabolic diseases, as demonstrated by developments in bioinformatics and microbiome sequencing over the next several years (Fan and Pedersen, 2021).

Both host traits and environmental conditions affect the gut microbiota's robustness and functionality. Lifestyle choices, particularly dietary habits, emerge as critical modifiers of the gut microbiota, contributing collectively to either a state of health or disease (Le Chatelier et al., 2013). In a state of health, there is typically a harmonious balance between the Bacteroidetes and Firmicutes phyla, which yields the production of beneficial metabolites essential for health. Bacteroidetes bacteria are often found in lower concentrations and Firmicutes bacteria in larger concentrations in individuals with metabolic problems. This imbalance has been associated with increased intestinal permeability, less diversity in gut flora, and lower production of SCFAs as compared to those without these problems (Qin et al., 2012).

Intermittent Fasting (IF): This diet intervention pattern targets a specific fasting period, which takes between a few hours and a few days and minimizes or eliminates the amount of calories. In recent years, the IF has attracted considerable attention and has been described as a potentially transformative paradigm for improving general health (Vasim et al., 2022). Different models of specific IF diet include limited feeding (TRF), alternate-day fasting (ADF), and 5:2 strategies (Dong et al., 2020). You have the option to select a fast lasting 16 hours with a period of 8 hours for nutrition, a 20-hour fast with a 4-hour window for nutrition, or other comparable variations in TRF. ADF, on the other hand, involves a 24-hour fast period, in which only 25% of the daily intake of energy is consumed, followed by a 24-hour eating period, which can be repeated several times a week. The 5:2 strategy includes two fast days and five non-restrictive days. Significantly, intermittent fasting triggers adaptive alterations in the body's metabolic, endocrine, and nervous systems to enhance overall physical performance and behavior. Numerous studies conducted over varying time periods consistently demonstrate the strong effectiveness of intermittent fasting in modifying disease outcomes by leveraging its interaction with gut microbiota (Guo et al., 2021). Beneficial gut microorganisms linked to health have regularly grown as a result of interventions, producing useful fermentation byproducts including lactate and acetate. These changes have led to a dramatic improvement in diseases such as hepatic steatosis, obesity, and insulin resistance (Li et al., 2017).

Mediterranean Diet: A remarkable dietary intervention strategy associated with more diverse and beneficial intestinal microorganisms is Mediterranean diet. Studies consistently demonstrate that following this dietary pattern contributes to an increase in microbial diversity and beneficial bacteria like bifidobacteria and lactobacillus. Simultaneously, it decreases potentially harmful bacteria such as Fusobacterium and Clostridium. Furthermore, following the Mediterranean diet has been linked to better metabolic health outcomes, such as a lower risk of obesity (Longo et al., 2023).

Low-Carbohydrate Diet: Another dietary strategy that merits attention is the low-carbohydrate diet. This approach restricts carbohydrate intake and emphasizes higher protein and fat consumption. Research has unveiled the potential of a low-carbohydrate diet to enhance gut microbiota diversity and reduce inflammation, ultimately leading to improvements in metabolic health. These effects encompass enhanced insulin sensitivity, reduced blood glucose levels, and improved lipid profiles. However, it is crucial to stress that research on the long-term reliability and effectiveness of low-carb diets is still underway (Longo et al., 2023).

High-Fiber Diet: The consumption of a high-fiber diet, rich in fiber-laden foods, also serves as a valuable dietary intervention. Research underscores the capacity of a high-fiber diet to bolster gut microbiota diversity while reducing inflammation, ultimately contributing to improved metabolic health. These advantages include lower blood glucose levels, better lipid profiles, and increased insulin sensitivity (Zhang et al., 2023). The evolving landscape of dietary interventions and their interactions with the gut microbiota presents a promising avenue for improving metabolic health and mitigating the risk of metabolic disorders. With ongoing research efforts, these dietary strategies may hold the key to fostering a balanced gut microbiota and optimizing metabolic well-being, thereby making strides in addressing one of the most pressing health challenges of our era.

5.6.3 Fecal Microbiota Transplantation and Other Therapies

5.6.3.1 Fecal Microbiota Transplantation

Transplanting fecal microbiota is being investigated extensively as a possible therapeutic option. In an attempt to reestablish a varied and harmonious balance of gut bacteria, fecal matter transplantation (FMT) transfers the feces of healthy donors to recipients. Numerous illnesses, including recurring Clostridium difficile infections, IBD, and other gastrointestinal problems, have been demonstrated to respond well to this therapy. Researchers are exploring different aspects of FMT including donor selection criteria, optimal delivery methods, safety considerations, and its effectiveness in addressing other health issues beyond gastrointestinal diseases. According to recent research, FMT may be a novel strategy for enhancing general gut health and perhaps treating a number of illnesses linked to disruptions in the balance of gut microbiota (Nowakowski et al., 2016).

The prevalence of obesity and type 2 diabetes is rising globally, endangering public health. Subgroup analysis and a single-variable meta-regression were carried out to look into possible causes of heterogeneity. Furthermore, researchers evaluated potential publication biases using the Egger test. The meta-analysis included data from nine studies involving a total of 303 participants. In the short term, specifically less than 6 weeks after undergoing FMT, patients in the FMT group exhibited decreased levels of glucose, glucose hemoglobin, and insulin in their blood compared to those in the placebo groups. Conversely, higher levels of HDL cholesterol were seen in the FMT group compared to the placebo group. These findings indicate that adjunct therapy with FMT is generally well-tolerated without causing significant adverse effects and holds promise for improving metabolic syndrome treatment outcomes. Although it has the potential to reduce HbA1c levels, improve insulin sensitivity, and raise HDL cholesterol levels, there were no discernible changes in weight reduction between the FMT and placebo groups (Qiu et al., 2023).

It is yet unclear how gut microbiota transfers affect intestinal bacterial development in people with metabolic syndrome. To get a deeper comprehension of FMT's effectiveness as a treatment for obesity and metabolic syndrome, a second comprehensive review utilizing meta-analysis has been conducted. FMT appears to provide potential benefits for individuals who are overweight and have high blood pressure, poor insulin and glucose control, and elevated blood lipid levels. Subsequent studies will likely focus on exploring metabolic aspects in obese patients to achieve a deeper comprehension of the potential benefits of FMT in this context (Zecheng et al., 2023).

Although prior studies have indicated the promise of FMT as a therapy strategy for type 2 diabetes (T2D), little is known about its underlying mechanism. The results showed that FMT improved hyperlipidemia and hyperglycemia levels, which had therapeutic benefits on T2D. Through analysis of 16S rRNA sequences and serum untargeted metabolic profiles, it was discovered that FMT restored imbalances within the gastrointestinal microbiota in T2DM mice. Moreover, certain molecules such as corticosterone, progesterone, and L-urine emerged as biomarkers following FMT treatment. According to bioinformatics analysis, the production of steroid hormones, the breakdown of arginine and proline, and the creation of unsaturated fatty acids could potentially act as regulatory mechanisms for FMT. In conclusion, this research presents substantial evidence that supports the therapeutic role of FMT in treating T2D. FMT shows promise as a viable approach for addressing metabolic disorders, T2D, and associated complications (Yang et al., 2023).

Antibiotic therapy is crucial to the treatment of infections, but it can disrupt a common bacterial population and increase the risk of subsequent disease, resulting in intestinal microbiosis as a potential contributor. In the study, scientists detailed the analysis of fecal samples and compared healthy people with sepsis patients. Patients with severe infections have a markedly different intestinal microbiota composition from healthy persons. This difference is both in pattern level and abundance, suggesting that Firmicutes are greatly decreased and Proteobacteria are overabundant. In order to investigate potential therapeutic approaches, researchers utilized a mouse model of sepsis induced by ventricular binding and puncture (known as CLP). Mice with imbalances in their gut microbial community have an increased susceptibility to death, inflammation, and organ dysfunction. Nevertheless, by controlling the number of particular bacterial species to levels similar to those observed in healthy mice, the injection of FMT and SCFA has been able to successfully attenuate these detrimental outcomes. Furthermore, FMT and SCFAs downregulate the expression of NLRP3 and GSDMD-N proteins while upregulating the expression of important intestinal proteins such as occludin. Finally, by inhibiting cell pyroptosis and lowering the synthesis of pro-inflammatory chemicals like IL-1 and IL-18, this has a protective effect against sepsis. These findings demonstrate the possibility of FMT and SCFA as effective therapies for sepsis, which in mice models promote beneficial microbe survival in this potentially fatal illness (Lou et al., 2022).

Although earlier research has shown that FMT is effective in treating T2DM patients' conditions, little is known about the specific processes behind this therapy strategy. This work clarified the effects and processes of FMT in T2DM by a thorough analysis utilizing a mouse model. When FMT was given to diabetic mice, a number of clinical markers improved, including serum insulin levels, oral glucose tolerance, and fasting plasma glucose. The study delved into the GM and serum metabolome using advanced techniques, revealing specific alterations in microbial taxa and metabolites associated with FMT. Correlation analysis demonstrated a link between structural GM changes and host metabolite levels. Furthermore, FMT has been shown to lessen inflammation, enhance the function of the gut barrier, and regulate the amount of immune cells in the bloodstream. All things considered, these data highlight the complex function that FMT plays in type 2 diabetes (T2DM), all being critical to its therapeutic effectiveness in halting the disease's progression (Chen et al., 2023).

5.6.3.2 Emerging Therapies

An increasing amount of research indicates that combining exercise with intermittent fasting (IF) presents a viable strategy for modifying gut microbiota for better metabolic health.

5.6.3.2.1 Effects of Intermittent Fasting on Gut Microbiota

Intermittent fasting has consistently demonstrated its ability to reshape the composition of gut microbes, promoting a healthier microbial ecosystem. Preclinical studies have revealed several notable findings:

- *Akkermansia muciniphila and Lactobacillus Bloom*: IF leads to a significant increase in Akkermansia muciniphila and Lactobacillus, which are associated with metabolic benefits (Cignarella et al., 2018). *A. muciniphila* has been linked to lowering the inflammation of illnesses caused by energy deficiencies, and disorders including hyperlipidemia, diabetes type 2, and fat liver are positively correlated with the low abundance of these microbes (Fan and Pedersen, 2021).
- *Reduction in Pro-Inflammatory Taxa*: Desulfovibrio and Turicibacter, two pro-inflammatory bacteria, are reduced by IF, which helps to create a less inflammatory gut environment.
- *Enhanced Antioxidative Microbial Metabolic Pathways*: IF enhances antioxidative microbial metabolic pathways, further promoting metabolic health (Cignarella et al., 2018).
- *Fasting-Induced Adipocyte Factor (FIAF)*: When fasting, lipoprotein lipase is significantly regulated by FIAF. The expression of FIAF is increased by probiotics. This enhances lipid metabolism and fortifies the body's defenses against diet-induced obesity (Wang et al., 2022).
- *Gut Epithelial Integrity*: According to a report, IF enhances the integrity of the intestinal epithelium, minimizing lipopolysaccharide (LPS) leakage and lowering systemic inflammation (Zhang et al., 2020). During fasting, this metabolic "switch" improves gut health and energy balance (Wang and Wu, 2022).
- *Circadian Rhythm Coordination*: Correctly executed fasting can synchronize the circadian rhythm's adaptive responses, including the suprachiasmatic nucleus in the brain and peripheral genetic clocks in many organs (Kaczmarek et al., 2017). Disrupted activity-rest cycles contribute to metabolic perturbations (Longo and Panda, 2016).
- *Intermittent Fasting and Liver Metabolism*: A decrease in hepatic glycogen and an increase in lipolysis caused by IF might result in the generation of β-hydroxybutyrate (β-HB). (Cignarella et al., 2018). β-HB is a crucial signaling mediator involved in various cellular functions, including lipolysis, oxidative stress, and metabolic homeostasis (Wang et al., 2021).
- *Metabolic Effects*: Fasting inhibits weight gain, increases energy expenditure by triggering non-shivering heat production in brown adipose tissue, and affects the expression of genes, surface cell receptors, and histone modifications (Moraes et al., 2017).

5.6.3.2.2 Influence of Physical Exercise on Gut Microbiota

Physical exercise is another integral component in the quest for better metabolic health, and its impact on gut microbiota cannot be understated:

- *Reduction in Obesity*: Regular and moderate physical activity is especially important for obese individuals to improve gut bacteria diversity and lower their risk of weight gain. This has led to favorable changes in the Firmicutes to Bacteroidetes ratio, which is closely associated with obesity (Evans et al., 2014).
- *Improving Gut Microbiota Composition*: Physical activity, such as endurance training, increases the number of butyrate-regulating bacterial species and stimulates the synthesis of propionate, butyrate, and acetate, among other SCFAs (Allen et al., 2018). These changes contribute to a healthier gut microbiota.
- *Impact on T2D*: Exercise has been linked to increases in insulin sensitivity and a decreased incidence of type 2 diabetes (T2D). As a result, the gut microbiota's makeup changes, favoring beneficial bacteria groups while suppressing pro-inflammatory ones (Motiani et al., 2020). Different intensities of exercise result in varying effects on specific gut microbiota groups (Torquati et al., 2023).
- *Addressing NAFLD*: Exercise has a beneficial effect on NAFLD via controlling inflammation, insulin sensitivity, and lipid metabolism. The integrity of the gut-liver axis is maintained by the enrichment of protective microbiota brought about by exercise (Abdelbasset et al., 2020).
- *Managing CVDs*: Cardiovascular diseases (CVDs) are linked to the gut microbiota. Regular exercise can enhance cardiovascular health by lowering triglyceride levels, improving endothelial function, and supporting a healthy gut microbiota (Lanter et al., 2014; Patel et al., 2015).

5.6.3.2.3 Synergy of Intermittent Fasting and Physical Exercise

The combined approach of intermittent fasting and physical exercise holds great promise for optimizing metabolic health. Experimental evidence has demonstrated several positive outcomes when both interventions are integrated:

- *Improved Metabolic Parameters*: Exercise and intermittent fasting work together to increase metabolic markers, such as glucose tolerance, to an exceptional degree. AMPK activity and GLUT4 protein expression play roles in this enhanced effect (Basilio et al., 2020).
- *Reducing Intrahepatic Triglycerides*: When aerobic exercise is combined with ADF, it can successfully lower intrahepatic triglycerides in people with NAFLD and obesity (Ezpeleta et al., 2023).
- *Altering Lipid Levels*: Fasting and physical activity combined have a considerable influence on lipid levels. For example, engaging in high-intensity interval exercise while fasting results in a notable decrease in body fat (Martínez-Rodríguez et al., 2021).
- *Favorable Effects on Fat-Free Mass*: In diet-induced obese mice, high-intensity interval training in conjunction with intermittent fasting decreases weight growth and enhances fat-free mass (Batitucci et al., 2022).

5.6.3.2.4 Uncharted Territory: The Gut Microbiota in the Synergy of IF and Physical Exercise

While the individual effects of intermittent fasting and physical exercise on gut microbiota are well-documented, their synergy remains an area of ongoing exploration. Some animal experiments have suggested that combining these interventions may lead to shifts in specific bacterial populations, but the broader implications for gut health and metabolic outcomes require further investigation (Figure 5.2) (Soares et al., 2021). Combining intermittent fasting with physical activity presents a comprehensive approach to regulating the gut microbiota and enhancing metabolic wellness. A fuller comprehension of the synergistic processes and their uses for clinical practice are predicted as this field of study advances. Table 5.1 demonstrates the summary of the advantages and disadvantages of various therapeutic strategies for metabolic health, including modulating the gut microbiota, dietary interventions, intermittent fasting, the Mediterranean diet, low-carbohydrate diet, high-fiber diet, Fecal Microbiota Transplantation (FMT), and antibiotics.

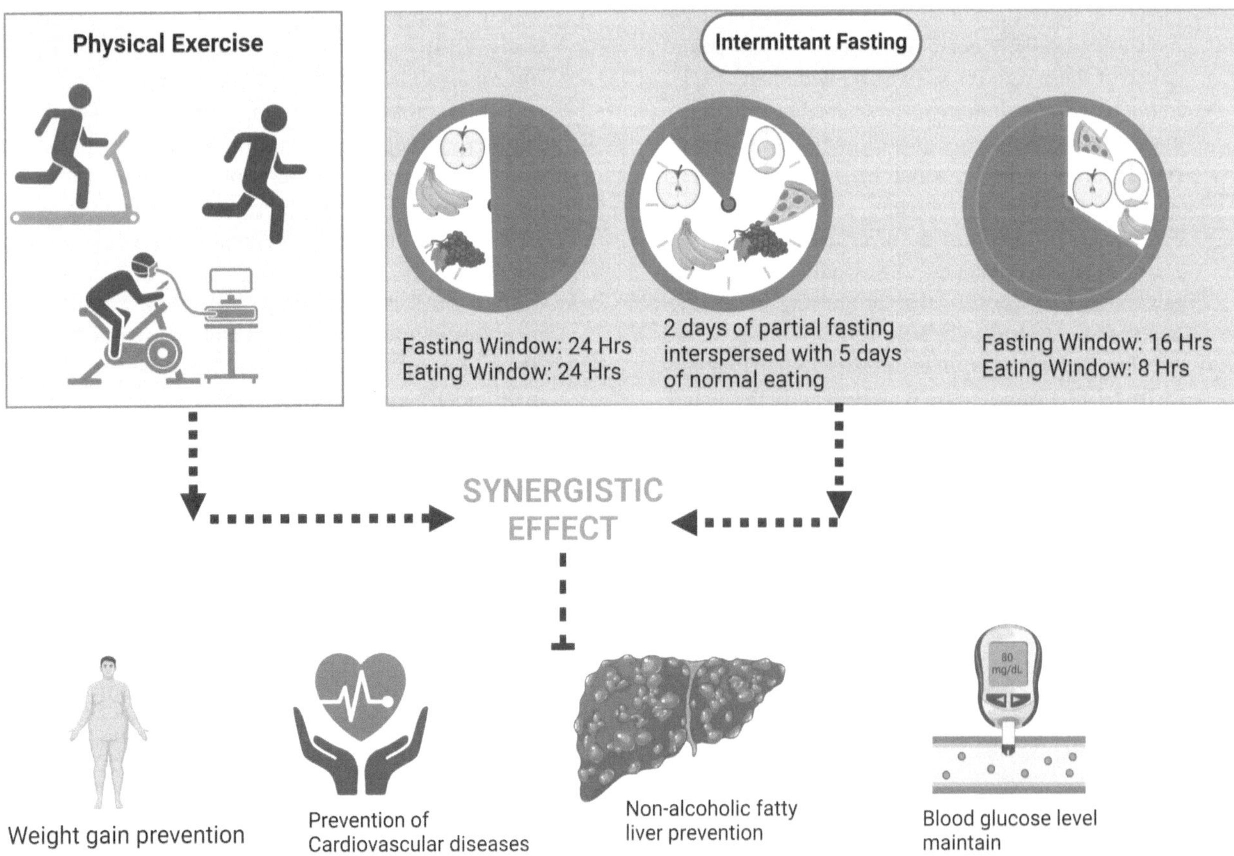

FIGURE 5.2 "Combining physical exercise and IF for preventing metabolic disorders." by Zhang et al., 2023 is licensed under CC BY 4.0.

TABLE 5.1
Comparison of Therapeutic Strategies for Metabolic Health

Strategy	Advantages	Disadvantages
Modulating Gut Microbiota	- Diverse methods (lifestyle, medical) (Longo et al., 2023)	- Long-term safety and efficacy need further research (Longo et al., 2023)
	- Dietary interventions show promise (Mediterranean diet, bariatric surgery) (Longo et al., 2023)	- Varying responses among individuals (Longo et al., 2023)
	- Potential for improving gut microbiota composition (Longo et al., 2023)	- Ongoing evolution of understanding (Longo et al., 2023)
Intermittent Fasting (IF)	- Multiple IF patterns with metabolic benefits (Vasim et al., 2022)	- Varying responses and effects on gut microbiota (Guo et al., 2021)
	- Enhances health-associated gut microbiota (Guo et al., 2021)	- Long-term effects require further study (Guo et al., 2021)
Mediterranean Diet	- Promotes diverse and beneficial gut microbiota (Longo et al., 2023)	- Causal relationship needs further research (Longo et al., 2023)
	- Linked to improved metabolic health (Longo et al., 2023)	- Ongoing investigation into safety and efficacy (Longo et al., 2023)
Low-Carbohydrate Diet	- Enhances gut microbiota diversity and reduces inflammation (Longo et al., 2023)	- Long-term safety and efficacy not fully established (Longo et al., 2023)
	- Improves insulin sensitivity and lipid profiles (Longo et al., 2023)	-
High-Fiber Diet	- Increases gut microbiota diversity and decreases inflammation (Zhang et al., 2023)	-
	- Improves insulin sensitivity and lipid profiles (Zhang et al., 2023)	-
Fecal Microbiota Transplantation (FMT)	- Restores balanced gut microbiota (Longo et al., 2023)	- Safety and efficacy in metabolic health need more research (Longo et al., 2023)
	- Promising in improving gut health and treating various conditions (Nowakowski et al., 2016)	- Limited data on long-term effects (Nowakowski et al., 2016)
Antibiotics	- Selective targeting of pathogenic bacteria (Longo et al., 2023)	- Overuse can lead to dysbiosis (Zhang et al., 2023)
	- Eliminates pathogenic bacteria within the gut microbiota (Longo et al., 2023)	- Potential adverse effects on metabolic health (Zhang et al., 2023)

5.7 CASE STUDIES AND CLINICAL EVIDENCE

Prebiotics are substrates that host bacteria specifically employ to promote health benefits and draw attention to their potential to improve metabolic health. Common prebiotics, such as inulin, fructosaccharides, and galactosaccharides, were evaluated in studies to evaluate their beneficial effects in metabolic diseases (Gibson et al., 2017). Specifically, the inclusion of Inulin or Inulin Propionate Ester has displayed potential in enhancing insulin resistance among individuals who are overweight or obese (Chambers et al., 2019). Furthermore, a meta-analysis offers strong proof that fructose of the inulin kind, particularly in individuals with type 2 diabetes and diabetes, has a favorable impact on important metabolic parameters (Wang et al., 2019).

Despite the accumulating body of evidence supporting the metabolic benefits of prebiotics, regulatory authorizations for prebiotic health claims remain limited (Gibson et al., 2017). Therefore, it is crucial to conduct additional research and thoroughly examine the impact of prebiotic effects on the host in order to achieve a thorough comprehension of their potential.

Probiotics, which are live microorganisms given in sufficient quantities to provide health advantages, offer an additional approach for improving metabolic well-being. While Bifidobacterium and Lactobacillus strains are frequently used as probiotics, specific health claims for probiotics have not been approved by the FDA and the EFSA (Hill et al., 2014). Nevertheless, randomized placebo-controlled trials, primarily employing species from the Lactobacillus and Bifidobacterium genera, have shown promise in improving glucose homeostasis in type 2 diabetic patients (Kocsis et al., 2020; Rittiphairoj et al., 2021; Tao et al., 2020). Even the effects of C. minuta on body weight in participants belonging to various weight groups are being studied in clinical trials (Yao et al., 2020).

Feeding live bacteria to the far end of the intestine presented challenges that needed advancements in storage, transportation, and transplantation technologies to enhance the beneficial impact of probiotics. Microencapsulation is a method of preventing organisms from adverse reactions during intestinal transport, such as oxygen exposure, low gastric pH, bile acids, and enzymes (Yao et al., 2020). Additionally, the realization that the benefits of probiotics may depend on bacterial engraftment within the intestine has prompted the exploration of synbiotics. Patients with type 2 diabetes have been studied for syncrotic treatments, which are characterized as mixtures of live bacteria and substrates that are particularly used by host microbes for beneficial effects on health. A 3-hour meal tolerance test was followed by a study that found that 12-week synbiotics improved glucose metabolism. Furthermore, the drug altered the proportions of A. muciniphila and B. infantis in the gut bacterial community (Perraudeau et al., 2020; Swanson et al., 2020).

Postbiotics, or inanimate microbial components or metabolites that provide health advantages, are a term introduced by the rapidly changing field of microbiota-based treatments (Salminen et al., 2021). Postbiotics have shown promise in the study of metabolic health. Specifically, the addition of butyrate, either on its own or combined with inulin, has yielded favorable outcomes regarding inflammatory status and cardiometabolic characteristics (Cleophas et al., 2019; Roshanravan et al., 2017). According to recent research, giving SCFA mixtures—like butyrate—through colonic infusions can raise plasma peptide YY levels, fat oxidation, and energy expenditure in men who are overweight or obese (Canfora et al., 2017). Nevertheless, there is not a uniform observation of metabolic advantages seen in all research studies when administering butyrate to individuals with metabolic syndrome (Bouter et al., 2018). This variance suggests that butyrate may exert localized effects within the colon, potentially improving host metabolism.

Microbiota-drug interactions are another dynamic facet of the microbiome's influence on metabolic health. Numerous treatments have been shown to alter the gut microbiota's makeup, indicating the possibility of developing pharmaceuticals that might positively alter the microbiome. These interactions represent a complex interplay in which drugs can modify the gut microbial composition, while microbes can enzymatically transform drugs, affecting their structure, bioavailability, bioactivity, and toxicity (Weersma et al., 2020). For example, in vitro screens have shown that drugs have a major impact on the formation of gut microbiota. Many medications with human objectives, such as the cholesterol-lowering medication simvastatin, prevented the development of a minimum of one variant of gut bacteria in vitro (Maier et al., 2018). Evidence also suggests that statins may modulate the gut microbial composition, potentially contributing to their effects (Vieira-Silva et al., 2020).

Metformin, a frequently prescribed medication for diabetes, is also known to impact the makeup of gut microbiota, potentially contributing to its therapeutic benefits (Forslund et al., 2015; Wu et al., 2017). A recent double-blind study showed significant alterations in the gut microbiome after four months of metformin treatment, potentially enhancing the production of SCFAs such as butyrate. Furthermore, compared to mice exposed to conventional microbiota, germ-free mice's glucose tolerance increased when they received stool specimens from people receiving metformin treatment (Wu et al., 2017). The positive benefits of metformin have been linked to a number of changes in metabolite profiles and microbial composition, highlighting the intricate interactions between medications and the microbiota of the gut (Sun et al., 2018). Additionally, studies have shown that metformin can influence the top portion of the small intestine's ability to detect nutrients, which can affect how much glucose is perceived through a route that involves GLP-1R and sodium-glucose cotransporter-1 (Bauer et al., 2018).

The bidirectional nature of drug-microbiota interactions emphasizes the importance of considering individual variations in gut microbial composition in drug therapy (Spanogiannopoulos et al., 2016). In some cases, modulating the gut microbiota before commencing a specific therapy may enhance treatment outcomes. A fascinating instance may be seen in cancer treatment, where patients who had not responded to anti-PD-1 medication in the past started to react after receiving FMT and then receiving anti-PD-1 therapy again (Baruch et al., 2021).

Furthermore, research has looked at the possibility of targeting particular microbial enzymes that are responsible for the synthesis of harmful compounds such as trimethylamine N-oxide (TMAO). Compounds similar in structure to choline, like 3,3-dimethyl-1-butanol, have displayed potential in inhibiting TMA lyases found in microbes. This inhibition results in decreased production of TMAO and a reduction in choline diet-induced atherosclerosis when tested on mice (Wang et al., 2015). Follow-up studies have identified second-generation inhibitors with increased potency and sustainability, offering the prospect of minimizing side effects (Roberts et al., 2018).

5.8 CHALLENGES AND FUTURE DIRECTIONS

5.8.1 Current Challenges in Gut Microbiota-Based Therapies

Microbiome-based therapies are a promising area of research for treating various diseases by manipulating and restoring the body's gut bacteria. However, there are several challenges that limit the widespread adoption of these therapies. These are a few of the present issues facing medicines based on gut microbiota:

- **Lack of clinical data**: Since the subject of microbiome research is still in its infancy, industry players often disagree and lack knowledge on how manipulation may affect the human microbiome and its potential to treat different diseases. Numerous individuals involved in this sector emphasize the need for further clinical evidence to support the use of this therapeutic method.
- **Reliability of diagnostic tools**: The reliability of diagnostic tools based on microbiome is a matter of concern due to the absence of FDA-approved therapies using this approach. At present, there are only limited treatment options available that can be effectively guided by personalized diagnostic tools.
- **Immunological consequences**: The use of microbiome transplantation therapy is currently at an early stage as a standard treatment option and its effectiveness in clinical trials has been limited.

It is crucial to carefully analyze the immunological consequences of these medicines in order to ensure their successful deployment.

- **Limited understanding of mechanisms**: Even with our limited understanding of the complex relationships that exist across the gut's microbiota and its host environment, it is becoming more and more important to investigate new treatment strategies that might influence the gut microbiota.
- **Dysbiosis**: Addressing the imbalance in microbiota composition poses a significant obstacle. It is becoming more and more important to establish a detailed knowledge of the diversity and metabolites involved with gut microbiota functionality within medical practice, given the critical role that gut microbiota plays in disease onset, diagnosis, and therapy.

5.8.2 Future Research Directions

Metabolic disorders show variability in their origin and clinical manifestations (Neeland et al., 2018; Tuomi et al., 2014). While diet has long been known to be associated with risk for many diseases, particularly when it comes to Western-style or high red meat intake, there is currently a renewed emphasis on the role the gut microbiota plays in defining metabolic health. The gut microbiota functions as an endocrine organ by metabolizing ingested nutrients and affecting the production and absorption of metabolites. Products and metabolites generated by gut bacteria impact a range of metabolic illnesses, including insulin resistance, adverse lipid profiles, elevated platelet reactivity, increased risk of blood clot formation, and chronic low-level inflammation. This implies that various causes of cardiometabolic illnesses may be influenced by the makeup of the gut microbiota (Cani et al., 2008; Haghikia et al., 2022; Koh et al., 2018; Zhu et al., 2016).

Numerous elements, such as genetic inclination, dietary patterns, levels of physical activity, tobacco use, stress levels, and the composition of gut microorganisms all intertwine to give rise to a distinct disease profile for every person. Recent studies have categorized patients into distinct clusters based on characteristics and risk of complications, offering opportunities for personalized treatment approaches (Ahlqvist et al., 2018; Wagner et al., 2021). Research should concentrate on developing therapies that are particular to patient subgroups rather than trying to find a treatment plan that works for everyone. For instance, pro- and synbiotics, as well as butyrate-containing supplements, may provide relief for those whose bodies lack the microorganisms necessary to create butyrate. On the other hand, inhibitors that precisely target the microbial enzymes responsible for creating these metabolites may be beneficial for individuals with increased levels of toxic metabolites like imidazole propionate and TMAO.

In order to account for the significant differences in how individuals respond to gut microbiota-targeted interventions as seen in previous studies, it is recommended that patients undergo a comprehensive assessment. Clinical data, host tissue transcriptomics, metagenomics, and metabolomics should all be analyzed as part of this assessment. The goal of this approach is to identify specific indicators that can predict how each patient will respond to treatment (Van Olden et al., 2021). Although previous studies have mainly examined cross-sectional data, it is crucial to conduct future prospective longitudinal studies. These upcoming investigations are needed in order to establish a causal relationship and ascertain whether microbiota or their byproducts can be used as diagnostic indicators (Zhou et al., 2019). These research investigations will provide further understanding of the differences in responses to various stressors and health conditions both within individuals and between individuals over time. To evaluate the efficacy and durability of gut microbiota modifications as a possible therapeutic or preventative approach for metabolic diseases, long-term research is essential. To achieve lasting effects, it is necessary to explore optimal approaches that take into account factors such as patient compliance and risk factors. Moreover, future studies have to concentrate on deciphering the intricate connection between nutrition, other risk factors, and gut bacteria.

Safety and drug interactions are critical considerations. It is essential for researchers to evaluate the possible negative consequences linked to various therapies aimed at targeting the gut microbiota. Furthermore, considering that individuals with metabolic disorders often take multiple medications, it is imperative to investigate how manipulating the gut microbiota may influence the effectiveness, activity level, and potential harm caused by these drugs. This includes exploring whether combination therapies involving gut microbiota-targeting interventions and common drugs can enhance therapeutic outcomes or if specific drug-microbiota combinations should be avoided.

5.9 CONCLUSION

In conclusion, research on the complex connection among the gut microbiota and metabolic conditions is becoming increasingly promising and might have a big impact on healthcare in the future. Metabolic diseases, characterized by their heterogeneity and multifaceted etiologies, challenge the development of universal treatment strategies. Instead, a personalized medicine approach, tailored to individual patient profiles, is becoming increasingly vital. Recent advancements in categorizing patients into distinct clusters based on characteristics and complications offer hope for precise interventions. Understanding how the gut microbiota affects important aspects of these conditions, such inflammation and insulin resistance, allows us to more effectively target patient subgroups. Long-term studies are necessary to assess the sustainability of gut microbiota manipulation, and in order to guarantee patient welfare, safety and medication interactions need to be carefully looked into. The future of metabolic disease research lies in unraveling the complexities of microbiota interactions, optimizing treatment strategies, and fostering tailored interventions. As we explore deeper into the mechanisms underlying these conditions, we move closer to a healthcare landscape where individualized treatment regimens are the norm, offering hope for more effective and targeted therapies. Researchers, clinicians, and patients must work together on this path in order to pave the way for a more individualized and health-conscious approach to treating metabolic illnesses.

REFERENCES

Abdelbasset, W. K., Tantawy, S. A., Kamel, D. M., Alqahtani, B. A., Elnegamy, T. E., Soliman, G. S., & Ibrahim, A. A. (2020). Effects of highintensity interval and moderate-intensity continuous aerobic exercise on diabetic obese patients with nonalcoholic fatty liver disease: A comparative randomized controlled trial. *Medicine*, 99(10), e19471. https://doi.org/10.1097/MD.0000000000019471

Abidi, A., & Rtibi, K. (2023). Editorial: Microbiota-hormones-gut axis as a therapeutic target for metabolic disorders. *Frontiers in Endocrinology*, 14, 1178222. https://doi.org/10.3389/fendo.2023.1178222

Agus, A., Clément, K., & Sokol, H. (2021). Gut microbiota-derived metabolites as central regulators in metabolic disorders. *Gut*, 70(6), 1174–1182. https://doi.org/10.1136/gutjnl-2020-323071

Ahlqvist, E., Storm, P., Käräjämäki, A., Martinell, M., Dorkhan, M., Carlsson, A., Vikman, P., Prasad, R. B., Aly, D. M., Almgren, P., Wessman, Y., Shaat, N., Spégel, P., Mulder, H., Lindholm, E., Melander, O., Hansson, O., Malmqvist, U., Lernmark, Å., . . . & Groop, L. (2018). Novel subgroups of adult-onset diabetes and their association with outcomes: A data-driven cluster analysis of six variables. *Lancet. Diabetes and Endocrinology*, 6(5), 361–369. https://doi.org/10.1016/S2213-8587(18)30051-2

Allen, J. M., Mailing, L. J., Niemiro, G. M., Moore, R., Cook, M. D., White, B. A., Holscher, H. D., & Woods, J. A. (2018). Exercise alters gut microbiota composition and function in lean and obese humans. *Medicine and Science in Sports and Exercise*, 50(4), 747–757. https://doi.org/10.1249/MSS.0000000000001495

Aron-Wisnewsky, J., Warmbrunn, M. V., Nieuwdorp, M., & Clément, K. (2021). Metabolism and metabolic disorders and the microbiome: The intestinal microbiota associated with obesity, lipid metabolism, and metabolic health-Pathophysiology and therapeutic strategies. *Gastroenterology*, 160(2), 573–599. https://doi.org/10.1053/j.gastro.2020.10.057

Bäckhed, F., Ding, H., Wang, T., Hooper, L. V., Koh, G. Y., Nagy, A., Semenkovich, C. F., & Gordon, J. I. (2004). The gut microbiota as an environmental factor that regulates fat storage. *Proceedings of the National Academy of Sciences of the United States of America*, 101(44), 15718–15723. https://doi.org/10.1073/pnas.0407076101

Bakaloudi, D. R., Halloran, A., Rippin, H. L., Oikonomidou, A. C., Dardavesis, T. I., Williams, J., Wickramasinghe, K., Breda, J., & Chourdakis, M. (2021). Intake and adequacy of the vegan diet: A systematic review of the evidence. *Clinical Nutrition*, 40(5), 3503–3521. https://doi.org/10.1016/j.clnu.2020.11.035

Baruch, E. N., Youngster, I., Ben-Betzalel, G., Ortenberg, R., Lahat, A., Katz, L., Adler, K., Dick-Necula, D., Raskin, S., Bloch, N., Rotin, D., Anafi, L., Avivi, C., Melnichenko, J., Steinberg-Silman, Y., Mamtani, R., Harati, H., Asher, N., Shapira-Frommer, R., . . . & Boursi, B. (2021). Fecal microbiota transplant promotes response in immunotherapy-refractory melanoma patients. *Science*, 371(6529), 602–609. https://doi.org/10.1126/science.abb5920

Basilio, P. G., Oliveira, A. P. C., Castro, A. C. F., Carvalho, M. R., Zagatto, A. M., Martinez, P. F., Okoshi, M. P., Okoshi, K., Ota, G. E., Reis, F. A. D., & Oliveira-Junior, S. A. (2020). Intermittent fasting attenuates exercise training-induced cardiac remodeling. *Arquivos Brasileiros de Cardiologia*, 115(2), 184–193. https://doi.org/10.36660/abc.20190349

Batitucci, G., Faria Junior, E. V., Nogueira, J. E., Brandão, C. F. C., Abud, G. F., Ortiz, G. U., Marchini, J. S., & Freitas, E. C. (2022). Impact of intermittent fasting combined with high-intensity interval training on body composition, metabolic biomarkers, and physical fitness in women with obesity. *Frontiers in Nutrition*, 9, 884305. https://doi.org/10.3389/fnut.2022.884305

Bauer, P. V., Duca, F. A., Waise, T. M. Z., Rasmussen, B. A., Abraham, M. A., Dranse, H. J., Puri, A., O'Brien, C. A., & Lam, T. K. T. (2018). Metformin alters upper small intestinal microbiota that impact a glucoseSGLT1-sensing glucoregulatory pathway. *Cell Metabolism*, 27(1), 101–117.e5. https://doi.org/10.1016/j.cmet.2017.09.019

Bianchetti, G., De Maio, F., Abeltino, A., Serantoni, C., Riente, A., Santarelli, G., Sanguinetti, M., Delogu, G., Martinoli, R., Barbaresi, S., Spirito, M., & Maulucci, G. (2023). Unraveling the gut microbiome-diet connection: Exploring the impact of digital precision and personalized nutrition on microbiota composition and host physiology. *Nutrients*, 15(18), 3931. https://doi.org/10.3390/nu15183931

Bouter, K., Bakker, G. J., Levin, E., Hartstra, A. V., Kootte, R. S., Udayappan, S. D., Katiraei, S., Bahler, L., Gilijamse, P. W., Tremaroli, V., Stahlman, M., Holleman, F., van Riel, N. A. W., Verberne, H. J., Romijn, J. A., Dallinga-Thie, G. M., Serlie, M. J., Ackermans, M. T., Kemper, E. M., . . . & Nieuwdorp, M. (2018). Differential metabolic effects of oral butyrate treatment in lean versus metabolic syndrome subjects. *Clinical and Translational Gastroenterology*, 9(5), 155. https://doi.org/10.1038/s41424-018-0025-4

Boutriq, S., González-González, A., Plaza-Andrades, I., Laborda-Illanes, A., Sánchez-Alcoholado, L., Peralta-Linero, J., Domínguez-Recio, M. E., Bermejo-Pérez, M. J., Lavado-Valenzuela, R., Alba, E., & Queipo-Ortuño, M. I. (2021) Gut and endometrial microbiome dysbiosis: A new emergent risk factor for endometrial cancer. *Journal of Personalized Medicine*, 11(7), 659. https://doi.org/10.3390/jpm11070659

Braunsdorf, C., Mailänder-Sánchez, D., & Schaller, M. (2016). Fungal sensing of host environment. *Cellular Microbiology*, 18(9), 1188–1200. https://doi.org/10.1111/cmi.12610

Brown, E. M., Clardy, J., & Xavier, R. J. (2023). Gut microbiome lipid metabolism and its impact on host physiology. *Cell Host and Microbe*, 31(2), 173–186. https://doi.org/10.1016/j.chom.2023.01.009

Brüssow, H. (2020). Problems with the concept of gut microbiota dysbiosis. *Microbial Biotechnology*, 13(2), 423–434. https://doi.org/10.1111/1751-7915.13479

Canfora, E. E., van der Beek, C. M., Jocken, J. W. E., Goossens, G. H., Holst, J. J., Olde Damink, S. W. M., Lenaerts, K., Dejong, C. H. C., & Blaak, E. E. (2017). Colonic infusions of short-chain fatty acid mixtures promote energy metabolism in overweight/obese men: A randomized crossover trial. *Scientific Reports*, 7(1), 2360. https://doi.org/10.1038/s41598-017-02546-x

Cani, P. D., Bibiloni, R., Knauf, C., Waget, A., Neyrinck, A. M., Delzenne, N. M., & Burcelin, R. (2008). Changes in gut microbiota control metabolic endotoxemia-induced inflammation in high-fat diet-induced obesity and diabetes in mice. *Diabetes*, 57(6), 1470–1481. https://doi.org/10.2337/db07-1403

Chambers, E. S., Byrne, C. S., Morrison, D. J., Murphy, K. G., Preston, T., Tedford, C., Garcia-Perez, I., Fountana, S., Serrano-Contreras, J. I., Holmes, E., Reynolds, C. J., Roberts, J. F., Boyton, R. J., Altmann, D. M., McDonald, J. A. K., Marchesi, J. R., Akbar, A. N., Riddell, N. E., Wallis, G. A., &

Frost, G. S. (2019). Dietary supplementation with inulin-propionate ester or inulin improves insulin sensitivity in adults with overweight and obesity with distinct effects on the gut microbiota, plasma metabolome and systemic inflammatory responses: A randomised cross-over trial. *Gut*, 68(8), 1430–1438. https://doi.org/10.1136/gutjnl-2019-318424

Chen, L., Guo, L., Feng, S., Wang, C., Cui, Z., Wang, S., Lu, Q., Chang, H., Hang, B., Snijders, A. M., Mao, J. H., Lu, Y., & Ding, D. (2023, May 1). Fecal microbiota transplantation ameliorates type 2 diabetes via metabolic remodeling of the gut microbiota in db/db mice. *BMJ Open Diabetes Research and Care*, 11(3), e003282. https://doi.org/10.1136/bmjdrc-2022-003282

Choi, Y., Park, E., Kim, S., Ha, J., Oh, H., Kim, Y., Lee, Y., Seo, Y., Kang, J., Lee, S., Lee, H., Yoon, Y., & Choi, K. H. (2021). Alleviation of periodontal disease using *Lactobacillus curvatus* SMFM2016-NK. *Journal of Functional Foods*, 83, 104531. https://doi.org/10.1016/j.jff.2021.104531

Cignarella, F., Cantoni, C., Ghezzi, L., Salter, A., Dorsett, Y., Chen, L., Phillips, D., Weinstock, G. M., Fontana, L., Cross, A. H., Zhou, Y., & Piccio, L. (2018). Intermittent fasting confers protection in CNS autoimmunity by altering the gut microbiota. *Cell Metabolism*, 27(6), 1222–1235.e6. https://doi.org/10.1016/j.cmet.2018.05.006

Cleophas, M. C. P., Ratter, J. M., Bekkering, S., Quintin, J., Schraa, K., Stroes, E. S., Netea, M. G., & Joosten, L. A. B. (2019). Effects of oral butyrate supplementation on inflammatory potential of circulating peripheral blood mononuclear cells in healthy and obese males. *Scientific Reports*, 9(1), 775. https://doi.org/10.1038/s41598-018-37246-7

Clerbaux, L. A., Fillipovska, J., Muñoz, A., Petrillo, M., Coecke, S., Amorim, M. J., & Grenga, L. (2022). Mechanisms leading to gut dysbiosis in COVID-19: Current evidence and uncertainties based on adverse outcome pathways. *Journal of Clinical Medicine*, 11(18), 5400. https://doi.org/10.3390/jcm11185400

daSilva, T. F., Casarotti, S. N., de Oliveira, G. L. V., & Penna, A. L. B. (2021). The impact of probiotics, prebiotics, and Synbiotics on the biochemical, clinical, and immunological markers, as well as on the gut microbiota of obese hosts. *Critical Reviews in Food Science and Nutrition*, 61(2), 337–355. https://doi.org/10.1080/10408398.2020.1733483

Dong, T. A., Sandesara, P. B., Dhindsa, D. S., Mehta, A., Arneson, L. C., Dollar, A. L., Taub, P. R., & Sperling, L. S. (2020). Intermittent fasting: A heart healthy dietary pattern? *American Journal of Medicine*, 133(8), 901–907. https://doi.org/10.1016/j.amjmed.2020.03.030

Evans, C. C., LePard, K. J., Kwak, J. W., Stancukas, M. C., Laskowski, S., Dougherty, J., Moulton, L., Glawe, A., Wang, Y., Leone, V., Antonopoulos, D. A., Smith, D., Chang, E. B., & Ciancio, M. J. (2014). Exercise prevents weight gain and alters the gut microbiota in a mouse model of high fat diet-induced obesity. *PLOS One*, 9(3), e92193. https://doi.org/10.1371/journal.pone.0092193

Ezpeleta, M., Gabel, K., Cienfuegos, S., Kalam, F., Lin, S., Pavlou, V., Song, Z., Haus, J. M., Koppe, S., Alexandria, S. J., Tussing-Humphreys, L., & Varady, K. A. (2023). Effect of alternate day fasting combined with aerobic exercise on non-alcoholic fatty liver disease: A randomized controlled trial. *Cell Metabolism*, 35(1), 56–70.e3. https://doi.org/10.1016/j.cmet.2022.12.001

Fan, Y., Qin, M., Zhu, J., Chen, X., Luo, J., Chen, T., Sun, J., Zhang, Y., & Xi, Q. (2022). MicroRNA sensing and regulating microbiota-host crosstalk via diet motivation. *Critical Reviews in Food Science and Nutrition*, 1–18. https://doi.org/10.1080/10408398.2022.2139220

Fan, Y., & Pedersen, O. (2021). Gut microbiota in human metabolic health and disease. *Nature Reviews. Microbiology*, 19(1), 55–71. https://doi.org/10.1038/s41579-020-0433-9

Forslund, K., Hildebrand, F., Nielsen, T., Falony, G., Le Chatelier, E., Sunagawa, S., Prifti, E., Vieira-Silva, S., Gudmundsdottir, V., Pedersen, H. K., Arumugam, M., Kristiansen, K., Voigt, A. Y., Vestergaard, H., Hercog, R., Costea, P. I., Kultima, J. R., Li, J., Jørgensen, T., . . . & Pedersen, O. (2015). Disentangling type 2 diabetes and metformin treatment signatures in the human gut microbiota. *Nature*, 528(7581), 262–266. https://doi.org/10.1038/nature15766

Genua, F., Raghunathan, V., Jenab, M., Gallagher, W. M., & Hughes, D. J. (2021). The role of gut barrier dysfunction and microbiome dysbiosis in colorectal cancer development. *Frontiers in Oncology*, 11, 626349. https://doi.org/10.3389/fonc.2021.626349

Gesper, M., Nonnast, A. B. H., Kumowski, N., Stoehr, R., Schuett, K., Marx, N., & Kappel, B. A. (2021). Gut-derived metabolite indole-3-propionic acid modulates mitochondrial function in cardiomyocytes and alters cardiac function. *Frontiers in Medicine*, 8, 648259. https://doi.org/10.3389/fmed.2021.648259

Gibson, G. R., Hutkins, R., Sanders, M. E., Prescott, S. L., Reimer, R. A., Salminen, S. J., Scott, K., Stanton, C., Swanson, K. S., Cani, P. D., Verbeke, K., & Reid, G. (2017). Expert consensus document: The International Scientific Association for Probiotics and Prebiotics (ISAPP) consensus statement on the definition and scope of prebiotics. *Nature Reviews. Gastroenterology and Hepatology*, 14(8), 491–502. https://doi.org/10.1038/nrgastro.2017.75

Giovannini, M. G., Lana, D., Traini, C., & Vannucchi, M. G. (2021). The microbiota-gut-brain axis and Alzheimer disease. From dysbiosis to neurodegeneration: Focus on the central nervous system glial cells. *Journal of Clinical Medicine*, 10(11), 2358. https://doi.org/10.3390/jcm10112358

Glorieux, G., Gryp, T., & Perna, A. (2020). Gut-derived metabolites and their role in immune dysfunction in chronic kidney disease. *Toxins*, 12(4), 245. https://doi.org/10.3390/toxins12040245

Gomaa, E. Z. (2020). Human gut microbiota/microbiome in health and diseases: A review. *Antonie van Leeuwenhoek*, 113(12), 2019–2040. https://doi.org/10.1007/s10482-020-01474-7

Gungor, O., Ulu, S., Hasbal, N. B., Anker, S. D., & Kalantar-Zadeh, K. (2021). Effects of hormonal changes on sarcopenia in chronic kidney disease: Where are we now and what can we do? *Journal of Cachexia, Sarcopenia and Muscle*, 12(6), 1380–1392. https://doi.org/10.1002/jcsm.12839

Guo, Y., Luo, S., Ye, Y., Yin, S., Fan, J., & Xia, M. (2021). Intermittent fasting improves cardiometabolic risk factors and alters gut microbiota in metabolic syndrome patients. *Journal of Clinical Endocrinology and Metabolism*, 106(1), 64–79. https://doi.org/10.1210/clinem/dgaa644

Haghikia, A., Zimmermann, F., Schumann, P., Jasina, A., Roessler, J., Schmidt, D., Heinze, P., Kaisler, J., Nageswaran, V., Aigner, A., Ceglarek, U., Cineus, R., Hegazy, A. N., van der Vorst, E. P. C., Döring, Y., Strauch, C. M., Nemet, I., Tremaroli, V., Dwibedi, C., Kränkel, N., Landmesser, U. (2022). Propionate attenuates atherosclerosis by immune-dependent regulation of intestinal cholesterol metabolism. *European Heart Journal*, *43*(6), 518–533. https://doi.org/10.1093/eurheartj/ehab644

Han, H., Su, Y., & Yin, J. (2023). Editorial: Gut microbial response to host metabolic phenotypes, volume II. *Frontiers in Nutrition*, *10*, 1136510. https://doi.org/10.3389/fnut.2023.1136510

Hill, C., Guarner, F., Reid, G., Gibson, G. R., Merenstein, D. J., Pot, B., Morelli, L., Canani, R. B., Flint, H. J., Salminen, S., Calder, P. C., & Sanders, M. E. (2014). Expert consensus document. The International Scientific Association for probiotics and prebiotics consensus statement on the scope and appropriate use of the term probiotic. *Nature Reviews. Gastroenterology and Hepatology*, 11(8), 506–514. https://doi.org/10.1038/nrgastro.2014.66

Hrncir, T. (2022). Gut microbiota dysbiosis: Triggers, consequences, diagnostic and therapeutic options. *Microorganisms*, 10(3), 578. https://doi.org/10.3390/microorganisms10030578

Iadanza, E., Fabbri, R., Bašić-ČiČak, D., Amedei, A., & Telalovic, J. H. (2020). Gut microbiota and artificial intelligence approaches: A scoping review. *Health and Technology*, 10(6), 1343–1358. https://doi.org/10.1007/s12553-020-00486-7

Jia, X., Lu, S., Zeng, Z., Liu, Q., Dong, Z., Chen, Y., Zhu, Z., Hong, Z., Zhang, T., Du, G., Xiang, J., Wu, D., Bai, W., Yang, B., Li, Y., Huang, J., Li, H., Safadi, R., & Lu, Y. (2020). Characterization of gut microbiota, bile acid metabolism, and cytokines in intrahepatic cholangiocarcinoma. *Hepatology*, 71(3), 893–906. https://doi.org/10.1002/hep.30852

Kaczmarek, J. L., Thompson, S. V., & Holscher, H. D. (2017). Complex interactions of circadian rhythms, eating behaviors, and the gastrointestinal microbiota and their potential impact on health. *Nutrition Reviews*, 75(9), 673–682. https://doi.org/10.1093/nutrit/nux036

Karl, J. P. (2021). Gut microbiota-targeted interventions for reducing the incidence, duration, and severity of respiratory tract infections in healthy non-elderly adults. *Military Medicine*, 186(3–4), e310–e318. https://doi.org/10.1093/milmed/usaa261

Kim, M. H., Yun, K. E., Kim, J., Park, E., Chang, Y., Ryu, S., Kim, H. L., & Kim, H. N. (2020). Gut microbiota and metabolic health among overweight and obese individuals. *Scientific Reports*, 10(1), 19417. https://doi.org/10.1038/s41598-020-76474-8

Kim, S., Kang, J. Y., Balance, W. C., Sutton, B. P., Shin, D. H., Jang, K. H., Shin, M., Kong, H., & Kim, J. W. (2021). Fabrication of cell penetrating peptide-conjugated bacterial cellulose nanofibrils with remarkable skin adhesion and water retention performance. *International Journal of Pharmaceutics*, 600, 120476. https://doi.org/10.1016/j.ijpharm.2021.120476

Kocsis, T., Molnár, B., Németh, D., Hegyi, P., Szakács, Z., Bálint, A., Garami, A., Soós, A., Márta, K., & Solymár, M. (2020). Probiotics have beneficial metabolic effects in patients with type 2 diabetes mellitus: A meta-analysis of randomized clinical trials. *Scientific Reports*, 10(1), 11787. https://doi.org/10.1038/s41598-020-68440-1

Koh, A., Molinaro, A., Ståhlman, M., Khan, M. T., Schmidt, C., Mannerås-Holm, L., Wu, H., Carreras, A., Jeong, H., Olofsson, L. E., Bergh, P. O., Gerdes, V., Hartstra, A., de Brauw, M., Perkins, R., Nieuwdorp, M., Bergström, G., & Bäckhed, F. (2018). Microbially produced imidazole propionate impairs insulin signaling through mTORC1. *Cell*, 175(4), 947–961.e17. https://doi.org/10.1016/j.cell.2018.09.055

Lanter, B. B., Sauer, K., & Davies, D. G. (2014). Bacteria present in carotid arterial plaques are found as biofilm deposits which may contribute to enhanced risk of plaque rupture. *mBio*, 5(3), e01206–e01214. https://doi.org/10.1128/mBio.01206-14

LeChatelier, E., Nielsen, T., Qin, J., Prifti, E., Hildebrand, F., Falony, G., Almeida, M., Arumugam, M., Batto, J. M., Kennedy, S., Leonard, P., Li, J., Burgdorf, K., Grarup, N., Jørgensen, T., Brandslund, I., Nielsen, H. B., Juncker, A. S., Bertalan, M., . . . & Pedersen, O. (2013). Richness of human gut microbiome correlates with metabolic markers. *Nature*, 500(7464), 541–546. https://doi.org/10.1038/nature12506

Leonard, M. M., Silvester, J. A., Leffler, D., Fasano, A., Kelly, C. P., Lewis, S. K., Goldsmith, J. D., Greenblatt, E., Kwok, W. W., McAuliffe, W. J., Galinsky, K., Siegelman, J., Chow, I. T., Wagner, J. A., Sapone, A., & Smithson, G. (2021). Evaluating responses to gluten challenge: A randomized, double-blind, 2-dose gluten challenge trial. *Gastroenterology*, 160(3), 720–733.e8. https://doi.org/10.1053/j.gastro.2020.10.040

Li, D., Li, Y., Yang, S., Lu, J., Jin, X., & Wu, M. (2022). Diet-gut microbiota-epigenetics in metabolic diseases: From mechanisms to therapeutics. *Biomedicine and Pharmacotherapy*, 153, 113290. https://doi.org/10.1016/j.biopha.2022.113290

Li, G., Xie, C., Lu, S., Nichols, R. G., Tian, Y., Li, L., Patel, D., Ma, Y., Brocker, C. N., Yan, T., Krausz, K. W., Xiang, R., Gavrilova, O., Patterson, A. D., & Gonzalez, F. J. (2017). Intermittent fasting promotes white adipose browning and decreases obesity by shaping the gut microbiota. *Cell Metabolism*, 26, 672–685.e4.

Litvak, Y., Byndloss, M. X., & Bäumler, A. J. (2018). Colonocyte metabolism shapes the gut microbiota. *Science*, 362(6418), eaat9076. https://doi.org/10.1126/science.aat9076

Liu, J. H., Ma, Q. H., Xu, Y., Chen, X., & Pan, C. W. (2020). Metabolic syndrome and 5-year incident hyperuricemia among older Chinese adults: A community-based cohort study. *Diabetes, Metabolic Syndrome and Obesity: Targets and Therapy*, 13, 4191–4200. https://doi.org/10.2147/DMSO.S278542

Longo, S., Rizza, S., & Federici, M. (2023, April 14). Microbiota-gut-brain axis: Relationships among the vagus nerve, gut microbiota, obesity, and diabetes. *Acta Diabetologica*, 60(8), 1007–1017. https://doi.org/10.1007/s00592-023-02088-x

Longo, V. D., & Panda, S. (2016). Fasting, circadian rhythms, and time-restricted feeding in healthy lifespan. *Cell Metabolism*, 23(6), 1048–1059. https://doi.org/10.1016/j.cmet.2016.06.001

Lou, X., Xue, J., Shao, R., Yang, Y., Ning, D., Mo, C., Wang, F., & Chen, G. (2022). Fecal microbiota transplantation and short-chain fatty acids reduce sepsis mortality by remodeling antibiotic-induced gut microbiota disturbances. *Frontiers in Immunology*, 13, 1063543. https://doi.org/10.3389/fimmu.2022.1063543

Ma, J., Meng, X., Liu, Y., Yin, C., Zhang, T., Wang, P., Park, Y. K., & Jung, H. W. (2020). Effects of a rhizome aqueous extract of Dioscorea batatas and its bioactive compound, allantoin in high fat diet and streptozotocin-induced diabetic mice and the regulation of liver, pancreas and skeletal muscle dysfunction. *Journal of Ethnopharmacology*, 259, 112926. https://doi.org/10.1016/j.jep.2020.112926

Maier, L., Pruteanu, M., Kuhn, M., Zeller, G., Telzerow, A., Anderson, E. E., Brochado, A. R., Fernandez, K. C., Dose, H., Mori, H., Patil, K. R., Bork, P., & Typas, A. (2018). Extensive impact of non-antibiotic drugs on human gut bacteria. *Nature*, 555(7698), 623–628. https://doi.org/10.1038/nature25979

Marco, M. L., Hill, C., Hutkins, R., Slavin, J., Tancredi, D. J., Merenstein, D., & Sanders, M. E. (2020). Should there be a recommended daily intake of microbes? *Journal of Nutrition*, 150(12), 3061–3067. https://doi.org/10.1093/jn/nxaa323

Marco, M. L., Sanders, M. E., Gänzle, M., Arrieta, M. C., Cotter, P. D., De Vuyst, L., Hill, C., Holzapfel, W., Lebeer, S., Merenstein, D., Reid, G., Wolfe, B. E., & Hutkins, R. (2021). The International Scientific Association for Probiotics and Prebiotics (ISAPP) consensus statement on fermented foods. *Nature Reviews. Gastroenterology and Hepatology*, 18(3), 196–208. https://doi.org/10.1038/s41575-020-00390-5

Martínez-Rodríguez, A., Rubio-Arias, J. A., García-De Frutos, J. M., Vicente-Martínez, M., & Gunnarsson, T. P. (2021). Effect of high-intensity interval training and intermittent fasting on body composition and physical performance in active women. *International Journal of Environmental Research and Public Health*, 18(12), 6431. https://doi.org/10.3390/ijerph18126431

Montanari, C., Parolisi, S., Borghi, E., Putignani, L., Bassanini, G., Zuvadelli, J., Bonfanti, C., Tummolo, A., Dionisi Vici, C., Biasucci, G., Burlina, A., Carbone, M. T., & Verduci, E. (2021). Dysbiosis, host metabolism, and non-communicable diseases: Trialogue in the inborn errors of metabolism. *Frontiers in Physiology*, 12, 716520. https://doi.org/10.3389/fphys.2021.716520

Moraes, R. C. M., Portari, G. V., Ferraz, A. S. M., da Silva, T. E. O., & Marocolo, M. (2017). Effects of intermittent fasting and chronic swimming exercise on body composition and lipid metabolism. *Applied Physiology, Nutrition and Metabolism*, 42(12), 1341–1346. https://doi.org/10.1139/apnm-2017-0435

Motiani, K. K., Collado, M. C., Eskelinen, J. J., Virtanen, K. A., Löyttyniemi, E., Salminen, S., Nuutila, P., Kalliokoski, K. K., & Hannukainen, J. C. (2020). Exercise training modulates gut microbiota profile and improves endotoxemia. *Medicine and Science in Sports and Exercise*, 52(1), 94–104. https://doi.org/10.1249/MSS.0000000000002112

Neeland, I. J., Poirier, P., & Després, J. P. (2018). Cardiovascular and metabolic heterogeneity of obesity: Clinical challenges and implications for management. *Circulation*, 137(13), 1391–1406. https://doi.org/10.1161/CIRCULATIONAHA.117.029617

Nowakowski, M. E., McCabe, R. E., Rowa, K., Pellizzari, J., Surette, M. G., Moayyedi, P., & Anglin, R. (2016, May 1). The gut microbiome: Potential innovations for the understanding and treatment of psychopathology. *Canadian Psychology / Psychologie Canadienne*, 57(2), 67–75. https://doi.org/10.1037/cap0000038

Pasdar, Y., Darbandi, M., Niazi, P., Hamzeh, B., Nachvak, M. S., & Barzegar, A. (2017). Risk factors of metabolic syndrome among food suppliers. *Srpski Arhiv za Celokupno Lekarstvo*, 145(5–6), 289–293. https://doi.org/10.2298/SARH160315034P

Patel, P. N., Shah, R. Y., Ferguson, J. F., & Reilly, M. P. (2015). Human experimental endotoxemia in modeling the pathophysiology, genomics, and therapeutics of innate immunity in complex cardiometabolic diseases. *Arteriosclerosis, Thrombosis, and Vascular Biology*, 35(3), 525–534. https://doi.org/10.1161/ATVBAHA.114.304455

Perraudeau, F., McMurdie, P., Bullard, J., Cheng, A., Cutcliffe, C., Deo, A., Eid, J., Gines, J., Iyer, M., Justice, N., Loo, W. T., Nemchek, M., Schicklberger, M., Souza, M., Stoneburner, B., Tyagi, S., & Kolterman, O. (2020). Improvements to postprandial glucose control in subjects with type 2 diabetes: A multicenter, double blind, randomized placebo-controlled trial of a novel probiotic formulation. *BMJ Open Diabetes Research and Care*, 8(1), e001319. https://doi.org/10.1136/bmjdrc-2020-001319

Peverill, M., Dirks, M. A., Narvaja, T., Herts, K. L., Comer, J. S., & McLaughlin, K. A. (2021). Socioeconomic status and child psychopathology in the United States: A meta-analysis of population-based studies. *Clinical Psychology Review*, 83, 101933. https://doi.org/10.1016/j.cpr.2020.101933

Pisoschi, A. M., Pop, A., Iordache, F., Stanca, L., Predoi, G., & Serban, A. I. (2021). Oxidative stress mitigation by antioxidants-an overview on their chemistry and influences on health status. *European Journal of Medicinal Chemistry*, 209, 112891. https://doi.org/10.1016/j.ejmech.2020.112891

Pizarroso, N. A., Fuciños, P., Gonçalves, C., Pastrana, L., & Amado, I. R. (2021). A review on the role of food-derived bioactive molecules and the microbiota-gut-brain axis in satiety regulation. *Nutrients*, 13(2), 632. https://doi.org/10.3390/nu13020632

Qin, J., Li, Y., Cai, Z., Li, S., Zhu, J., Zhang, F., Liang, S., Zhang, W., Guan, Y., Shen, D., Peng, Y., Zhang, D., Jie, Z., Wu, W., Qin, Y., Xue, W., Li, J., Han, L., Lu, D., . . . & Wang, J. (2012). A metagenome-wide association study of gut microbiota in type 2 diabetes. *Nature*, 490(7418), 55–60. https://doi.org/10.1038/nature11450

Qiu, B., Liang, J., & Li, C. (2023, July 20). Effects of fecal microbiota transplantation in metabolic syndrome: A meta-analysis of randomized controlled trials. *PLOS One*, 18(7), e0288718. https://doi.org/10.1371/journal.pone.0288718

Raposo, M. A., Armiliato, G. N. A., Guimarães, N. S., Caram, C. A., Silveira, R. D. S., & Tupinambás, U. (2017). Metabolic disorders and cardiovascular risk in people living with HIV/AIDS without the use of antiretroviral therapy. *Revista da Sociedade Brasileira de Medicina Tropical*, 50(5), 598–606. https://doi.org/10.1590/0037-8682-0258-2017

Rath, E., Moschetta, A., & Haller, D. (2018). Mitochondrial function-Gatekeeper of intestinal epithelial cell homeostasis. *Nature Reviews. Gastroenterology and Hepatology*, 15(8), 497–516. https://doi.org/10.1038/s41575-018-0021-x

Régnier, M., Van Hul, M., Knauf, C., & Cani, P. D. (2021). Gut microbiome, endocrine control of gut barrier function and metabolic diseases. *Journal of Endocrinology*, 248(2), R67–R82. https://doi.org/10.1530/JOE-20-0473

Reque, P. M., & Brandelli, A. (2021). Encapsulation of probiotics and nutraceuticals: Applications in functional food industry. *Trends in Food Science and Technology*, 114, 1–10. https://doi.org/10.1016/j.tifs.2021.05.022

Rittiphairoj, T., Pongpirul, K., Janchot, K., Mueller, N. T., & Li, T. (2021). Probiotics contribute to glycemic control in patients with type 2 diabetes mellitus: A systematic review and meta-analysis. *Advances in Nutrition*, 12(3), 722–734. https://doi.org/10.1093/advances/nmaa133

Roberts, A. B., Gu, X., Buffa, J. A., Hurd, A. G., Wang, Z., Zhu, W., Gupta, N., Skye, S. M., Cody, D. B., Levison, B. S., Barrington, W. T., Russell, M. W., Reed, J. M., Duzan, A., Lang, J. M., Fu, X., Li, L., Myers, A. J., Rachakonda, S., . . . & Hazen, S. L. (2018). Development of a gut microbe targeted nonlethal therapeutic to inhibit thrombosis potential. *Nature Medicine*, 24(9), 1407–1417. https://doi.org/10.1038/s41591-018-0128-1

Roshanravan, N., Mahdavi, R., Alizadeh, E., Jafarabadi, M. A., Hedayati, M., Ghavami, A., Alipour, S., Alamdari, N. M., Barati, M., & Ostadrahimi, A. (2017). Effect of butyrate and inulin supplementation on glycemic status, lipid profile and glucagon-like peptide 1 level in patients with type 2 diabetes: A randomized double-blind, placebo-controlled trial. *Hormone and Metabolic Research*, 49(11), 886–891. https://doi.org/10.1055/s-0043-119089

Safarimosavi, S., Mohebbi, H., & Rohani, H. (2021). High-intensity interval vs. continuous endurance training: Preventive effects on hormonal changes and physiological adaptations in prediabetes patients. *Journal of Strength and Conditioning Research*, 35(3), 731–738. https://doi.org/10.1519/JSC.0000000000002709

Salminen, S., Collado, M. C., Endo, A., Hill, C., Lebeer, S., Quigley, E. M. M., Sanders, M. E., Shamir, R., Swann, J. R., Szajewska, H., & Vinderola, G. (2021). The International Scientific Association of Probiotics and Prebiotics (ISAPP) consensus statement on the definition and scope of postbiotics. *Nature Reviews. Gastroenterology and Hepatology*, 18(9), 649–667. https://doi.org/10.1038/s41575-021-00440-6

Scannapieco, F. A., & Dongari-Bagtzoglou, A. (2021). Dysbiosis revisited: Understanding the role of the oral microbiome in the pathogenesis of gingivitis and periodontitis: A critical assessment. *Journal of Periodontology*, 92(8), 1071–1078. https://doi.org/10.1002/JPER.21-0120

Schoeler, M., & Caesar, R. (2019). Dietary lipids, gut microbiota and lipid metabolism. *Reviews in Endocrine and Metabolic Disorders*, 20(4), 461–472. https://doi.org/10.1007/s11154-019-09512-0

Schreiber, F., Arasteh, J. M., & Lawley, T. D. (2015). Pathogen resistance mediated by IL-22 signaling at the epithelial-microbiota interface. *Journal of Molecular Biology*, 427(23), 3676–3682. https://doi.org/10.1016/j.jmb.2015.10.013

Schreurs, M. P. H., de Vos van Steenwijk, P. J., Romano, A., Dieleman, S., & Werner, H. M. J. (2021). How the gut microbiome links to menopause and obesity, with possible implications for endometrial cancer development. *Journal of Clinical Medicine*, 10(13), 2916. https://doi.org/10.3390/jcm10132916

Shimizu, H., Ohue-Kitano, R., & Kimura, I. (2019). Regulation of host energy metabolism by gut microbiota-derived short-chain fatty acids. *Glycative Stress Research*, 6(3), 181–191.

Sjödin, K. S., Sjödin, A., Ruszczyński, M., Kristensen, M. B., Hernell, O., Szajewska, H., & West, C. E. (2023). Targeting the gut-lung axis by synbiotic feeding to infants in a randomized controlled trial. *BMC Biology*, 21(1), 38. https://doi.org/10.1186/s12915-023-01531-3

Soares, N. L., Dorand, V. A. M., Cavalcante, H. C., Batista, K. S., de Souza, D. M., Lima, M. D. S., Salvadori, M. G. D. S. S., Magnani, M., Alves, A. F., & Aquino, J. S. (2021). Does intermittent fasting associated with aerobic training influence parameters related to the gut-brain axis of Wistar rats? *Journal of Affective Disorders*, 293, 176–185. https://doi.org/10.1016/j.jad.2021.06.028

Spanogiannopoulos, P., Bess, E. N., Carmody, R. N., & Turnbaugh, P. J. (2016). The microbial pharmacists within us: A metagenomic view of xenobiotic metabolism. *Nature Reviews. Microbiology*, 14(5), 273–287. https://doi.org/10.1038/nrmicro.2016.17

Stolfi, C., Maresca, C., Monteleone, G., & Laudisi, F. (2022). Implication of intestinal barrier dysfunction in gut dysbiosis and diseases. *Biomedicines*, 10(2), 289. https://doi.org/10.3390/biomedicines10020289

Sun, L., Xie, C., Wang, G., Wu, Y., Wu, Q., Wang, X., Liu, J., Deng, Y., Xia, J., Chen, B., Zhang, S., Yun, C., Lian, G., Zhang, X., Zhang, H., Bisson, W. H., Shi, J., Gao, X., Ge, P., . . . & Jiang, C. (2018). Gut microbiota and intestinal FXR mediate the clinical benefits of metformin. *Nature Medicine*, 24(12), 1919–1929. https://doi.org/10.1038/s41591-018-0222-4

Swanson, K. S., Gibson, G. R., Hutkins, R., Reimer, R. A., Reid, G., Verbeke, K., Scott, K. P., Holscher, H. D., Azad, M. B., Delzenne, N. M., & Sanders, M. E. (2020). The International Scientific Association for Probiotics and Prebiotics (ISAPP) consensus statement on the definition and scope of synbiotics. *Nature Reviews. Gastroenterology and Hepatology*, 17(11), 687–701. https://doi.org/10.1038/s41575-020-0344-2

Tanes, C., Bittinger, K., Gao, Y., Friedman, E. S., Nessel, L., Paladhi, U. R., Chau, L., Panfen, E., Fischbach, M. A., Braun, J., Xavier, R. J., Clish, C. B., Li, H., Bushman, F. D., Lewis, J. D., & Wu, G. D. (2021). Role of dietary fiber in the recovery of the human gut microbiome and its metabolome. *Cell Host and Microbe*, 29(3), 394–407.e5. https://doi.org/10.1016/j.chom.2020.12.012

Tao, Y. W., Gu, Y. L., Mao, X. Q., Zhang, L., & Pei, Y. F. (2020). Effects of probiotics on type II diabetes mellitus: A meta-analysis. *Journal of Translational Medicine*, 18(1), 30. https://doi.org/10.1186/s12967-020-02213-2

Tomasova, L., Grman, M., Ondrias, K., & Ufnal, M. (2021). The impact of gut microbiota metabolites on cellular bioenergetics and cardiometabolic health. *Nutrition and Metabolism*, 18(1), 72. https://doi.org/10.1186/s12986-021-00598-5

Torquati, L., Gajanand, T., Cox, E. R., Willis, C. R. G., Zaugg, J., Keating, S. E., & Coombes, J. S. (2023). Effects of exercise intensity on gut microbiome composition and function in people with type 2 diabetes. *European Journal of Sport Science*, 23(4), 530–541. https://doi.org/10.1080/17461391.2022.2035436

Tuomi, T., Santoro, N., Caprio, S., Cai, M., Weng, J., & Groop, L. (2014). The many faces of diabetes: A disease with increasing heterogeneity. *Lancet*, 383(9922), 1084–1094. https://doi.org/10.1016/S0140-6736(13)62219-9

VanBest, N., Rolle-Kampczyk, U., Schaap, F. G., Basic, M., Olde Damink, S. W. M., Bleich, A., Savelkoul, P. H. M., von Bergen, M., Penders, J., & Hornef, M. W. (2020). Bile acids drive the newborn's gut microbiota maturation. *Nature Communications*, 11(1), 3692. https://doi.org/10.1038/s41467-020-17183-8

VanOlden, C. C., Van de Laar, A. W., Meijnikman, A. S., Aydin, O., Van Olst, N., Hoozemans, J. B., De Brauw, L. M., Bruin, S. C., Acherman, Y. I. Z., Verheij, J., Pyykkö, J. E., Hagedoorn, M., Sanderman, R., Bosma, N. C., Tremaroli, V., Lundqvist, A., Olofsson, L. E., Herrema, H., . . . & Gerdes, V. E. A. (2021). A systems biology approach to understand gut microbiota and host metabolism in morbid obesity: Design of the BARIA Longitudinal Cohort Study. *Journal of Internal Medicine*, 289(3), 340–354. https://doi.org/10.1111/joim.13157

Vandenplas, Y., Carnielli, V. P., Ksiazyk, J., Luna, M. S., Migacheva, N., Mosselmans, J. M., Picaud, J. C., Possner, M., Singhal, A., & Wabitsch, M. (2020). Factors affecting early-life intestinal microbiota development. *Nutrition*, 78, 110812. https://doi.org/10.1016/j.nut.2020.110812

Vasim, I., Majeed, C. N., & DeBoer, M. D. (2022). Intermittent fasting and metabolic health. *Nutrients*, 14(3), 631. https://doi.org/10.3390/nu14030631

Vernocchi, P., Del Chierico, F., & Putignani, L. (2020). Gut microbiota metabolism and interaction with food components. *International Journal of Molecular Sciences*, 21(10), 3688. https://doi.org/10.3390/ijms21103688

Vieira-Silva, S., Falony, G., Belda, E., Nielsen, T., Aron-Wisnewsky, J., Chakaroun, R., Forslund, S. K., Assmann, K., Valles-Colomer, M., Nguyen, T. T. D., Proost, S., Prifti, E., Tremaroli, V., Pons, N., Le Chatelier, E., Andreelli, F., Bastard, J. P., Coelho, L. P., Galleron, N., . . . & Raes, J. (2020). Statin therapy is associated with lower prevalence of gut microbiota dysbiosis. *Nature*, 581(7808), 310–315. https://doi.org/10.1038/s41586-020-2269-x

Wagner, R., Heni, M., Tabák, A. G., Machann, J., Schick, F., Randrianarisoa, E., Hrabě de Angelis, M., Birkenfeld, A. L., Stefan, N., Peter, A., Häring, H. U., & Fritsche, A. (2021). Pathophysiology-based subphenotyping of individuals at eldiabetes. *Nature Medicine*, 27(1), 49–57. https://doi.org/10.1038/s41591-020-1116-9

Wang, L., Chen, P., & Xiao, W. (2021). β-hydroxybutyrate as an antiaging metabolite. *Nutrients*, 13, 3420.

Wang, L., Yang, H., Huang, H., Zhang, C., Zuo, H. X., Xu, P., Niu, Y. M., & Wu, S. S. (2019). Inulin-type fructans supplementation improves glycemic control for the prediabetes and type 2 diabetes populations: Results from a GRADE-assessed systematic review and dose-response meta-analysis of 33 randomized controlled trials. *Journal of Translational Medicine*, 17(1), 410. https://doi.org/10.1186/s12967-019-02159-0

Wang, Y., Ai, Z., Xing, X., Fan, Y., Zhang, Y., Nan, B., Li, X., Wang, Y., & Liu, J. (2022). The ameliorative effect of probiotics on diet-induced lipid metabolism disorders: A review. *Critical Reviews in Food Science and Nutrition*, 1–17. https://doi.org/10.1080/10408398.2022.2132377

Wang, Y., & Wu, R. (2022). The effect of fasting on human metabolism and psychological health. *Disease Markers*, 2022, 5653739. https://doi.org/10.1155/2022/5653739

Wang, Z., Roberts, A. B., Buffa, J. A., Levison, B. S., Zhu, W., Org, E., Gu, X., Huang, Y., Zamanian-Daryoush, M., Culley, M. K., DiDonato, A. J., Fu, X., Hazen, J. E., Krajcik, D., DiDonato, J. A., Lusis, A. J., & Hazen, S. L. (2015). Non-lethal inhibition of gut microbial trimethylamine production for the treatment of atherosclerosis. *Cell*, 163(7), 1585–1595. https://doi.org/10.1016/j.cell.2015.11.055

Weersma, R. K., Zhernakova, A., & Fu, J. (2020). Interaction between drugs and the gut microbiome. *Gut*, 69(8), 1510–1519. https://doi.org/10.1136/gutjnl-2019-320204

West, R., Michie, S., Rubin, G. J., & Amlôt, R. (2020). Applying principles of behaviour change to reduce SARS-CoV-2 transmission. *Nature Human Behaviour*, 4(5), 451–459. https://doi.org/10.1038/s41562-020-0887-9

Wu, H., Esteve, E., Tremaroli, V., Khan, M. T., Caesar, R., Mannerås-Holm, L., Ståhlman, M., Olsson, L. M., Serino, M., Planas-Fèlix, M., Xifra, G., Mercader, J. M., Torrents, D., Burcelin, R., Ricart, W., Perkins, R., Fernàndez-Real, J. M., & Bäckhed, F. (2017). Metformin alters the gut microbiome of individuals with treatment-naive type 2 diabetes, contributing to the therapeutic effects of the drug. *Nature Medicine*, 23(7), 850–858. https://doi.org/10.1038/nm.4345

Xiao, H., & Kang, S. (2020). The role of the gut microbiome in energy balance with a focus on the gut-adipose tissue axis. *Frontiers in Genetics*, 11, 297. https://doi.org/10.3389/fgene.2020.00297

Xie, Y., Hu, F., Xiang, D., Lu, H., Li, W., Zhao, A., Huang, L., & Wang, R. (2020, January 2). The metabolic effect of gut microbiota on drugs. *Drug Metabolism Reviews*, 52(1), 139–156. https://doi.org/10.1080/03602532.2020.1718691

Yang, W., Xia, Z., Zhu, Y., Tang, H., Xu, H., Hu, X., Lin, C., Jiang, T., He, P., & Shen, J. (2023, December 31). Comprehensive study of untargeted metabolomics and 16S rRNA reveals the mechanism of fecal microbiota transplantation in improving a mouse model of T2D. *Diabetes, Metabolic Syndrome and Obesity: Targets and Therapy*, 16, 1367–1381. https://doi.org/10.2147/DMSO.S404352

Yao, M., Xie, J., Du, H., McClements, D. J., Xiao, H., & Li, L. (2020). Progress in microencapsulation of probiotics: A review. *Comprehensive Reviews in Food Science and Food Safety*, 19(2), 857–874. https://doi.org/10.1111/1541-4337.12532

Zecheng, L., Donghai, L., Runchuan, G., Yuan, Q., Qi, J., Yijia, Z., Shuaman, R., Xiaoqi, L., Yi, W., Ni, M., Yijin, Q., Liang, P., & Jun, W. (2023, June 24). Fecal microbiota transplantation in obesity metabolism: A meta analysis and systematic review. *Diabetes Research and Clinical Practice*, 202, 110803. https://doi.org/10.1016/j.diabres.2023.110803

Zhang, L., Wang, Y., Sun, Y., & Zhang, X. (2023, May 11). Intermittent fasting and physical exercise for preventing metabolic disorders through interaction with gut microbiota: A review. *Nutrients*, 15(10), 2277. https://doi.org/10.3390/nu15102277

Zhang, M., Hou, Z. K., Huang, Z. B., Chen, X. L., & Liu, F. B. (2021). Dietary and lifestyle factors related to gastroesophageal reflux disease: A systematic review. *Therapeutics and Clinical Risk Management*, 17, 305–323. https://doi.org/10.2147/TCRM.S296680

Zhang, X., Zhao, Y., Xu, J., Xue, Z., Zhang, M., Pang, X., Zhang, X., & Zhao, L. (2015). Modulation of gut microbiota by berberine and metformin during the treatment of high-fat diet-induced obesity in rats. *Scientific Reports*, 5(1), 14405. https://doi.org/10.1038/srep14405

Zhang, X., Zou, Q., Zhao, B., Zhang, J., Zhao, W., Li, Y., Liu, R., Liu, X., & Liu, Z. (2020). Effects of alternate-day fasting, time-restricted fasting and intermittent energy restriction DSS-induced on colitis and behavioral disorders. *Redox Biology*, 32, 101535. https://doi.org/10.1016/j.redox.2020.101535

Zheng, L., Wen, X. L., & Duan, S. L. (2022). Role of metabolites derived from gut microbiota in inflammatory bowel disease. *World Journal of Clinical Cases*, 10(9), 2660–2677. https://doi.org/10.12998/wjcc.v10.i9.2660

Zhou, W., Sailani, M. R., Contrepois, K., Zhou, Y., Ahadi, S., Leopold, S. R., Zhang, M. J., Rao, V., Avina, M., Mishra, T., Johnson, J., Lee-McMullen, B., Chen, S., Metwally, A. A., Tran, T. D. B., Nguyen, H., Zhou, X., Albright, B., Hong, B. Y., . . . & Snyder, M. (2019). Longitudinal multiomics of host-microbe dynamics in prediabetes. *Nature*, 569(7758), 663–671. https://doi.org/10.1038/s41586-019-1236-x

Zhu, C., Wang, X., Li, J., Jiang, R., Chen, H., Chen, T., & Yang, Y. (2022). Determine independent gut microbiota-diseases association by eliminating the effects of human lifestyle factors. *BMC Microbiology*, 22(1), 4. https://doi.org/10.1186/s12866-021-02414-9

Zhu, W., Gregory, J. C., Org, E., Buffa, J. A., Gupta, N., Wang, Z., Li, L., Fu, X., Wu, Y., Mehrabian, M., Sartor, R. B., McIntyre, T. M., Silverstein, R. L., Tang, W. H. W., DiDonato, J. A., Brown, J. M., Lusis, A. J., & Hazen, S. L. (2016). Gut microbial metabolite TMAO enhances platelet hyperreactivity and thrombosis risk. *Cell*, 165(1), 111–124. https://doi.org/10.1016/j.cell.2016.02.011

Zou, R., Xu, F., Wang, Y., Duan, M., Guo, M., Zhang, Q., Zhao, H., & Zheng, H. (2020). Changes in the gut microbiota of children with autism spectrum disorder. *Autism Research*, 13(9), 1614–1625. https://doi.org/10.1002/aur.2358

6 The Impact of Probiotic and Synbiotic Supplementation on Oxidative Stress and Inflammation

Himanshu Sharma, Sanjesh Kumar, Sumel Ashique, Pratibha Bhowmick, Radheshyam Pal, Arshad Farid, Roomah Javed, Farzad Taghizadeh-Hesary, and Subhajit Mandal

6.1 INTRODUCTION (INCLUDES PROBIOTIC, PREBIOTIC AND SYNBIOTIC, ROS, AND INFLAMMATION)

The significance of gut health has become increasingly understood in recent years in maintaining overall well-being [1]. Often called the "second brain," the gut is the home of an intricate microbial ecosystem that affects our metabolism, immune system, and even mental well-being. Within this intricate microbial ecosystem, probiotics, prebiotics, and synbiotics have gained widespread recognition as useful tools for improving gut health and lowering reactive oxygen species (ROS) and inflammation. Probiotics are living microorganisms, mostly beneficial bacteria, that give humans two health benefits when consumed in the right amount [2]. They are referred to as "friendly bacteria" and have gained popularity because of their ability to maintain a balanced gut flora. Probiotics create substances that promote gut health and squelch harmful organisms, assisting in the preservation of a balanced microbial ecosystem. On the other hand, prebiotics are indigestible materials found in some diets, such as high-fiber fruits and vegetables. These materials nourish the stomach's beneficial microorganisms. Prebiotics are essentially the fuel that supports the growth of a robust microbial community and keeps probiotics alive. They provide a means of promoting the development of beneficial bacteria, which ultimately maintains a balanced gut flora [3]. Combining probiotics and prebiotics results in synbiotic partnerships. Synbiotics are made to maximize the beneficial bacteria in the gut's ability to survive and proliferate by working in concert with prebiotics and probiotics. The combined approach aims to enhance the benefits of gut microbiota health, including its capacity to reduce inflammation and oxidative stress. Oxygen atoms left over from the body's numerous metabolic activities combine to form highly reactive molecules known as reactive oxygen species, or ROS [4]. However, ROS are necessary for numerous physiological processes, including immunological response and cell communication, excessive ROS production can result in oxidative stress. In consequence, oxidative stress can harm cellular constituents such as proteins, lipids, and DNA, which can lead to several illnesses such as cancer, heart disease, and neurological problems. Inflammation is a fundamental immune response to a disease, trauma, or outside intruders [5]. Increased blood flow, the recruitment of immune cells, and the production of signaling molecules to address the problem are its defining features. On the other hand, uncontrolled or chronic inflammation is associated with a range of health problems, such as atherosclerosis, illnesses connected to obesity, and chronic inflammatory diseases. One important component of the complex interaction between ROS and inflammation is the gut [6]. The composition and balance of gut bacteria have an important effect on ROS levels and the degree of systemic inflammation [7]. Prebiotics, probiotics, and synbiotics (combination of pre- and probiotics) are very useful to decrease the oxidative stress and inflammation by altering the gut flora. Through the promotion of a healthy gut microbiota, these treatments can aid in the preservation of the body's optimal balance, which affects not only immune system performance and overall health but also digestive health. The dynamic interplay between probiotics, prebiotics, and synbiotics as well as their capacity to manage ROS and inflammation will be examined in this discussion, providing insight into how these strategies might be used to support and enhance general health [8].

6.2 SOURCE OF ROS IN THE HUMAN BODY

ROS, or molecules containing oxygen that are very reactive, are naturally created as byproducts of several physiological metabolic processes. Depending on their concentration and the context in which they are created, these chemicals may have both positive and negative impacts [9]. The human body produces ROS from the following common sources. Organic Circuits Oxidative phosphorylation in the mitochondria produces most of the body's ROS. This procedure is how these organelles produce energy. While cellular energy depends on the synthesis of ademosin triphosphate (ATP), this process also produces ROS, including radicals like superoxide and hydrogen peroxide. When there is inflammation, the immune system produces ROS.

DOI: 10.1201/9781032702438-6

Similar to neutrophils and macrophages, phagocytic cells release ROS in an attempt to fight invasive infections. On the other hand, prolonged inflammation can lead to an increase in ROS generation, which can cause tissue damage [10]. In reaction to external stimuli including radiation, air pollution, and certain chemicals, the body may manufacture more ROS [11]. This process is necessary for the synthesis of energy, but it can also cause oxidative stress. When some medications, poisons, and xenobiotics break down in the liver and other organs, more ROS are produced. This may cause cellular damage and contribute to certain illnesses [12]. Exposure to ionizing radiation, such as X-rays and gamma rays, can generate ROS, which can damage cells and alter DNA [13]. ROS can arise in the skin as a result of UV radiation from the sun, which can cause photoaging and skin damage. Moreover, ROS may be produced by the body's normal chemical activities, such as the disintegration of certain molecules. ROS have been connected to numerous diseases and health issues suchas cancer, neurological disorders, and cardiovascular disease. They are engaged in several physiological processes. On the other hand, oxidative stress can result from excessive or unregulated ROS production [14]. To combat the negative effects of ROS, the body contains built-in antioxidant defense systems. Maintaining the proper balance between ROS production and antioxidant defenses is essential for general health (Figure 6.1) [15].

6.3 INTERLINK BETWEEN ROS AND INFLAMMATION IN VARIOUS CONDITIONS

ROS and inflammation are linked in several physiological and pathological situations. ROS may both cause and be caused by inflammation, leading to a complex interplay. This is an overview of the several scenarios in which inflammation and ROS interact. Pathogens, such as bacteria or viruses, cause an immune response. Immune cells like neutrophils and macrophages produce ROS as a protective strategy to get rid of invading microorganisms [17]. When the body is infected, ROS are produced by the body to help with the inflammatory process. Persistent inflammation is linked to chronic inflammatory disorders, such as inflammatory bowel disease and rheumatoid arthritis. This persistent inflammation may result in the formation of ROS continuing [18]. ROS can activate pro-inflammatory signaling pathways, which can worsen inflammation and destroy tissue. Atherosclerosis is a condition where plaque builds up in the arteries, and it is associated with chronic inflammation. The generation of ROS inside blood vessel walls can lead to oxidative modification of proteins and lipids, which can worsen inflammation and hasten the onset of atherosclerosis [19]. In the central nervous system, ROS are produced during neuroinflammation, often as a consequence of microglial activation. The brain conditions such as Parkinson's and Alzheimer's have been linked to ROS. Internal inflammatory disorders, especially chronic inflammation, can contribute to the development and spread of cancer. Because ROS may damage and mutate DNA, they may have a role in the development of cancer [20]. ROS generation rises in situations where there is decreased blood flow (ischemia) and then a restoration of blood flow (reperfusion), as in heart attacks and strokes [21]. The injury may worsen as a result of this surge of ROS following reperfusion, which can lead to more tissue damage and inflammation. Numerous ailments, including asthma and COPD, are linked with elevated ROS levels in chronic lung inflammation [21]. ROS can cause lung injury by triggering inflammatory pathways. Meta-inflammation, a chronic low-grade inflammatory state, is one of the characteristics of obesity. ROS have a role in the development of insulin resistance and metabolic dysfunction as well as the inflammation linked to obesity [22]. Inflammation and ROS are intimately related in a number of circumstances. ROS have the capacity to behave as signaling molecules that initiate inflammatory responses, which in turn can increase ROS production. This feedback loop can accelerate the development of many illnesses and cause tissue damage [23]. Controlling oxidative stress and inflammation is essential to treating these diseases [24]. In order to lessen the detrimental effects of ROS and inflammation in certain disease states, antioxidants and anti-inflammatory techniques are frequently used [25].

6.4 DESCRIBE THE BACTERIAL METABOLITES (SCFAS, BILE ACID, ETC.)

Bacterial metabolites are produced by a range of microorganisms, particularly gut bacteria, during the fermentation and digestion of dietary substrates in the GI tract. These metabolites have a critical role in maintaining intestinal health, controlling host physiology, and improving overall health [26]. The two primary classes of metabolites that bacteria create are SCFAs and bile acids [27].

6.4.1 Short-Chain Fatty Acids (SCFAs)

Together with acetate, the stomach also produces butyrate and propionate, which are the other two major SCFAs. It is readily absorbed by the host and can function as a metabolic substrate for the generation of energy [28]. Propionate is another SCFA that is vital to metabolism. After being absorbed, the liver may use it as a gluconeogenic precursor [29]. This suggests that it might be converted into glucose, which helps regulate blood sugar levels. Butyrate is arguably the most well-known SCFA due to its numerous health benefits. For colonocytes, it serves as their main source of energy [30]. It's critical to lower inflammation and preserve the gut barrier's integrity. Additionally, butyrate has been linked to a lower incidence of inflammatory bowel illnesses and colon cancer [31].

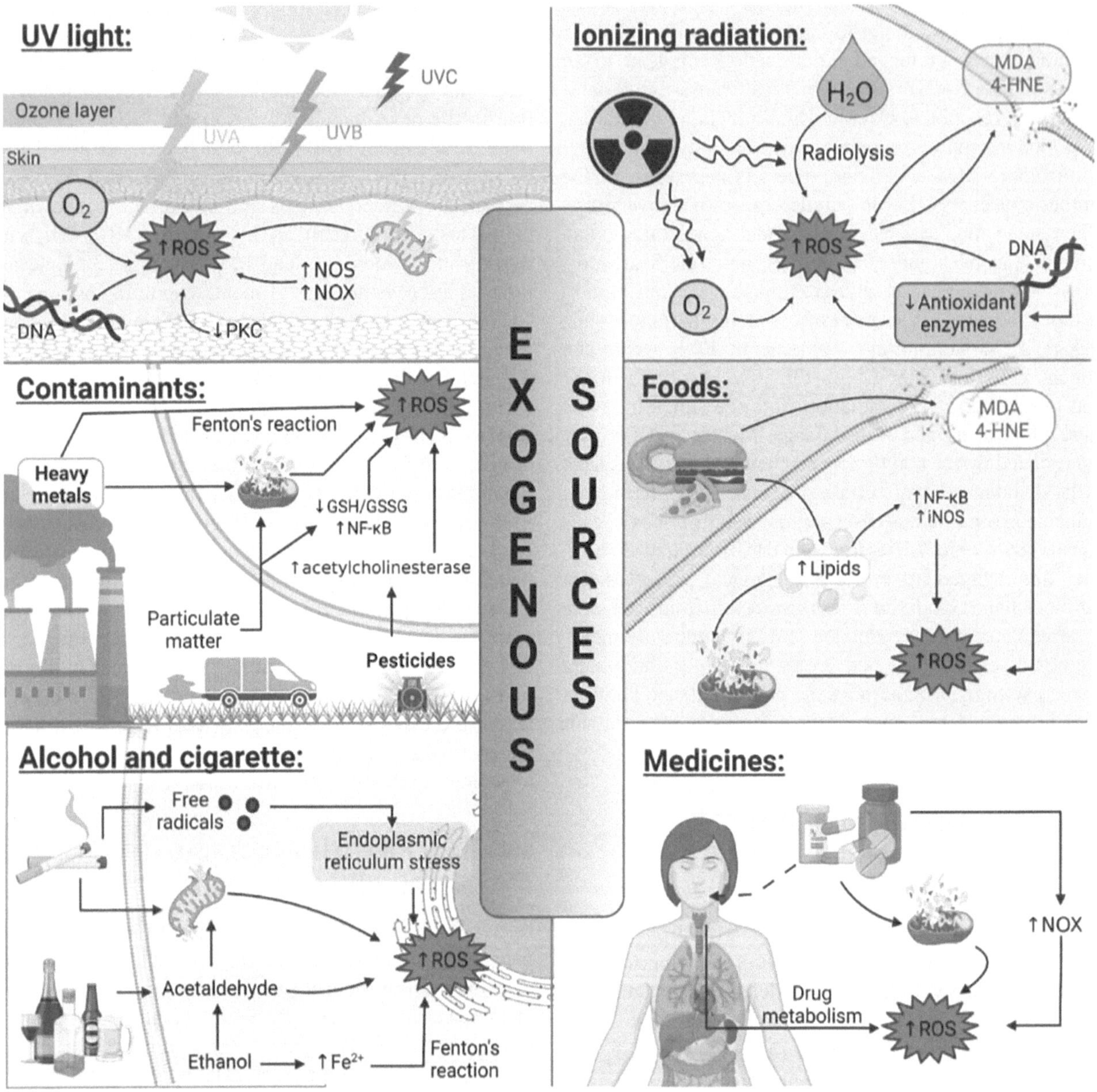

FIGURE 6.1 Oxidative stress, which damages lipids and DNA, is brought on by external sources of reactive oxygen species through a number of mechanisms, including radiation, pollution, and alcohol. This open access article is subject to the conditions and limitations of the Creative Commons Attribution (CC BY) license [16] (https://creativecommons.org/licenses/by/4.0/).

6.4.2 Bile Acids

Liver forms bile acids that are reserved in the gallbladder. Dietary lipids are delivered into the small intestine to aid in their breakdown and absorption [32]. By a process known as deconjugation and dihydroxylation, gut bacteria transform primary bile acids into secondary bile acids. [33]. Once entered the bloodstream, the secondary bile acids have a variety of physiological effects. One secondary bile acid that has been connected to the breakdown of dietary lipids and cholesterol is deoxycholic acid. Lithocholic acid is another secondary bile acid that has been linked to a number of impacts on host metabolism and health; this may have an impact on the makeup of the gut microbiota [34].

Additionally, bile acids are involved in signaling pathways that control the metabolism of glucose and fat. The physiology and well-being of the host are impacted in many ways by these bacterial metabolites, SCFAs, and bile acids. They have an impact on intestinal health. Butyrate helps to lower the inflammation and preserve the unification of the intestinal barrier. They can lower the chance of illnesses and enhance intestinal motility [35]. SCFAs and bile acids are essential for the host's energy metabolism and have an effect on lipid and glucose balance [36]. They could affect insulin sensitivity, body weight, and metabolic disease risk factors, such as diabetes and obesity [37]. SCFAs contain immunomodulatory properties and the ability to influence immune cell activity, which help to control the host's immunological response. These metabolites have the ability to reduce stomach and other bodily tissue inflammation [38]. Increased inflammation and inflammatory disorders have been linked to the dysregulation of these metabolites. A lower incidence of colorectal cancer has been associated with butyrate and secondary bile acids; this is probably due to their anti-inflammatory and colonocyte-promoting qualities. In summary, two forms of bacterial metabolites that are essential for immunity, metabolism, gut health, and general well-being are bile acids and SCFAs. Understanding how the gut microbiota creates and utilizes these metabolites is necessary to determine their potential therapeutic and preventative applications in a variety of medical conditions [39].

6.5 MECHANISM OF PROBIOTICS AND SYNBIOTICS TO CONTROL ROS AND INFLAMMATION

A wealth of research evidence demonstrates the complex and interrelated mechanisms via which probiotics and synbiotics control inflammation and ROS, illustrating their diverse effects on health and disease [40]. Particularly, probiotics and synbiotics have significant effects on each of these pathways, which include the production of antioxidants, the inhibition of ROS-generating enzymes, the strengthening of the gut barrier, the modulation of immunological responses, and the change of the gut microbiota [41].

6.5.1 Modulation of Gut Microbiota

Pattern recognition receptors identify microbial-associated molecular patterns and probiotics by interacting with gut epithelial cells. Probiotics are generally composed of live beneficial microorganisms like Lactobacillus and Bifidobacterium species. Interleukin-10 is suppressed, whereas pro-inflammatory cytokines are increased and mitogen-activated protein kinase pathways are activated as a result of this interaction's activation of signaling cascades [42].

6.5.2 Immune Regulation

The gut epithelial cells interact with probiotics, which are mainly composed of live beneficial microorganisms like Lactobacillus and Bifidobacterium species, by recognizing microbial-associated molecular patterns, such as toll-like receptors, employing pattern recognition receptors. This relationship increases the production of anti-inflammatory cytokines such as interleukin-10 and inhibits the release of pro-inflammatory cytokines such as tumor necrosis factor-alpha and interleukin-6. It also activates the pathways for nuclear factor-kappa and MAPK [43]. In a model of aging mice, a synbiotic formulation including Lactobacillus casei and inulin reduced the formation of ROS and inflammation by helping the development of valuable bacteria and the formation of SCFAs like butyrate [44] in SCFAs are well recognized for their anti-inflammatory characteristics; according to research, they can reduce inflammation, alter immune cell G protein-coupled receptors, and inhibit histone deacetylases [45]. Probiotics interfere with pattern recognition receptors, also known as toll-like receptors, upsetting the delicate balance between pro- and anti-inflammatory mediators.

6.5.3 Strengthening the Gut Barrier

Research has shown that some probiotic strains improve the integrity of the intestinal barrier by upregulating the expression of tight junction proteins [46]. By reducing the production of ROS and boosting the appearance of tight junction proteins in the intestinal epithelium, Lactobacillus plantarum, for instance, has shown antioxidative properties in mice. Because the gut barrier keeps bacterial products and endotoxins out of the circulation, maintaining it is essential for lowering systemic inflammation. [47].

6.5.4 Production of Antioxidants

Antioxidant molecules such as superoxide dismutase and catalase can be directly produced by probiotics. By scavenging ROS, these enzymes aggressively combat harmful ROS and shield cells from oxidative damage [48]. Probiotics have been demonstrated to increase the synthesis of gastrointestinal mucins, which act as a barrier to lessen inflammatory reactions and shield the gut epithelium from luminal antigens [49].

6.5.5 Inhibition of ROS-Generating Enzymes

Probiotics and synbiotics affect immune cells and the gut epithelium via supporting the development of favorable microbes and preventing the evolution of dangerous species [50]. By changing the ratio of pro-to-anti-inflammatory chemicals secreted in the gut, this microbial change can further reduce inflammation and the generation of ROS. Nitric oxide synthases and NADPH oxidases are two important enzymes that contribute to the production of ROS in immune cells, and probiotics can directly regulate these enzymes [51]. By dramatically lowering the generation of ROS, inhibiting these enzymes gradually decreases oxidative stress. In a mouse model of colitis, for instance, Bifidobacterium longum has been demonstrated to raise antioxidant enzyme activity and reduce ROS formation [52]. A portion of this impact is attained by altering the gut microbiota's composition [53].

6.5.6 Synbiotics and Their Synergistic Effects

These anti-inflammatory and antioxidant properties are strengthened by synbiotics, which blend probiotics with prebiotics. Prebiotics that increase the metabolic activity of probiotic bacteria include fructo oligosaccharides and insulin [54]. These anti-inflammatory and antioxidant properties are strengthened by synbiotics, which blend probiotics with prebiotics. Prebiotics that increase the metabolic activity of

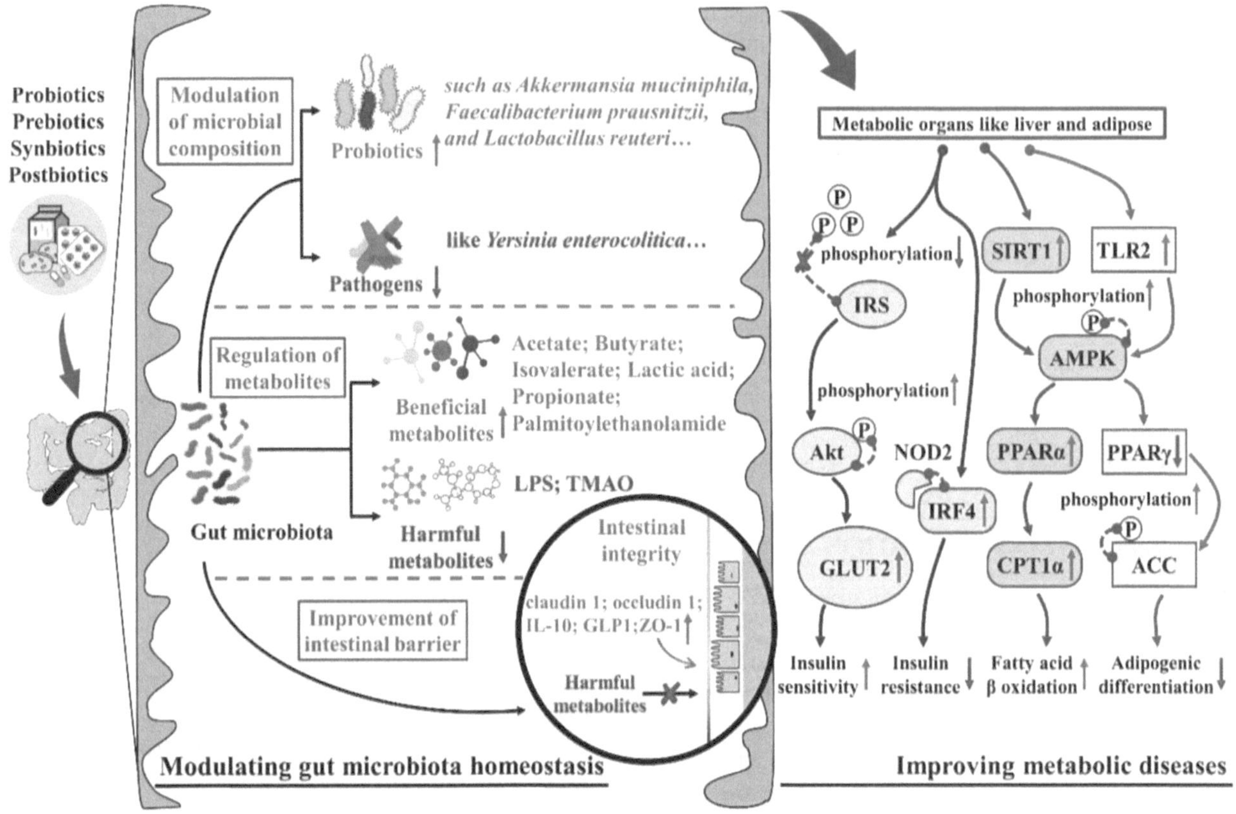

FIGURE 6.2 Probiotics, prebiotics, and synbiotics influence metabolic diseases by modulating bacterial populations, regulating the gut microbiota, improving the intestinal barrier, and metabolite production. These activities enhance the metabolic system overall via many molecular pathways [56]. The conditions and restrictions of Creative Commons Attribution license have focused in this open access article (https://creativecommons.org/licenses/by/4.0/).

probiotic bacteria include fructo oligosaccharides and insulin. These interrelated pathways show the potential of probiotics and synbiotics as therapeutic agents for inflammatory diseases and illnesses linked to oxidative stress, with beneficial implications for human health and well-being. These treatments provide an all-encompassing strategy for reducing inflammation and oxidative stress, with effects ranging from immune response modulation and gut microbiota management to antioxidant synthesis, gut barrier fortification, and inhibition of ROS-generating enzymes [55] (Figure 6.2).

6.6 APPLICATION OF PROBIOTIC/SYNBIOTIC TO INHIBIT ROS AND INFLAMMATION

Synbiotics, or the combination of prebiotics and probiotics, are a comprehensive and effective way to lower ROS and inflammation in a range of medical conditions (Table 6.1). Synbiotics provide a potent way to promote health and treat sickness by utilizing the complementing qualities of probiotics, which often comprise helpful bacteria like Lactobacillus and Bifidobacterium strains, and prebiotics, which act as probiotics' development substrates. Probiotics have shown great promise in maintaining the intestinal barrier, modifying the composition of gut flora, and controlling immunological responses in gastrointestinal illnesses. Reducing inflammation and oxidative damage in the gut environment requires this modulation. Synbiotics have proven to be very effective in treating inflammatory bowel illnesses, including Crohn's disease and ulcerative colitis [57]. Prebiotic substances that have been synthesized provide bacteria with the growth factors they need to produce butyrate and other SCFAs. By modifying G protein-coupled receptors on immune cells and preventing histone deacetylase activity, SCFAs have anti-inflammatory properties that reduce inflammation [58]. Using synbiotics may be beneficial for metabolic illnesses such as obesity, diabetes, and metabolic syndrome. These therapies improve insulin sensitivity and decrease systemic inflammation by changing the gut microbiota's makeup. Under these conditions, probiotics encourage the development of beneficial bacteria and the synthesis of SCFAs, which lower oxidative stress and inflammation. Among other things, they have been shown to reduce body weight, enhance insulin resistance, and enhance glucose regulation. It has been demonstrated that probiotic supplements reduce oxidative stress and inflammation when respiratory conditions like allergic rhinitis and asthma are present [59]. Prebiotics are essential for the synthesis of probiotics as well as for boosting their immune-modulating properties [60]. People with these conditions may experience fewer symptoms and a higher quality of life as a result of this immune system control. There is particular promise in the use of synbiotics to treat neurological illnesses such as neurodegenerative disorders and neuro-inflammation. Synbiotics have the ability to modify the gut–brain axis, which in turn impacts inflammation and oxidative stress inside the CNSA new study suggests that the beginning and progression of neuroinflammatory and neurodegenerative illnesses may be influenced by changes in the gut flora [61]. This immune system regulation may result in a decrease of symptoms and an increase in the quality of life for people with these illnesses. Treatment for neurological ailments such as neuroinflammatory diseases and neurodegenerative disorders may benefit particularly from the use of synbiotics. Synbiotics disturb the inflammation and oxidative stress in CNS by fluctuating GBA [62]. According to recent studies, alterations in the gut microbiota may have an effect on the development and progression of neuroinflammatory and neurodegenerative illnesses. Research has looked into the possibility of using synbiotics to change the immune system and lower the severity of rheumatoid arthritis. It has been shown that taking synbiotics lowers inflammation and oxidative stress in heart conditions including atherosclerosis and hypertension. The onset and course of cardiovascular disease are associated with these factors [63]. Because synbiotics can regulate immune response, preserve the gut barrier, and alter gut microbiota, they have great potential for enhancing cardiovascular health. Taking synbiotics may help lower blood pressure and arterial stiffness, according to certain studies [64]. When it comes to ailments like bacterial vaginosis and vulvovaginal candidiasis, synbiotics may also help reduce inflammation and oxidative stress. Certain gynecological disorders may occur less frequently if the vaginal microbiome is altered and the microbial environment is healthy. Synbiotics may have an anti-inflammatory effect on dermatological conditions such as atopic dermatitis and acne by influencing the skin microbiota and strengthening the skin barrier. Recent studies suggest that many dermatological disorders may be influenced by the skin microbiome, and that using synbiotics to treat it may have positive therapeutic effects [65]. Interest in the use of synbiotics has grown in connection to the central nervous system. An increasing amount of research indicates that in treating a range of neurological and neuropsychiatric conditions, the gut–brain axis is the two-way communication channel between the stomach and the central nervous system. It affects a variety of conditions, including anxiety, depression, and neurodegenerative diseases like Parkinson's and Alzheimer's. In these situations, probiotics can successfully treat oxidative stress and inflammation by altering the gut microbiota and regulating neurotransmitter synthesis [66]. Recent research suggests that synbiotics may enhance mood, memory, and general brain health. To sum up, the diverse array of uses for synbiotics indicates their promise as a practical approach to managing ROS and inflammation see Tables 6.1 and 6.2.

6.7 FUTURE PROSPECTIVE OF PROBIOTICS/SYNBIOTICS AS THERAPEUTICS INTERVENTION TO INHIBIT ROS AND INFLAMMATION

It is optimistic for the future because probiotics and synbiotics have the potential to be used as medicinal therapies to lower inflammation and ROS. Probiotics, such as strains of Lactobacillus and Bifidobacterium, have shown promise in improving the gut barrier and changing the makeup of the gut microbiota, which in turn controls immunological responses. Complex biological interactions, including the activation of toll-like receptors and other pattern recognition receptors on gut epithelial cells, are linked to these roles. These receptors identify microbe-associated molecular patterns, which set off signaling cascades that decrease pro-inflammatory cytokines and raise anti-inflammatory cytokines [79]. Yan et al. (2011), for instance, demonstrated that probiotic Lactobacillus rhamnosus GG inhibited pro-inflammatory cytokines by means of toll-like receptor 2 signaling pathways in a mouse model of colitis. Probiotics also directly influence the enzymes that produce ROS and encourage the synthesis of antioxidants. Kong et al. have been reported that Lactobacillus casei Shirota can increase the production of endogenous antioxidant enzymes and also decrease the oxidative stress in the liver of mice by increasing the nuclear factor-kappa B pathway [80]. Furthermore, there's growing interest in the interaction between probiotics and prebiotics in synbiotics. Probiotic bacteria manufacture other SCFAs and Butyrate. Research from 2021 by Carretta et al. demonstrates the strong anti-inflammatory qualities of SCFAs [81]. They can also change the G protein-coupled receptors on immune cells, reduce inflammation, and affect histone deacetylases [82]. Probiotics interact with pattern recognition receptors, which include TLRs, to assist manage the delicate equilibrium among pro- and anti-inflammatory mediators in health and illness. This interference suppresses pro-inflammatory pathways and reduces the formation of ROS. This process includes disorders of the CNS, in which the gut–brain axis is crucial. Murai et al. (2023) and Castelli et al. (2023) suggest that probiotic-regulated gut microbiota may influence oxidative stress and central nervous system inflammation, thereby providing new avenues for treating conditions such as anxiety, depression, Parkinson's disease, and Alzheimer's disease (2021) [83, 84]. Future research should look at the possible application of probiotics and synbiotics, which are beneficial in treating oxidative stress and inflammation-related cardiovascular diseases. According to a study by Ghorbani et al. (2022), these drugs may be used to treat or prevent conditions including hypertension and atherosclerosis by regulating immune responses, maintaining the gut barrier, and managing gut flora [85]. Although their effects on metabolic illnesses such as diabetes and obesity are still being investigated, they have the potential to significantly change the gut microbiota and reduce systemic inflammation. They may be

TABLE 6.1
Using Probiotics to Reduce Inflammation and ROS

Name	Composition	Target Diseases	Mechanisms	Main Effects	References
			Probiotics		
Lactobacillus rhamnosus GG	Lactobacillus rhamnosus GG	Inflammatory bowel disease	Modulation of gut microbiota, immunomodulation, antioxidant	Reduced inflammation and oxidative stress	[67]
Bifidobacterium breve M-16V	Bifidobacterium breve M-16V	IBD, colitis, obesity	ROS scavenging, modulation of gut microbiota, anti-inflammatory	Reduced oxidative stress and inflammation	[68]
Lactobacillus casei Shirota	Lactobacillus casei Shirota	Liver diseases, metabolic disorders	Enhanced antioxidant enzyme production, immunomodulation	Mitigated oxidative stress, improved metabolic health	[69]
Lactobacillus acidophilus and Bifidobacterium bifidum	Lactobacillus and Bifidobacterium strains	Ulcerative colitis	Modulation of gut microbiota, reinforced gut barrier	Improved gut barrier function, reduced inflammation	[70]

TABLE 6.2
Application of Synbiotics for Inhibiting ROS and Involved Mechanism

Synbiotics	Composition	Target Diseases	Mechanisms	Main Effects	References
Synbiotic formulation containing Lactobacillus casei and inulin	Lactobacillus casei and inulin	Aging, oxidative stress-related disorders	Promotion of beneficial bacteria, SCFA production, immunomodulation	Reduced ROS production, decreased inflammation	[71]
Synbiotic formulation containing Lactobacillus acidophilus and inulin	Lactobacillus acidophilus and inulin	Obesity, metabolic disorders	Enhanced growth of beneficial bacteria, SCFA production	Improved insulin sensitivity, reduced inflammation	[72]
Synbiotic formulation containing Bifidobacterium longum BB536 and galactooligosaccharides	Bifidobacterium longum BB536 and galactooligosaccharides	Colitis	Modulation of gut microbiota, inhibition of ROS generation	Reduced oxidative stress, improved gut health	[73]
Synbiotic formulation containing Lactobacillus plantarum 299v and inulin	Lactobacillus plantarum 299v and inulin	Inflammatory bowel disease	Modulation of gut microbiota, increased expression of tight junction proteins	Reinforced gut barrier, reduced inflammation	[74]
Synbiotic combination of Lactobacillus and Bifidobacterium strains with inulin	Lactobacillus, Bifidobacterium, and inulin	Gastrointestinal disorders, metabolic disorders	Modulation of gut microbiota, enhanced production of SCFAs	Reduced inflammation, improved metabolic health	[75]
Synbiotic formulation containing Lactobacillus rhamnosus GG and galactooligosaccharides	Lactobacillus rhamnosus GG and galactooligosaccharides	Inflammatory bowel disease	Modulation of gut microbiota, immunomodulation	Reduced inflammation and oxidative stress	[76]
Synbiotic formulation containing Bifidobacterium breve M-16V and galactooligosaccharides	Bifidobacterium breve M-16V and galactooligosaccharides	IBD, obesity	ROS scavenging, modulation of gut microbiota	Reduced oxidative stress and inflammation	[77]
Synbiotic formulation containing Lactobacillus casei Shirota and oligofructose-enriched inulin	Lactobacillus casei Shirota and inulin	Liver diseases, metabolic disorders	Enhanced antioxidant enzyme production, immunomodulation	Mitigated oxidative stress, improved metabolic health	[78]

used to treat conditions pertaining to the neurological, cardiovascular, pulmonary, metabolic, and digestive systems, etc. Immunological modulation changed gut microbiota, inflammation, and ROS management, and GBA combine to develop novel therapy paths for complex CNS diseases and neuroinflammatory illnesses. As research into the functions of probiotics and synbiotics progresses, these supplements may prove to be therapeutic treatments that affect several aspects of human health and well-being.

6.8 CHALLENGES AND LIMITATIONS

Probiotics and synbiotics have a lot of potential as therapeutic remedies to lower ROS and inflammation, but they also have certain disadvantages [86]. One significant challenge is the complexity of the gut flora, which varies greatly across individuals. The effectiveness of probiotics and synbiotics may be impacted by this inter-individual variation, making precise results hard to forecast [87]. Additionally, probiotic strains may face competition for survival and colonization in the gut from environmental factors and the established gut microbiota, which might diminish their efficacy. Anti-inflammatory and antioxidant qualities are associated with probiotics and synbiotics, albeit their precise modes of action are yet unclear. Even though data suggests that it has immunomodulatory and antioxidant properties, advance research is still required to completely understand the complex cellular interactions and specific molecular processes [88]. There is also subtle information on their potential effects on the CNS, where the complex GBA is involved in the treatment of conditions including anxiety, depression, and neurodegenerative disorders [89]. Mechanisms and interplay of oxidative stress, central nervous system inflammation, and gut microbiota modulation remain largely unknown to research [90]. The selection of probiotic strains and the makeup of synbiotics are crucial elements in determining their effectiveness [91]. It might be challenging to identify which strains are optimal and at what dose for a certain purpose since different strains may have varied effects on health conditions. Furthermore, the lack of defined strategies for the usage of probiotics and synbiotics in clinical settings poses a barrier to their broad usage as therapeutic medicines [92]. Probiotics and synbiotics may not always be the best option for individuals with compromised immune systems due to the possibility of infection. Drug interactions can occur, therefore those who take medication or have underlying medical conditions should also proceed with caution. Additionally, more investigation is required to ascertain the probiotics' and synbiotics' long-term safety as well as any potential adverse effects [93]. Regulation and quality assurance of probiotic and synbiotic products are further topics of study. The viability and stability of live microorganisms in commercial items might differ, which may have an impact on the efficacy of the products. These products have to meet stringent quality and safety standards in order to be used therapeutically. In conclusion, even though probiotics and synbiotics have a great deal of potential to treat inflammation and ROS, using them as therapeutic interventions is challenging due to a variety of factors, including individual variability, complex mechanisms, strain selection, survival and colonization of strains, a lack of standardization, safety concerns, and product quality control [93].

6.9 CONCLUSION

Exciting and active research has properly been done on the special effects of probiotic and the mixture of probiotics and prebiotics on inflammation and oxidative stress. It has been demonstrated that probiotics include various Bifidobacterium and Lactobacillus strains that have the ability to alter the gut microbiota by activating PRRs like TLRs that can detect MAMPs and start signaling cascades. This activation results in the production of interleukin-10, an anti-inflammatory cytokine, which also suppresses tumor necrosis factor-alpha and interleukin-6. Investigations have demonstrated the specific molecular interactions Lactobacillus rhamnosus GG employs to downregulate pro-inflammatory cytokines through toll-like receptor 2 signaling pathways. Furthermore, as demonstrated by the Lactobacillus casei Shirota investigation, probiotics have been shown to modulate the oxidative stress directly by blocking NF-κB pathway and stimulating the production of antioxidant enzymes. These complex mechanisms also function in synbiotics, where probiotics living on prebiotics like inulin and fructooligosaccharides create SCFAs. By interfering with histone deacetylases and G protein-coupled receptors, which both have anti-inflammatory properties, the probiotics produce these SCFAs. Probiotics and synbiotics have many potential therapeutic advantages, but there are also a number of drawbacks and restrictions that need to be understood. Predictability is complicated by the possibility that individual differences in the makeup of their gut flora might lead to different reactions to probiotics. The various habitats in the stomach that probiotic bacteria may colonize and live in can potentially account for this discrepancy in results. The lack of specific guidelines for using probiotic and synbiotic supplements in therapeutic settings is another barrier to their widespread usage. Awareness of safety issues and possible drug interactions should be exercised, especially for people whose immune systems are weakened. In order to ensure long-term safety and minimize any negative effects, more study is required. However, promising directions for further research on probiotics and synbiotics are already being investigated. The complex interaction between these therapies and CNS is essential where GBA is responsible for their effects on pro- and anti-inflammatory mediators. According to a recent study, altering gut microbiota may have an effect on inflammation and oxidative stress in the central nervous system, providing novel treatment options for disorders including anxiety, depression, and neurodegenerative illnesses. Additionally, there is growing interest in the possible use of probiotics and synbiotics in the management of metabolic disorders and cardiovascular illnesses. Numerous studies have shown that these interventions' ability to modify gut microbiota, strengthen the gut barrier, and control immune responses may prove invaluable in the prevention and management of these conditions, given that oxidative stress and inflammation are major factors in the pathophysiology of many diseases. In conclusion, there are several approaches to managing inflammation and oxidative stress offered by the constantly developing field of probiotics and synbiotics. Despite the difficulties and restrictions, research is continuing to identify feasible remedies and broaden the range of illnesses for which they may be applied, including metabolic, cardiovascular, and central nervous system ailments. With the advancement of probiotic and synbiotic research, these state-of-the-art technologies have the potential to drastically change how we think about health and well-being.

ACKNOWLEDGMENT

None.

CONFLICT OF INTEREST

None.

FUNDING

None.

REFERENCES

1. Zheng, H. J., Guo, J., Jia, Q., Huang, Y. S., Huang, W. J., Zhang, W., Zhang, F., Liu, W. J., & Wang, Y. (2019). The effect of probiotic and synbiotic supplementation on biomarkers of inflammation and oxidative stress in diabetic patients: A systematic review and meta-analysis of randomized controlled trials. *Pharmacological Research*, *142*, 303–313. https://doi.org/10.1016/j.phrs.2019.02.016
2. Naseri, K., Saadati, S., Ghaemi, F., Ashtary-Larky, D., Asbaghi, O., Sadeghi, A., Afrisham, R., & de Courten, B. (2023). The effects of probiotic and synbiotic supplementation on inflammation, oxidative stress, and circulating adiponectin and leptin concentration in subjects with prediabetes and type 2 diabetes mellitus: A GRADE-assessed systematic review, meta-analysis, and meta-regression of randomized clinical trials. *European Journal of Nutrition*, *62*(2), 543–561. https://doi.org/10.1007/s00394-022-03012-9
3. Ton, A. M. M., Campagnaro, B. P., Alves, G. A., Aires, R., Côco, L. Z., Arpini, C. M., Guerra E Oliveira, T., Campos-Toimil, M., Meyrelles, S. S., Pereira, T. M. C., & Vasquez, E. C. (2020). Oxidative stress and dementia in alzheimer's patients: Effects of synbiotic supplementation. *Oxidative Medicine and Cellular Longevity*, 2020, 2638703. https://doi.org/10.1155/2020/2638703
4. Pourrajab, B., Fatahi, S., Sohouli, M. H., Găman, M. A., & Shidfar, F. (2022). The effects of probiotic/synbiotic supplementation compared to placebo on biomarkers of oxidative stress in adults: A systematic review and meta-analysis of randomized controlled trials. *Critical Reviews in Food Science and Nutrition*, *62*(2), 490–507. https://doi.org/10.1080/10408398.2020.1821166
5. Ghavami, A., Khorvash, F., Khalesi, S., Heidari, Z., & Askari, G. (2021). The effects of synbiotic supplementation on oxidative stress and clinical symptoms in women with migraine: A double-blind, placebo-controlled, randomized trial. *Journal of Functional Foods*, *86*, 104738. https://doi.org/10.1016/j.jff.2021.104738
6. Heshmati, J., Farsi, F., Shokri, F., Rezaeinejad, M., Almasi-hashiani, A., Vesali, S., & Sepidarkish, M. (2018). A systematic review and meta-analysis of the probiotics and Synbiotics effects on oxidative stress. *Journal of Functional Foods*, *46*, 66–84. https://doi.org/10.1016/j.jff.2018.04.049
7. Kooshki, A., Tofighiyan, T., & Miri, M. (2019). A synbiotic supplement for inflammation and oxidative stress and lipid abnormalities in hemodialysis patients. *Hemodialysis International. International Symposium on Home Hemodialysis*, *23*(2), 254–260. https://doi.org/10.1111/hdi.12748
8. Mehrabani, S., Khorvash, F., Heidari, Z., Tajabadi-Ebrahimi, M., & Amani, R. (2023). The effects of synbiotic supplementation on oxidative stress markers, mental status, and quality of life in patients with Parkinson's disease: A double-blind, placebo-controlled, randomized controlled trial. *Journal of Functional Foods*, *100*, 105397. https://doi.org/10.1016/j.jff.2022.105397
9. Amirani, E., Milajerdi, A., Mirzaei, H., Jamilian, H., Mansournia, M. A., Hallajzadeh, J., & Ghaderi, A. (2020). The effects of probiotic supplementation on mental health, biomarkers of inflammation and oxidative stress in patients with psychiatric disorders: A systematic review and meta-analysis of randomized controlled trials. *Complementary Therapies in Medicine*, *49*, 102361. https://doi.org/10.1016/j.ctim.2020.102361
10. Nguyen, T. T. U., Kim, H. W., & Kim, W. (2021). Effects of probiotics, prebiotics, and Synbiotics on uremic toxins, inflammation, and oxidative stress in hemodialysis patients: A systematic review and meta-analysis of randomized controlled trials. *Journal of Clinical Medicine*, *10*(19), 4456. https://doi.org/10.3390/jcm10194456
11. Karamali, M., Nasiri, N., Taghavi Shavazi, N., Jamilian, M., Bahmani, F., Tajabadi-Ebrahimi, M., & Asemi, Z. (2018). The effects of synbiotic supplementation on pregnancy outcomes in gestational diabetes. *Probiotics and Antimicrobial Proteins*, *10*(3), 496–503. https://doi.org/10.1007/s12602-017-9313-7
12. Bakhtiary, M., Morvaridzadeh, M., Agah, S., Rahimlou, M., Christopher, E., Zadro, J. R., & Heshmati, J. (2021). Effect of probiotic, prebiotic, and synbiotic supplementation on cardiometabolic and oxidative stress parameters in patients with chronic kidney disease: A systematic review and meta-analysis. *Clinical Therapeutics*, *43*(3), e71–e96. https://doi.org/10.1016/j.clinthera.2020.12.021
13. Zare Javid, A., Aminzadeh, M., Haghighi-Zadeh, M. H., & Jamalvandi, M. (2020). The effects of synbiotic supplementation on glycemic status, lipid profile, and biomarkers of oxidative stress in type 1 diabetic patients. A placebo-controlled, double-blind, randomized clinical trial. *Diabetes, Metabolic Syndrome and Obesity: Targets and Therapy*, *13*, 607–617. https://doi.org/10.2147/DMSO.S238867
14. Vasquez, E. C., Pereira, T. M. C., Peotta, V. A., Baldo, M. P., & Campos-Toimil, M. (2019). Probiotics as beneficial dietary supplements to prevent and treat cardiovascular diseases: Uncovering their impact on oxidative stress. *Oxidative Medicine and Cellular Longevity*, *2019*, 3086270. https://doi.org/10.1155/2019/3086270
15. Tabrizi, R., Ostadmohammadi, V., Akbari, M., Lankarani, K. B., Vakili, S., Peymani, P., Kariminik, A., & Asemi, Z. (2019). The effects of probiotic supplementation on clinical symptom, weight loss, glycemic control, lipid and hormonal profiles, biomarkers of inflammation, and oxidative stress in women with polycystic ovary syndrome: A systematic review and meta-analysis of randomized controlled trials. *Probiotics and Antimicrobial Proteins*, 1–10.
16. Aranda-Rivera, A. K., Cruz-Gregorio, A., Arancibia-Hernández, Y. L., Hernández-Cruz, E. Y., & Pedraza-Chaverri, J. (2022). RONS and oxidative stress: An overview of basic concepts. *Oxygen*, *2*(4), 437–478. https://doi.org/10.3390/oxygen2040030

17. Soleimani, A., Motamedzadeh, A., Zarrati Mojarrad, M., Bahmani, F., Amirani, E., Ostadmohammadi, V., Tajabadi-Ebrahimi, M., & Asemi, Z. (2019). The effects of synbiotic supplementation on metabolic status in diabetic patients undergoing hemodialysis: A randomized, double-blinded, placebo-controlled trial. *Probiotics and Antimicrobial Proteins*, *11*(4), 1248–1256. https://doi.org/10.1007/s12602-018-9499-3
18. Jamilian, M., Amirani, E., & Asemi, Z. (2019). The effects of vitamin D and probiotic co-supplementation on glucose homeostasis, inflammation, oxidative stress and pregnancy outcomes in gestational diabetes: A randomized, double-blind, placebo-controlled trial. *Clinical Nutrition*, *38*(5), 2098–2105. https://doi.org/10.1016/j.clnu.2018.10.028
19. Karamali, M., Eghbalpour, S., Rajabi, S., Jamilian, M., Bahmani, F., Tajabadi-Ebrahimi, M., Keneshlou, F., Mirhashemi, S. M., Chamani, M., Hashem Gelougerdi, S., & Asemi, Z. (2018). Effects of probiotic supplementation on hormonal profiles, biomarkers of inflammation and oxidative stress in women with polycystic ovary syndrome: A randomized, doubleblind, placebo-controlled trial. *Archives of Iranian Medicine*, *21*(1), 1–7.
20. Zamani, B., Farshbaf, S., Golkar, H. R., Bahmani, F., & Asemi, Z. (2017). Synbiotic supplementation and the effects on clinical and metabolic responses in patients with rheumatoid arthritis: A randomised, double-blind, placebo-controlled trial. *British Journal of Nutrition*, *117*(8), 1095–1102. https://doi.org/10.1017/S000711451700085X
21. Bohlouli, J., Namjoo, I., Borzoo-Isfahani, M., Hojjati Kermani, M. A., Balouch Zehi, Z., & Moravejolahkami, A. R. (2021). Effect of probiotics on oxidative stress and inflammatory status in diabetic nephropathy: A systematic review and meta-analysis of clinical trials. *Heliyon*, *7*(1), e05925. https://doi.org/10.1016/j.heliyon.2021.e05925
22. Jamilian, M., Mansury, S., Bahmani, F., Heidar, Z., Amirani, E., & Asemi, Z. (2018). The effects of probiotic and selenium co-supplementation on parameters of mental health, hormonal profiles, and biomarkers of inflammation and oxidative stress in women with polycystic ovary syndrome. *Journal of Ovarian Research*, *11*, 1.
23. Badehnoosh, B., Karamali, M., Zarrati, M., Jamilian, M., Bahmani, F., Tajabadi-Ebrahimi, M., Jafari, P., Rahmani, E., & Asemi, Z. (2018). The effects of probiotic supplementation on biomarkers of inflammation, oxidative stress and pregnancy outcomes in gestational diabetes. *Journal of Maternal-Fetal and Neonatal Medicine*, *31*(9), 1128–1136. https://doi.org/10.1080/14767058.2017.1310193
24. Kuskunov, T., Tilkiyan, E., Doykov, D., Boyanov, K., Bivolarska, A., & Hristov, B. (2023). The effect of synbiotic supplementation on uremic toxins, oxidative stress, and inflammation in hemodialysis patients-Results of an uncontrolled prospective single-arm study. *Medicina*, *59*(8), 1383. https://doi.org/10.3390/medicina59081383
25. Wang, Z., Li, W., Lyu, Z., Yang, L., Wang, S., Wang, P., Song, F., Chen, K., & Huang, Y. (2022). Effects of probiotic/prebiotic/synbiotic supplementation on blood glucose profiles: A systematic review and meta-analysis of randomized controlled trials. *Public Health*, *210*, 149–159. https://doi.org/10.1016/j.puhe.2022.06.012
26. Tamtaji, O. R., Milajerdi, A., Reiner, Ž., Asemi, Z., Dadgostar, E., Heidari-Soureshjani, R., Mamsharifi, P., Amirani, E., Mirzaei, H., Hallajzadeh, J., & Ghaderi, A. (2020). A systematic review and meta-analysis: The effects of probiotic supplementation on metabolic profile in patients with neurological disorders. *Complementary Therapies in Medicine*, *53*, 102507. https://doi.org/10.1016/j.ctim.2020.102507
27. Salehi-Abargouei, A., Ghiasvand, R., & Hariri, M. (2017). Prebiotics, prosynbiotics and Synbiotics: Can they reduce plasma oxidative stress parameters? A systematic review. *Probiotics and Antimicrobial Proteins*, *9*(1), 1–11. https://doi.org/10.1007/s12602-016-9248-4
28. Fallah, F., & Mahdavi, R. (2023). l-carnitine and synbiotic co-supplementation: Beneficial effects on metabolic-endotoxemia, meta-inflammation, and oxidative-stress biomarkers in obese patients: A double blind, randomized, controlled clinical trial. *Food and Function*, *14*(4), 2172–2187. https://doi.org/10.1039/d2fo03348h
29. Firouzi, S., & Haghighatdoost, F. (2018). The effects of prebiotic, probiotic, and synbiotic supplementation on blood parameters of renal function: A systematic review and meta-analysis of clinical trials. *Nutrition*, *51–52*, 104–113. https://doi.org/10.1016/j.nut.2018.01.007
30. Zheng, H. J., Guo, J., Wang, Q., Wang, L., Wang, Y., Zhang, F., Huang, W. J., Zhang, W., Liu, W. J., & Wang, Y. (2021). Probiotics, prebiotics, and Synbiotics for the improvement of metabolic profiles in patients with chronic kidney disease: A systematic review and meta-analysis of randomized controlled trials. *Critical Reviews in Food Science and Nutrition*, *61*(4), 577–598. https://doi.org/10.1080/10408398.2020.1740645
31. Shamasbi, S. G., Ghanbari-Homayi, S., & Mirghafourvand, M. (2020). The effect of probiotics, prebiotics, and Synbiotics on hormonal and inflammatory indices in women with polycystic ovary syndrome: A systematic review and meta-analysis. *European Journal of Nutrition*, *59*(2), 433–450. https://doi.org/10.1007/s00394-019-02033-1
32. Borzabadi, S., Oryan, S., Eidi, A., Aghadavod, E., Daneshvar Kakhaki, R., Tamtaji, O. R., Taghizadeh, M., & Asemi, Z. (2018). The effects of probiotic supplementation on gene expression related to inflammation, insulin and lipid in patients with Parkinson's disease: A randomized, double-blind, placebocontrolled trial. *Archives of Iranian Medicine*, *21*(7), 289–295.
33. Sheng, K., He, S., Sun, M., Zhang, G., Kong, X., Wang, J., & Wang, Y. (2020). Synbiotic supplementation containing Bifidobacterium infantis and xylooligosaccharides alleviates dextran sulfate sodium-induced ulcerative colitis. *Food and Function*, *11*(5), 3964–3974. https://doi.org/10.1039/d0fo00518e
34. Asemi, Z., Khorrami-Rad, A., Alizadeh, S. A., Shakeri, H., & Esmaillzadeh, A. (2014). Effects of synbiotic food consumption on metabolic status of diabetic patients: A double-blind randomized cross-over controlled clinical trial. *Clinical Nutrition*, *33*(2), 198–203. https://doi.org/10.1016/j.clnu.2013.05.015
35. Ashique, S. A., Faruk, A., Ahmad, F. J., Khan, T., Mishra, N., Azhar, E. I., Chouayekh, H.,. . . Chouayekh, H. (2023). It is all about probiotics to control cervical cancer. Bacillus species as direct-fed microbial antibiotic alternatives for monogastric production. *Probiotics and Antimicrobial Proteins*, *15*(1), 1–16. https://doi.org/10.1007/s12602-022-09909-5
36. Akram, N., Saeed, F., Afzaal, M., Shah, Y. A., Qamar, A., Faisal, Z., Ghani, S., Ateeq, H., Akhtar, M. N., Tufail, T., Hussain, M., Asghar, A., Rasheed, A., & Jbawi, E. A. (2023). Gut microbiota and synbiotic foods: Unveiling

the relationship in COVID-19 perspective. *Food Science and Nutrition*, *11*(3), 1166–1177. https://doi.org/10.1002/fsn3.3162
37. Kim, Y. A., Keogh, J. B., & Clifton, P. M. (2018). Probiotics, prebiotics, synbiotics and insulin sensitivity. *Nutrition Research Reviews*, *31*(1), 35–51. https://doi.org/10.1017/S095442241700018X
38. Ardeshirlarijani, E., Tabatabaei-Malazy, O., Mohseni, S., Qorbani, M., Larijani, B., & Baradar Jalili, R. (2019). Effect of probiotics supplementation on glucose and oxidative stress in type 2 diabetes mellitus: A meta-analysis of randomized trials. *Daru*, *27*(2), 827–837. https://doi.org/10.1007/s40199-019-00302-2
39. Kiernan, D. P., O'Doherty, J. V., & Sweeney, T. (2023). The effect of maternal probiotic or synbiotic supplementation on sow and offspring gastrointestinal microbiota, health, and performance. Animals: *An Open Access Journal from MDPI*, *13*(19), 2996. https://doi.org/10.3390/ani13192996
40. Sangouni, A. A., & Ghavamzadeh, S. (2019). A review of synbiotic efficacy in non-alcoholic fatty liver disease as a therapeutic approach. *Diabetes and Metabolic Syndrome*, *13*(5), 2917–2922. https://doi.org/10.1016/j.dsx.2019.07.063
41. Li, H. Y., Zhou, D. D., Gan, R. Y., Huang, S. Y., Zhao, C. N., Shang, A., Xu, X. Y., & Li, H. B. (2021). Effects and mechanisms of probiotics, prebiotics, Synbiotics, and postbiotics on metabolic diseases targeting gut microbiota: A narrative review. *Nutrients*, *13*(9), 3211. https://doi.org/10.3390/nu13093211
42. Hevia, A., Delgado, S., Sánchez, B., & Margolles, A. (2015). Molecular players involved in the interaction between beneficial bacteria and the immune system. *Frontiers in Microbiology*, *6*, 1285. https://doi.org/10.3389/fmicb.2015.01285
43. Sanders, M. E., Benson, A., Lebeer, S., Merenstein, D. J., & Klaenhammer, T. R. (2018). Shared mechanisms among probiotic taxa: Implications for general probiotic claims. *Current Opinion in Biotechnology*, *49*, 207–216. https://doi.org/10.1016/j.copbio.2017.09.007
44. Yousefi, B., Eslami, M., Ghasemian, A., Kokhaei, P., Salek Farrokhi, A., & Darabi, N. (2019). Probiotics importance and their immunomodulatory properties. *Journal of Cellular Physiology*, *234*(6), 8008–8018. https://doi.org/10.1002/jcp.27559
45. Llewellyn, A., & Foey, A. (2017). Probiotic modulation of innate cell pathogen sensing and signaling events. *Nutrients*, *9*(10), 1156. https://doi.org/10.3390/nu9101156
46. Nabavi-Rad, A., Sadeghi, A., Asadzadeh Aghdaei, H., Yadegar, A., Smith, S. M., & Zali, M. R. (2022). The double-edged sword of probiotic supplementation on gut microbiota structure in Helicobacter pylori management. *Gut Microbes*, *14*(1), 2108655. https://doi.org/10.1080/19490976.2022.2108655
47. Rose, E. C., Odle, J., Blikslager, A. T., & Ziegler, A. L. (2021). Probiotics, prebiotics and epithelial tight junctions: A promising approach to modulate intestinal barrier function. International *Journal of Molecular Sciences*, *22*(13), 6729. https://doi.org/10.3390/ijms22136729
48. Gou, H. Z., Zhang, Y. L., Ren, L. F., Li, Z. J., & Zhang, L. (2022). How do intestinal probiotics restore the intestinal barrier? *Frontiers in Microbiology*, *13*, 929346. https://doi.org/10.3389/fmicb.2022.929346
49. Ali, S. S., Ahsan, H., Zia, M. K., Siddiqui, T., & Khan, F. H. (2020). Understanding oxidants and antioxidants: Classical team with new players. *Journal of Food Biochemistry*, *44*(3), e13145. https://doi.org/10.1111/jfbc.13145
50. Amoroso, C., Perillo, F., Strati, F., Fantini, M. C., Caprioli, F., & Facciotti, F. (2020). The role of gut microbiota biomodulators on mucosal immunity and intestinal inflammation. *Cells*, *9*(5), 1234. https://doi.org/10.3390/cells9051234
51. Zhu, R., Lang, T., Yan, W., Zhu, X., Huang, X., Yin, Q., & Li, Y. (2021). Gut microbiota: Influence on carcinogenesis and modulation strategies by drug delivery systems to improve cancer therapy. *Advanced Science*, *8*(10), 2003542. https://doi.org/10.1002/advs.202003542
52. Gómez-Guzmán, M., Toral, M., Romero, M., Jiménez, R., Galindo, P., Sánchez, M., Zarzuelo, M. J., Olivares, M., Gálvez, J., & Duarte, J. (2015). Antihypertensive effects of probiotics Lactobacillus strains in spontaneously hypertensive rats. *Molecular Nutrition and Food Research*, *59*(11), 2326–2336. https://doi.org/10.1002/mnfr.201500290
53. Averina, O. V., Poluektova, E. U., Marsova, M. V., & Danilenko, V. N. (2021). Biomarkers and utility of the antioxidant potential of probiotic lactobacilli and bifidobacteria as representatives of the human gut microbiota. *Biomedicines*, *9*(10), 1340. https://doi.org/10.3390/biomedicines9101340
54. Ashique, S., Garg, A., Bhatt, S., Sirohi, E., Fatima, N., Bajwa, N., & Mishra, N. (2023). Synbiotics in cervical cancer. In *Synbiotics for the management of cancer* (pp. 135–155). Springer Nature Singapore.
55. Olas, B. (2020). Probiotics, prebiotics and Synbiotics-A promising strategy in prevention and treatment of cardiovascular diseases? *International Journal of Molecular Sciences*, *21*(24), 9737. https://doi.org/10.3390/ijms21249737
56. Li, H. Y., Zhou, D. D., Gan, R. Y., Huang, S. Y., Zhao, C. N., Shang, A., Xu, X. Y., & Li, H. B. (2021). Effects and mechanisms of probiotics, prebiotics, Synbiotics, and postbiotics on metabolic diseases targeting gut microbiota: A narrative review. *Nutrients*, *13*(9), 3211. https://doi.org/10.3390/nu13093211
57. Akutko, K., & Stawarski, A. (2021). Probiotics, prebiotics and Synbiotics in inflammatory bowel diseases. *Journal of Clinical Medicine*, *10*(11), 2466. https://doi.org/10.3390/jcm10112466
58. Plaza-Díaz, J., Ruiz-Ojeda, F. J., Vilchez-Padial, L. M., & Gil, A. (2017). Evidence of the anti-inflammatory effects of probiotics and Synbiotics in intestinal chronic diseases. *Nutrients*, *9*(6), 555. https://doi.org/10.3390/nu9060555
59. Zheng, H. J., Guo, J., Jia, Q., Huang, Y. S., Huang, W. J., Zhang, W., Zhang, F., Liu, W. J., & Wang, Y. (2019). The effect of probiotic and synbiotic supplementation on biomarkers of inflammation and oxidative stress in diabetic patients: A systematic review and meta-analysis of randomized controlled trials. *Pharmacological Research*, *142*, 303–313. https://doi.org/10.1016/j.phrs.2019.02.016
60. Heshmati, J., Farsi, F., Shokri, F., Rezaeinejad, M., Almasi-hashiani, A., Vesali, S., & Sepidarkish, M. (2018). A systematic review and meta-analysis of the probiotics and Synbiotics effects on oxidative stress. *Journal of Functional Foods*, *46*, 66–84. https://doi.org/10.1016/j.jff.2018.04.049
61. Goyal, D., Ali, S. A., & Singh, R. K. (2021). Emerging role of gut microbiota in modulation of neuroinflammation and neurodegeneration with emphasis on Alzheimer's disease. *Progress in Neuro-Psychopharmacology and Biological Psychiatry*, *106*, 110112. https://doi.org/10.1016/j.pnpbp.2020.110112
62. Iddir, M., Brito, A., Dingeo, G., Fernandez Del Campo, S. S., Samouda, H., La Frano, M. R., & Bohn, T. (2020). Strengthening the immune system and reducing inflammation and oxidative stress through diet and nutrition: Considerations during the COVID-19 crisis. *Nutrients*, *12*(6), 1562. https://doi.org/10.3390/nu12061562

63. Hadi, A., Pourmasoumi, M., Kazemi, M., Najafgholizadeh, A., & Marx, W. (2022). Efficacy of synbiotic interventions on blood pressure: A systematic review and meta-analysis of clinical trials. *Critical Reviews in Food Science and Nutrition*, *62*(20), 5582–5591. https://doi.org/10.1080/10408398.2021.1888278
64. Basavaprabhu, H. N., Sonu, K. S., & Prabha, R. (2020). Mechanistic insights into the action of probiotics against bacterial vaginosis and its mediated preterm birth: An overview. *Microbial Pathogenesis*, *141*, 104029. https://doi.org/10.1016/j.micpath.2020.104029
65. Szántó, M., Dózsa, A., Antal, D., Szabó, K., Kemény, L., & Bai, P. (2019). Targeting the gut-skin axis-Probiotics as new tools for skin disorder management? *Experimental Dermatology*, *28*(11), 1210–1218. https://doi.org/10.1111/exd.14016
66. Yadav, H., Jaldhi, R., Bhardwaj, R., Anamika, S., Bakshi, A., Gupta, S., & Maurya, S. K. (2023). Unveiling the role of gut-brain axis in regulating neurodegenerative diseases: A comprehensive review. *Life Sciences*, 330, 122022. https://doi.org/10.1016/j.lfs.2023.122022
67. Cristofori, F., Dargenio, V. N., Dargenio, C., Miniello, V. L., Barone, M., & Francavilla, R. (2021). Anti-inflammatory and immunomodulatory effects of probiotics in gut inflammation: A door to the body. *Frontiers in Immunology*, *12*, 578386. https://doi.org/10.3389/fimmu.2021.578386
68. Patole, S. K., Rao, S. C., Keil, A. D., Nathan, E. A., Doherty, D. A., & Simmer, K. N. (2016). Benefits of Bifidobacterium breve M-16V supplementation in preterm neonates-a retrospective cohort study. *PLOS ONE*, *11*(3), e0150775. https://doi.org/10.1371/journal.pone.0150775
69. Koebnick, C., Wagner, I., Leitzmann, P., Stern, U., & Zunft, H. J. (2003). Probiotic beverage containing Lactobacillus casei Shirota improves gastrointestinal symptoms in patients with chronic constipation. *Canadian Journal of Gastroenterology and Hepatology*, *17*(11), 655–659. https://doi.org/10.1155/2003/654907
70. Ashour, Z., Shahin, R., Ali-Eldin, Z., El-Shayeb, M., El-Tayeb, T., & Bakr, S. (2022). Potential impact of gut Lactobacillus acidophilus and Bifidobacterium bifidum on hepatic histopathological changes in non-cirrhotic hepatitis C virus patients with different viral load. *Gut Pathogens*, *14*(1), 25. https://doi.org/10.1186/s13099-022-00501-4
71. Maftei, N. M., Iancu, A. V., Goroftei Bogdan, R. E., Gurau, T. V., Ramos-Villarroel, A., & Pelin, A. M. (2023). A novel symbiotic beverage based on sea buckthorn, soy milk and inulin: Production, characterization, probiotic viability, and sensory acceptance. *Microorganisms*, *11*(3), 736. https://doi.org/10.3390/microorganisms11030736
72. Rangel-Torres, B. E., García-Montoya, I. A., Rodríguez-Tadeo, A., & Jiménez-Vega, F. (2022). The symbiosis between Lactobacillus acidophilus and inulin: Metabolic benefits in an obese murine model. *Probiotics and Antimicrobial Proteins*, 1–9. https://doi.org/10.1007/s12602-022-10012-y
73. Alam, Z., Shang, X., Effat, K., Kanwal, F., He, X., Li, Y., Xu, C., Niu, W., War, A. R., & Zhang, Y. (2022). The potential role of prebiotics, probiotics, and Synbiotics in adjuvant cancer therapy especially colorectal cancer. *Journal of Food Biochemistry*, *46*(10), e14302. https://doi.org/10.1111/jfbc.14302
74. Taweerodjanakarn, S., Kongnum, K., & Hongpattarakere, T. (2023). Persistence of maternal milk derived Lactobacillus plantarum in the infant feces and its antagonistic activity against Escherichia coli O157: H7. *Food Science and Biotechnology*, *32*(8), 1079–1089. https://doi.org/10.1007/s10068-023-01243-y
75. García-Gamboa, R., Domínguez-Simi, M. Á., Gradilla-Hernández, M. S., Bravo-Madrigal, J., Moya, A., & González-Avila, M. (2022). Antimicrobial and antibiofilm effect of inulin-type fructans, used in synbiotic combination with Lactobacillus spp. against Candida albicans. *Plant Foods for Human Nutrition*, *77*(2), 212–219. https://doi.org/10.1007/s11130-022-00966-3
76. Kaewarsar, E., Chaiyasut, C., Lailerd, N., Makhamrueang, N., Peerajan, S., & Sirilun, S. (2023). Optimization of mixed inulin, fructooligosaccharides, and galactooligosaccharides as prebiotics for stimulation of probiotics growth and function. *Foods*, *12*(8), 1591. https://doi.org/10.3390/foods12081591
77. Abdul Kalam Saleena, L., Chang, S. K., Simarani, K., Arunachalam, K. D., Thammakulkrajang, R., How, Y. H., & Pui, L. P. (2023). A comprehensive review of Bifidobacterium spp: As a probiotic, application in the food and therapeutic, and forthcoming trends. *Critical Reviews in Microbiology*, 1–17. https://doi.org/10.1080/1040841X.2023.2243617
78. Khursheed, R., Gulati, M., Wadhwa, S., Vishwas, S., Sharma, D. S., Corrie, L., Alam, A., Alnasser, S. M., Aba Alkhayl, F. F., Parveen, Z., Nammi, S., Chellappan, D. K., Gupta, G., Zacconi, F., Steel, A., Adams, J., Jha, N. K., Dua, K., & Singh, S. K. (2022). Multifaceted role of Synbiotics as nutraceuticals, therapeutics and carrier for drug delivery. *Chemico-Biological Interactions*, *368*, 110223. https://doi.org/10.1016/j.cbi.2022.110223
79. Petruzziello, C., Saviano, A., & Ojetti, V. (2023). Probiotics, the immune response and acute appendicitis: A review. *Vaccines*, *11*(7), 1170. https://doi.org/10.3390/vaccines11071170
80. Ashique, S., Mishra, N., Garg, A., Sibuh, B. Z., Taneja, P., Rai, G., Djearamane, S., Wong, L. S., Al-Dayan, N., Roychoudhury, S., Kesari, K. K., Slama, P., Roychoudhury, S., & Gupta, P. K. (2023). Recent updates on correlation between reactive oxygen species and Synbiotics for effective management of ulcerative colitis. *Frontiers in Nutrition*, *10*, 1126579. https://doi.org/10.3389/fnut.2023.1126579
81. Kong, Y., Olejar, K. J., On, S. L. W., & Chelikani, V. (2020). The potential of Lactobacillus spp. for modulating oxidative stress in the gastrointestinal tract. *Antioxidants*, *9*(7), 610. https://doi.org/10.3390/antiox9070610
82. Carretta, M. D., Quiroga, J., López, R., Hidalgo, M. A., & Burgos, R. A. (2021). Participation of short-chain fatty acids and their receptors in gut inflammation and colon cancer. *Frontiers in Physiology*, *12*, 662739. https://doi.org/10.3389/fphys.2021.662739
83. Murai, T., & Matsuda, S. (2023). Therapeutic implications of probiotics in the gut microbe-modulated neuroinflammation and progression of Alzheimer's disease. *Life*, *13*(7), 1466. https://doi.org/10.3390/life13071466
84. Jain, M., Agarwal, A., Singh, K., & Jarouliya, U. (2024). Probiotics and immune response in disease prevention and treatment. In *Immune-boosting nutraceuticals for better human health* (pp. 99–129). Apple Academic Press.

85. Ghorbani, Z., Kazemi, A., U P Bartolomaeus, T., Martami, F., Noormohammadi, M., Salari, A., Löber, U., Balou, H. A., K Forslund, S., & Mahdavi-Roshan, M. (2023). The effect of probiotic and synbiotic supplementation on lipid parameters among patients with cardiometabolic risk factors: A systematic review and meta-analysis of clinical trials. *Cardiovascular Research*, *119*(4), 933–956. https://doi.org/10.1093/cvr/cvac128
86. Arun., K. B., Nisha, P., & Finamore, A. Emerging perspectives on probiotics, prebiotics, and Synbiotics for prevention and management of chronic disease. (2023). *Frontiers in Nutrition*, *10*, 1309140. https://doi.org/10.3389/fnut.2023.1309140
87. Dahiya, D., & Nigam, P. S. (2022). Probiotics, prebiotics, Synbiotics, and fermented foods as potential biotics in nutrition improving health via microbiome-gut-brain axis. *Fermentation*, *8*(7), 303. https://doi.org/10.3390/fermentation8070303
88. Zhao, Z., Xiao, G., Xia, J., Guo, H., Yang, X., Jiang, Q., Wang, H., Hu, J., & Zhang, C. (2023). Effectiveness of probiotic/prebiotic/synbiotic treatments on anxiety: A systematic review and meta-analysis of randomized controlled trials. *Journal of Affective Disorders*, *343*, 9–21. https://doi.org/10.1016/j.jad.2023.09.018
89. Shivakoti, R., Laughton, B., Shafiq, M., Schoeman, E., Glashoff, R. H., Barnabas, S., Fry, S., Leu, C. S., Wang, S., Bode, L., Aldrovandi, G., Kuhn, L., & Slogrove, A. L. (2023). Feasibility study of a Powder-Based Supplement Intervention for a future Synbiotic Trial in Breastfed Children from South Africa. *Research Square*. https://doi.org/10.21203/rs.3.rs-2842773/v1
90. Wolfe, W., Xiang, Z., Yu, X., Li, P., Chen, H., Yao, M., Fei, Y., Huang, Y., Yin, Y., & Xiao, H. (2023). The challenge of applications of probiotics in gastrointestinal diseases. *Advanced Gut and Microbiome Research*, 2023, 1–10. https://doi.org/10.1155/2023/1984200
91. Bilal, M., Ashraf, S., & Zhao, X. (2022). Dietary component-induced inflammation and its amelioration by prebiotics, probiotics, and Synbiotics. *Frontiers in Nutrition*, *9*, 931458. https://doi.org/10.3389/fnut.2022.931458
92. Gu, Q., Yin, Y., Yan, X., Liu, X., Liu, F., & McClements, D. J. (2022). Encapsulation of multiple probiotics, Synbiotics, or nutrabiotics for improved health effects: A review. *Advances in Colloid and Interface Science*, 309, 102781. https://doi.org/10.1016/j.cis.2022.102781
93. Han, D., Żulewska, J., Xiong, K., & Yang, Z. (2022). Synergy between oligosaccharides and probiotics: From metabolic properties to beneficial effects. *Critical Reviews in Food Science and Nutrition*, 1–23. https://doi.org/10.1080/10408398.2022.2139218

7 Correlation and Successive Role of Synbiotics to Manage Blood Pressure

Himanshu Sharma, Monika Kaushik, Venishaa S, Rashmi Pathak, Arshad Farid, and Mithun Bhowmick

7.1 INTRODUCTION

Hypertension, sometimes referred to as high blood pressure, affects millions of individuals globally and is a significant risk factor for cardiovascular diseases. Environmental, behavioral, and genetic factors all have a complicated role in the development and exacerbation of hypertension. Recent research has explored the possibility of synbiotics, which are a combination of probiotics and prebiotics, to regulate gut microbiota and enhance blood pressure management (Chavda et al., 2021). The human gut has a diverse community of bacteria known as the gut microbiota, which is vital to maintaining overall health. Variations in the balance of these microorganisms have been linked to certain health conditions, such as hypertension. Given that they mix probiotics and prebiotics to support and maintain a healthy gut flora, synbiotics provide a novel approach to blood pressure management. Because probiotics include live beneficial bacteria, they increase the amount of good microflora in the stomach (Khursheed et al., 2022). These microorganisms produce beneficial compounds such as short-chain fatty acids, which have been connected to improved cardiovascular health. Because probiotics promote the production of nitric oxide, a vasodilator that helps regulate blood vessel tone, they may potentially have an impact on blood pressure. On the other hand, probiotics need prebiotics as fuel to continue growing and functioning. These indigestible substances, which are often heavy in fiber, enter the colon undigested and are fermented by gut bacteria (see Figure 7.1). Fermentation produces metabolites that have been linked to cardiovascular health and may aid in blood pressure regulation (Requena & Pérez Martínez, 2022).

7.1.1 Background

The primary indicator of hypertension, a condition that continues to be a major global health issue with serious implications for cardiovascular health, is elevated blood pressure. Even with advancements in pharmacological

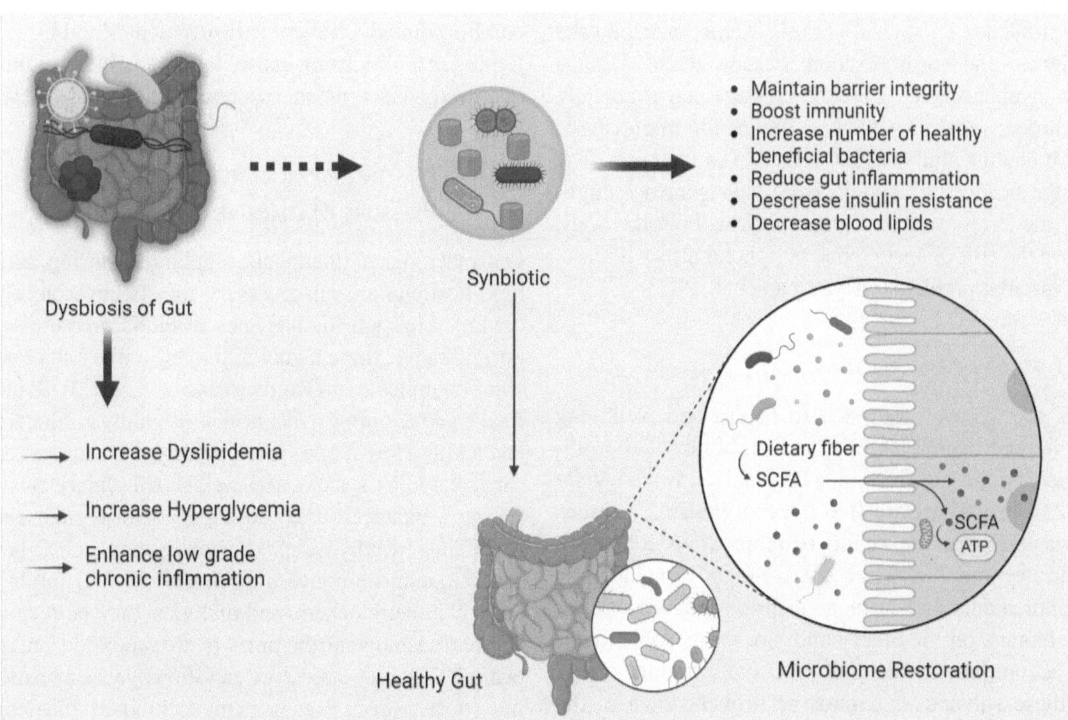

FIGURE 7.1 Role of synbiotics to manage blood pressure (Núñez-Sánchez et al., 2021) 2214–7993/ã 2021 The Authors. Published by Elsevier Ltd. This is an open access article under the CC BY license (http://creativecommons.org/licenses/by/4.0/).

DOI: 10.1201/9781032702438-7

therapy, a multifactorial approach is typically necessary due to the complicated nature of hypertension. The intricate connection between blood pressure regulation and gut flora has come to light recently, underscoring the promise of synbiotics as a workable therapeutic approach (Pyle, 2022). The gut microbiota is a dynamic colony of bacteria that reside in the gastrointestinal system and are now known to have a significant influence on several aspects of human health. Variations in its structure and function have been linked to inflammatory processes, metabolic issues, and cardiovascular diseases including hypertension. Synbiotics combine the advantageous properties of probiotics and prebiotics to address the intricate link between the gut flora and blood pressure management (Maioli et al., 2022).

7.1.2 Significance of Blood Pressure Management

Blood pressure regulation is crucial for public health since it directly avoids cardiovascular diseases and the effects they bring (Gyawali et al., 2019). Being the "silent killer," hypertension typically exhibits no outward symptoms, making it imperative to recognized and address any potential side effects. First and foremost, heart failure, stroke, and coronary artery disease (CAD) are among the cardiovascular disorders for which hypertension significantly increases the risk (Rodríguez-García et al., 2005). High blood pressure puts excessive strain on the walls of the arteries, which in turn causes atherosclerosis, or the hardening and narrowing of the arteries. This increases the risk of heart attacks and strokes. People's risk of these potentially fatal cardiovascular events can be significantly reduced by controlling their blood pressure (Kordvarkane et al., 2023). In addition, hypertension has a negative influence on several organ systems, including the brain, kidneys, and cardiovascular system. Renal damage brought on by unchecked high blood pressure may eventually result in chronic renal disease. It is one of the main causes of cognitive decline and vascular dementia in the brain. The systemic significance of blood pressure management is highlighted by the strain on blood arteries throughout the body, which raises the risk of aneurysms, peripheral artery disease, and other vascular problems (Aljuraiban et al., 2023).

7.1.3 Overview of Synbiotics

Synbiotics are a novel approach to health and wellbeing that combine the beneficial effects of prebiotics and probiotics to modify the gut flora in a favorable way (del Valle et al., 2023). Probiotics are live microorganisms, primarily bacteria, that provide health benefits when consumed in appropriate amounts. They are frequently included in dietary supplements and fermented foods (Suastika et al., 2023). Prebiotics, on the other hand, are indigestible materials that accompany meals and are usually dietary fibers. Because these substances cannot be broken down in the upper gastrointestinal tract, they go to the colon, where gut bacteria ferment them. This fermentation process produces short-chain fatty acids and other byproducts that contribute to the establishment of a favorable environment for the growth and activity of beneficial bacteria. Synbiotics are symbiotic interactions formed by the cooperation of probiotics and prebiotics. Probiotics thrive and perform better when they have nourishment from prebiotics (see Figure 7.2). An increasingly recognized benefit of maintaining overall health is the cultivation of a diverse and well-balanced gut microbiota, which is facilitated by this cooperative interaction (Zepeda-Hernández et al., 2021).

7.2 UNDERSTANDING BLOOD PRESSURE

Blood pressure, a vital physiological indicator, shows the force that blood flow applies to the walls of arteries. The diastolic pressure, or the force the heart produces in between beats, and the systolic pressure, or the force the heart experiences during a cardiac contraction and blood pumping, are the two values that represent it (Naseri et al., 2022). Typically, the value is expressed as systolic over diastolic, for example, 120/80 mmHg, where "mmHg" stands for millimeters of mercury, the unit of measurement. Although ideal levels may vary depending on factors including age, sex, and general health, normal blood pressure is typically thought to be about 120/80 mmHg (Khursheed et al., 2022). When the force of blood on the arterial walls is continuously too great, it is known as hypertension or high blood pressure. The fact that this illness is frequently asymptomatic has earned it the nickname "silent killer," since it can go years without presenting any clear symptoms. Prolonged high blood pressure puts stress on the arteries, which narrows blood vessels, causes atherosclerosis, and raises the risk of heart attacks and strokes, among other catastrophic cardiovascular events. Hypotension, on the other hand, is a condition in which there is insufficient blood flow to essential organs, which can cause lightheadedness, fainting, and, in extreme circumstances, shock (Yang et al., 2021).

7.2.1 Existing Approaches to Blood Pressure Management

Pharmacological treatments, regular monitoring, and lifestyle modifications are all necessary for effective blood pressure control. Through maintenance of blood pressure within the normal range, these tactics aim to lower the risk of cardiovascular complications (Kordvarkane et al., 2023). Reducing salt intake and adopting a diet heavy in healthy grains, fruits, vegetables, and low-fat dairy. Regular exercise supports a healthy cardiovascular system and weight (M. Jafari et al., 2020). Eating a balanced diet and engaging in regular exercise to maintain a healthy weight. Various drugs, such as beta-blockers, Angiotensin-converting enzyme (ACE) inhibitors, calcium channel blockers, and diuretics, may be recommended as pharmacological therapies to reduce blood pressure (Wu et al., 2023). Blood pressure elevation may be a result of ongoing stress. Stress management techniques like yoga, deep breathing exercises, and meditation might be helpful. To monitor changes and evaluate the success of therapies, regular blood pressure checks are crucial. More and more people are recommending home blood pressure monitoring to get a more

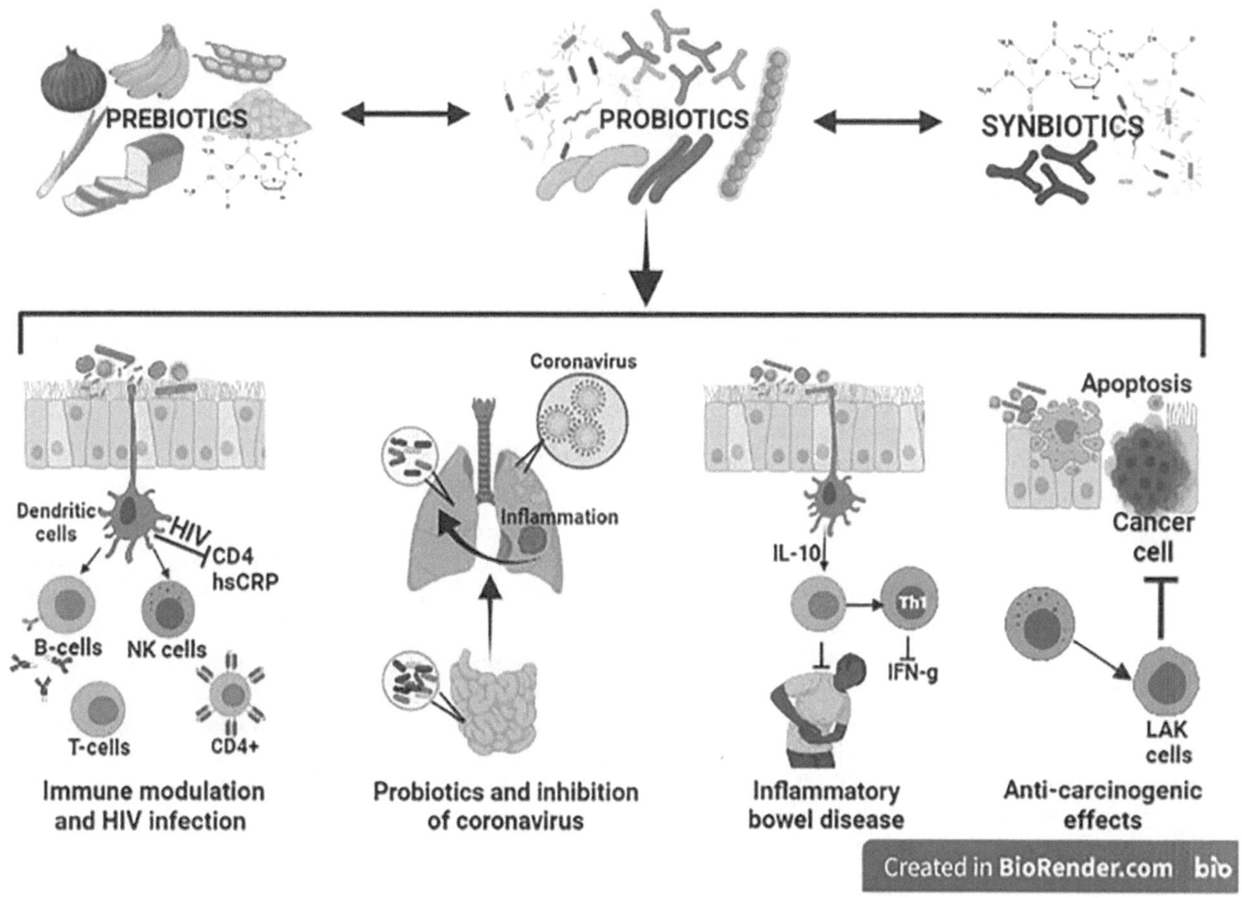

FIGURE 7.2 The microbiome of the gut and potential molecular pathways associated with illnesses of the heart and metabolism. FXR stands for farnesoid X receptor; GLP for glucagon-like peptide; GPR for G-protein–coupled receptor; LPS for lipopolysaccharide; PYY for peptide YY; TLR for toll-like receptor; TMA for trimethylamine; and TMAO for trimethylamine N-oxide are the acronyms for brown adipose tissue (Tang et al., 2017).

complete picture. Blood pressure increase may be caused by excessive alcohol and caffeine use. For the general health of your heart, you must stop smoking. Tobacco products include compounds that over time can cause blood vessel damage and elevated blood pressure. Continual evaluation and modification of blood pressure control tactics depend on routine visits with medical professionals (Mitsnefes et al., 2023).

7.2.2 Introduction to Synbiotics

Combining the beneficial effects of probiotics and prebiotics to promote a balanced and robust gut flora, synbiotics represent a cutting-edge and rapidly developing discipline in the field of health and wellbeing (Z. Wang et al., 2022). Probiotics are living microorganisms, mostly bacteria, that provide health benefits when taken in enough amounts. Common bacteria found in fermented foods like yogurt and nutritional supplements include Lactobacillus and Bifidobacterium. Prebiotics are indigestible fibers that nourish healthy bacteria in the stomach, supporting probiotics in the process (Riasatian et al., 2023). Frequently obtained from foods such as onions, garlic, and bananas, these substances evade digestion in the upper gastrointestinal tract and make their way to the colon, where they specifically promote the development and function of probiotics. The idea that probiotics and prebiotics work in concert to improve the survival and efficacy of probiotic bacteria is the basis for the notion of synbiotics (Geng et al., 2023). This combination aims to maximize the gut microbial habitat by fostering a diverse and well-balanced ecosystem within the gastrointestinal tract. Research demonstrates their role in immune system control, improved absorption of nutrients, and potential benefits for cardiovascular and metabolic health. Due to the intricate relationships that synbiotics have with the gut flora, they provide a potential therapeutic alternative for a range of conditions, including digestive issues and cardiovascular disease (Musazadeh et al., 2022).

7.2.3 Previous Research on Synbiotics and Blood Pressure

Lei et al. (2023) investigated probiotics or synbiotics in addition to conventional drugs in a meta-analysis that included ten research on the treatment of CAD. The results showed that there was an increase in nitric oxide and high-density lipoprotein cholesterol and a substantial decrease in low-density lipoprotein cholesterol, fasting glucose, and hypersensitive

C-reactive protein levels. On the other hand, there was no discernible change in lipid levels, systolic, or diastolic blood pressure (SBP and DBP). This implies a possible synergistic function for probiotics or synbiotics in augmenting the efficacy of traditional CAD therapies, namely, in regulating inflammatory indicators, glucose metabolism, and lipid profiles (Lei et al., 2023). Arabi et al. (2022) investigated that meta-analysis over five studies with 1049 patients, the synbiotic therapies showed notable benefits in a range of cardiovascular and metabolic parameters. Significantly, the synbiotic intervention decreased body weight, systolic blood pressure, waist circumference, triglycerides, total cholesterol, and low-density lipoprotein cholesterol. High-density lipoprotein cholesterol levels increased together with a drop in serum interleukin-6 concentrations, which is suggestive of anti-inflammatory actions. The delivery of synbiotics did not, however, significantly alter serum C-reactive protein concentrations, body mass index, DBP, heart rate, insulin resistance, or fasting plasma glucose levels. These results demonstrate the potential benefits of synbiotics for improving cardiovascular and metabolic parameters (Arabi et al., 2022). Rahimi et al. (2022) investigated comparison to a placebo, our experiment shows that taking synbiotics along with instruction on nutrition and a healthy lifestyle significantly lowers fasting blood glucose (FBG). This implies that improving metabolic syndrome (MetS) indicators involve both modifying the gut flora and caloric restriction. The all-encompassing strategy of education, lifestyle modification, and synbiotics shows promise in treating the broader metabolic variables linked to MetS in addition to FBG levels. This study emphasizes the potential of synbiotics as a comprehensive approach to metabolic health management and emphasizes the value of integrated therapies in fostering general wellbeing (Rahimi et al., 2022).

7.3 MECHANISMS OF BLOOD PRESSURE REGULATION

In order to preserve the proper perfusion of organs while preventing damage to blood vessels, blood pressure control is a complicated physiological process requiring multiple systems. Local factors inside blood arteries, the RAAS, and the nervous system are the main players in blood pressure control (Hasan et al., 2022). The sympathetic and parasympathetic branches of the autonomic nervous system are essential. Stress or physical exertion can cause sympathetic activation, which raises blood pressure by narrowing blood vessels and speeding up the heart rate. By encouraging relaxation and vasodilation, parasympathetic activity has the opposite effect (Pingali & Hunter, 2023). Blood pressure and fluid balance are controlled by the RAAS, a hormonal system. The kidneys release renin when blood flow to them declines, which starts a chain reaction that produces angiotensin II. Angiotensin II promotes salt and water retention by constricting blood vessels and stimulating the production of aldosterone, which eventually raises blood pressure (Sherwood et al., 2003). Blood pressure control is also influenced by local elements found in blood arteries, such as endothelial cells. Vasodilation is brought on by nitric oxide, which is generated by endothelial cells and lowers blood pressure. Furthermore, the vasoconstrictor endothelin and the vasodilator prostacyclin affect vascular tone. Major arteries include baroreceptors, which sense variations in blood pressure and alert the brainstem's cardiovascular centers to modify heart rate and vascular tone appropriately. Furthermore, by regulating blood volume through the retention or excretion of water and salt, the kidneys play a critical role in the long-term management of blood pressure (Ribeiro-Silva et al., 2023).

7.3.1 Role of Gut Microbiota in Cardiovascular Health

One important factor affecting cardiovascular health is the gut microbiota, a varied collection of bacteria that live in the gastrointestinal system (Hamjane et al., 2024). Research on the complex interactions between the gut microbiota and the cardiovascular system is constantly evolving, elucidating many ways by which gut microorganisms influence the preservation or compromise of cardiovascular health (Hemmati et al., 2023). Modulation of host metabolism by gut bacteria is one such pathway. Dietary fibers are fermented by microorganisms to create SCFAs such as butyrate, propionate, and acetate, which have been linked to cardiovascular advantages (Roessler et al., 2022). SCFAs are essential for cardiovascular health because they improve lipid metabolism, boost insulin sensitivity, and reduce inflammation. Furthermore, the gut microbiota has a role in the conversion of some dietary components, such phosphatidylcholine and choline, into TMA. Afterward, TMA is converted by the liver to trimethylamine-N-oxide (TMAO) (Jain et al., 2024). Elevated TMAO levels have been linked to increased cardiovascular risk and atherosclerosis, underscoring the influence of gut bacteria on systemic processes. One characteristic that sets cardiovascular diseases apart is inflammation, which is controlled by the gut microbiota. Bacterial products might be able to enter the bloodstream more easily if the gut barrier were to become more porous due to dysbiosis, an imbalance in the gut microbial ecology. Consequently, an inflammatory response is triggered, potentially contributing to the development and progression of cardiovascular disorders (Zhao et al., 2023). The balance of pro- and anti-inflammatory cytokines and the development of regulatory T cells are all impacted by the gut microbiota's interactions with the immune system. Because persistent inflammation plays a major role in the development of atherosclerosis and other cardiovascular diseases, this immune regulation has consequences for cardiovascular health (Li et al., 2023). Lu et al. (2023) studied that dietary decisions have a major influence on the metabolism of bile acid (BA) and microbiota. Increased production of bile salt hydrolase and 7α-dehydroxylase causes high-fat diets to boost secondary and unconjugated BAs. BA excretion is aided by diets high in fiber and polyphenols. It's possible that inaccurate dietary assessment led to the lack of dietary relationships with serum BAs (SBAs) in this research of individuals with recently diagnosed diabetes. FXR is a crucial nuclear receptor that controls metabolic activities, and it is activated by unconjugated BAs. Although genome-wide studies on CHD and stroke did not demonstrate relevance, maybe because of ethnic and diabetic variations, FXR polymorphisms, such as rs56163822 and rs17030295, were associated to CVD in diabetic subjects, suggesting a potential involvement. The significance of FXR polymorphisms on cardiovascular health requires more investigation (Lu et al., 2023). Chai et al. (2023) investigated that chronic exposure to DEHP has been demonstrated to cause cardiovascular damage, which includes decreased heart rate, increased cholesterol and blood glucose levels, inflammation, fibrosis, and cardiac malfunction. The cardiovascular system of obese mice was shown to be more vulnerable than that of normal mice in an animal model that reflected ecologically relevant amounts of DEHP. DEHP-induced cardiovascular risk was associated with changes in the gut microbial ecology and arachidonic acid (AA) metabolic balance, as revealed by multi-omics data. The correlation between *F. rodentium* and AA metabolism was validated by in vitro tests, as seen in Figure 7.3. These results clarify the mechanism by which exposure to DEHP causes cardiovascular disease in obese people, highlighting the possible involvement of AA metabolism in gut microbiome. Investigating the in vivo relationship between AA metabolism and F. rodentium as well as possible pathways needs more study (Chai et al., 2023).

Figure 7.3. The microbiome of the gut and potential molecular pathways associated with illnesses of the heart and metabolism. FXR stands for farnesoid X receptor; GLP for glucagon-like peptide; GPR for G-protein–coupled receptor; LPS for lipopolysaccharide; PYY for peptide YY; TLR for toll-like receptor; TMA for trimethylamine; and TMAO for trimethylamine N-oxide are the acronyms for brown adipose tissue (Tang et al., 2017).

7.3.2 Synbiotics: Definition and Components

Synbiotics are a symbiotic blend of prebiotics and probiotics that work together to improve the balance and overall

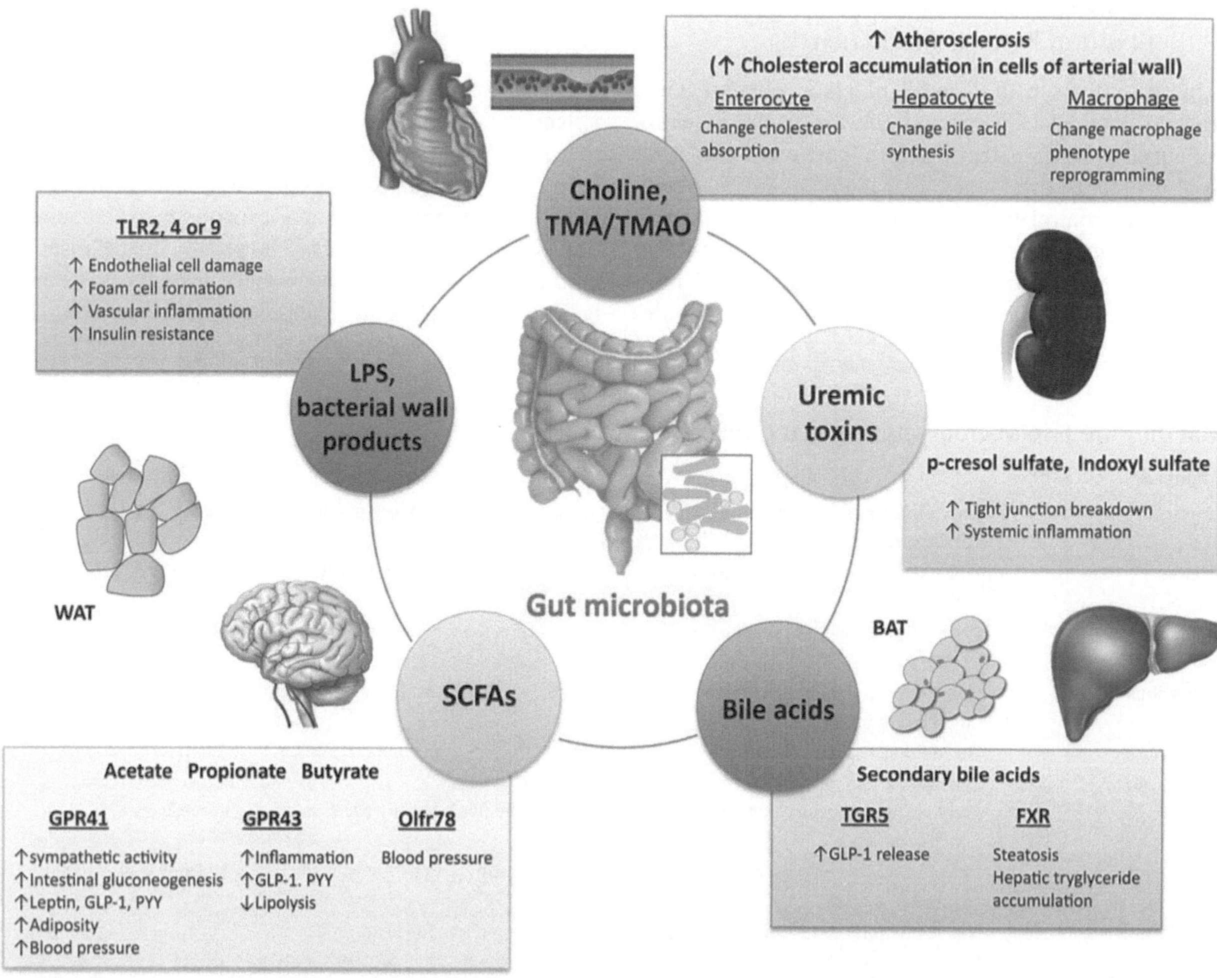

FIGURE 7.3 The microbiome of the gut and potential molecular pathways associated with illnesses of the heart and metabolism. FXR stands for farnesoid X receptor; GLP for glucagon-like peptide; GPR for G-protein–coupled receptor; LPS for lipopolysaccharide; PYY for peptide YY; TLR for toll-like receptor; TMA for trimethylamine; and TMAO for trimethylamine N-oxide are the acronyms for brown adipose tissue (Tang et al., 2017).

health of the gut flora. By combining the advantages of both elements, this arrangement improves the habitat for beneficial microorganisms. When ingested in sufficient quantities, probiotics live microorganisms, mostly bacteria produce health benefits (Chan & Liu, 2022). Probiotic strains that are commonly found in fermented foods such as yogurt, kefir, and sauerkraut are Lactobacillus and Bifidobacterium. Probiotics enhance gut health via modulating several aspects of the host's immune and metabolic systems, producing bioactive compounds, and promoting the growth of beneficial bacteria (van der Schoot et al., 2022). Prebiotics are indigestible fibers or substances that feed probiotics, encouraging their development and activity within the digestive system. FOS, GOS, and inulin are a few types of prebiotics. These materials make it past the upper gastrointestinal system without being broken down, arriving in the colon undigested, where probiotic bacteria ferment them (Coleman et al., 2022). Table 7.1 shows that the fermentation process generates SCFAs and other metabolites that support gut health and general wellbeing.

7.3.3 Potential Mechanisms of Synbiotics in Blood Pressure Regulation

Synbiotics influence the control of blood pressure via a variety of methods. By encouraging the establishment of advantageous gut flora, they produce short-chain fatty acids that affect blood vessel tone (X. Wang et al., 2023). Neural circuits that control blood pressure may be impacted by modulations in the gut–brain axis. Taking synbiotics helps prevent chronic inflammation, which raises blood pressure, by lowering inflammatory cytokines. Some strains of probiotics increase the generation of nitric oxide, which causes vasodilation. Furthermore, synbiotics increase metabolism, which affects lipid profiles and glucose metabolism (Núñez-Sánchez et al., 2021). Table 7.2 illustrates the several methods via which synbiotics might support cardiovascular health and blood pressure balance.

7.4 CORRELATION BETWEEN SYNBIOTICS AND BLOOD PRESSURE

Because of the possible impact of gut microbiota regulation on cardiovascular health, the relationship between synbiotics and blood pressure has received attention. Synbiotics, which include probiotics and prebiotics, may help regulate blood pressure through a number of methods, according to recent study (Khursheed et al., 2022). A crucial element is the effect of synbiotics on the makeup of the gut flora. Changes in the gut microbial community have been connected to diseases like hypertension, while a balanced and diversified community has been linked to cardiovascular health (Keulers et al., 2022). Synbiotics may create an environment that is favorable for ideal blood pressure by encouraging the development of helpful bacteria and generating bioactive chemicals. Another factor is the anti-inflammatory properties of synbiotics. Synbiotics have demonstrated the capacity to modify inflammatory indicators, and chronic inflammation is linked to hypertension (Askari et al., 2021). Synbiotics may help to keep blood pressure readings within normal ranges by lowering systemic inflammation. Furthermore, synbiotics have been linked to improvements in glucose metabolism and lipid profiles, among other metabolic markers. Since metabolic dysfunction and hypertension are linked, treating these

TABLE 7.1
Probiotics Are Live Microorganisms That Confer Health Benefits

Component	Definition	Function	References
Probiotics	Living microbes, often strains of yeast or bacterium	Restore and preserve a balanced population of gut microbiota	(Jan et al., 2023)
Prebiotics	Fibers that are not digested, usually oligosaccharides	Offer a growing medium for the benevolent bacteria	(X. Liu et al., 2024)
Synbiotic blend	Probiotic and prebiotic combination	Combined action to increase probiotic survival	(Chauhan & Sharma, 2023)
Lactobacillus	Commonly seen in fermented foods, this kind of bacteria	Support the equilibrium of the intestinal microbiota	(Cheng et al., 2023)
Bifidobacterium	An additional species of bacteria possessing probiotic qualities	Supports the control of the immune system and intestinal health	(Amoah et al., 2023)
Inulin	Prebiotic fiber obtained from the roots of chicory	Encourages the colon's healthy bacteria to proliferate	(Rezende et al., 2021)
Fructo-oligosaccharides	Prebiotic substances present in a variety of fruits	Encourage a healthy gut environment and eat probiotics	(Mohanty et al., 2018)
Colony-forming units	Viable probiotic cell measurement	Number of living microorganisms in the product	(Yin et al., 2024)
Symbiosis	Probiotics and prebiotics' interactions	Establishes a favorable environment for the development of microorganisms	(Devi et al., 2023)
Gastrointestinal health	General health of the digestive tract	Enhanced by encouraging a healthy gut microbiome	(Woźniak et al., 2021)

TABLE 7.2
Possible Ways That Synbiotics Regulate Blood Pressure

Mechanism	Description	Reference
Microbial metabolites	Synbiotics increase the synthesis of SCFAs, especially butyrate, by encouraging the development of beneficial bacteria. By affecting blood vessel tone and function, SCFAs influence vasodilation and blood pressure regulation	(Sircana et al., 2019)
Modulation of the gut–brain axis	The gut–brain axis facilitates bidirectional communication between the gut bacteria and the central nervous system. Synbiotics may affect the release of neurotransmitters and neuropeptides from brain circuits that regulate blood pressure	(Guo et al., 2019)
Inflammatory modulation	Synbiotics have the ability to reduce chronic low-grade inflammation by modulating the production of inflammatory cytokines through their impact on the gut flora. This anti-inflammatory action could help control blood pressure	(Sumida et al., 2023)
Nitric oxide production	Synbiotics contain some probiotic strains that have been linked to higher NO production. Blood vessel tone can be regulated by NO, a vasodilator, which may enhance vascular function and lower blood pressure	(Mahdavi-Roshan et al., 2022)
Metabolic effects	Metabolic indicators such as glucose metabolism and lipid profiles have been shown to improve with the use of synbiotics. Taking synbiotics may help regulate blood pressure indirectly since metabolic dysfunction is linked to hypertension	(Ofosu et al., 2021)

conditions may have an impact on blood pressure management (Scorletti et al., 2020). Naseri et al. (2022) investigated encouraging patients with type 2 diabetes mellitus (T2DM) to utilize probiotics and synbiotics as helpful adjuncts in controlling cardiovascular risk factors. Weight, blood pressure, and lipid profiles all showed improvements. Larger and longer-term trials are necessary to determine their therapeutic importance in lowering cardiovascular morbidity and mortality, even if these advantages were minor and should be used with caution. Probiotic therapies for type 2 diabetes must also be refined by identifying the best bacterial strains, dosages, and therapy durations. Probiotics appear to be a generally promising adjuvant therapy for complete risk factor control in individuals with type 2 diabetes (Naseri et al., 2022). Yang et al. (2021) investigated that the ability of a unique symbiosis, called SBT, which includes prebiotics (GOS and stachyose), probiotics (B. lactis, L. acidophilus, L. rhamnosus, and L. plantarum), and CS to relieve constipation with less adverse effects than chemical medications. Consuming SBT improved intestinal propulsive performance, increased fecal moisture content, and dramatically shortened the time to first black stool defection. With an emphasis on the gut microbiota and metabolome, the study investigated the processes behind SBT's mitigating effectiveness on constipation. Administration of SBT raised blood concentrations of excitatory neurotransmitters (GAS, MTL, VIP, and SP), which are known to improve defecation and gastrointestinal motility. Moreover, SBT administration increased serum 5-HT levels, which encouraged the contraction of colonic smooth muscle and improved the efficacy of intestinal propulsive activity. The results highlight the possibility of SBT as a therapeutic treatment for constipation, highlighting its complex effects on neurotransmitters and the gastrointestinal tract. It is necessary to conduct more studies to determine the ideal dosage, length of time, and possible therapeutic uses (Yang et al., 2021).

7.5 SUCCESSIVE ROLE OF SYNBIOTICS IN BLOOD PRESSURE MANAGEMENT

Through a number of interrelated pathways involving the gut microbiota, inflammation, and metabolic processes, the subsequent involvement of synbiotics in blood pressure (Hellebois et al., 2020). Probiotics and prebiotics are examples of synbiotics, which work together to enhance the GI's environment and promote overall cardiovascular health. A diverse and well-balanced gut microbiome is supported by the growth of beneficial bacteria, which is encouraged by the modification of the gut microbiota synbiotics (Khursheed et al., 2019). The fermentation of prebiotics and the synthesis of bioactive chemicals are two metabolic pathways in which this microbial population is essential. Microbial metabolites, such as short-chain fatty acids, are produced as a consequence. These metabolites influence blood pressure management by improving blood vessel function and vasodilation. Chronic low-grade inflammation reduction is a major contributor to hypertension. By altering the makeup of the gut microbiota, synbiotics have shown anti-inflammatory benefits (Kaur et al., 2021). This control of inflammation may be systemic in nature, affecting inflammation outside the stomach and aiding in blood pressure regulation. Benefits in lipid profiles and glucose metabolism have been linked to improvements in metabolic parameters brought about by synbiotics. Resolving metabolic dysfunction is essential for managing hypertension, and synbiotics may have a beneficial effect on these parameters, helping to control blood pressure. Endothelial function and the generation of nitric oxide improved endothelial function and higher nitric oxide generation have been associated with specific probiotic strains found in synbiotics (Tembhre et al., 2023). An essential feature of hypertension is endothelial dysfunction, and NO functions as a vasodilator to assist control of blood vessel tone. Improved vascular health and lowered blood pressure may be facilitated by synbiotics through increased NO production. Apart from their immediate physiological benefits, synbiotics are frequently used in conjunction with diet and lifestyle education programs. In addition to promoting dietary modifications, frequent exercise, and stress reduction, this holistic approach also helps people regulate their blood pressure (Santos-Marcos et al., 2019).

7.5.1 Short-term Effects

Growing interest has been shown in the short-term effects of synbiotics on blood pressure because of the body's quick reaction to therapies that alter the gut microbiota and related physiological (Dai et al., 2023). The gut microbiota's dynamic synbiotics has the short-term capacity to rapidly modify the composition and activity of the gut microbiota. Probiotics quickly establish themselves thanks to prebiotics, which provide them with the necessary growth substrate. This modification may result in the production of bioactive compounds such as short-chain fatty acids, which can influence blood pressure regulation (Evariste et al., 2023). Vasodilation and tone of blood vessels of certain probiotic strains used in synbiotics have shown promise in improving vasodilation by generating nitric oxide. Improved blood vessel function and quick changes in blood pressure can result from this transient impact. Activities that reduce inflammation. Inflammatory indicators may be quickly affected by brief synbiotic treatments (Nan et al., 2024). Syncrotizing the gut microbiota can affect the release of pro-inflammatory cytokines, which can help reduce systemic inflammation linked to hypertension quickly. Synbiotics with metabolic reactions have the potential to temporarily alter lipid profiles and glucose metabolism, among other metabolic parameters. These quick reactions may have an impact on blood pressure management, especially in people who have metabolic dysregulation. The start of brief synbiotic treatments frequently corresponds with the beginning of lifestyle modifications. Blood pressure can immediately, if modestly, improve with education on healthy eating, exercise, and stress management (Z. Liu et al., 2024).

7.5.1.1 Immediate Impact on Blood Pressure

The rapid effects of synbiotics on blood pressure are a reflection of the gut microbiotas and related physiological processes' quick reactions. While certain effects could become apparent over time, some effects can appear sooner and affect blood pressure right away after ingestion (Button et al., 2023). With the introduction of advantageous bacteria and the provision of prebiotics to aid in their development, synbiotics swiftly alter the gut microbiome. Changes in the gut environment can be triggered by this quick microbial adjustment, which can impact the synthesis of bioactive substances that are involved in blood pressure regulation. Synbiotics contain some probiotic strains that have been shown to improve vasodilation by upregulating the production of NO (Satessa et al., 2020). Blood vessel tone is immediately affected by NO, a vasodilator that relaxes blood vessels, which may possibly lower blood pressure. Synbiotics have the ability to quickly affect inflammatory pathways by altering the gut microbiome. Synbiotics may help prevent systemic inflammation—which is connected to blood pressure regulation—immediately by lowering the generation of inflammatory cytokines. Metabolic parameters can alter quickly as a result of short-term synbiotic therapy. This might lead to changes in glucose metabolism and lipid profiles, which are important variables that affect blood pressure regulation. The central nervous system and the gut bacteria may communicate quickly thanks to the gut–brain axis. Through the production of neuroactive chemicals by gut bacteria, synbiotics may have an immediate impact on neuronal circuits that regulate blood pressure (Harikumar & Krishanan, 2022).

7.5.1.2 Influencing Factors

The initial effect of synbiotics on blood pressure is influenced by many variables. These variables include the dynamic interactions of host physiology, the gut microbiota, and environmental influences. Changes may occur more quickly in those whose microbiota is less balanced or diversified (Pyle, 2022). Specificity of probiotic strains within synbiotics, various probiotic strains may exhibit differing rates of colonization and metabolic activity. The particular strains involved may have an effect on how quickly favorable effects on blood pressure manifest. Prebiotics are essential for probiotic development because they provide a prebiotic substrate (Downs et al., 2022). Adequate consumption of prebiotics facilitates the fast growth of advantageous bacteria in the body, which instantly lowers blood pressure. Individual variability: The physiological reaction to synbiotics might differ depending on a person's health overall, their genetic makeup, and any underlying medical issues. The type and intensity of the reaction might vary depending on the host's metabolism and gut flora makeup. The immediate effects of synbiotics are influenced by lifestyle and dietary variables in addition to each other. When combined with a healthy lifestyle, a high-fiber, low-processed diet can improve the efficacy of synbiotic therapies on blood pressure (Mahdavi-Roshan et al., 2022).

7.5.2 Long-term Effects

Beyond short-term impacts, lasting changes in gut microbiota composition, vascular health, and metabolic control are among the long-term effects of synbiotics on blood pressure. Long-term use of synbiotics can result in long-lasting changes that support a comprehensive strategy for blood pressure control (Button et al., 2023). A stable and well-balanced gut flora is encouraged by long-term synbiotic usage. Regular supplementation increases the good bacteria population, which supports the development of an environment that improves blood pressure management. Reduction of chronic inflammation extended use of synbiotics helps to maintain a decrease in chronic low-grade inflammation, which is a major cause of hypertension (Baritugo et al., 2023). Over time, adjusting the gut flora contributes to preserving the equilibrium of systemic inflammation. Glucose metabolism and lipid profiles are two metabolic indicators that are significantly impacted by metabolic homeostasis synbiotics. The parameters linked to long-term blood pressure regulation are positively impacted by these persistent metabolic changes (Dangi et al., 2023). Maintaining vascular health in order to maintain healthy blood vessel tone and flexibility both of which are essential for long-term blood pressure regulation long-term synbiotic supplementation may enhance endothelial function and the synthesis of nitric oxide. Nutritional and lifestyle choices synbiotics support healthy lifestyle modifications when they are included in long-term health programs (Ishiguro et al., 2023).

7.5.3 Sustained Blood Pressure Reduction

Long-term synbiotic usage is related with a sustained drop in blood pressure, which is linked to extensive changes in a variety of physiological and microbiological variables (Rashid et al., 2023). These enduring effects are in favor of a thorough, long-term blood pressure treatment plan. Persistent low-grade inflammation is a significant component in the development of hypertension. By promoting a balanced inflammatory state over time, the long-acting anti-inflammatory qualities of synbiotics help to provide long-lasting reductions in blood pressure (Hadi et al., 2019). Long-term synbiotic usage is associated with persistent improvements in metabolic markers, such as glucose metabolism and lipid profiles. By treating the underlying causes of hypertension, these metabolic improvements help to regulate blood pressure generally. Endothelial function and continuous NO generation are supported by long-term synbiotic treatments (Chaturvedi et al., 2021). A healthy blood vessel's tone and flexibility are essential for controlling blood pressure, and these characteristics help to maintain them over time. Positive lifestyle modifications are reinforced by the use of synbiotics in a long-term health plan. Sustained education on stress management, physical exercise, and a balanced diet promotes cardiovascular health overall and lowers blood pressure over time. Better lipid metabolism, glucose management, and vascular health are only a few of the many cardiovascular advantages that come from synbiotics' multifarious actions (Singh et al., 2019).

7.5.4 Maintenance Strategies

A combination of regular supplementation, dietary integration, lifestyle education, monitoring, and customized methods are effective maintenance techniques for long-term synbiotic usage in blood pressure management (X. Wang et al., 2023). The objective of these techniques is to establish a comprehensive structure that provides long-term, sustainable advantages. Regular augmentation maintaining the ongoing presence of beneficial probiotics and prebiotics requires regular and persistent use of synbiotic supplements (Lou et al., 2024). This guarantees continuous assistance for the gut flora and related physiological mechanisms that aid in the management of blood pressure. To maintain the benefits of synbiotics, dietary integration is essential for promoting a diet high in foods high in prebiotics. Natural sources of prebiotics include fruits, vegetables, and fiber. These foods promote microbial development and enhance the synergistic effects of synbiotic supplementation. Education on leading a healthy lifestyle is essential (Zhou et al., 2024). This includes encouraging heart-healthy practices, stress reduction strategies, and frequent physical activity. The overall effectiveness of synbiotic therapies in the control of blood pressure is strongly influenced by lifestyle choices. It is possible to evaluate the efficacy of synbiotic therapies by routine blood pressure monitoring (Jamshidi et al., 2022). Blood pressure regulation can be optimized by modifying the synbiotic composition or dose in accordance with individual responses and changing health situations. Individualized techniques acknowledge that people respond differently to synbiotics; hence, it's important to use individualized strategies. Customizing synbiotic formulations and therapies according to individual health concerns, genetic makeup, and response patterns strengthens the strategy's personalized aspect. It is essential to include synbiotics into comprehensive cardiovascular therapy in a coordinated manner. Working together with healthcare providers guarantees that synbiotics successfully complement other therapies, which adds to a comprehensive strategy for managing blood pressure (Anggeraini et al., 2021).

7.6 SYNBIOTICS IN SPECIAL POPULATIONS

Synbiotics have demonstrated promise in treating specific health issues and enhancing general wellbeing in a variety of distinct groups (Zhang et al., 2023). Adapting therapies to the requirements of varied populations requires an understanding of how synbiotics might be used in these particular circumstances. During gestation, synbiotics could benefit both the mother and the developing fetus. It has been investigated if modifying the mother's gut microbiota using synbiotics might have advantages such as lowering inflammation and preventing gestational diabetes (Castillo-Escandón et al., 2023). The influence of a mother's gut health on the development of her infant's microbiome is also a topic of increasing attention. Microbiota development is very important throughout the early stages of life. Research has examined the potential of supplementing newborns and children with probiotics to prevent and manage illnesses such as respiratory infections, allergies, and eczema. Certain studies have shown beneficial effects on the development of the immune system and a decreased risk of atopic illnesses (Zhou et al., 2024). The gut microbiota is known to alter with age, and chronic disease risk is also known to rise. The potential of synbiotics to enhance immune system performance, lower inflammatory response, and promote gastrointestinal health in the elderly has been studied. These therapies might lead to improved general health and wellbeing in older people. People with metabolic disorders including type 2 diabetes and MetS may benefit from taking supplements (Z. Wang et al., 2022). These benefits support overall metabolic health in people with particular metabolic difficulties. The use of antibiotics may upset the gut microbiota's equilibrium, resulting in digestive problems. Probiotics and prebiotics combined in synbiotics may help reestablish microbial equilibrium and lessen disruptions brought on by antibiotics, thus supporting gastrointestinal health both during and after antibiotic therapy (Chan & Liu, 2022).

7.6.1 Geriatric Population

The geriatric population, defined as those 65 years of age and above, has particular health issues connected to aging, such as altered gut microbiota, heightened vulnerability to infections, and chronic illnesses related to aging (Núñez-Sánchez et al., 2021). In order to address particular health issues and enhance general wellbeing in the elderly population, synbiotics have emerged as a potentially effective strategy (Askari et al., 2021). Dysbiosis, a condition marked by changes in the makeup of the gut microbiota, is linked to aging. Synbiotics provide a way to modify and replenish a more balanced microbial habitat in the aging gut through the combination of probiotics and prebiotics (Fernandes et al., 2017). Maintaining the health of the digestive system and nutrition absorption depends on this regulation. Immune system deterioration with age frequently results in heightened vulnerability to infections and weakened defenses. The potential of synbiotics to strengthen the immune system in the elderly has been investigated. This might lead to a reduced frequency and severity of illnesses as well as a greater defense against pathogens (Sah et al., 2023). Constipation and irritable bowel syndrome (IBS) are among the digestive problems that elderly people frequently face. Synbiotics can help with these problems by encouraging regular bowel movements, lowering gut inflammation, and enhancing gastrointestinal health in general (Montoya-Uribe et al., 2022).

7.6.2 Pediatric Population

Among children, synbiotics have drawn interest due to their capacity to enhance several areas of health and have a good impact on the microbiota's development. Children's distinct physiological traits, developing immune systems, and particular health issues must all be taken into account in order to fully comprehend the significance of synbiotics in children (Hughes & Holscher, 2021). The development and maturity of the gut microbiota are largely dependent on the early years of life. Synbiotics, which include probiotics and prebiotics, may help create a diversified and robust microbial community, which would provide the groundwork for general wellbeing (Mealey & Long, 2018). Childhood is a critical period for the immune system's development. Research has been done on the potential of synbiotics to modify the immune system and support a responsive and balanced immune system. The potential of early life synthetic therapies to prevent allergies and atopic disorders has been investigated. Evidence exists to show that synbiotics may aid in the immune system's development, hence lowering the incidence of atopic illnesses and allergic responses (El-Sahhar & Varga-Weisz, 2022). Gastrointestinal problems in children, such as diarrhea, constipation, and colic, are common. By improving general gastrointestinal health, lowering inflammation, and fostering a healthy gut flora, synbiotics may help alleviate these problems. The gut microbiome of children receiving antibiotic therapy may be disturbed. Synbiotics have demonstrated potential in reducing antibiotic-associated disruptions, assisting in the restoration of microbial balance, and averting gastrointestinal problems linked to the use of antibiotics (Ibrahem, 2015). Certain pediatric conditions, such as inflammatory bowel disease (IBD) and IBS, may benefit from synbiotic interventions. According to research, children with certain diseases may benefit from using synbiotics to help with symptom management and gut health (Qiao et al., 2023).

7.6.3 Individuals with Comorbidities

In those with type 2 diabetes, the use of synbiotics helps to improve glycemic control (Nauta et al., 2013). Syncrotics may help regulate blood sugar levels by modifying the gut flora and treating underlying inflammation. Synbiotics may be beneficial for those with MetS, a group of risk factors for cardiovascular disease. Studies suggest that blood pressure control, cholesterol profiles, and other metabolic health-related parameters may improve (Montoya-Uribe et al., 2022). Ruiz et al. (2024) findings presented provide evidence that the effects of spices on energy expenditure, fat balance, and body adiposity reduction are similar in fish and mammals. Furthermore, there are a number of ways via which improvements in gut immunological conditions are seen. According to these findings, including a variety of spices in one's diet may be a useful nutritional tactic. The adverse effects that are frequently linked to fish oil decreases in fish feeds may be lessened with the use of such supplements. This highlights the potential of spices as a useful element in enhancing general health and wellbeing in aquatic animals, with benefits similar to those shown in land mammals (Ruiz et al., 2024). Nikpayam et al. (2023) investigated that SBP and DBP, as well as TC, LDL-C, HDL-C, and TG, show a significant reduction when chia product supplementation is used. However, anthropometric measurements, glycemic-related parameters, and inflammatory variables show no discernible effect. The results indicate encouraging cardiovascular benefits, but they also emphasize the need for more RCTs with bigger sample numbers and longer durations to improve the precision of the results and confirm these effects (Nikpayam et al., 2023). IBD symptoms, such as ulcerative colitis and Crohn's disease, have been promisingly treated using synbiotics. They might be used as an adjuvant treatment in the management of IBD because of their anti-inflammatory properties and support for gut health.

With synbiotic therapies, people with IBS, a functional gastrointestinal illness, may find relief from symptoms including bloating and changed bowel patterns (Dhopatkar et al., 2023). Reducing symptoms may be aided by altering the gut microbiome. Through their beneficial effects on blood pressure management, lipid profiles, and general cardiovascular health, synbiotics show cardiovascular advantages. For those who already have cardiovascular disease or are at risk, these consequences may be especially important. Dysregulation of the immune system can occur in several autoimmune diseases. Because of their immune-modulatory properties, synbiotics may affect an autoimmune patient's immunological responses and lower inflammation (Ooi et al., 2019).

7.7 PRACTICAL APPLICATIONS AND RECOMMENDATIONS

A comprehensive strategy is used to enhance general health and wellbeing in practical applications and suggestions for integrating synbiotics into daily life (Paul et al., 2022). Discussions with medical specialists people, especially those with underlying medical issues or on medication, should speak with healthcare providers before starting synbiotic supplementation. Selecting the right formulation and synbiotic compatibility will be aided by a comprehensive assessment of health state. Personalized synbiotic formulations with targeted supplementation are essential (Reehana et al., 2021). Targeted supplementation can be more successful if particular probiotic strains and prebiotic types are taken into account according to health goals and circumstances. Prebiotic-rich foods including fruits, vegetables, whole grains, and fermented foods like yogurt are encouraged to be consumed when included into dietary patterns. By fostering a varied and supportive habitat for the gut microbiota, this dietary integration enhances the benefits of synbiotic supplementation (Illanes & Guerrero, 2016). For optimal effects, it is important to maintain long-term consistency in the usage of synbiotics. To see consistent benefits in immune response, gut health, and other related outcomes, long-term supplementation could be required. Adopting a more holistic lifestyle approach should include both lifestyle adjustments and synbiotic therapies (S. Jafari et al., 2023). Promote the adoption of healthy behaviors in people, such as regular exercise, stress reduction, and a balanced diet, as these elements all work together to improve overall wellbeing. Synbiotic strategy can be adjusted based on individual responses when health measures, such as gut health markers and related biomarkers, are regularly monitored (Douglas & Sanders, 2008).

7.7.1 Dietary Guidelines for Synbiotic Intake

The consumption of probiotic-rich foods, prebiotic sources, and, when needed, synbiotic supplements are all combined in a balanced and varied manner according to dietary guidelines for synbiotic intake. Incorporate a range of foods high in probiotics into your diet, including fermented foods like miso, kimchi, kefir, sauerkraut, and yogurt (X. Wang et al., 2023). Live beneficial bacteria found in these foods naturally support intestinal health. Eat a variety of meals high in prebiotics to encourage the development and activity of good bacteria in the stomach. Fruits (bananas, apples), vegetables (garlic, onions), whole grains, and legumes are good sources. The focus should be on a plant-based diet that includes a variety of fruits, vegetables, whole grains, and nuts (Hersi et al., 2023). Plant-based diets supply vital nutrients and help create an environment that is conducive to a varied gut bacterium. Make sure you are getting enough dietary fiber because it is a prebiotic substrate that helps good bacteria grow. Good sources of dietary fiber that promote intestinal health are fruits, vegetables, beans, whole grains, and legumes (Sobotik et al., 2021). Limit your intake of sugary and highly processed meals, as they might have a bad effect on your digestive system. Whole, minimally processed foods include fiber and other elements that processed meals may not have. Consider taking a synbiotic pill if you think your diet may not contain enough of them. Those who take certain drugs, have particular health issues, or have trouble getting probiotics and prebiotics from whole foods should pay particular attention to this. Make sure your food is well-balanced and satisfies your needs for all nutrients. Integration of synbiotics into a nutrient-dense, well-rounded diet maximizes their advantages. Synbiotics are a component of a holistic approach to health (Zhang et al., 2023).

7.7.2 Integration into Clinical Practice

Clinical practitioners must use a thorough and patient-centered approach when integrating synbiotics into treatment, taking into account each patient's unique health needs as well as evidence-based recommendations and current research (Khursheed et al., 2019). Perform comprehensive patient evaluations to learn about each person's health, medical background, and unique issues. When recommending synbiotics, follow recommendations based on the most recent research and data. Think about which prebiotic and probiotic strains are most suited to each patient's desired health result. Tailor synbiotic treatments to the unique needs, preferences, and reactions of each patient (Chatterjee et al., 2022). Take into account variables including age, comorbidities, food preferences, and any drug interactions. Establish routine patient outcome monitoring, taking note of any negative effects, improvement in symptoms, and signs of gut health. To maximize benefits and meet changing health demands, modify synbiotic techniques as necessary. To guarantee a comprehensive approach, cooperate with experts in a variety of domains, such as nutrition, immunology, and gastrointestinal (Kurian et al., 2022). This partnership improves synbiotic therapies' efficacy, particularly in complicated patients. Inform patients on how using synbiotics can improve their overall health and intestinal health. To help patients take charge of their health, provide them clear information about the advantages, how to use it properly, and how to include it into their regular routines. For diseases including MetS, IBD, and IBS where gut health is important, include synbiotics in your treatment regimens. Make sure your therapy approaches work in unison. Stay up to date on the most recent findings in the synbiotic and gut microbiota fields of study. Evidence-based and current patient care is enhanced by ongoing learning and the incorporation of new discoveries into clinical practice (Sudheer et al., 2022).

7.8 FUTURE PERSPECTIVE

Based on new findings and a better comprehension of the complex connection between gut microbiota and cardiovascular health, the potential benefits of synbiotics in controlling blood pressure appear promising (van Duynhoven et al., 2013). It is envisaged that precision medicine techniques would customize synbiotic treatments according to a person's distinct gut microbiome, genetic makeup, and cardiovascular risk profile, maximizing the efficacy of these treatments. Further investigation is anticipated to reveal new strains of probiotics, combinations of prebiotics, and creative formulations that will augment the synergistic benefits of synbiotics. More focused and effective synbiotic products created especially for blood pressure-related pathways may result from this research (Hamjane et al., 2024). Future telemedicine solutions, wearable technology, and interactive applications may be used to include synbiotic suggestions into larger lifestyle and nutrition platforms. People may now include synbiotics into their regular activities and monitor and control their blood pressure in real-time thanks to this integration (Lu et al., 2023). A robust and long-lasting role for synbiotics in cardiovascular health strategies will be cemented by anticipated long-term clinical trials that evaluate their long-term effects on blood pressure control and related cardiovascular outcomes. It is anticipated that interdisciplinary cooperation among microbiologists, cardiologists, dietitians, and data scientists will advance knowledge of the intricate processes relating to the control of blood pressure and gut flora (Hemmati et al., 2023). Innovative research techniques and game-changing discoveries might result from this partnership. Future uses of synbiotics could center on their potential as a preventative measure, highlighting their part in early intervention plans to slow the onset of hypertension and lower the total burden of cardiovascular illnesses. In conclusion, synbiotics show potential in the changing environment as a personalized and all-encompassing strategy to blood pressure control in the pursuit of improved cardiovascular health (Domínguez-López et al., 2023).

7.9 CONCLUSION

In conclusion, there are significant implications for cardiovascular health from the dynamic and emerging issue of the link between synbiotics and their eventual role in blood pressure regulation. Based on the available studies, it seems that the intricate relationship between gut flora and blood pressure regulation offers a promising avenue for therapeutic interventions. Because they can alter crucial factors including inflammation, oxidative stress, and lipid metabolism, synbiotics have a complicated impact on blood pressure. The summarized data from clinical studies demonstrate positive outcomes, including reduced SBP and DBP, better lipid profiles, and good impacts on other cardiovascular risk factors. The outlook for synbiotics in the control of blood pressure is exciting: more interdisciplinary collaboration, novel formulations being investigated, precision medicine techniques, and interaction with digital platforms. By providing distinct and tailored methods for individuals with varying cardiovascular risk profiles, these advancements hold promise for enhancing the targeted efficacy of synbiotic treatments. As research into cardiovascular health continues, longer-term clinical studies and a deeper understanding of the underlying processes will contribute to the establishment of synbiotics as a durable and sustainable component of regimens. By acting as a preventive measure, synthetics can reduce the overall burden of hypertension and cardiovascular disease, particularly when employed in early intervention strategies. In summary, the shift from correlation to the eventual role of synbiotics in blood pressure management illustrates a trajectory marked by knowledge based on evidence and a commitment to tailored, comprehensive approaches. For people seeking effective and customized treatments to reach their optimal state of cardiovascular health.

ACKNOWLEDGMENT

The authors are thankful to the Principal, Department of Pharmacy, Teerthanker Mahaveer University, Moradabad, Uttar Pradesh for providing the necessary facilities and support.

COMPETING INTEREST STATEMENT

The authors declare no conflict of interest.

DISCLAIMER

None

REFERENCES

Aljuraiban, G. S., Gibson, R., Chan, D. S. M., Van Horn, L., & Chan, Q. (2023). The role of diet in the prevention of hypertension and management of blood pressure: A umbrella review of meta-analyses of interventional and observational studies. *Advances in Nutrition*, 100123. https://doi.org/https://doi.org/10.1016/j.advnut.2023.09.011

Amoah, K., Tan, B., Zhang, S., Chi, S., Yang, Q., Liu, H., Yang, Y., Zhang, H., & Dong, X. (2023). Host gut-derived Bacillus probiotics supplementation improves growth performance, serum and liver immunity, gut health, and resistive capacity against Vibrio harveyi infection in hybrid grouper (♀Epinephelus fuscoguttatus×♂Epinephelus lanceolatus). *Animal Nutrition*, *14*, 163–184. https://doi.org/https://doi.org/10.1016/j.aninu.2023.05.005

Anggeraini, A. S., Massi, M. N., Hamid, F., Ahmad, A., As'ad, S., & Bukhari, A. (2021). Effects of synbiotic supplement on body weight and fasting blood glucose levels in obesity: A randomized placebo-controlled trial. *Annals of Medicine and Surgery*, *68*, 102548. https://doi.org/https://doi.org/10.1016/j.amsu.2021.102548

Arabi, S. M., Bahrami, L. S., Rahnama, I., & Sahebkar, A. (2022). Impact of synbiotic supplementation on cardiometabolic and anthropometric indices in patients with metabolic syndrome: A systematic review and meta-analysis of randomized controlled trials. *Pharmacological Research*, *176*, 106061. https://doi.org/https://doi.org/10.1016/j.phrs.2022.106061

Askari, G., Ghavami, A., Shahdadian, F., & Moravejolahkami, A. R. (2021). Effect of synbiotics and probiotics supplementation on autoimmune diseases: A systematic review and meta-analysis of clinical trials. *Clinical Nutrition*, *40*(5), 3221–3234. https://doi.org/https://doi.org/10.1016/j.clnu.2021.02.015

Baritugo, K. A., Bakhsh, A., Kim, B., & Park, S. (2023). Perspectives on functional foods for improvement of canine health and treatment of diseases. *Journal of Functional Foods*, *109*, 105744. https://doi.org/https://doi.org/10.1016/j.jff.2023.105744

Button, J. E., Cosetta, C. M., Reens, A. L., Brooker, S. L., Rowan-Nash, A. D., Lavin, R. C., Saur, R., Zheng, S., Autran, C. A., Lee, M. L., Sun, A. K., Alousi, A. M., Peterson, C. B., Koh, A. Y., Rechtman, D. J., Jenq, R. R., & McKenzie, G. J. (2023). Precision modulation of dysbiotic adult microbiomes with a human-milk-derived synbiotic reshapes gut microbial composition and metabolites. *Cell Host & Microbe*, *31*(9), 1523–1538.e10. https://doi.org/https://doi.org/10.1016/j.chom.2023.08.004

Castillo-Escandón, V., Ramos-Clamont Montfort, G., Islas Rubio, A. R., Marszalek, J. E., Subiría-Cueto, R., & Fernández Michel, S. (2023). Development of healthy synbiotic corn-based snack: Nutritional composition and effect of agave fructan-alginate coating on survival of Lactobacillus acidophilus. *Journal of Cereal Science*, *114*, 103777. https://doi.org/https://doi.org/10.1016/j.jcs.2023.103777

Chai, X., Wen, L., Song, Y., He, X., Yue, J., Wu, J., Chen, X., Cai, Z., & Qi, Z. (2023). DEHP exposure elevated cardiovascular risk in obese mice by disturbing the arachidonic acid metabolism of gut microbiota. *Science of the Total Environment*, *875*, 162615. https://doi.org/https://doi.org/10.1016/j.scitotenv.2023.162615

Chan, M. Z. A., & Liu, S.-Q. (2022). Fortifying foods with synbiotic and postbiotic preparations of the probiotic yeast, Saccharomyces boulardii. *Current Opinion in Food Science*, *43*, 216–224. https://doi.org/https://doi.org/10.1016/j.cofs.2021.12.009

Chatterjee, G., Negi, S., Basu, S., Faintuch, J., O'Donovan, A., & Shukla, P. (2022). Microbiome systems biology advancements for natural well-being. *Science of the Total Environment*, *838*, 155915. https://doi.org/https://doi.org/10.1016/j.scitotenv.2022.155915

Chaturvedi, S., Khartad, A., & Chakraborty, S. (2021). The potential of non-dairy synbiotic instant beverage powder: Review on a new generation of healthy ready-to-reconstitute drinks. *Food Bioscience*, *42*, 101195. https://doi.org/https://doi.org/10.1016/j.fbio.2021.101195

Chauhan, J., & Sharma, R. K. (2023). Synbiotic formulations with microbial biofilm, animal derived (casein, collagen, chitosan) and plant derived (starch, cellulose, alginate) prebiotic polymers: A review. *International Journal of Biological Macromolecules*, *248*, 125873. https://doi.org/https://doi.org/10.1016/j.ijbiomac.2023.125873

Chavda, V., Chaurasia, B., Deora, H., & Umana, G. E. (2021). Chronic kidney disease and stroke: A bi-directional risk cascade and therapeutic update. *Brain Disorders*, *3*, 100017. https://doi.org/https://doi.org/10.1016/j.dscb.2021.100017

Cheng, S., Li, B., Ding, Y., Hou, B., Hung, W., He, J., Jiang, Y., Zhang, Y., & Man, C. (2023). The probiotic fermented milk of Lacticaseibacillus paracasei JY062 and Lactobacillus gasseri JM1 alleviates constipation via improving gastrointestinal motility and gut microbiota. *Journal of Dairy Science*. https://doi.org/https://doi.org/10.3168/jds.2023-24154

Coleman, J. L., Hatch-McChesney, A., Small, S. D., Allen, J. T., Sullo, E., Agans, R. T., Fagnant, H. S., Bukhari, A. S., & Karl, J. P. (2022). Orally ingested probiotics, prebiotics, and synbiotics as countermeasures for respiratory tract infections in nonelderly adults: A systematic review and meta-analysis. *Advances in Nutrition*, *13*(6), 2277–2295. https://doi.org/https://doi.org/10.1093/advances/nmac086

Dai, H., Han, J., Wang, T., Yin, W.-B., Chen, Y., & Liu, H. (2023). Recent advances in gut microbiota-associated natural products: Structures, bioactivities, and mechanisms. *Natural Product Reports*, *40*(6), 1078–1093. https://doi.org/https://doi.org/10.1039/d2np00075j

Dangi, P., Chaudhary, N., Chaudhary, V., Virdi, A. S., Kajla, P., Khanna, P., Jha, S. K., Jha, N. K., Alkhanani, M. F., Singh, V., & Haque, S. (2023). Nanotechnology impacting probiotics and prebiotics: A paradigm shift in nutraceuticals technology. *International Journal of Food Microbiology*, *388*, 110083. https://doi.org/https://doi.org/10.1016/j.ijfoodmicro.2022.110083

del Valle, J. C., Bonadero, M. C., & Fernández-Gimenez, A. V. (2023). Saccharomyces cerevisiae as probiotic, prebiotic, synbiotic, postbiotics and parabiotics in aquaculture: An overview. *Aquaculture*, *569*, 739342. https://doi.org/https://doi.org/10.1016/j.aquaculture.2023.739342

Devi, R., Sharma, E., Thakur, R., Lal, P., Kumar, A., Altaf, M. A., Singh, B., Tiwari, R. K., Lal, M. K., & Kumar, R. (2023). Non-dairy prebiotics: Conceptual relevance with nutrigenomics and mechanistic understanding of the effects on human health. *Food Research International*, *170*, 112980. https://doi.org/https://doi.org/10.1016/j.foodres.2023.112980

Dhopatkar, N., Keeler, J. L., Mutwalli, H., Whelan, K., Treasure, J., & Himmerich, H. (2023). Gastrointestinal symptoms, gut microbiome, probiotics and prebiotics in anorexia nervosa: A review of mechanistic rationale and clinical evidence. *Psychoneuroendocrinology*, *147*, 105959. https://doi.org/https://doi.org/10.1016/j.psyneuen.2022.105959

Domínguez-López, I., Arancibia-Riveros, C., Marhuenda-Muñoz, M., Tresserra-Rimbau, A., Toledo, E., Fitó, M., Ros, E., Estruch, R., & Lamuela-Raventós, R. M. (2023). Association of microbiota polyphenols with cardiovascular health in the context of a Mediterranean diet. *Food Research International*, *165*, 112499. https://doi.org/https://doi.org/10.1016/j.foodres.2023.112499

Douglas, L. C., & Sanders, M. E. (2008). Probiotics and prebiotics in dietetics practice. *Journal of the American Dietetic Association*, *108*(3), 510–521. https://doi.org/https://doi.org/10.1016/j.jada.2007.12.009

Downs, B. W., Banik, S. P., Bagchi, M., Banik Ghosh, R., Kushner, S., & Bagchi, D. (2022). Chapter 15- The microbiome, immunity, anaerobism, and inflammatory conditions: A multifaceted systems biology intervention. In D. Bagchi & B. W. B. T.- M. (eds.), *Downs*

Immunity, Digestive Health and Nutrition (pp. 205–216). Academic Press. https://doi.org/https://doi.org/10.1016/B978-0-12-822238-6.00024-8

El-Sahhar, S., & Varga-Weisz, P. (2022). Chapter Five - the gut microbiome in health and disease: Inflammatory bowel diseases. In D. A. Bohan & A. B. T.- A. in E. R. Dumbrell (eds.), *Functional Microbiomes* (Vol. 67, pp. 289–330). Academic Press. https://doi.org/https://doi.org/10.1016/bs.aecr.2022.09.005

Evariste, L., Mouchet, F., Pinelli, E., Flahaut, E., Gauthier, L., & Barret, M. (2023). Gut microbiota impairment following graphene oxide exposure is associated to physiological alterations in xenopus laevis tadpoles. *Science of the Total Environment*, *857*, 159515. https://doi.org/https://doi.org/10.1016/j.scitotenv.2022.159515

Fernandes, R., do Rosario, V. A., Mocellin, M. C., Kuntz, M. G. F., & Trindade, E. B. S. M. (2017). Effects of inulin-type fructans, galacto-oligosaccharides and related synbiotics on inflammatory markers in adult patients with overweight or obesity: A systematic review. *Clinical Nutrition*, *36*(5), 1197–1206. https://doi.org/https://doi.org/10.1016/j.clnu.2016.10.003

Geng, S., Zhang, T., Gao, J., Li, X., Chitrakar, B., Mao, K., & Sang, Y. (2023). In vitro screening of synbiotics composed of Lactobacillus paracasei VL8 and various prebiotics and mechanism to inhibits the growth of Salmonella Typhimurium. *LWT*, *180*, 114666. https://doi.org/https://doi.org/10.1016/j.lwt.2023.114666

Guo, R., Chen, L.-H., Xing, C., & Liu, T. (2019). Pain regulation by gut microbiota: Molecular mechanisms and therapeutic potential. *British Journal of Anaesthesia*, *123*(5), 637–654. https://doi.org/https://doi.org/10.1016/j.bja.2019.07.026

Gyawali, R., Nwamaioha, N., Fiagbor, R., Zimmerman, T., Newman, R. H., & Ibrahim, S. A. (2019). Chapter 12- The role of prebiotics in disease prevention and health promotion. In R. R. Watson & V. R. B. T.- D. I. in G. D. Preedy (eds.), *Dietary Interventions in Gastrointestinal Diseases* (pp. 151–167). Academic Press. https://doi.org/https://doi.org/10.1016/B978-0-12-814468-8.00012-0

Hadi, A., Sepandi, M., Marx, W., Moradi, S., & Parastouei, K. (2019). Clinical and psychological responses to synbiotic supplementation in obese or overweight adults: A randomized clinical trial. *Complementary Therapies in Medicine*, *47*, 102216. https://doi.org/https://doi.org/10.1016/j.ctim.2019.102216

Hamjane, N., Mechita, M. B., Nourouti, N. G., & Barakat, A. (2024). Gut microbiota dysbiosis -associated obesity and its involvement in cardiovascular diseases and type 2 diabetes. A systematic review. *Microvascular Research*, *151*, 104601. https://doi.org/https://doi.org/10.1016/j.mvr.2023.104601

Harikumar, G., & Krishanan, K. (2022). The growing menace of drug resistant pathogens and recent strategies to overcome drug resistance: A review. *Journal of King Saud University - Science*, *34*(4), 101979. https://doi.org/https://doi.org/10.1016/j.jksus.2022.101979

Hasan, A., Zerin, F., Menon, S. N., Alam, M. A., & Hasan, R. (2022). Mechanism of canagliflozin-induced vasodilation in resistance mesenteric arteries and the regulation of systemic blood pressure. *Journal of Pharmacological Sciences*, *150*(4), 211–222. https://doi.org/https://doi.org/10.1016/j.jphs.2022.09.004

Hellebois, T., Tsevdou, M., & Soukoulis, C. (2020). Chapter Five - functionalizing and bio-preserving processed food products via probiotic and synbiotic edible films and coatings. In A. G. da Cruz, E. S. Prudencio, E. A. Esmerino, & M. C. B. T.-A. in F. and N. R. da Silva (eds.), *Probiotic and Prebiotics in Foods: Challenges, Innovations and Advances* (Vol. 94, pp. 161–221). Academic Press. https://doi.org/https://doi.org/10.1016/bs.afnr.2020.06.004

Hemmati, M., Kashanipoor, S., Mazaheri, P., Alibabaei, F., Babaeizad, A., Asli, S., Mohammadi, S., Gorgin, A. H., Ghods, K., Yousefi, B., & Eslami, M. (2023). Importance of gut microbiota metabolites in the development of cardiovascular diseases (CVD). *Life Sciences*, *329*, 121947. https://doi.org/https://doi.org/10.1016/j.lfs.2023.121947

Hersi, M. A., Genc, E., Pipilos, A., & Keskin, E. (2023). Effects of dietary synbiotics and biofloc meal on the growth, tissue histomorphology, whole-body composition and intestinal microbiota profile of Nile tilapia (Oreochromis niloticus) cultured at different salinities. *Aquaculture*, *570*, 739391. https://doi.org/https://doi.org/10.1016/j.aquaculture.2023.739391

Hughes, R. L., & Holscher, H. D. (2021). Fueling gut microbes: A review of the interaction between diet, exercise, and the gut microbiota in athletes. *Advances in Nutrition*, *12*(6), 2190–2215. https://doi.org/https://doi.org/10.1093/advances/nmab077

Ibrahem, M. D. (2015). Evolution of probiotics in aquatic world: Potential effects, the current status in Egypt and recent prospectives. *Journal of Advanced Research*, *6*(6), 765–791. https://doi.org/https://doi.org/10.1016/j.jare.2013.12.004

Illanes, A., & Guerrero, C. (2016). Chapter 2- Functional foods and feeds: Probiotics, prebiotics, and synbiotics (A. Illanes, C. Guerrero, C. Vera, L. Wilson, R. Conejeros, & F. B. T.- L.-D. P. Scott (eds.), *Lactose-Derived Prebiotics* (pp. 35–86). Academic Press. https://doi.org/https://doi.org/10.1016/B978-0-12-802724-0.00002-0

Ishiguro, E., Haskey, N., & Campbell, K. (2023). Chapter 7- Targeting the gut microbiota for health (E. Ishiguro, N. Haskey, & K. B. T.- G. M. (Second E. Campbell (eds.), *Interactive Effects on Nutrition and Health* (pp. 179–221). Academic Press. https://doi.org/https://doi.org/10.1016/B978-0-323-91387-4.00005-3

Jafari, M., Desai, A., & Damani, R. (2020). Blood pressure management after mechanical thrombectomy in stroke patients. *Journal of the Neurological Sciences*, *418*, 117140. https://doi.org/https://doi.org/10.1016/j.jns.2020.117140

Jafari, S., Jafari, S. M., Ebrahimi, M., Kijpatanasilp, I., & Assatarakul, K. (2023). A decade overview and prospect of spray drying encapsulation of bioactives from fruit products: Characterization, food application and in vitro gastrointestinal digestion. *Food Hydrocolloids*, *134*, 108068. https://doi.org/https://doi.org/10.1016/j.foodhyd.2022.108068

Jain, H., Marsool, M. D. M., Goyal, A., Sulaiman, S. A., Fatima, L., Idrees, M., Sharma, B., Borra, V., Gupta, P., Nadeem, A., Jain, J., Ali, H., & Sohail, A. H. (2024). Unveiling the relationship between gut microbiota and heart failure: Recent understandings and insights. *Current Problems in Cardiology*, *49*(1, Part C), 102179. https://doi.org/https://doi.org/10.1016/j.cpcardiol.2023.102179

Jamshidi, S., Masoumi, S. J., Abiri, B., Sarbakhsh, P., Sarrafzadeh, J., Nasimi, N., & Vafa, M. (2022). The effect of synbiotic and vitamin D co-supplementation on body composition and quality of life in middle-aged overweight and obese women:

A randomized controlled trial. *Clinical Nutrition ESPEN*, *52*, 270–276. https://doi.org/https://doi.org/10.1016/j.clnesp.2022.09.005

Jan, T., Negi, R., Sharma, B., Kour, D., Kumar, S., Rai, A. K., Rustagi, S., Singh, S., Sheikh, M. A., Kumar, K., Ahmed, N., & Yadav, A. N. (2023). Diversity, distribution and role of probiotics for human health: Current research and future challenges. *Biocatalysis and Agricultural Biotechnology*, *53*, 102889. https://doi.org/https://doi.org/10.1016/j.bcab.2023.102889

Kaur, S., Thukral, S. K., Kaur, P., & Samota, M. K. (2021). Perturbations associated with hungry gut microbiome and postbiotic perspectives to strengthen the microbiome health. *Future Foods*, *4*, 100043. https://doi.org/https://doi.org/10.1016/j.fufo.2021.100043

Keulers, L., Dehghani, A., Knippels, L., Garssen, J., Papadopoulos, N., Folkerts, G., Braber, S., & van Bergenhenegouwen, J. (2022). Probiotics, prebiotics, and synbiotics to prevent or combat air pollution consequences: The gut-lung axis. *Environmental Pollution*, *302*, 119066. https://doi.org/https://doi.org/10.1016/j.envpol.2022.119066

Khursheed, R., Gulati, M., Wadhwa, S., Vishwas, S., Sharma, D. S., Corrie, L., Alam, A., Alnasser, S. M., Aba Alkhayl, F. F., Parveen, Z., Nammi, S., Chellappan, D. K., Gupta, G., Zacconi, F., Steel, A., Adams, J., Jha, N. K., Dua, K., & Singh, S. K. (2022). Multifaceted role of synbiotics as nutraceuticals, therapeutics and carrier for drug delivery. *Chemico-Biological Interactions*, *368*, 110223. https://doi.org/https://doi.org/10.1016/j.cbi.2022.110223

Khursheed, R., Singh, S. K., Wadhwa, S., Kapoor, B., Gulati, M., Kumar, R., Ramanunny, A. K., Awasthi, A., & Dua, K. (2019). Treatment strategies against diabetes: Success so far and challenges ahead. *European Journal of Pharmacology*, *862*, 172625. https://doi.org/https://doi.org/10.1016/j.ejphar.2019.172625

Kordvarkane, Z., Oshvandi, K., Mohammadi, Y., & Azizi, A. (2023). Effect of education based on the Common-Sense Model of Self-Regulation on blood pressure and self-management of hypertensive patients: A clinical trial study. *International Journal of Nursing Sciences*, *10*(3), 294–301. https://doi.org/https://doi.org/10.1016/j.ijnss.2023.06.009

Kurian, S. J., Baral, T., Sekhar M, S., & Rao, M. (2022). *Chapter 28- Role of probiotics and prebiotics in digestion, metabolism, and immunity* (D. Bagchi & S. E. B. T.- N. and F. F. in B. D. Ohia Metabolism and Immune Health (eds.); pp. 501–522). Academic Press. https://doi.org/https://doi.org/10.1016/B978-0-12-821232-5.00026-4

Lei, Y., Xu, M., Huang, N., & Yuan, Z. (2023). Meta-analysis of the effect of probiotics or synbiotics on the risk factors in patients with coronary artery disease. *Frontiers in Cardiovascular Medicine*, *10*.

Li, L., Yan, S., Liu, S., Wang, P., Li, W., Yi, Y., & Qin, S. (2023). In-depth insight into correlations between gut microbiota and dietary fiber elucidates a dietary causal relationship with host health. *Food Research International*, *172*, 113133. https://doi.org/https://doi.org/10.1016/j.foodres.2023.113133

Liu, X., Hu, K. K. Y., & Haritos, V. S. (2024). Enzymatic production of cello-oligosaccharides with potential human prebiotic activity and release of polyphenols from grape marc. *Food Chemistry*, *435*, 137562. https://doi.org/https://doi.org/10.1016/j.foodchem.2023.137562

Liu, Z., Liu, M., Meng, J., Wang, L., & Chen, M. (2024). A review of the interaction between diet composition and gut microbiota and its impact on associated disease. *Journal of Future Foods*, *4*(3), 221–232. https://doi.org/https://doi.org/10.1016/j.jfutfo.2023.07.004

Lou, J., Cui, S., Huang, N., Jin, G., Chen, C., Fan, Y., Zhang, C., & Li, J. (2024). Efficacy of probiotics or synbiotics in critically ill patients: A systematic review and meta-analysis. *Clinical Nutrition ESPEN*, *59*, 48–62. https://doi.org/https://doi.org/10.1016/j.clnesp.2023.11.003

Lu, Q., Chen, J., Jiang, L., Geng, T., Tian, S., Liao, Y., Yang, K., Zheng, Y., He, M., Tang, H., Pan, A., & Liu, G. (2023). Gut microbiota-derived secondary bile acids, bile acids receptor polymorphisms, and risk of cardiovascular disease in individuals with newly diagnosed type 2 diabetes: a cohort study. *The American Journal of Clinical Nutrition*. https://doi.org/https://doi.org/10.1016/j.ajcnut.2023.08.023

Mahdavi-Roshan, M., Salari, A., Kheirkhah, J., & Ghorbani, Z. (2022). The Effects of Probiotics on Inflammation, Endothelial Dysfunction, and Atherosclerosis Progression: A Mechanistic Overview. *Heart, Lung and Circulation*, *31*(5), e45–e71. https://doi.org/https://doi.org/10.1016/j.hlc.2021.09.006

Maioli, T. U., Trindade, L. M., Souza, A., Torres, L., Andrade, M. E. R., Cardoso, V. N., & Generoso, S. V. (2022). Non-pharmacologic strategies for the management of intestinal inflammation. *Biomedicine & Pharmacotherapy*, *145*, 112414. https://doi.org/https://doi.org/10.1016/j.biopha.2021.112414

Mealey, R. H., & Long, M. T. (2018). *Chapter 1- Mechanisms of Disease and Immunity* (S. M. Reed, W. M. Bayly, & D. C. B. T.- E. I. M. (Fourth E. Sellon (eds.); pp. 3–78). W.B. Saunders. https://doi.org/https://doi.org/10.1016/B978-0-323-44329-6.00001-2

Mitsnefes, M. M., Maltenfort, M., Denburg, M. R., Flynn, J. T., Schuchard, J., Dixon, B. P., Patel, H. P., Claes, D., Dickinson, K., Chen, Y., Gluck, C., Leonard, M., Verghese, P. S., & Forrest, C. B. (2023). Derivation of paediatric blood pressure percentiles from electronic health records. *EBioMedicine*, *98*, 104885. https://doi.org/https://doi.org/10.1016/j.ebiom.2023.104885

Mohanty, D., Misra, S., Mohapatra, S., & Sahu, P. S. (2018). Prebiotics and synbiotics: Recent concepts in nutrition. *Food Bioscience*, *26*, 152–160. https://doi.org/https://doi.org/10.1016/j.fbio.2018.10.008

Montoya-Uribe, V., Glibetic, N., Aan, F. J., & Matter, M. L. (2022). 2.24- *The Gut Microbiota, Nutrition, and Long-Term Disease Risk: A Mother and Child Perspective* (M. B. T.- C. G. M. Glibetic (ed.); pp. 289–307). Elsevier. https://doi.org/https://doi.org/10.1016/B978-0-12-819265-8.00068-1

Musazadeh, V., Faghfouri, A. H., Kavyani, Z., & Dehghan, P. (2022). Synbiotic as an adjunctive agent can be useful in the management of hyperglycemia in adults: An umbrella review and meta-research of meta-analysis studies. *Journal of Functional Foods*, *99*, 105355. https://doi.org/https://doi.org/10.1016/j.jff.2022.105355

Nan, G., Zhao, H., Wu, Q., Liu, L., Guan, Z., Li, C., Wu, H., Xiang, D., & Wu, Q. (2024). Comparative study of the effects of Tartary buckwheat seed and sprout consumption on the physiological indices and gut microbiota of C57BL/6J mice. *Food Science and Human Wellness*, *13*(2), 791–800. https://doi.org/https://doi.org/10.26599/FSHW.2022.9250067

Naseri, K., Saadati, S., Yari, Z., Asbaghi, O., Hezaveh, Z. S., Mafi, D., Hoseinian, P., Ashtary-Larky, D., Hekmatdoost, A., & de Courten, B. (2022). Beneficial effects of probiotic and synbiotic supplementation on some cardiovascular risk factors among individuals with prediabetes and type 2 diabetes mellitus: A grade-assessed systematic review, meta-analysis, and meta-regression of randomized clinica. *Pharmacological Research*, *182*, 106288. https://doi.org/https://doi.org/10.1016/j.phrs.2022.106288

Nauta, A. J., Ben Amor, K., Knol, J., Garssen, J., & van der Beek, E. M. (2013). Relevance of pre- and postnatal nutrition to development and interplay between the microbiota and metabolic and immune systems123. *The American Journal of Clinical Nutrition*, *98*(2), 586S–593S. https://doi.org/https://doi.org/10.3945/ajcn.112.039644

Nikpayam, O., Jafari, A., Safaei, E., Naghshi, N., Najafi, M., & Sohrab, G. (2023). Effect of chia product supplement on anthropometric measures, blood pressure, glycemic-related parameters, lipid profile and inflammatory indicators: A systematic and meta-analysis. *Journal of Functional Foods*, *110*, 105867. https://doi.org/https://doi.org/10.1016/j.jff.2023.105867

Núñez-Sánchez, M. A., Herisson, F. M., Cluzel, G. L., & Caplice, N. M. (2021). Metabolic syndrome and synbiotic targeting of the gut microbiome. *Current Opinion in Food Science*, *41*, 60–69. https://doi.org/https://doi.org/10.1016/j.cofs.2021.02.014

Ofosu, F. K., Mensah, D.-J. F., Daliri, E. B.-M., Lee, B.-H., & Oh, D.-H. (2021). Chapter 14- Probiotics, diet, and gut microbiome modulation in metabolic syndromes prevention (D. Dhanasekaran & A. B. T.- A. in P. Sankaranarayanan (eds.); pp. 217–231). Academic Press. https://doi.org/https://doi.org/10.1016/B978-0-12-822909-5.00014-9

Ooi, S. L., Correa, D., & Pak, S. C. (2019). Probiotics, prebiotics, and low FODMAP diet for irritable bowel syndrome - What is the current evidence? *Complementary Therapies in Medicine*, *43*, 73–80. https://doi.org/https://doi.org/10.1016/j.ctim.2019.01.010

Paul, P., Kaul, R., Harfouche, M., Arabi, M., Al-Najjar, Y., Sarkar, A., Saliba, R., & Chaari, A. (2022). The effect of microbiome-modulating probiotics, prebiotics and synbiotics on glucose homeostasis in type 2 diabetes: A systematic review, meta-analysis, and meta-regression of clinical trials. *Pharmacological Research*, *185*, 106520. https://doi.org/https://doi.org/10.1016/j.phrs.2022.106520

Pingali, H., & Hunter, S. D. (2023). Exploring mechanisms of blood pressure regulation in response to device-guided and non-device-guided slow breathing: A mini review. *Autonomic Neuroscience*, *244*, 103050. https://doi.org/https://doi.org/10.1016/j.autneu.2022.103050

Pyle, S. (2022). *2.23- Human Gut Microbiota and the Influence of Probiotics, Prebiotics, and Micronutrients* (M. B. T.- C. G. M. Glibetic (ed.); pp. 271–288). Elsevier. https://doi.org/https://doi.org/10.1016/B978-0-12-819265-8.00076-0

Qiao, L., Dou, X., Song, X., Chang, J., Yi, H., & Xu, C. (2023). Targeting mitochondria with antioxidant nutrients for the prevention and treatment of postweaning diarrhea in piglets. *Animal Nutrition*, *15*, 275–287. https://doi.org/https://doi.org/10.1016/j.aninu.2023.09.002

Rahimi, F., Pasdar, Y., Kaviani, M., Abbasi, S., Fry, H., Hekmatdoost, A., Nikpayam, O., Sohrab, G., Rezaei, M., & Nachvak, S. M. (2022). Efficacy of the synbiotic supplementation on the metabolic factors in patients with metabolic syndrome: A randomized, triple-blind, placebo-controlled trial. *International Journal of Clinical Practice*, *2022*.

Rashid, H., Zaidi, A., Anwar, M. A., & Tariq, M. (2023). A synbiotic made of an autochthonous Enterococcus durans strain and microbial polysaccharides improves broiler chicken health. *Journal of Agriculture and Food Research*, *14*, 100812. https://doi.org/https://doi.org/10.1016/j.jafr.2023.100812

Reehana, N., Mohamed Imran, M. Y., Thajuddin, N., & Dhanasekaran, D. (2021). Chapter 10- Synbiotics in nutrition (D. Dhanasekaran & A. B. T.- A. in P. Sankaranarayanan (eds.); pp. 149–161). Academic Press. https://doi.org/https://doi.org/10.1016/B978-0-12-822909-5.00010-1

Requena, T., & Pérez Martínez, G. (2022). *3.14- Probiotics, Prebiotics, Synbiotics, Postbiotics and Other Biotics. What's Next?* (M. B. T.- C. G. M. Glibetic (ed.); pp. 197–210). Elsevier. https://doi.org/https://doi.org/10.1016/B978-0-12-819265-8.00094-2

Rezende, E. S. V., Lima, G. C., & Naves, M. M. V. (2021). Dietary fibers as beneficial microbiota modulators: A proposed classification by prebiotic categories. *Nutrition*, *89*, 111217. https://doi.org/https://doi.org/10.1016/j.nut.2021.111217

Riasatian, M., Mazloomi, S. M., Ahmadi, A., Derakhshan, Z., & Rajabi, S. (2023). Benefits of fermented synbiotic soymilk containing Lactobacillus acidophilus, Bifidobacterium lactis, and inulin towards lead toxicity alleviation. *Heliyon*, *9*(6), e17518. https://doi.org/https://doi.org/10.1016/j.heliyon.2023.e17518

Ribeiro-Silva, J. C., Tavares, C. A. M., & Girardi, A. C. C. (2023). The blood pressure lowering effects of glucagon-like peptide-1 receptor agonists: A mini-review of the potential mechanisms. *Current Opinion in Pharmacology*, *69*, 102355. https://doi.org/https://doi.org/10.1016/j.coph.2023.102355

Rodríguez-García, J. L., Botia, E., de La Sierra, A., Villanueva, M. A., & González-Spínola, J. (2005). Significance of elevated blood pressure and its management on the short-term outcome of patients with acute ischemic stroke. *American Journal of Hypertension*, *18*(3), 379–384. https://doi.org/https://doi.org/10.1016/j.amjhyper.2004.10.004

Roessler, J., Leistner, D. M., Landmesser, U., & Haghikia, A. (2022). Modulatory role of gut microbiota in cholesterol and glucose metabolism: Potential implications for atherosclerotic cardiovascular disease. *Atherosclerosis*, *359*, 1–12. https://doi.org/https://doi.org/10.1016/j.atherosclerosis.2022.08.018

Ruiz, A., Sanahuja, I., Andree, K. B., Furones, D., Holhorea, P. G., Calduch-Giner, J. A., Pastor, J. J., Viñas, M., Pérez-Sánchez, J., Morais, S., & Gisbert, E. (2024). Supplementation of gilthead seabream (Sparus aurata) diets with spices as a functional strategy to control excess adiposity through lipid, cholesterol and bile acid metabolism, and to induce an immunomodulatory intestinal regulation. *Aquaculture*, *581*, 740378. https://doi.org/https://doi.org/10.1016/j.aquaculture.2023.740378

Sah, R. K., Nandan, A., Athira, K., Prashant, S., Sathianarayanan, S., Jose, A., Venkidasamy, B., & Nile, S. H. (2023). Decoding the role of the gut microbiome in gut-brain axis, stress-resilience, or stress-susceptibility: A review. *Asian Journal of Psychiatry*, 103861. https://doi.org/https://doi.org/10.1016/j.ajp.2023.103861

Santos-Marcos, J. A., Perez-Jimenez, F., & Camargo, A. (2019). The role of diet and intestinal microbiota in the development of metabolic syndrome. *The Journal of Nutritional Biochemistry*, *70*, 1–27. https://doi.org/https://doi.org/10.1016/j.jnutbio.2019.03.017

Satessa, G. D., Kjeldsen, N. J., Mansouryar, M., Hansen, H. H., Bache, J. K., & Nielsen, M. O. (2020). Effects of alternative feed additives to medicinal zinc oxide on productivity, diarrhoea incidence and gut development in weaned piglets. *Animal*, *14*(8), 1638–1646. https://doi.org/https://doi.org/10.1017/S1751731120000154

Scorletti, E., Afolabi, P. R., Miles, E. A., Smith, D. E., Almehmadi, A., Alshathry, A., Childs, C. E., Del Fabbro, S., Bilson, J., Moyses, H. E., Clough, G. F., Sethi, J. K., Patel, J., Wright, M., Breen, D. J., Peebles, C., Darekar, A., Aspinall, R., Fowell, A. J., ... Byrne, C. D. (2020). Synbiotics alter fecal microbiomes, but not liver fat or fibrosis, in a randomized trial of patients with nonalcoholic fatty liver disease. *Gastroenterology*, *158*(6), 1597–1610.e7. https://doi.org/https://doi.org/10.1053/j.gastro.2020.01.031

Sherwood, A., Hughes, J. W., & McFetridge, J. (2003). Ethnic differences in the hemodynamic mechanisms of ambulatory blood pressure regulation. *American Journal of Hypertension*, *16*(4), 270–273. https://doi.org/https://doi.org/10.1016/S0895-7061(02)03269-7

Singh, S. K., Tiwari, V. K., Chadha, N. K., Munilkumar, S., Prakash, C., & Pawar, N. A. (2019). Effect of dietary synbiotic supplementation on growth, immune and physiological status of Labeo rohita juveniles exposed to low pH stress. *Fish & Shellfish Immunology*, *91*, 358–368. https://doi.org/https://doi.org/10.1016/j.fsi.2019.05.023

Sircana, A., De Michieli, F., Parente, R., Framarin, L., Leone, N., Berrutti, M., Paschetta, E., Bongiovanni, D., & Musso, G. (2019). Gut microbiota, hypertension and chronic kidney disease: Recent advances. *Pharmacological Research*, *144*, 390–408. https://doi.org/https://doi.org/10.1016/j.phrs.2018.01.013

Sobotik, E. B., Ramirez, S., Roth, N., Tacconi, A., Pender, C., Murugesan, R., & Archer, G. S. (2021). Evaluating the effects of a dietary synbiotic or synbiotic plus enhanced organic acid on broiler performance and cecal and carcass Salmonella load. *Poultry Science*, *100*(12), 101508. https://doi.org/https://doi.org/10.1016/j.psj.2021.101508

Suastika, A. V, Widiana, G. R., Fatmawati, N. N. D., Suastika, K., Paulus, I. B., & Sujaya, I. N. (2023). The role of probiotics and synbiotics on treatment of gestational diabetes: systematic review and meta-analysis. *AJOG Global Reports*, 100285. https://doi.org/https://doi.org/10.1016/j.xagr.2023.100285

Sudheer, S., Gangwar, P., Usmani, Z., Sharma, M., Sharma, V. K., Sana, S. S., Almeida, F., Dubey, N. K., Singh, D. P., Dilbaghi, N., Khayat Kashani, H. R., Gupta, V. K., Singh, B. N., Khayatkashani, M., & Nabavi, S. M. (2022). Shaping the gut microbiota by bioactive phytochemicals: An emerging approach for the prevention and treatment of human diseases. *Biochimie*, *193*, 38–63. https://doi.org/https://doi.org/10.1016/j.biochi.2021.10.010

Sumida, K., Pierre, J. F., Yuzefpolskaya, M., Colombo, P. C., Demmer, R. T., & Kovesdy, C. P. (2023). Gut microbiota-targeted interventions in the management of chronic kidney disease. *Seminars in Nephrology*, *43*(2), 151408. https://doi.org/https://doi.org/10.1016/j.semnephrol.2023.151408

Tang, W. H. W., Kitai, T., & Hazen, S. L. (2017). Gut Microbiota in Cardiovascular Health and Disease. *Circulation Research*, *120*(7), 1183–1196. https://doi.org/10.1161/CIRCRESAHA.117.309715

Tembhre, M. K., Shipra, Imran, S., & Jaiswal, K. (2023). *Chapter 4- The Modulatory Approaches of Microbiome Therapeutics* (N. S. Chauhan & S. B. T.- M. T. Kumar (eds.); pp. 95–126). Academic Press. https://doi.org/https://doi.org/10.1016/B978-0-323-99336-4.00013-6

van der Schoot, A., Helander, C., Whelan, K., & Dimidi, E. (2022). Probiotics and synbiotics in chronic constipation in adults: A systematic review and meta-analysis of randomized controlled trials. *Clinical Nutrition*, *41*(12), 2759–2777. https://doi.org/https://doi.org/10.1016/j.clnu.2022.10.015

van Duynhoven, J., Vaughan, E. E., van Dorsten, F., Gomez-Roldan, V., de Vos, R., Vervoort, J., van der Hooft, J. J. J., Roger, L., Draijer, R., & Jacobs, D. M. (2013). Interactions of black tea polyphenols with human gut microbiota: implications for gut and cardiovascular health1234. *The American Journal of Clinical Nutrition*, *98*(6), 1631S–1641S. https://doi.org/https://doi.org/10.3945/ajcn.113.058263

Wang, X., Ma, Y., Wu, X., Chen, B., Fang, X., Zhong, Q., Liao, Z., Wang, J., & Wang, L. (2023). The dietary intervention of synbiotic preparation promotes the bioconversion of soy isoflavones to equol and its metabolic mechanism. *Journal of Functional Foods*, *109*, 105784. https://doi.org/https://doi.org/10.1016/j.jff.2023.105784

Wang, Z., Li, W., Lyu, Z., Yang, L., Wang, S., Wang, P., Song, F., Chen, K., & Huang, Y. (2022). Effects of probiotic/prebiotic/synbiotic supplementation on blood glucose profiles: A systematic review and meta-analysis of randomized controlled trials. *Public Health*, *210*, 149–159.

Woźniak, D., Cichy, W., Przysławski, J., & Drzymała-Czyż, S. (2021). The role of microbiota and enteroendocrine cells in maintaining homeostasis in the human digestive tract. *Advances in Medical Sciences*, *66*(2), 284–292. https://doi.org/https://doi.org/10.1016/j.advms.2021.05.003

Wu, P., Bai, Z., Xu, L., Wang, P., Chen, X., Du, L., Li, X., Zhao, Z., & Fang, Z. (2023). New approaches for rapid setpoint determination and uninterrupted tracking in non-invasive continuous blood pressure monitoring based on volume-clamp method. *Biomedical Signal Processing and Control*, *86*, 105305. https://doi.org/https://doi.org/10.1016/j.bspc.2023.105305

Yadav, M. K., Kumari, I., Singh, B., Sharma, K. K., & Tiwari, S. K. (2022). Probiotics, prebiotics and synbiotics: Safe options for next-generation therapeutics. *Applied Microbiology and Biotechnology*, *106*(2), 505–521. https://doi.org/10.1007/s00253-021-11646-8

Yang, Z., Ye, S., Xu, Z., Su, H., Tian, X., Han, B., Shen, B., Liao, Q., Xie, Z., & Hong, Y. (2021). Dietary synbiotic ameliorates constipation through the modulation of gut microbiota and its metabolic function. *Food Research International*, *147*, 110569. https://doi.org/https://doi.org/10.1016/j.foodres.2021.110569

Yin, M., Chen, M., Yuan, Y., Liu, F., & Zhong, F. (2024). Encapsulation of Lactobacillus rhamnosus GG in whey protein isolate-shortening oil and gum Arabic by complex coacervation: Enhanced the viability of probiotics during spray drying and storage. *Food Hydrocolloids*, *146*, 109252. https://doi.org/https://doi.org/10.1016/j.foodhyd.2023.109252

Zepeda-Hernández, A., Garcia-Amezquita, L. E., Requena, T., & García-Cayuela, T. (2021). Probiotics, prebiotics, and synbiotics added to dairy products: Uses and applications to manage type 2 diabetes. *Food Research International*, *142*, 110208. https://doi.org/https://doi.org/10.1016/j.foodres.2021.110208

Zhang, C., Fang, T., Shi, L., Wang, Y., Deng, X., Wang, J., & Zhou, Y. (2023). The synbiotic combination of probiotics and inulin improves NAFLD though modulating gut microbiota. *The Journal of Nutritional Biochemistry*, 109546. https://doi.org/https://doi.org/10.1016/j.jnutbio.2023.109546

Zhao, J., Zhao, F., Yuan, J., Liu, H., & Wang, Y. (2023). Gut microbiota metabolites, redox status, and the related regulatory effects of probiotics. *Heliyon*, *9*(11), e21431. https://doi.org/https://doi.org/10.1016/j.heliyon.2023.e21431

Zhou, S., Wang, M., Li, W., Zhang, Y., Zhao, T., Song, Q., & Cong, J. (2024). Comparative efficacy and tolerability of probiotic, prebiotic, and synbiotic formulations for adult patients with mild-moderate ulcerative colitis in an adjunctive therapy: A network meta-analysis. *Clinical Nutrition*, *43*(1), 20–30. https://doi.org/https://doi.org/10.1016/j.clnu.2023.11.010

8 Synbiotics
A Novel Paradigm for Phenylketonuria Management by Targeting Gut–Microbiota and Gut–Brain Axes

Sana Fatima, Muhammad Muzammal, Shaista Naz, Muzammil Ahmad Khan, Alamgir Khan, Arshad Farid, and Wasim Shah

8.1 INTRODUCTION

One of the biggest interfaces among hosts, its antigens, and the environmental factors can be represented by human's gastrointestinal (GI) tract. All the food that a person eats will pass from GI tract in their lifetime. This food not only carries the nutrients but also carries microbes that it carries from the outer environment into the body. These external microbes passing through GI tract will pose a great impact on the integrity of the gut's health [1]. All the microbes (bacteria, eukarya, and archaea) that make up the colonies in the gut of a host are called gut microbiota in a mutualism relationship where both the host and the microbiota gain benefits [2,3].

There are many benefits provided by gut microbiota by using their various functions, i.e., integrity of gut health by maintaining and fortifying its health along with maintenance of mucous epithelium of the intestine [4], harvesting energy [5] from the food, providing, and regulating immunity [6].

The GI tract is layered by mucous from the inside which becomes more thicker as it proceeds toward the colon [7]. This layer of mucous in the colon provides a medium between the host and microbes residing in the colon. Colonies of microbes formed over a long period of time will produce a normal intestinal mucous [8]. The mucous in the colon can be divided into two layers depending on the thickness and permeability. The inner layer of the mucous is extremely dense which makes it impermeable while the outer layer is loosely packed thus it's more permeable for bacteria. This is why, the denser layer is sterile while the outer layer being permeable suits the colonization of bacteria. This layer also has the energy source for the residing bacteria in the form of mucin proteins having *O*-glycans. The mucin proteins also provide a binding site for the microbiota [9,10]. The mucous layer is packed loosely and shows a versatile range of arrangement which makes a niche for a versatile range of microbes that show a range of proliferation as well as energy utilization patterns [11].

The natural microbiota can be diversified also through mutations as well as gene transfer [12]. This diversification produces a variation in the microbial niche that will lead to more diversification consequently. Along with this, introduction of new microbes into the gut can also produce colonization of diverse range of microbes shaping a community that provides benefits to the host [13,14].

8.2 HOW MICROBIAL POPULATION IS INFLUENCED

The gut microbes show various features throughout various phases of life. During the early phases of host's life, the microbial community is rather simple, and it becomes more diverse with the colonization of new bacteria as the host ages. This diversification and complexity in the gut microbiota of the host can be due to influences of environment, genetics as well as physiology, i.e., lifestyle, hormonal balance, diet, immune system as well as the feedback among the gut and brain [15]. In the case of humans, the community of microbes in the gut can also be varied based on where the person is living.

Trillions of microbes reside in the intestine and all these microbes can be divided into six phyla, i.e., Bacteroidetes, Firmicutes, Actinobacteria, Fusobacteria, Verrucomicrobia, and Proteobacteria. Although the constitution of the microbiome varies from person to person, the most of the microbes (60%) that constitute the gut microbiota belong to the phylum Firmicutes, i.e., *Enterococcus, Ruminococcus, Lactobacillus,* and *Clostridium* [16,17].

8.3 MODULATION OF GUT MICROBIOME VIA DIET

Various studies in humans show that alterations are observed in the gut microbiota induced by alterations in the diet and this alteration is reproducible [18]. This is also observed that the diversity in gut microbiota is rather less due to simple diets while the urban areas as they provide variety in diet, people show more diversification in gut microbiota among themselves [19].

The interaction among nutrients and microbes can be either direct where the nutrients provide the necessary

DOI: 10.1201/9781032702438-8

elements for bacterial growth or do not provide these elements, or this interaction can be indirect where the microbes indirectly affect the metabolism of the host as well as their immune responses which can either protect or disrupt the intestinal barriers providing health benefits or prompting diseases, respectively [20].

The quality of diet as well as its composition, in studies, show the composition of microbial communities that resulted due to swapping protein-rich diets with protein fermentation in comparison to plant-based diet with carbohydrate fermentation [21]. Also, consuming healthy diet is shown to be related with the gene richness of the microbiota in humans [22].

The abundance of various bacterial communities in the GI tract is also related to the health conditions of the host as well as the effect of bacterial metabolism on different communities. For instance, association of *Ruminococcus gnavus* produces pro-inflammatory carbohydrates in hosts that are suffering from Chron's disease [23]. Bacterial communities of the genus *Clostridia* produce various toxic compounds, which produce a negative effect on Lactic acid bacteria reproduction [24]. However, Faecalibacterium prausnitzii generates short-chain fatty acids (SCFA) that serve as indicators of gut health due to their immunosuppressive properties [25].

Also, the effect of bacterial populations of various species is very important as it acts as a marker for the host's health. For instance, if a person has a balance between Firmicutes and Bacteroidetes, it acts as a marker of the host's obesity and a higher BMI [26]. On the other hand, a lower ratio of these bacterial populations produces a negative response to the host's BMI. For such a case, diet changes like a high-fiber diet may help in weight loss by reduction in extracted energy from the food [27].

Although the correlation between diet and microbiota and their effect on various health conditions of the host is an interesting topic of research, there is still some difficulty due to a range of variables that affect both in favor and in opposition for the host's health. Therefore, extensive research is needed to anticipate the effect of changes in diet as well as introduction or removal of bacterial communities in the GI tract. Nonetheless, the effect of various nutrients has been shown to alter the microbiota with no doubt [28–30].

Table 8.1 depicts the effect of various micro and macro nutrients along with the most commonly used additives that show an interaction with microbiota of the GI tract. This table also summarizes the effect of abundance of various bacterial species/genus and their interaction that affect the host's health (both beneficial and disadvantageous) [20].

8.4 GUT–BRAIN AXIS

One more captivating subject concerning the crosstalk among the GI tract microbes and the central nervous system (CNS) is in its early stages with respect to the understanding of the intricate procedures as well as the amount of medical research. The GI tract microbes can interact with CNS five diverse ways:

- Neuroanatomical pathway
- Neuroendocrine-hypothalamic–pituitary–adrenal axis pathway
- The immune system
- Gut microbiota metabolism pathway
- Intestinal mucosal barrier and blood-brain barrier [43]

This drift of communication among the microbes and CNS can go in both directions, i.e.,

- Bottom-up: that goes from the bottom, i.e., microbes from GI tract to the top, i.e., the brain.
- Top-down from the top; the brain to down; microbes of the GI tract.

TABLE 8.1
Association among Diet and Probable Variations in Microbial Population

Nutrients		Function	Gut Microbiota Alteration	Refs.
Sugars	Glycogen, starches, and fibers	SCFA (short-chain fatty acid) manufacture through microbial fermentation	Upsurge of population in Bacteroidetes, Bifidobacterium, *Clostridium*, *Prevotella*, and *Akkermansia*	[31] [32] [33] [34]
	Sweeteners (artificial)	Develop the danger of intolerance toward glucose	Upsurge in the population of *Bacteroides* as well as Clostridiales	[35]
Proteins		Improve the function of intestinal mucous barrier along with exertion of significant part in responses of the immune system and against oxidative	Reduction in the population of Bifidobacterium along with upsurge in the population ratio among Bacteroidetes and Firmicutes	[36] [37] [38] [39]
Lipids	Saturated lipids	Amplified intestinal penetrability	Amplified population of gram-negative bacteria	[40]
	Unsaturated lipids	Secondary relation with the GI microbes	Upsurge in the population of *Lactobacillus* and *Akkermansia*	[41] [42]

The first type of messaging mostly transpires via neuroendocrine as well as neuroimmune systems, with the involvement of the cells of enteroendocrine as well as enterochromaffin from the GI system, the mucous intestinal barrier, along with blood-brain barrier. The metabolites that are produced by the microbes of the gut, include tryptophan, SCFAs, and secondary bile acids, act as significant troupes intermediating the communication from the gut microbes toward the brain [44,45].

On the contrary, the communication that goes from the brain toward the gut microbes, i.e., the top-down pathway, transpires via the mucous intestinal barrier regulation, neuroanatomical pathway, and on the releasing neurotransmitters (e.g., 5-HT and catecholamines) [46,47].

Cells of the immune system (e.g., dendritic cells and macrophages) along with enteric glial cells (EGCs) continuously check the microbes-related chemicals formed within the gut. In providing a response toward these internal stimuli produced via microbial communities, neuro-modulatory chemicals are released locally that direct the enteric nerves. After this simulation of the enteric nerves is done, in response, they can cause an effect toward the brain as well as the spinal cord (CNS) by transmission through vagus nerves. Once the chemicals or other types of stimuli spread into the neurons, CNS, astrocytes, and microglia will respond via altering their transcriptional program, which will either support or inhibit the compulsive settings. Growing information is now putting light toward the procedures in fundamentals of microbes–brain–gut axis in various diseases, like psychiatric diseases along with neurodegenerative as well as metabolic disorders [48,49].

At the level of GI tract, motility as well as the permeability of gut regulation, bile secretions, mucous as well as the mucosal immunity system is under the control of the autonomic nervous system [50]. Furthermore, this nervous system can impact the integrity of mucous intestinal barrier will alter the penetrability of the epithelium cells of the intestine as well as modulate the mucous layer of the intestine. The role of some bacteria like lactobacilli are described to cause improvement in the enteric nervous system along with activation of vagus nerve [51], whereas some other lactobacilli are reported to be related in the production of neurotransmitters, that are related to the regulation of the intestinal transportation [52].

The role of SCFAs is mostly researched subject in the modulation of gut microbes, secreted via the microbes of the intestine, that is the key product obtained by the fermentation of un-digestible nutritional fibers as well as hard starch. SCFAs are distributed systematically through the blood and can cross the barrier between the brain and blood and play various important functions that include neuroactive properties. The precise procedure by which SCFAs perform their functions is basically unfamiliar but numerous animal research have revealed an impact on significant neurological as well as behavioral procedures which might show involvement in developmental and degenerative disorders of the nervous system [53,54].

Intestinal microbes characterize a crucial bioreactor system that changes nutritional chemicals into secondary metabolites having a vital part in a range of physical mechanisms. SCFAs act as one of the richest products that are produced by the process of fermentation done by the microbes present in the intestine [55]. A communication from the microbes toward the brain, mainly via the products produced by nutrient fermentation that engage various cellular receptors that are present on the epithelium cells of the GI tract, can control central as well as peripheral properties by altering metabolism of host [56]. The other way around, regulation through the brain toward the intestinal microbes is primarily intermediated via the vagal nerve, which can control the intestinal environment by reduction of mobility in the intestine along with permeability of the intestinal cells as well as exerting anti-inflammatory functions.

Thus, the diet of a person has a crucial part, particularly when a person is under dietetic extremes due to their lifestyle as well as in case of a disease that takes into account a restricted diet, on the mode of action of the gut–brain axis processes. Furthermore, important mediators are present as well, depending on the nutritional behaviors, endure the communication that goes along the gut–brain axis. Additionally, the gut microbes have the capacity to control the integrity of the barrier both inside the intestine as well as between the blood and brain, along with partial absorption of nutrient through the surface of mucous membrane [57].

8.5 MODULATION OF MICROBIOTA FOR THERAPY

Prodigious attention, nowadays, has been positioned toward the probable involvement of the gut microbes in the pathogenesis of a disease along with its clinical indicators, which makes it an attractive target for the cure of particular disorders. For instance, in such a case that a person is suffering from a metabolic syndrome, there will be co-related disorders that will show their effects like insulin resistance, obesity, diabetes, heart disease, and liver disease, the studies are presently concentrating toward the investigation of bacterial population arrangement as well as on the association of these bacterial communities with various diseases. Also, the studies are focusing on explaining the various pathways as well as secondary metabolites stimulated and formed by these bacterial communities, to comprehend their effects associated to metabolic syndrome [58]. The research shows that some nutrients can be advantageous for gut microbes, even though they go undigested from humans. This idea has shown sustenance in the increase of prebiotics, undigested nutrients that prove advantageous for stimulation of the growth or the action, or in some cases; both, selectively, of various microbial types inhabiting the GI tract, that will consequently prove beneficent by improvement of human health [59].

Prebiotics are substances that might provide positive feedback for the probiotics. These probiotics are produced on an

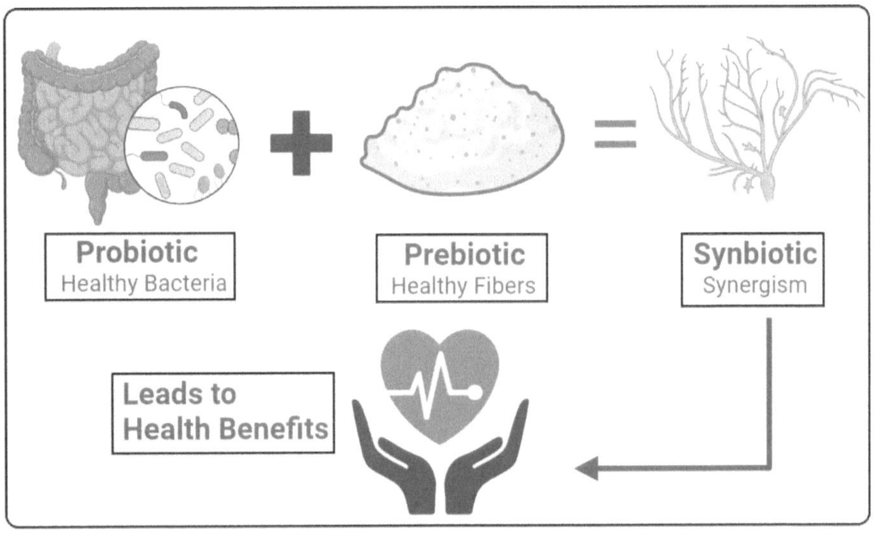

FIGURE 8.1 Use of synbiotics leading to health benefits.

industrial level and are available in the form of supplements. If properly combined (prebiotic and probiotic) they are called synbiotics. When taken as synbiotics, they can even provide greater benefits on the health of the host [60] (Figure 8.1).

Even though more research is essential beforehand the use of synbiotics for the benefit of host successfully, it still seems there are potentially strong signs that this method can be advantageous. For instance, the use of synbiotics and their metabolites have proved helpful for host's health in various neurodevelopmental disorders [61] as well as neurological disorders [62], diabetes [63], obesity [64], and metabolic syndrome [65]. Damage to bacterial diversity signifies the primary step toward an alteration in the environment of microbes, increasing the host's vulnerability toward various diseases.

Recently, in a review, Green et al. [66] reported the characteristics of synbiotics in metabolic disorders and obesity. The GI microbiota shows involvement in genesis of diseases, even though the interaction of the various features that are involved is still not understood fully. The literature available implicates dysbiosis of gut will lead to various metabolic disorders and wealth of available literature strongly implicates that gut dysbiosis is a key contributor to obesity development and associated metabolic anomalies, in addition to regulation of the microbiome via consumption of synbiotics signify a path for probable therapeutic involvements.

For instance, integration of either the fermentable sugars, or the integration of various strains of *Bifidobacterium/Lactobacillus*, or in some cases, integration of both, in the host's diet will not only facilitate progress toward ideal body weight as well as adiposeness but also apply additional positive properties on glycemic regulation, inflammations in the host, along with the intake of energy [66] (Figure 8.2).

It's thus imperative to study continuation on populations of affected host, particularly in incidence of disorders like the inherited errors of metabolism (IEMs), in which case, the patients are frequently taking an altered dietary routine that is continued over a long period of time, that can even last for a lifetime, suffering from various consequences.

Preliminary analysis of such diseases has already been led, selecting to increase the knowledge which will eventually permit scientists to provide a personalized plan for the use of synbiotics to treat various IEMs.

8.6 ASSOCIATION AMONG IEMS AND GUT MICROBIOME

As far as IEMs are concerned, during the past few years, there has been an upsurge in the research and the publishing of data that is related to the effect of the dietary routine of a person on their gut microbiota, because of the statistics that clinical intervention in affected people of such diseases happens by taking a specifically personalized dietetic routine.

These disorders, which are caused by the absence or deficiency of action of a specific enzyme, present great genetic as well as epigenetic heterogeneousness, and thus, they correspondingly show diverse responses among affected people having a similar genotype like; phenylketonuria (PKU) [67].

8.7 PHENYLKETONURIA

PKU (OMIM # 261600) also recognized as deficiency of phenylalanine hydroxylase (PAH) as well as Følling disease. It's an inherited error that leads to metabolism of an amino acid called phenylalanine (Phe). This disorder is triggered by mutations that are pathogenetic in the PAH gene. The function of this gene is to convert phenylalanine to tyrosine in the presence of tetrahydrobiopterin (BH4) that act as a co-substrate (data accessed from OMIM on 24/10/2023) (Figure 8.3).

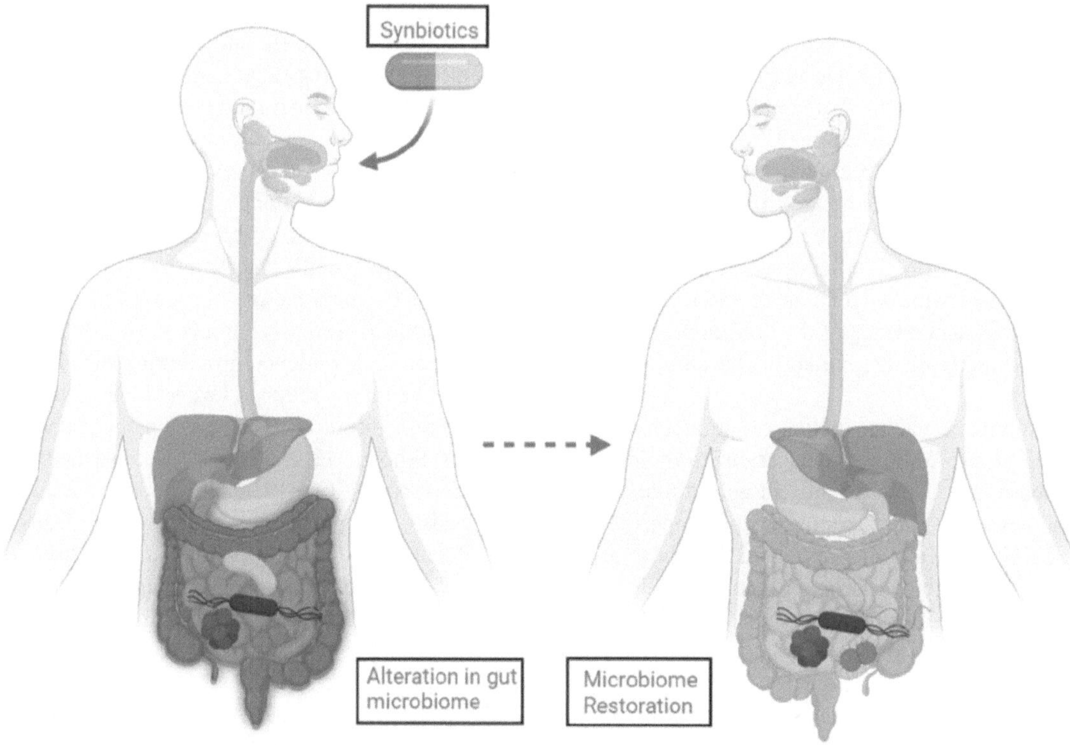

FIGURE 8.2 Restoration of Gut's microbial population via usage of synbiotics.

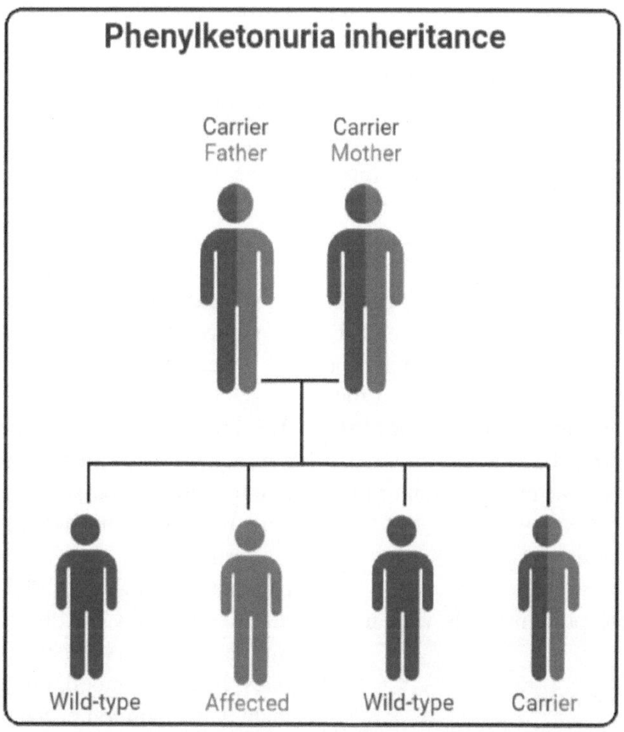

FIGURE 8.3 Inheritance pattern of PKU.

In case of patients suffering from PKU and are not treated, the concentration of phenylalanine increases in blood strikingly, consequently forming phenyl-ketone particles that can be noticed in the excreted urine; on the other hand, concentration of tyrosine becomes relatively lower.

8.8 MANAGEMENT OF PKU VIA DIET

The above discussion shows that the most logical step forward for the management of such a disease would be to control the dietary routine of the person suffering in which the consumption of the amino acid phenylalanine is reduced or even absent. This reduced diet to control the intake of this amino acid has proved to be a potential step for the management of PKU and a huge health improvement has been observed in the patient. This outcome not only helps the patients of PKU but also can be utilized for other inherited metabolic disorders. Treatment via limiting diet for PKU has been extremely great, and the reason behind it is that this amino acid can only be taken into the body via food and cannot be formed in the body on its own. That is why phenylalanine is included as an essential amino acid, which means that dependence of the concentration of phenylalanine is directly on the intake of the amino acid via food [68].

Even though the restriction in diet with reduced or absent Phe has been proven to be very successful in the management of disease, it still doesn't present an optimal way for treating the disorder. For example, when comparing children with PKU who were on a restricted diet for treatment of the disease to healthy children without PKU, the treated children showed a relatively higher incidence of decreased executive functions, impaired learning abilities, and attention deficit hyperactivity disorder [69].

As these children age, there is seen a loss in control of metabolism along with potentially negative effects on mood, memory, attention, and executive functions. In some of the patients, there is also an observance of seizure attacks along with development of lower extremity spasticity if the patients do not seek or do not adhere to the treatment in the adult stages [70]. Development of encephalopathy has been reported to occur once a prolonged loss of metabolic control in a person is seen along with in affected people in primary presentation of the disorder [71,72]. The occurrence of encephalopathy as a consequence of PKU also shows response to restricted diet plan. Additionally, visual aberrations have also been documented to arise through adult age when the affected person doesn't adhere to diet plan or to stop following the diet once the diet is re-introduced [71]. This data seems to be relevant with the deficits in the vision of those children who were suffering with PKU, and they did not adhere to the restricted diet in comparison to the adults who were PKU patients [73,74].

The restricted diet provided for the management of PKU includes:

- Reduced intake of Phe
- Intake of supplements for protein needs with no Phe
- A low-protein diets

The intake of phenylalanine is the only possible way for management of PKU and as it doesn't produce in the body on its own, by restricting the intake of Phe, the blood concentration will also be lowered consequently. Now, the amount of Phe reduction in the diet varies from person to person depending on the requirement of Phe for the total protein synthesis of a person. For instance, the growth of a person dependent on his/her age will require a certain amount of Phe to be healthy. Similarly, to maintain a balance between catabolism and anabolism requires a certain amount of Phe during illness. Also, if the person has a deficiency of PAH enzyme, the severity of this deficiency will also put an effect on the total extent of diet restriction [75].

When a person is on a restricted protein diet, only Phe intake is not lowered, along with Phe, intake of other essential amino acids is also compromised along with the reduction in the constituents obtained through natural diet that is involved in the manufacture of proteins like; various minerals, carnitine as well as vitamins.

Thus, in PKU patients, providing a substitute protein to compensate for the reduced levels of Phe is very important. The protein mixture given as supplementary diet for the patients although lacks Phe must be enriched in substitute protein tyrosine (Tyr). In healthy people, the metabolism of Phe leads to the production of Tyr which means that when Phe is reduced, it will consequently reduce the levels of Tyr. Thus, PKU patients are provided with Tyr so that the balance is not disturbed. Similarly, other macronutrients are also added to the supplementary diet that are present in the normal diet anyways.

The third restriction for PKU patients is that they consume a low-protein diet that re-enriched in other nutrients like lipids and carbs. This carb and lipid-rich diet is very important to meet the energy needs of the patient and also the diet mimics the food habits of a normal person [75].

Although, the main effect of PKU when untreated is metabolic defect, it consequentially causes an impairment of behavioral as well as neurological activities. Even though, the effects of PKU are heterogenous, the treatment of the disease follows only some approaches like.

- A therapy to replace enzymes so that enzymes that are reduced are replenished
- Therapy to reduce substrate
- Treatment via diet management to reduce the accumulated toxic materials [76].

The effect of dietary changes restricts various nutrients, consequently, the restriction causes dysbiosis of GI tract, malnutrition, diabetes, obesity, inflammatory bowel disorders, liver disorders, autism, and cancer.

Furthermore, another aspect that is considered in patients suffering from PKU is the potential effect of these diseases on the CNS due to the variations in metabolism. Similarly, the CNS also shows an effect on the metabolic rates, behavior, mood, coordination, temperature management, and cognition of the patients.

In untreated PKU and in propionic and methylmalonic acidaemia, for instance, neurological and behavioral impairment are highly variable, while liver disease is commonly developed in tyrosinemia type 1 and urea cycle disorders. Despite such heterogeneity, treatment approaches generally include one of the following: (I) enzyme replacement therapy, to replenish the deficient enzyme; (II) substrate reduction therapy; or (III) dietary treatment (or organ transplantation in selected cases) [77]. The purpose of the dietary treatment in IEMs is to reduce the target toxic compound that accumulates in the body, but contemporarily it may cause either dangerous overload, deficiencies of certain food groups and nutrients, or both [78]. Examples are diets that result in restricted or are excessively rich in certain nutrients and that may prompt intestinal dysbiosis with systemic effects such as malnutrition, obesity, type 1 or type 2 diabetes, inflammatory bowel disease, liver disease, symptoms of autism spectrum disorders, and even cancer.

Another aspect that needs to be taken into account in IEMs is the susceptibility of the CNS and the liver due to their high metabolic rate [79]. A few publications indicate how the microbiota may influence the CNS and consequently exert unwanted effects on metabolism [80], coordination [81], cognition [82], temperature control, and sensation [83].

8.9 MICROBES AND THEIR ROLE IN MANAGEMENT OF PKU

8.9.1 Pre-clinical Studies

The role of the use of synbiotics for the treatment of PKU has been studied the most out of all the inherited metabolic disorders. There are some clinical studies that have reported to give data on the processes that involve the use of microbes for the treatment of PKU in various animal models along with shedding light on how various approaches can be used for the usage of microbes that may benefit PKU patients.

Primarily, the research was published by Sawin et al. [84] in 2015 on the analysis of the role of the use of synbiotics on the modulation of PKU. The research shed light on the role of glycomacropeptide (GMP) which is a highly glycosylated protein that is manufactured in the body naturally. It is made up of a peptide chain having 64 aa and is obtained during the process of the manufacture of cheese. This protein is now being considered as a substitute for the Phe amino acid for patients that have restricted diet. GMP is considered as a prebiotic. The study reported that in the presence of GMP (prebiotic) the population of probiotics, e.g., Bifidobacterium increased in model mice within a time of 3 days only after they were provided with the treatment. The research was conducted in normal/healthy mice as control and mice having PKU (*Pah*^{enu2}). The evaluation of the results after treatment of the mice with GMP as a prebiotic by the analysis of fecal as well as caecal material and the population of microbial population along with the immune responses of the host and the production of short-chain fatty acids (SCFA). As we know, the fecal and caecal composition is basically dependent on diet of the host, thus it can be deduced that the changes in these are directly dependent on changes in diet. Thus, when GMP was added to the diet of PKU patients, there was observed a reduction in *Desulfovibrio* as well as *Proteobacteria* in both the control and the mice having PKU. The bacteria from the genus *Desulfovibrio* were observed to be in a relation for the manufacture of HSO_4^-, ion which has cytotoxic characteristics, found in higher concentration in patients that are suffering from colon ulcers. Additionally, upon analysis of the caecal material of mice models, it was observed that the level of SCFAs, butyrate as well as acetate to be heightened in those mice that were treated with GMP as compared to other inflammatory biomarkers that were reduced in treated mice without having any effect on the concentration of Phe [84].

In a more recent study, an investigation was performed in a pre-clinical trial on the effect of synbiotics on the presence of tetrahydrobiopterin (BH_4) which is influenced by the probiotics that produce tetrahydrobiopterin (BH_4). In the study, the comparison of mice with GTP cyclohydrolase 1-deficient hyperphenylalaninaemia-1 (hph-1) and normal mice was performed in the existence of these probiotics. These BH_4-generating probiotics release an enzyme called 6-pyruvoyltetrahydropterin synthase (PTPS-2). In the study, levels of this enzyme were measured to check the effect of the treatment on mice models. It was observed that in normal mice, in the presence of these probiotics, there was a higher level of PTPS-2 enzyme in the feces. In treated hph-1 mice, the production of this enzyme after treatment was observed and the probiotic identified to generate the enzymes were identified to be *Aldercreutzia equolifaciens* and *Microbacterium schleiferi*. In human feces, similar results were observed that there were higher levels of this enzyme, and the bacteria associated with the production of these enzymes were identified to be species of bacteria related to phylum Actinobacteria [85].

Furthermore, in pre-clinical studies, the analysis of use of synbiotics was observed using GMP-based products in the artificial model of colon. The model generated feces in both the wild type (healthy) as well as weakened model (not suffering from PKU). The GMP-based prebiotic was reported to maintain the development and growth of probiotics like *Clostridium* and *Coprococcus*. There was an upsurge in the level of these probiotics in the feces in the treated model in comparison to the control chemical/lactose used instead of GMP-based chemicals. On the other hand, in the presence of lactose, the fermentation of lactose led to upsurge in the population of Proteobacteria which showed that depending on what type of substrate is being used, the relative abundance of various microbes in the GI tract while commercial GMP particularly was observed to increase the growth of beneficial bacteria in healthy colon models [86].

There are reported approaches that show the potential of genetically modified organisms (GMOs) inside the gut of affected people. These GMOs were described to potentially degrade phenyl alanine taken in through diet before it gets absorbed in the blood. These GMOs act as probiotics and are engineered by taking out gene that codes for Phe degrading enzyme from *Anabaena variabilis*; a cyanobacteria, and the gene is then cloned in a vector that is added to Lactobacillus *reuteri*, which then expresses the engineered gene. The results were then confirmed in vitro to check the expression of gene to produce a functional enzyme via Lactobacillus *reuteri*. After the confirmation, the GMO probiotic was tested in PKU mice models that were homozygous for PKU abnormality. The results of the treatment showed that Phe levels in the blood were reduced after treatment just after 3–4 days. This effect of the probiotic use was checked with a continued experiment for 1–2 weeks where the previous results were confirmed with a continued lowered level of Phe in the blood [87].

Like the study with the use of GMOs, another study was performed in *E. coli* as GM probiotic. The gene that coded for phenylalanine metabolism was taken out and from GI tract of mammals was added to *E. coli*. This enzyme uses various metabolism pathways to produce non-toxic chemicals like trans-cinnamic acid that again gets metabolized inside the liver to produce hippurate which is then excreted out via urine. Homozygous mice for PKU were tested with the GM probiotic (*E. coli*) and the association of lowered concentration of Phe in the blood was documented after treatment. In wild-type mice, after treatment, 38% lowered concentration of Phe was observed in comparison to control wild-type mice models. A similar experiment was also conducted in monkey models which further gave evidence for similar results [88].

In another pre-clinical study, Murine models for PKU were used to analyze the effect of treatment given with probiotic (E. coli) engineered genetically to produce phenylalanine lysis enzyme on the reduction of Phe in serum of the models, after a day of treatment. The results of the study showed that after a day of treatment, there were 50% lowered levels of Phe in the serum depending on the design of GMOs as well as the severity of PKU [89] (Table 8.2).

8.9.2 Clinical Studies

Many studies have been performed on the association between the use of various synbiotics and their effect on PKU. In a study performed by MacDonald et al. [90], focused on the same aim by the use of prebiotics. The purpose of the study was to analyze the results of usage of oligosaccharides (scGOS/lcFOS) as prebiotics used as a mixture of metabolic formula to manage PKU in children. The children chosen for the study were restricted only to being fed breast milk. The study was hypothesized on the theory that breast milk that lack the presence of oligosaccharides that might be present normally, may lead to an increase pH in the feces of the child along with lowered levels of bifidobacteria which leaves the patients more at risk of further infections. The study postulated that by treatment via probiotic strains, this effect could be mitigated. The results of the study showed that by the use of dominant probiotic strains, levels of oligosaccharides could be maintained that in turn maintain the population of bifidobacteria as well as pH in the feces. The same bacteria additionally maintained the levels of phenylalanine. The results presented a potential effect of the use of probiotics in PKU patients for disease treatment. After the observation period ended, the patients showed a normal level of bifidobacteria, enterococcus, and lactobacillus bacterial population as a healthy person proving the above-mentioned results [90].

One of the primary research studies done for the management of PKU via synbiotics, young patients (age 4) suffering from PKU were taken as subjects which showed that the patient had lowered population of various beneficial bacteria. The results of the study presented that the composition of bacterial population in the GI tract varied among patients suffering from PKU in comparison to healthy patients. This differentiation might be associated with dietary restrictions provided to PKU patients for disease management. For instance, caloric percentages obtained from carbs, proteins, and fats, protein concentration taken in that provide varied amino acid levels as well as the level of Phe in the blood. The researchers described that this variation might be due to the diseased condition of the subjects that have varied Phe levels which might have altered the population of gut microbes that is the consequence of dietary restrictions or both [91].

In PKU patients, analysis for the prediction of microbial genes presented an upsurged expression of genes related to biosynthesis of lipo-polysaccharides which may be related to the inflammation in the patients. Because of the daily ingestion of proteins, the levels of Phe in the circulating blood are supposed to have added to the population shift in the GI tract [92].

Additionally, research in the model animals, association of the role of GMP, has been shown in PKU patients.

TABLE 8.2
Use of Various Synbiotic Products in Pre-clinical Studies for Treatment of PKU Patients

Product Used	Results	Refs.
GMP prebiotic	Reduction in *Desulfovibrio* as well as *Proteobacteria* Upsurge in level of SCFAs, butyrate and acetate	[84]
BH_4 generating probiotics	Higher level of PTPS-2 enzyme	[85]
GMP-based products	Maintained the development and growth of probiotics like *Clostridium* and *Coprococcus*	[86]
Genetically modified organisms (GMOs) *Lactobacillus reuteri*	Phe levels in the blood were reduced after treatment just after 3–4 days	[87]
E. coli as GMO	38% lowered concentration of Phe	[88]
E. coli as GMO	50% lowered levels of Phe in the serum	[89]

TABLE 8.3
Use of Various Synbiotic Products in Clinical Studies for Treatment of PKU Patients

Product Used	Results	Refs.
Oligosaccharides (scGOS/lcFOS)	maintained the levels of population of bifidobacteria and phenylalanine	[90]
GMP/GMP products	GMP usage as alternative to Phe	[93]
GMP	Maintenance of Trp levels	[94]
GMP or other GMP-based chemicals	Reduction in deoxycarnitine in the plasma of PKU patients	[95]
Restricted diet	Negative correlation showing reduction in butyrate levels as well as probiotics	[96]
Restricted diet	Negative correlation with fiber intake and glycemic index as well as variation in GI tract microbiota	[97]

The concentration of Phe that is provided by the use of GMP or GMP products as prebiotics proves that addition of these prebiotics in the diet can be potentially used as an alternative to Phe. This usage proved to be successful especially in PKU patients nowadays [93].

In another clinical trial, usage of GMP was documented by Ney et al. [94], during research that analyzed the use of various proteins that were taken by subjects as alternatives to other proteins on the monoamine metabolites as well as their precursors in PKU patients. The metabolic analysis showed the degradative compounds that are produced from tyrosine and tryptophan were upsurged in PKU patients ingesting free proteins compared to those that took GMP-based products as an alternative. The hypothesis of the study stated that the normal proteins didn't have enough Tyr due to the reasons that the residual Tyr was degraded even more by the microbes in the GI tract in comparison to those that took alternatives like GMP or other GMP-based chemicals. On the other hand, there was no substantial effect on the degradation of Trp. Nonetheless, Trp metabolism was still affected which was linked to the inflammation in patients [94] (Table 8.3).

Furthermore, lipid metabolism in the presence of GMP was studied in adult PKU patients who were on a restricted diet taking natural amino acids, GMP, or other GMP-based chemicals as an alternate. This study was based on the hypothesis that an alteration in lipid metabolism on neuronal level, there is an observation of an upsurged oxidation as well as rate of inflammation which might consequentially will produce a negative modulation of cognition in patients suffering from PKU. Although this research didn't directly measure the results of various alternatives of proteins on the population of bacteria in the gut, it still insinuated that there was a reduction in deoxycarnitine in the plasma of PKU patients which consequentially will reduce the biosynthesis of carnitine. PKU patients who take free proteins receive a higher concentration of carnitine in comparison to the patients who take GMP alternatives. The patients also show a higher level of urine due to higher carnitine metabolism that may be a result of more availability of carnitine in patients taking GMP products [95].

To analyze a more precise results on the variation of the GI tract microbes by variation in the diet of patients suffering from PKU. A study was performed on children suffering from PKU who were on a restricted diet in comparison to children on unrestricted diet having a mild PKU. Diseased patients showed a significant reduction in butyrate levels in the feces along with reduction in some bacteria that produce butyrate, and the results show a healthy status in PKU patients [96].

In a follow-up of above-mentioned research, another study was conducted with a deeper analysis of the composition of gut microbial population dependent on variations in the diet of two populations. The study showed that microbes from the phylum Bacteroidetes as well as Firmicutes were enriched in patients of PKU while *Veillonellaceae* was found to be reduced. In patients with mild PKU abundance of *Clostridium*, *Blautia*, and *Blautia*. Whereas the effect of diet on the gut microbiota in patients suffering from hyper PKU showed a negative correlation of *Faecalibacterium* with fiber intake along with glycemic levels.

In a similar manner, in mild PKU, a negative correlation was observed with *Ruminococcaceae* and glycemic index as well as fiber intake whereas, a positive correlation was observed via *Lachnospiraceae* with both the glycemic index and fiber intake. The results of this study imply that not only does the amino acid intake affect the management of PKU but also the intake of other nutritional substances like carbohydrates that are allowed to be taken during a restricted diet. Also, the previous data and the data obtained via this study, the gene sequencing of the probiotic bacteria showed that the members of *Ruminococcus* that degrade starch act as indicator species in patients suffering from PKU. The results of this study indicate the importance of the use of synbiotics in patients with PKU along with the importance of a dietary regimen to be observed strictly in patients suffering from PKU [97].

8.10 CONCLUSION

The conclusion of the above-mentioned discussion shows the role of microbial population that is continuously under study for the management of IEMs like PKU. There are a range of factors that affect the disease management which is why a personalized approach could be used which should prove beneficial. Various diet regimens are kept under study to deduce the association among diet and microbiota modulation. A reduction in the diversity of microbes in GI tract led to reduction of SCFAs as well as butyrate along with an upsurge in inflammation. The usage of synbiotics has been studied critically and the results show that by intake of synbiotics, the microbiota of the host can be restored. Various approaches can be applied for the treatment of PKU in the future like the use of GMOs and other pharmacological products.

ACKNOWLEDGMENTS

We would like to acknowledge all the lab members working in the Lab of Human Molecular Genetics, Gomal Centre of Biochemistry and Biotechnology, Gomal University, Dera Ismail khan, Pakistan, for their help in finding the required literature.

ETHICAL APPROVAL

Not applicable.

AUTHORS' CONTRIBUTION

S.F. and M.M. collected the data and drafted the manuscript; M.A.K. helped in figure drafting; W.S. supervision; A.F., S.N., and A.K. helped in English language and drafting the manuscript.

FUNDING

Not applicable.

CONFLICT OF INTEREST

Not declared by the authors.

DATA AVAILABILITY STATEMENT

All the data presented here is save in password-protected laptop of M.M and will be available on request.

REFERENCES

1. Bengmark, S. (1998). Ecological control of the gastrointestinal tract. The role of probiotic flora. *Gut*, *42*(1), 2–7. https://doi.org/10.1136/gut.42.1.2
2. Bäckhed, F., Ley, R. E., Sonnenburg, J. L., Peterson, D. A., & Gordon, J. I. (Hosts). (2005). Host-bacterial mutualism in the human intestine. *Science*, *307*(5717), 1915–1920. https://doi.org/10.1126/science.1104816
3. Round, J. L., & Mazmanian, S. K. (2010). Inducible Foxp3+ regulatory T-cell development by a commensal bacterium of the intestinal microbiota. *Proceedings of the National Academy of Sciences of the United States of America*, *107*(27), 12204–12209. https://doi.org/10.1073/pnas.0909122107
4. Natividad, J. M. M., & Verdu, E. F. (2013). Modulation of intestinal barrier by intestinal microbiota: Pathological and therapeutic implications. *Pharmacological Research*, *69*(1), 42–51. https://doi.org/10.1016/j.phrs.2012.10.007
5. Den Besten, G., Van Eunen, K., Groen, A. K., Venema, K., Reijngoud, D. J., & Bakker, B. M. (2013). The role of short-chain fatty acids in the interplay between diet, gut microbiota, and host energy metabolism. *Journal of Lipid Research*, *54*(9), 2325–2340. https://doi.org/10.1194/jlr.R036012
6. Gensollen, T., Iyer, S. S., Kasper, D. L., & Blumberg, R. S. (2016). How colonization by microbiota in early life shapes the immune system. *Science*, *352*(6285), 539–544. https://doi.org/10.1126/science.aad9378
7. Gustafsson, J. K., Ermund, A., Johansson, M. E. V., Schütte, A., Hansson, G. C., & Sjövall, H. (2012). An ex vivo method for studying mucus formation, properties, and thickness in human colonic biopsies and mouse small and large intestinal explants. American Journal of Physiology. Gastrointestinal and Liver Physiology, 302(4), G430–G438. https://doi.org/10.1152/ajpgi.00405.2011
8. Johansson, M. E. V., Jakobsson, H. E., Holmén-Larsson, J., Schütte, A., Ermund, A., Rodríguez-Piñeiro, A. M., Arike, L., Wising, C., Svensson, F., Bäckhed, F., & Hansson, G. C. (2015). Normalization of host intestinal mucus layers requires long-term microbial colonization. *Cell Host and Microbe*, *18*(5), 582–592. https://doi.org/10.1016/j.chom.2015.10.007
9. Juge, N. (2012). Microbial adhesins to gastrointestinal mucus. Trends in Microbiology, *20*(1), 30–39. https://doi.org/10.1016/j.tim.2011.10.001
10. Tailford, L. E., Crost, E. H., Kavanaugh, D., & Juge, N. (2015). Mucin glycan foraging in the human gut microbiome. Frontiers in Genetics, *6*, 81. https://doi.org/10.3389/fgene.2015.00081
11. Li, H., Limenitakis, J. P., Fuhrer, T., Geuking, M. B., Lawson, M. A., Wyss, M., Brugiroux, S., Keller, I., Macpherson, J. A., Rupp, S., Stolp, B., Stein, J. V., Stecher, B., Sauer, U., McCoy, K. D., & Macpherson, A. J. (2015). The outer mucus layer hosts a distinct intestinal microbial niche. *Nature Communications*, *6*, 8292. https://doi.org/10.1038/ncomms9292
12. Foster, P. L. (2007). Stress-induced mutagenesis in bacteria. Critical Reviews in Biochemistry and Molecular Biology, *42*(5), 373–397. https://doi.org/10.1080/10409230701648494
13. Svanbäck, R., & Bolnick, D. I. (2007). Intraspecific competition drives increased resource use diversity within a natural population. Proceedings. Biological Sciences, 274(1611), 839–844. https://doi.org/10.1098/rspb.2006.0198
14. Emerson, B. C., & Kolm, N. (2005). Species diversity can drive speciation. *Nature*, *434*(7036), 1015–1017. https://doi.org/10.1038/nature03450
15. Kundu, P., Blacher, E., Elinav, E., & Pettersson, S. (2017). Our gut microbiome: The evolving inner self. *Cell*, *171*(7), 1481–1493. https://doi.org/10.1016/j.cell.2017.11.024
16. Eckburg, P. B., Bik, E. M., Bernstein, C. N., Purdom, E., Dethlefsen, L., Sargent, M., Gill, S. R., Nelson, K. E., & Relman, D. A. (2005). Diversity of the human intestinal microbial flora. *Science*, *308*(5728), 1635–1638. https://doi.org/10.1126/science.1110591
17. Lopez-Legarrea, P., Fuller, N. R., Zulet, M. A., Martinez, J. A., & Caterson, I. D. (2014). The influence of Mediterranean, carbohydrate and high protein diets on gut microbiota composition in the treatment of obesity and associated inflammatory state. Asia Pacific Journal of Clinical Nutrition, *23*(3), 360–368. https://doi.org/10.6133/apjcn.2014.23.3.16
18. David, L. A., Maurice, C. F., Carmody, R. N., Gootenberg, D. B., Button, J. E., Wolfe, B. E., Ling, A. V., Devlin, A. S., Varma, Y., Fischbach, M. A., Biddinger, S. B., Dutton, R. J., & Turnbaugh, P. J. (2014). Diet rapidly and reproducibly alters the human gut microbiome. *Nature*, *505*(7484), 559–563. https://doi.org/10.1038/nature12820

19. Kolodziejczyk, A. A., Zheng, D., & Elinav, E. (2019). Diet-microbiota interactions and personalized nutrition. *Nature Reviews. Microbiology*, *17*(12), 742–753. https://doi.org/10.1038/s41579-019-0256-8
20. Zmora, N., Suez, J., & Elinav, E. (2019). You are what you eat: Diet, health and the gut microbiota. *Nature Reviews. Gastroenterology and Hepatology*, *16*(1), 35–56. https://doi.org/10.1038/s41575-018-0061-2
21. Muegge, B. D., Kuczynski, J., Knights, D., Clemente, J. C., González, A., Fontana, L., Henrissat, B., Knight, R., & Gordon, J. I. (2011). Diet drives convergence in gut microbiome functions across mammalian phylogeny and within humans. *Science*, *332*(6032), 970–974. https://doi.org/10.1126/science.1198719
22. Cotillard, A., Kennedy, S. P., Kong, L. C., Prifti, E., Pons, N., Le Chatelier, E., Almeida, M., Quinquis, B., Levenez, F., Galleron, N., Gougis, S., Rizkalla, S., Batto, J. M., Renault, P., ANR MicroObes consortium, Doré, J., Zucker, J. D., Clément, K., & Ehrlich, S. D. (2013). Dietary intervention impact on gut microbial gene richness. *Nature*, *500*(7464), 585–588. https://doi.org/10.1038/nature12480
23. Henke, M. T., Kenny, D. J., Cassilly, C. D., Vlamakis, H., Xavier, R. J., & Clardy, J. (2019). Ruminococcus gnavus, a member of the human gut microbiome associated with Crohn's disease, produces an inflammatory polysaccharide. Proceedings of the National Academy of Sciences of the United States of America, *116*(26), 12672–12677. https://doi.org/10.1073/pnas.1904099116
24. Nowak, A., & Libudzisz, Z. (2006). Influence of phenol, p-cresol and indole on growth and survival of intestinal lactic acid bacteria. *Anaerobe*, *12*(2), 80–84. https://doi.org/10.1016/j.anaerobe.2005.10.003
25. Forbes, J. D., Van Domselaar, G., & Bernstein, C. N. (2016). The gut microbiota in immune-mediated inflammatory diseases. Frontiers in Microbiology, 7, 1081. https://doi.org/10.3389/fmicb.2016.01081
26. Verdam, F. J., Fuentes, S., De Jonge, C., Zoetendal, E. G., Erbil, R., Greve, J. W., Buurman, W. A., De Vos, W. M., & Rensen, S. S. (2013). Human intestinal microbiota composition is associated with local and systemic inflammation in obesity. *Obesity*, *21*(12), E607–E615. https://doi.org/10.1002/oby.20466
27. Ley, R. E., Bäckhed, F., Turnbaugh, P., Lozupone, C. A., Knight, R. D., & Gordon, J. I. (2005). Obesity alters gut microbial ecology. Proceedings of the National Academy of Sciences of the United States of America, *102*(31), 11070–11075. https://doi.org/10.1073/pnas.0504978102
28. Tompkins, G. R., O'Dell, N. L., Bryson, I. T., & Pennington, C. B. (2001). The effects of dietary ferric iron and iron deprivation on the bacterial composition of the mouse intestine. *Current Microbiology*, *43*(1), 38–42. https://doi.org/10.1007/s002840010257
29. Werner, T., Wagner, S. J., Martínez, I., Walter, J., Chang, J. S., Clavel, T., Kisling, S., Schuemann, K., & Haller, D. (2011). Depletion of luminal iron alters the gut microbiota and prevents Crohn's disease-like ileitis. *Gut*, *60*(3), 325–333. https://doi.org/10.1136/gut.2010.216929
30. Dostal, A., Chassard, C., Hilty, F. M., Zimmermann, M. B., Jaeggi, T., Rossi, S., & Lacroix, C. (2012). Iron depletion and repletion with ferrous sulfate or electrolytic iron modifies the composition and metabolic activity of the gut microbiota in rats. *Journal of Nutrition*, *142*(2), 271–277. https://doi.org/10.3945/jn.111.148643
31. De Vadder, F., Kovatcheva-Datchary, P., Goncalves, D., Vinera, J., Zitoun, C., Duchampt, A., Bäckhed, F., & Mithieux, G. (2014). Microbiota-generated metabolites promote metabolic benefits via gut-brain neural circuits. Cell, 156(1–2), 84–96. https://doi.org/10.1016/j.cell.2013.12.016
32. Tan, J., McKenzie, C., Potamitis, M., Thorburn, A. N., Mackay, C. R., & Macia, L. (2014). The role of short-chain fatty acids in health and disease. *Advances* in Immunology, 121, 91–119. https://doi.org/10.1016/B978-0-12-800100-4.00003-9
33. Sandhu, K. V., Sherwin, E., Schellekens, H., Stanton, C., Dinan, T. G., & Cryan, J. F. (2017). Feeding the microbiota-gut-brain axis: Diet, microbiome, and neuropsychiatry. Translational Research: The Journal of Laboratory and Clinical Medicine, *179*, 223–244. https://doi.org/10.1016/j.trsl.2016.10.002
34. Sonnenburg, J. L., & Bäckhed, F. (2016). Diet-microbiota interactions as moderators of human metabolism. *Nature*, *535*(7610), 56–64. https://doi.org/10.1038/nature18846
35. Suez, J., Korem, T., Zeevi, D., Zilberman-Schapira, G., Thaiss, C. A., Maza, O., Israeli, D., Zmora, N., Gilad, S., Weinberger, A., Kuperman, Y., Harmelin, A., Kolodkin-Gal, I., Shapiro, H., Halpern, Z., Segal, E., & Elinav, E. (2014). Artificial sweeteners induce glucose intolerance by altering the gut microbiota. *Nature*, *514*(7521), 181–186. https://doi.org/10.1038/nature13793
36. Conlon, M. A., & Bird, A. R. (2014). The impact of diet and lifestyle on gut microbiota and human health. *Nutrients*, *7*(1), 17–44. https://doi.org/10.3390/nu7010017
37. Koh, A., De Vadder, F., Kovatcheva-Datchary, P., & Bäckhed, F. (2016). From dietary fiber to host physiology: Short-chain fatty acids as key bacterial metabolites. *Cell*, *165*(6), 1332–1345. https://doi.org/10.1016/j.cell.2016.05.041
38. Yang, Z., & Liao, S. F. (2019). Physiological effects of dietary amino acids on gut health and functions of swine. Frontiers in Veterinary Science, 6, 169. https://doi.org/10.3389/fvets.2019.00169
39. Alves, A., Bassot, A., Bulteau, A. L., Pirola, L., & Morio, B. (2019). Glycine metabolism and its alterations in obesity and metabolic diseases. Nutrients, 11(6). https://doi.org/10.3390/nu11061356
40. Caesar, R., Tremaroli, V., Kovatcheva-Datchary, P., Cani, P. D., & Bäckhed, F. (2015). Crosstalk between gut microbiota and dietary lipids aggravates WAT inflammation through TLR signaling. *Cell Metabolism*, *22*(4), 658–668. https://doi.org/10.1016/j.cmet.2015.07.026
41. Mani, V., Hollis, J. H., & Gabler, N. K. (2013). Dietary oil composition differentially modulates intestinal endotoxin transport and postprandial endotoxemia. Nutrition and Metabolism, 10(1), 6. https://doi.org/10.1186/1743-7075-10-6
42. Bailey, M. A., & Holscher, H. D. (2018). Microbiome-mediated effects of the Mediterranean diet on inflammation. Advances in Nutrition, *9*(3), 193–206. https://doi.org/10.1093/advances/nmy013
43. Bercik, P., Collins, S. M., & Verdu, E. F. (2012). Microbes and the gut-brain axis. *Neurogastroenterology and Motility*, *24*(5), 405–413. https://doi.wiley.com/10.1111/j.1365-2982.2012.01906.x. https://doi.org/10.1111/j.1365-2982.2012.01906.x
44. Bonaz, B., Bazin, T., & Pellissier, S. (2018). The vagus nerve at the interface of the microbiota-gut-brain axis. Frontiers in Neuroscience, 12, 49. https://doi.org/10.3389/fnins.2018.00049

45. Allen, A. P., Dinan, T. G., Clarke, G., & Cryan, J. F. (2017). A psychology of the human brain-gut-microbiome axis. Social and Personality Psychology Compass, 11(4), e12309. https://doi.org/10.1111/spc3.12309
46. Mayer, E. A., Savidge, T., & Shulman, R. J. (2014). Brain-gut microbiome interactions and functional bowel disorders. *Gastroenterology*, *146*(6), 1500–1512. https://doi.org/10.1053/j.gastro.2014.02.037
47. Santos, J., Saperas, E., Nogueiras, C., Mourelle, M., Antolín, M., Cadahia, A., & Malagelada, J. R. (1998). Release of mast cell mediators into the jejunum by cold pain stress in humans. *Gastroenterology*, *114*(4), 640–648. https://doi.org/10.1016/S0016-5085(98)70577-3
48. Erny, D., & Prinz, M. (2020). How microbiota shape microglial phenotypes and epigenetics. *Glia*, *68*(8), 1655–1672. https://doi.org/10.1002/glia.23822
49. Szőke, H., Kovács, Z., Bókkon, I., Vagedes, J., Szabó, A. E., Hegyi, G., Sterner, M. G., Kiss, Á., & Kapócs, G. (2020). Gut dysbiosis and serotonin: Intestinal 5-HT as a ubiquitous membrane permeability regulator in host tissues, organs, and the brain. Reviews in the Neurosciences, *31*(4), 415–425. https://doi.org/10.1515/revneuro-2019-0095
50. Wehrwein, E. A., Orer, H. S., & Barman, S. M. (2016). Overview of the anatomy, physiology, and pharmacology of the autonomic nervous system. *Comprehensive Physiology*, *6*(3), 1239–1278. https://doi.org/10.1002/CPHY.C150037
51. Perez-Burgos, A., Mao, Y. K., Bienenstock, J., & Kunze, W. A. (2014). The gut-brain axis rewired: Adding a functional vagal nicotinic "sensory synapse." *FASEB Journal*, *28*(7), 3064–3074. https://doi.org/10.1096/fj.13-245282
52. Yarullina, D. R., Mikheeva, R. O., Sabirullina, G. I., Zelenikhin, P. V., Ilinskaya, O. N., & Sitdikova, G. F. (2016). Role of nitric oxide produced by lactobacilli in relaxation of intestinal smooth muscles. Bulletin of Experimental Biology and Medicine, *160*(3), 343–346. https://doi.org/10.1007/s10517-016-3166-z
53. Fung, T. C., Olson, C. A., & Hsiao, E. Y. (2017). Interactions between the microbiota, immune and nervous systems in health and disease. *Nature Neuroscience*, *20*(2), 145–155. https://doi.org/10.1038/nn.4476
54. Silva, Y. P., Bernardi, A., & Frozza, R. L. (2020). The role of short-chain fatty acids from gut microbiota in gut-brain communication. Frontiers in Endocrinology *(*Lausanne*)*, 11, 25. https://doi.org/10.3389/fendo.2020.00025
55. Canfora, E. E., Meex, R. C. R., Venema, K., & Blaak, E. E. (2019). Gut microbial metabolites in obesity, NAFLD and T2DM. *Nature Reviews. Endocrinology*, *15*(5), 261–273. https://doi.org/10.1038/s41574-019-0156-z
56. Torres-Fuentes, C., Schellekens, H., Dinan, T. G., & Cryan, J. F. (2017). The microbiota-gut-brain axis in obesity. *Lancet. Gastroenterology and Hepatology*, *2*(10), 747–756. https://doi.org/10.1016/S2468-1253(17)30147-4
57. Tuohy, K. M., Venuti, P., Cuva, S., Furlanello, C., Gasperotti, M., Mancini, A., Ceppa, F., Cavalieri, D., de Filippo, C., Vrhovsek, U., Mena, P., Del Rio, D., & Fava, F. (2014). Diet and the gut microbiota - How the gut: Brain axis impacts on autism. Diet-Microbe Interactions *in the* Gut Effects *on* Hum*an* Health *and* Disease. https://doi.org/10.1016/B978-0-12-407825-3.00015-0
58. Shapiro, H., Suez, J., & Elinav, E. (2017). Personalized microbiome-based approaches to metabolic syndrome management and prevention. *Journal of Diabetes*, *9*(3), 226–236. https://doi.org/10.1111/1753-0407.12501
59. Guarino, M. P. L., Altomare, A., Emerenziani, S., Di Rosa, C., Ribolsi, M., Balestrieri, P., Iovino, P., Rocchi, G., & Cicala, M. (2020). Mechanisms of action of prebiotics and their effects on gastro-intestinal disorders in adults. Nutrients, 12(4). https://doi.org/10.3390/nu12041037
60. Markowiak, P., & Ślizewska, K. (2017). Effects of probiotics, prebiotics, and Synbiotics on human health. Nutrients, 9(9). https://doi.org/10.3390/nu9091021
61. Borghi, E., & Vignoli, A. (2019). Rett syndrome and other neurodevelopmental disorders share common changes in gut microbial community: A descriptive review. International Journal of Molecular Sciences, 20(17). https://doi.org/10.3390/ijms20174160
62. Gómez-Eguílaz, M., Ramón-Trapero, J. L., Pérez-Martínez, L., & Blanco, J. R. (2018). The beneficial effect of probiotics as a supplementary treatment in drug-resistant epilepsy: A pilot study. *Beneficial Microbes*, *9*(6), 875–881. https://doi.org/10.3920/BM2018.0018
63. Miraghajani, M., Zaghian, N., Dehkohneh, A., Mirlohi, M., & Ghiasvand, R. (2019). Probiotic soy milk consumption and renal function among type 2 diabetic patients with nephropathy: A randomized controlled clinical trial. Probiotics and Antimicrobial Proteins, *11*(1), 124–132. https://doi.org/10.1007/s12602-017-9325-3
64. Huang, C. H., Ho, C. Y., Chen, C. T., Hsu, H. F., & Lin, Y. H. (2019). Probiotic BSH activity and anti-obesity potential of lactobacillus plantarum strain TCI378 isolated from Korean Kimchi. Preventive Nutrition and Food Science, *24*(4), 434–441. https://doi.org/10.3746/pnf.2019.24.4.434
65. Turnbaugh, P. J., Hamady, M., Yatsunenko, T., Cantarel, B. L., Duncan, A., Ley, R. E., Sogin, M. L., Jones, W. J., Roe, B. A., Affourtit, J. P., Egholm, M., Henrissat, B., Heath, A. C., Knight, R., & Gordon, J. I. (2009). A core gut microbiome in obese and lean twins. *Nature*, *457*(7228), 480–484. https://doi.org/10.1038/nature07540
66. Green, M., Arora, K., & Prakash, S. (2020). Microbial medicine: Prebiotic and probiotic functional foods to target obesity and metabolic syndrome. International Journal of Molecular Sciences, 21(8). https://doi.org/10.3390/ijms21082890
67. Krga, I., & Glibetic, M. (2022). 2.16 Gut microbiota in health and diseases. *Comprehensive. Gut Microbiota*. https://doi.org/10.1016/B978-0-12-819265-8.00045-0
68. MacLeod, E. L., & Ney, D. M. (2010). Nutritional management of phenylketonuria. Annales Nestle [English Ed.], *68*(2), 58–69. https://doi.org/10.1159/000312813
69. Skonieczna-Żydecka, K., Grochans, E., Maciejewska, D., Szkup, M., Schneider-Matyka, D., Jurczak, A., Łoniewski, I., Kaczmarczyk, M., Marlicz, W., Czerwińska-Rogowska, M., Pełka-Wysiecka, J., Dec, K., & Stachowska, E. (2018). Faecal short chain fatty acids profile is changed in polish depressive women. Nutrients, 10(12). https://doi.org/10.3390/nu10121939
70. Thompson, A. J., Smith, I., Brenton, D., Youl, B. D., Rylance, G., Davidson, D. C., Kendall, B., & Lees, A. J. (1990). Neurological deterioration in young adults with phenylketonuria. *Lancet*, *336*(8715), 602–605. https://doi.org/10.1016/0140-6736(90)93401-A
71. Rubin, S., Piffer, A. L. L., Rougier, M. B., Delyfer, M. N., Korobelnik, J. F., Redonnet-Vernhet, I., Marchal, C., Goizet, C., Mesli, S., Gonzalez, C., Gin, H., & Rigalleau, V. (2013). Sight-threatening phenylketonuric encephalopathy in a young adult, reversed by diet. JIMD Reports, 10, 83–85. https://doi.org/10.1007/8904_2012_207

72. Jaulent, P., Charriere, S., Feillet, F., Douillard, C., Fouilhoux, A., & Thobois, S. (2020). Neurological manifestations in adults with phenylketonuria: New cases and review of the literature. *Journal of Neurology*, *267*(2), 531–542. https://doi.org/10.1007/s00415-019-09608-2
73. Kornguth, S., Gilbert-Barness, E., Langer, E., & Hegstrand, L. (1992). Golgi-Kopsch silver study of the brain of a patient with untreated phenylketonuria, seizures, and cortical blindness. American Journal of Medical Genetics, *44*(4), 443–448. https://doi.org/10.1002/ajmg.1320440412
74. Leuzzi, V., Rinalduzzi, S., Chiarotti, F., Garzia, P., Trasimeni, G., & Accornero, N. (1998). Subclinical visual impairment in phenylketonuria. A neurophysiological study (VEP-P) with clinical, biochemical, and neuroradiological (MRI) correlations. Journal of Inherited Metabolic Disease, *21*(4), 351–364. https://doi.org/10.1023/A:1005346422918
75. MacDonald, A., van Wegberg, A. M. J., Ahring, K., Beblo, S., Bélanger-Quintana, A., Burlina, A., Campistol, J., Coşkun, T., Feillet, F., Giżewska, M., Huijbregts, S. C., Leuzzi, V., Maillot, F., Muntau, A. C., Rocha, J. C., Romani, C., Trefz, F., & van Spronsen, F. J. (2020). PKU dietary handbook to accompany PKU guidelines. Orphanet Journal of Rare Diseases, 15(1). https://doi.org/10.1186/s13023-020-01391-y
76. Rocha, J. C., & MacDonald, A. (2016). Dietary intervention in the management of phenylketonuria: Current perspectives. Pediatric Health, Medicine and Therapeutics, *7*, 155–163. https://doi.org/10.2147/PHMT.S49329
77. Ferreira, C. R., van Karnebeek, C. D. M., Vockley, J., & Blau, N. (2019). A proposed nosology of inborn errors of metabolism. Genetics in Medicine, *21*(1), 102–106. https://doi.org/10.1038/s41436-018-0022-8
78. Boyer, S. W., Barclay, L. J., & Burrage, L. C. (2015). Inherited metabolic disorders: Aspects of chronic nutrition management. Nutrition in Clinical Practice, *30*(4), 502–510. https://doi.org/10.1177/0884533615586201
79. Sahoo, S., Franzson, L., Jonsson, J. J., & Thiele, I. (2012). A compendium of inborn errors of metabolism mapped onto the human metabolic network. *Molecular Biosystems*, *8*(10), 2545–2558. https://doi.org/10.1039/c2mb25075f
80. Montagner, A., Korecka, A., Polizzi, A., Lippi, Y., Blum, Y., Canlet, C., Tremblay-Franco, M., Gautier-Stein, A., Burcelin, R., Yen, Y. C., Je, H. S., Al-Asmakh, M., Mithieux, G., Arulampalam, V., Lagarrigue, S., Guillou, H., Pettersson, S., & Wahli, W. (2016). Hepatic circadian clock oscillators and nuclear receptors integrate microbiome-derived signals. Scientific Reports, 6, 20127. https://doi.org/10.1038/srep20127
81. Sampson, T. R., Debelius, J. W., Thron, T., Janssen, S., Shastri, G. G., Ilhan, Z. E., Challis, C., Schretter, C. E., Rocha, S., Gradinaru, V., Chesselet, M. F., Keshavarzian, A., Shannon, K. M., Krajmalnik-Brown, R., Wittung-Stafshede, P., Knight, R., & Mazmanian, S. K. (2016). Gut microbiota regulate motor deficits and neuroinflammation in a model of Parkinson's disease. *Cell*, *167*(6), 1469–1480.e12. https://doi.org/10.1016/j.cell.2016.11.018
82. Steenbergen, L., Sellaro, R., van Hemert, S., Bosch, J. A., & Colzato, L. S. (2015). A randomized controlled trial to test the effect of multispecies probiotics on cognitive reactivity to sad mood. *Brain, Behavior, and Immunity*, *48*, 258–264. https://doi.org/10.1016/j.bbi.2015.04.003
83. Chevalier, C., Stojanović, O., Colin, D. J., Suarez-Zamorano, N., Tarallo, V., Veyrat-Durebex, C., Rigo, D., Fabbiano, S., Stevanović, A., Hagemann, S., Montet, X., Seimbille, Y., Zamboni, N., Hapfelmeier, S., & Trajkovski, M. (2015). Gut microbiota orchestrates energy homeostasis during cold. *Cell*, *163*(6), 1360–1374. https://doi.org/10.1016/j.cell.2015.11.004
84. Sawin, E. A., De Wolfe, T. J., Aktas, B., Stroup, B. M., Murali, S. G., Steele, J. L., & Ney, D. M. (2015). Glycomacropeptide is a prebiotic that reduces Desulfovibrio bacteria, increases cecal short-chain fatty acids, and is anti-inflammatory in mice. *American Journal of Physiology. Gastrointestinal and Liver Physiology*, *309*(7), G590–G601. https://doi.org/10.1152/ajpgi.00211.2015
85. Belik, J., Shifrin, Y., Arning, E., Bottiglieri, T., Pan, J., Daigneault, M. C., & Allen-Vercoe, E. (2017). Intestinal microbiota as a tetrahydrobiopterin exogenous source in hph-1 mice. *Scientific Reports*, *7*, 39854. https://doi.org/10.1038/srep39854
86. Ntemiri, A., Chonchúir, F. N., O'Callaghan, T. F., Stanton, C., Ross, R. P., & O'Toole, P. W. (2017). Glycomacropeptide sustains microbiota diversity and promotes specific taxa in an artificial colon model of elderly gut microbiota. Journal of Agricultural and Food Chemistry, 65(8), 1836–1846. https://doi.org/10.1021/acs.jafc.6b05434
87. Durrer, K. E., Allen, M. S., & Hunt von Herbing, I. H. (2017). Genetically engineered probiotic for the treatment of phenylketonuria (PKU); Assessment of a novel treatment in vitro and in the PAHenu2 mouse model of PKU. PLOS ONE, 12(5), e0176286. https://doi.org/10.1371/journal.pone.0176286
88. Isabella, V. M., Ha, B. N., Castillo, M. J., Lubkowicz, D. J., Rowe, S. E., Millet, Y. A., Anderson, C. L., Li, N., Fisher, A. B., West, K. A., Reeder, P. J., Momin, M. M., Bergeron, C. G., Guilmain, S. E., Miller, P. F., Kurtz, C. B., & Falb, D. (2018). Development of a synthetic live bacterial therapeutic for the human metabolic disease phenylketonuria. *Nature Biotechnology*, *36*(9), 857–864. https://doi.org/10.1038/nbt.4222
89. Crook, N., Ferreiro, A., Gasparrini, A. J., Pesesky, M. W., Gibson, M. K., Wang, B., Sun, X., Condiotte, Z., Dobrowolski, S., Peterson, D., & Dantas, G. (2019). Adaptive strategies of the candidate probiotic E. coli Nissle in the mammalian gut. Cell Host and Microbe, *25*(4), 499–512.e8. https://doi.org/10.1016/j.chom.2019.02.005
90. MacDonald, A., Cochrane, B., Wopereis, H., & Loveridge, N. (2011). Specific prebiotics in a formula for infants with phenylketonuria. Molecular Genetics and Metabolism, 104 *Suppl.*, S55–S59. https://doi.org/10.1016/j.ymgme.2011.09.015
91. Pinheiro de Oliveira, F. P., Mendes, R. H., Dobbler, P. T., Mai, V., Pylro, V. S., Waugh, S. G., Vairo, F., Refosco, L. F., Roesch, L. F. W., & Schwartz, I. V. D. (2016). Phenylketonuria and gut microbiota: A controlled study based on next-generation sequencing. PLOS ONE, 11(6), e0157513. https://doi.org/10.1371/journal.pone.0157513
92. Deon, M., Sitta, A., Faverzani, J. L., Guerreiro, G. B., Donida, B., Marchetti, D. P., Mescka, C. P., Ribas, G. S., Coitinho, A. S., Wajner, M., & Vargas, C. R. (2015). Urinary biomarkers of oxidative stress and plasmatic inflammatory profile in phenylketonuric treated patients. International Journal of Developmental Neuroscience, *47*(B), 259–265. https://doi.org/10.1016/j.ijdevneu.2015.10.001
93. Daly, A., Evans, S., Chahal, S., Santra, S., & MacDonald, A. (2017). Glycomacropeptide in children with phenylketonuria: Does its phenylalanine content affect blood phenylalanine control? Journal of Human Nutrition and Dietetics, *30*(4), 515–523. https://doi.org/10.1111/jhn.12438

94. Ney, D. M., Murali, S. G., Stroup, B. M., Nair, N., Sawin, E. A., Rohr, F., & Levy, H. L. (2017). Metabolomic changes demonstrate reduced bioavailability of tyrosine and altered metabolism of tryptophan via the kynurenine pathway with ingestion of medical foods in phenylketonuria. Molecular Genetics and Metabolism, *121*(2), 96–103. https://doi.org/10.1016/j.ymgme.2017.04.003
95. Stroup, B. M., Nair, N., Murali, S. G., Broniowska, K., Rohr, F., Levy, H. L., & Ney, D. M. (2018). Metabolomic markers of essential fatty acids, carnitine, and cholesterol metabolism in adults and adolescents with phenylketonuria. *Journal of Nutrition*, *148*(2), 194–201. https://doi.org/10.1093/jn/nxx039
96. Verduci, E., Moretti, F., Bassanini, G., Banderali, G., Rovelli, V., Casiraghi, M. C., Morace, G., Borgo, F., & Borghi, E. (2018). Phenylketonuric diet negatively impacts on butyrate production. Nutrition, Metabolism, and Cardiovascular Diseases, *28*(4), 385–392. https://doi.org/10.1016/j.numecd.2018.01.004
97. Bassanini, G., Ceccarani, C., Borgo, F., Severgnini, M., Rovelli, V., Morace, G., Verduci, E., & Borghi, E. (2019). Phenylketonuria diet promotes shifts in Firmicutes populations. Frontiers in Cellular and Infection Microbiology, 9, 101. https://doi.org/10.3389/fcimb.2019.00101

9 Synbiotic
Potential Role in Hemochromatosis Management

Monika Kaushik, Himanshu Sharma, Prathap Madeswaraguptha, Venishaa S., Murugesan, and Vananga Mudi

9.1 INTRODUCTION

9.1.1 SYNBIOTICS

Nutrition today does more than provide the body with essential nutrients to grow and thrive. These duties include health and illness prevention. Food safety and content are prioritized in highly processed food. Today's main health issues include food poisoning, obesity, allergies, cardiovascular disease, and cancer, so food quality is vital. Scientific research suggests probiotics, prebiotics, and synbiotics promote health. Medications and functional meals are options. The Greek word "probiotic" means "for life". Probiotics are the living strains of entirely chosen microbes that, when given in sufficient quantities, benefit the host (Markowiak et al. 2017).

To supplement probiotics, prebiotics can be used for health benefits, numerous research has shown. A blend of prebiotics and probiotics that function together is called "synbiotic" (Gibson et al. 2004). Since "synbiotic" implies synergy, it should only be used for goods where a prebiotic component favorably selects a probiotic bacteria (Markowiak et al. 2017).

Here we present a model for hepatocyte's HFE-mediated hepcidin signaling pathway. (a) HFE is bound to TfR1 and other proteins linked to hepcidin remain silent at low plasma iron levels; (b) HFE is displaced from TfR1 and iron absorption occurs as plasma iron levels rise. HFE, TfR2, BMPs (such as BMP-2, BMP-4, and BMP-9) and their receptor BMPR form a putative 'iron-sensing' complex, which activates hepcidin transcription via Smad proteins. Cellular and systemic signals regulate iron metabolism in the hepatocyte (Pantopoulos, 2008).

Synbiotics are beneficial when prebiotics and probiotics work together to achieve their intended purpose (Figure 9.1 and Table 9.1). Although there has been a recent increase in teeth cleanliness, prebiotics, and probiotics have long been linked to improved gut and tooth health. The purpose of synbiotics is to increase probiotic survival in microhabitats like the mouth. Probiotic viability during upper gastrointestinal tract transit may be enhanced by synbiotics. Intestinal balance and health are maintained by colon implantation made possible by probiotics, common bacteria, and their stimulating actions (Markowiak et al. 2017). By stopping infections like Streptococcus mutans and Candida spp. from colonizing the mouth, synbiotics may also help preserve the oral microbiota (Johnston et al. 2006).

Some of the positive benefits that synbiotics have on people are as follows (Zhang et al. 2010):

1. Enhanced Lactobacillus and Bifidobacterium genus count and maintained intestinal microbiota balance
2. Improved cirrhosis hepatic function
3. Improved immunomodulation
4. Reduced nosocomial infections in post-surgical procedures and interventions.

Translocation brings LPSs, ethanol, and SFCAs from bacteria to the liver. SCFs boost hepatic triacylglycerol production and storage. Detoxicating the liver may increase IHTG storage and steatosis. A synbiotic with five probiotics (L. plantarum, L. delbrueckii spp. bulgaricus, L. acidophilus, *L. rhamnosus*, and B. bifidum) and insulin as a prebiotic decreased IHTG in NASH adults within 6 months. LPSs cause insulin resistance and inflammatory cell uptake in NAFLD by inducing proinflammatory cytokines like TNF-α (Markowiak et al. 2017). A synbiotic product with a blend of probiotics (L. casei, L. rhamnosus, S. thermophilus, B. breve, B. acidophilus, B. longum, and L. bulgaricus) and fructooligosacc showed suppression of NF-κB and lower TNF-α production in 52 adults. L. rhamnosus, B. lactis, inulin, and oligofructose prebiotics enhanced rats' intestinal IgA. Synbiotics lower cholesterol and blood pressure (Socha et al. 2002). Synbiotics increase calcium, magnesium, and phosphorus absorption, improving liver function (Pérez-Conesa et al. 2006). Danq et al.'s (2013) meta-analysis examined pro/prebiotics/synbiotics for eczema prevention, including bacterial strain efficacy and allergy status changes in children. The probiotic did not affect systemic sensitization (Dan et al. 2013). SYN1, L. rhamnosus GG, and B. animalis subsp. lactis Bb12 were studied on colorectal cancer patients (Markowiak et al. 2017).

DOI: 10.1201/9781032702438-9

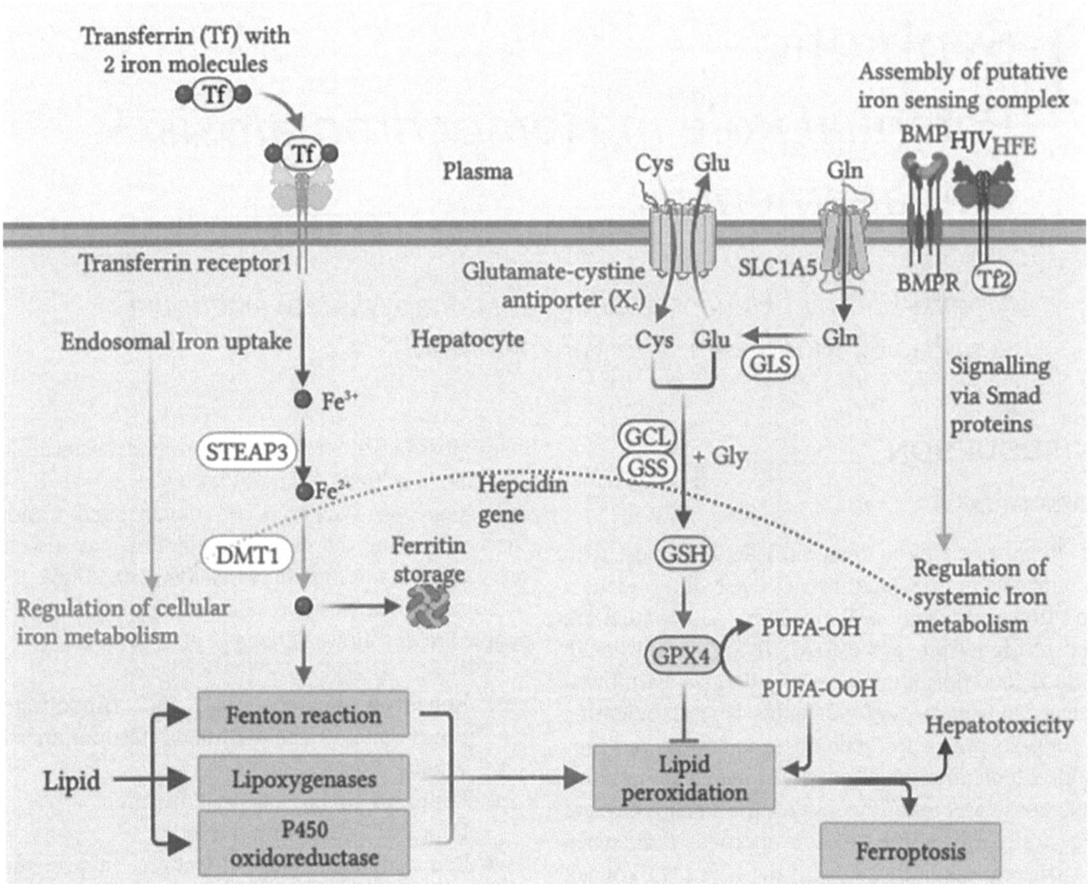

FIGURE 9.1 Modulation of iron levels by hepcidin.

9.1.2 Hemochromatosis

The inherited condition known as hereditary hemochromatosis is characterized by an autosomal recessive inheritance pattern. This condition is characterized by a lack in hepcidin, which is a protein that regulates iron balance. Controlling the amount of iron that is absorbed by the digestive tract is the primary mechanism that regulates what the body stores. In addition to menstruation and the shedding of senescent cells, there are no other physiological mechanisms that are responsible for the outflow of iron. When an excessive amount of iron is deposited into parenchymal cells, it causes damage to the tissues there and ultimately leads to organ failure. Among the organs that are most frequently affected, the liver, pancreas, joints, heart, skin, and pituitary glands are the most frequently affected. The aim of this chapter is to discuss the causes of hereditary hemochromatosis and other kinds of iron overload, as well as their diagnostic and therapeutic implications using synbiotics (Kane et al. 2021).

9.2 SELECTION CRITERIA FOR SYNBIOTICS

Hemochromatosis, a hereditary condition that causes iron excess, offers a complicated issue for healthcare providers. While phlebotomy remains the core of treatment, new study shows that synbiotics, a mix of probiotics and prebiotics, may give extra benefits in treating hemochromatosis. Yet, not all synbiotics are made comparable, and thorough research is required to enhance efficacy while minimizing possible hazards. The topic covers critical criteria for selecting synbiotics for hemochromatosis treatment, with the goal of informing healthcare practitioners and supporting optimum patient care. The human gut microbiome is critical for iron homeostasis. As a result, while selecting synbiotics for hemochromatosis therapy, the influence on the gut microbiota composition ought to be considered. Lactobacillus and Bifidobacterium strains with shown ability to modify iron absorption should be picked. Additionally, synbiotics formulations should include prebiotics that preferentially encourage the development of beneficial bacteria involved in iron metabolism (Zakrzewska et al. 2022).

Choose synbiotics comprising human-derived or clinically proven strains with a high safety profile in iron overload circumstances. Avoid innovative or experimental strains with minimal safety data. Some prebiotics, such as galactooligosaccharides (GOS), can produce bloating or gas. Consider synbiotics that contain prebiotics that have been shown to be well tolerated by patients with iron excess, such as inulin or fructo-oligosaccharides (FOS) (Markowiak and Śliżewska 2017). The recommended synbiotics should have a good safety profile, particularly

TABLE 9.1
Synbiotics and their Impact on Human Health

Mouth Flora Diversity	Synbiotic Make-Up	Positive Aspects	Major Impacts	References
Synbiotics	S. boulardii, B. lactis, and Bacillus plantarum. Kefir, kimchi, sauerkraut, and yogurt	Prevent hemochromatosis and reduce the body's sorption of iron	With the use of probiotics and dietary changes, like consuming more fiber and reducing iron-rich meals	Botta et al. (2021)
Synbiotics	Arabinose, xylose, and xylitol Lactobacillus species, L. fermentum, L. plantarum, and L. paracasei Lactobacilli spp.	Biofilm-breaking and antimicrobial properties against cancer-causing microorganisms	Minimize P. gingivalis, S. mutans, and Candida albicans biofilm development Rich supply of bacteriocin, a bacteriostatic factor	Fuad et al. (2022)
Synbiotics	L. casei, L. rhamnosus, S. thermophilus, B. breve, B. longum, FOS, L. plantarum, L. delbrueckii spp. bulgaricus, L. acidophilus, inulin	Illness of the non-alcoholic fatty liver	Reduction in IHTG content. TNF-α decrease and NF-κB inhibition	Markowiak et al. (2017)
Synbiotics	Psyllium, B. longum	Gastrointestinal issues	Receiving probiotic or prebiotic therapy, compared to patients with UC receiving synbiotic therapy saw larger improvements in their quality of life.	Markowiak et al. (2017)
Synbiotics	B. lactis Bb12, L. rhamnosus GG, and inulin	Many forms of cancer	Increased fecal L. rhamnosus and B. lactis, decreased C. perfringens, inhibits polypectomized patients' increased IL-2 secretion, and protects cancer patient's increased interferon-γ production	Markowiak et al. (2017)
Synbiotics	CGMCC1.3,724, L. rhamnosus, inulin	Obesity	Leptin levels drop along with weight loss, but Lachnospiraceae levels rise	Markowiak et al. (2017)
Synbiotics	L. bulgaricus, B. breve, L. acidophilus, B. longum, L. casei, L. rhamnosus, S. thermophilus, and FOS	Syndrome of insulin resistance	Insulin resistance and fasting blood sugar levels both markedly improved	Markowiak et al. (2017)
Synbiotics	S. thermophilus, FOS, B. breve, B. longum, L. acidophilus, L. casei, L. rhamnosus, L. bulgaricus, and S. thermophilus	Type 2 diabetes	Elevated TGL and HOMA-IR plasma levels; decreased serum CRP levels	Markowiak et al. (2017)

for persons with hemochromatosis who may already have poor health owing to iron overload. The lack of unwanted effects, allergic reactions, or combinations with existing drugs should be rigorously evaluated. Any possible dangers connected with the use of synbiotics must be balanced by their demonstrable advantages in the management of hemochromatosis. Iron levels should be checked regularly while using synbiotics. While synbiotics may be beneficial, they should not be used in place of phlebotomy or other proven iron-reduction techniques. When choosing a synbiotic, consider unique patient considerations such as age, comorbidities, and eating preferences. Consult a healthcare expert for specific advice. Keep up to speed on the latest synbiotics and hemochromatosis research. The area is continually changing, and new discoveries may influence subsequent selection requirements. Synbiotics are used in hemochromatosis treatment to rebalance the microbial environment of the stomach. This not only promotes microbial balance but also increases the synthesis of beneficial short-chain fatty acids, resulting in a better gut environment and less inflammation. Despite the chronic nature of hemochromatosis, the long-term effects of synbiotic usage on iron metabolism should be carefully explored. Constant tracking of blood levels of iron, inflammatory indicators, and gut microbiota composition will give an understanding of the long-term influence of synbiotics on the general health of people with hemochromatosis (Osterholm and Georgieff 2015).

9.3 RESEARCH AND CLINICAL EVIDENCE

Probiotics are living bacteria and yeasts that provide a variety of health advantages when ingested on a regular basis. These "good" bacteria live predominantly in the gut, where they aid in digestion and immunological function. Certain probiotic strains have been demonstrated in studies to have an anti-inflammatory impact on the body, which can assist to alleviate Hemochromatosis symptoms. Probiotics were discovered to play a function in regulating iron levels in the body, in addition to anti-inflammatory qualities. Hemochromatosis is a disorder characterized by excessive iron buildup in the body, which can cause organ damage and other issues (Huo et al. 2022). According to research, probiotics may assist to reduce iron absorption in the stomach, decreasing total iron levels in the body and perhaps improving results for those with Hemochromatosis (Seyoum, Baye, and Humblot 2021).

Although there are a lot of various types of probiotics on the market, not all of them are made equal when it comes of their efficiency in controlling Hemochromatosis conditions. Lactobacillus plantarum, Bifidobacterium lactis, and Saccharomyces boulardii are among the most efficient probiotic strains for Hemochromatosis.

Probiotics have been demonstrated in studies to help reduce iron absorption in the body, which is useful for those with hemochromatosis. In addition to probiotics, dietary adjustments such as limiting iron-rich meals and boosting fiber intake might help control discomfort (Hoppe et al. 2015). It is quite simple to incorporate probiotics into your Hemochromatosis therapy strategy. Begin by including probiotic-rich foods in your diet, such as yogurt, kefir, sauerkraut, and kimchi. You may also benefit from taking a high-quality probiotic supplement on a daily basis, as suggested by the doctor. It's critical to carefully follow the dose directions and to give your body time to react to the new probiotic routine. Both probiotic pills and fermented foods can help with Hemochromatosis symptoms. Probiotic supplements, on the other hand, may be more convenient and contain a larger concentration of helpful bacteria than fermented meals (https://casadesante.com/blogs/probiotics/best-probiotic-for-hemochromatosis). Furthermore, some people may find fermented foods difficult to tolerate due to their strong taste or texture.

Hemochromatosis upsets the delicate balance of gut microorganisms, which can result in inflammation and decreased iron absorption control. Probiotics promote helpful strains, restoring microbial balance and generating an environment that is less conductive to iron absorption (You et al. 2022).

Fermented foods, on the other hand, contain a greater diversity of helpful bacteria types than probiotic pills. This diversity of bacteria can assist enhance gut health and stimulate the immune system, which is especially significant for Hemochromatosis patients. Fermented foods also include elements such as vitamins and minerals that probiotic pills do not. Probiotics ferment dietary fiber, resulting in the formation of beneficial SCFAs. These fatty acids improve gut health by lowering inflammation, increasing nutrient absorption, and fortifying the gut barrier. SCFAs may also have a role in hemochromatosis by potentially altering iron transport inside the body, targeting reserves that are inaccessible by phlebotomy (Markowiak-Kopeć and Śliżewska 2020). Hemochromatosis is frequently associated with comorbidities such as liver disease and diabetes. Probiotics may help manage these illnesses by moderating intestinal inflammation and boosting metabolic health, according to research. This might increase general well-being and possibly lower the chance of problems. It is critical to select the correct probiotic strain. Prioritize strains with demonstrated iron-binding and gut-modulating capabilities that are appropriate for people with iron excess. Probiotics have intriguing promise in the treatment of hemochromatosis (Santa et al. 2023). These microorganisms provide a new frontier in optimizing iron management and enhancing general well-being for persons with this complex illness, from lowering iron absorption to altering the gut flora and controlling comorbidities. While more study is needed, continued advances in the area hold out hope for a future in which probiotics become a vital weapon in the battle against iron overload, providing hope for a better future for people plagued by Hemochromatosis.

9.4 MECHANISM OF ACTION OF SYNBIOTICS

Given that prebiotics mostly exert their effects in the large intestine and probiotics primarily function in both the small and large intestines, it is reasonable to assume that the two may work together synergistically (Markowiak et al. 2017). Intestinal transit, fermentation, and the formation of probiotic strains are the primary uses of prebiotics. Probiotic microbes may develop a greater tolerance to oxygenation, pH, and temperature in the colon of a specific organism when prebiotics are used, according to some research (Sekhon et al. 2010). Tolerance to these conditions can be increased by using an additional energy source, but the exact mechanism by which this works remains unclear. In the right setting, that mix of ingredients can have a beneficial effect on the host's health, and the result is microbiological dietary supplements that really work (Markowiak et al. 2017) (Figure 9.2).

The two modes of action that are known to be associated with synbiotics are as follows:

1. Action through the enhancement of the viability of probiotic microorganisms;
2. Action through the provision of certain health effects.

Intestinal metabolic activity is modulated, beneficial bacteria are developed, and potential gastrointestinal tract infections are inhibited when prebiotics are used to stimulate probiotics. This leads to the preservation of intestinal biostructure. By destroying harmful molecules including nitrosamines and cancer-causing compounds, synbiotics lower amounts of unwanted metabolites. The usage of these compounds raises concentrations of some compounds that may have beneficial effects on the host's health, including carbon disulfides, methyl acetates, short-chain fatty acids, and ketones (Manigandan et al. 2012).

Antibacterial, anticancerogenic, and anti-allergic actions are among the desirable qualities of synbiotics, in terms of their therapeutic usefulness. They stop both constipation and diarrhea in their tracks and fight

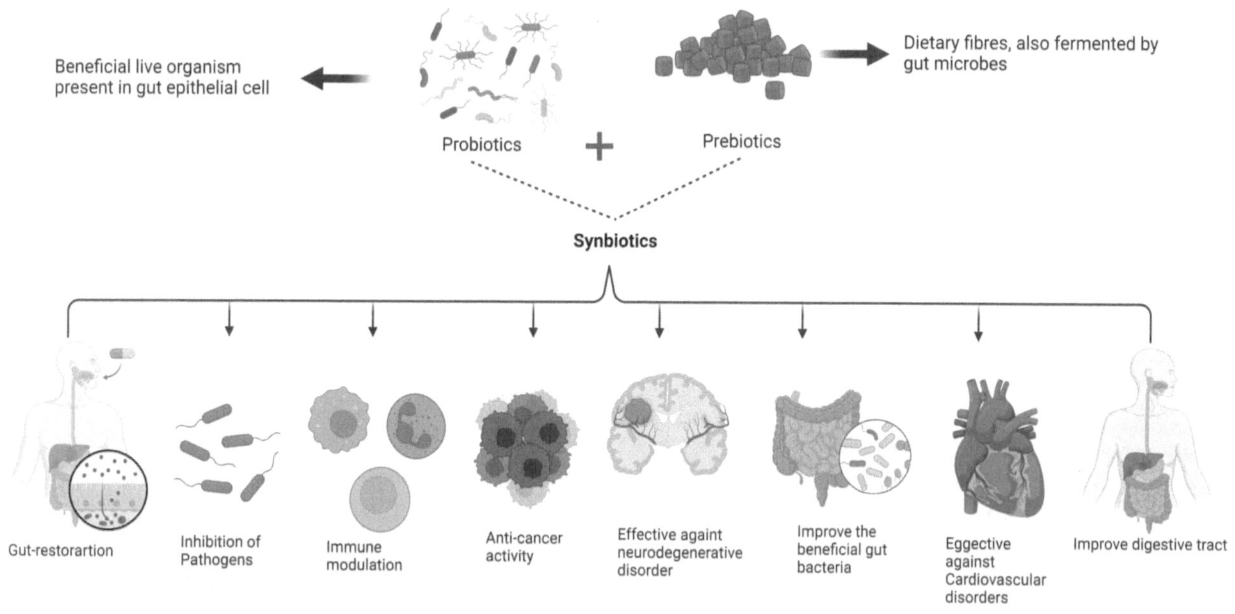

FIGURE 9.2 Effects of synbiotics and the mechanisms by which they exert their influence.

against gastrointestinal deterioration. According to recent research, synbiotics have the potential to effectively cure neurological illnesses linked to improper liver function, regulate the immune system, reduce blood fat and sugar levels, and prevent osteoporosis (Pandey et al. 2015). Figure 9.1 illustrates the notion of synbiotic action mechanisms, which are based on the remodeling of intestinal microbiota with probiotic bacteria and correctly selected prebiotics as their substrates. These mechanisms are featured in the presentation (Markowiak et al. 2017).

9.5 INTRODUCTION OF IRON

Iron is an essential element for almost all living organisms as it participates in a wide variety of metabolic processes, including oxygen transport, deoxyribonucleic acid (DNA) synthesis, and electron transport. Iron is the biologically essential component of every living organism. A primary function of iron lies in its involvement in oxygen transport particularly in higher organisms. The incorporation of iron into hemoglobin, the protein residing in red blood cells, facilitating the binding and transport of oxygen from the lungs to tissues and organs. The participation of iron in DNA processes, including replication and repair, indicates its significance in cell division, growth, and preservation of genetic integrity. Iron emerges as a central player in the electron transport chain. As an integral component of various proteins and enzymes participating in this chain, iron facilitates the ordered flow of electrons, ultimately culminating in the generation of adenosine triphosphate (ATP), the primary currency of cellular energy. The two natures of iron as both an essential nutrient and a potential toxicant underscores the balance in cellular processes (Aisen et al. 2001). The four classes of iron-containing proteins carry out these reactions in the mammalian system: (i) iron-containing nonenzymatic proteins (hemoglobin and myoglobin), (ii) iron-sulfur enzymes, (iii) heme-containing enzymes and (iv) iron-containing enzymes that are noniron-sulfur, nonheme enzymes iron-containing molecules either as part of the prosthetic group of hemoglobin within red blood cells.

9.5.1 Hemoglobin Formation

Hemoglobin is a vital component, this protein is primarily found in red blood cells and has importance in the transport of oxygen from the lungs to various tissues and organs. The inbuilt ability of hemoglobin to bind and release oxygen is fundamental to cellular respiration and to produce energy. The inbuilt ability of hemoglobin to bind and release oxygen is fundamental to cellular respiration and to produce energy (Rodgers et al. 2019). Hemoglobin is synthesized in the bone marrow in a process that involves multiple steps. First, the marrow produces erythroblasts, which are immature red blood cells. These cells then mature and begin to produce hemoglobin. The hemoglobin is composed of two main parts heme and globin, the heme portion imparts red color and oxygen binding ability, whereas the globin part has two types alpha-globin and beta-globin. This arrangement enables hemoglobin to bind with oxygen molecules and enables transport of oxygen throughout body.

9.5.2 Myoglobin Function

Myoglobin plays a crucial role in facilitating oxygen transport and storage within muscle cells. The primary functions are oxygen binding and storage, myoglobin is a protein that consists heme group with presence of iron at its core, which has capacity to bind to oxygen. During the high availability of oxygen, myoglobin binds with oxygen and stores it within muscle cells. When the requirement of oxygen increases due to physical factors, myoglobin releases the stored oxygen, which in turn allows maintaining an adequate supply of blood. By acting as oxygen reservoir, myoglobin helps prevent oxygen deprivation in muscle tissues (Abbaspour et al. 2014). The ability of myoglobin to store and release oxygen is crucial for sustaining muscle function, particularly in tissues that experience fluctuations in oxygen availability. This makes myoglobin an essential component for supporting aerobic respiration in muscle cells, where oxygen is necessary for energy production.

9.5.3 Oxygen Transport

One of the primary functions of iron is its involvement in oxygen transport. In higher organisms, such as humans, iron is a key component of hemoglobin, the protein responsible for binding and transporting oxygen from the lungs to tissues and organs throughout the body. This process is vital for cellular respiration and energy production. Iron plays a crucial role in our body's energy production. Iron is key player in a team, specifically in cellular respiration—the process that creates energy in our cells. Iron is part of proteins that make up electron transport chains in the mitochondria, the cell's powerhouses. The importance of iron in energy metabolism has been highlighted in various studies.

9.5.4 Energy Metabolism

Iron plays a crucial role in the electron transport chain process where energy is produced within mitochondria in the form of ATP. Iron-containing proteins such as cytochromes participate in electron transfer process. Iron is essential for the function of enzymes involved in various pathways, enzymes with iron cofactors aiding in carbohydrates, fats, and proteins. These metabolic flows are one of the fundamental steps to acquire energy from the nutrients we consume, if the iron levels are low, it will lead to decrease in energy production, and maintaining adequate iron levels is crucial for sustaining the energy needed for the body's proper functioning and overall well-being (Goswami et al. 2002).

9.5.5 Immune System Function

Iron is crucial for the normal functioning of the immune system, mainly in the proliferation and activation of immune cells (Soyano et al. 1999). Adequate iron levels are necessary to support the rapid multiplication of immune cells during an immune response. Iron contributes to the immune response by participating in the production of reactive oxygen species (ROS). In the fenton reaction, iron interacts with hydrogen peroxide to generate highly reactive and toxic ROS. Iron-binding proteins, such as transferrin and lactoferrin, are main components of iron sequestration strategy, as these proteins have higher affinity for iron, bind, and form stable complexes. This stable binding makes the accessibility of iron less toward pathogens. Transferrin, found in blood, binds to the iron dietary sources which create complex that prevents free iron from being readily available to microbes. Lactoferrin, present in bodily secretions such as saliva and milk, serves similar purpose (Gafter-Gvili et al. 2019).

9.5.6 Neurotransmitter Synthesis

Iron serves as a cofactor for enzymes involved in the synthesis of neurotransmitters, particularly dopamine and serotonin. In the synthesis of dopamine, iron is involved in the conversion step which is tyrosine to L-DOPA, a precursor of dopamine. At the same time, iron participates in the synthesis of serotonin from tryptophan and norepinephrine from dopamine. The fluctuations in iron levels can have impact on neurotransmitter function, giving rise to spectrum of neurological conditions (Jenkins et al. 2016).

9.5.7 DNA Synthesis and Repair

Iron serves as redox cofactor in enzymes that play a key role in DNA metabolism. These enzymes are necessary in various stages of DNA synthesis, repair, and maintenance. Enzymes such as DNA polymerases, primase, helicases, nucleases, glycosylases, and ribonucleotide reductases depend on iron for their proper functioning in DNA metabolism. The dual role of iron acting as cofactor for essential enzymes and a potential source of oxidative stress describes balance for maintaining proper DNA functioning. Despite its capability to generate ROS, such as hydroxyl radicals through the fenton reaction, iron is indispensable for the activity of various enzymes involved in DNA processes (Puigl et al. 2017).

9.5.8 Absorption/Intake of Iron from Diet

Iron, obtained from our diet, is stored in cells called enterocytes in the intestines. When the body needs iron, it gets released into the bloodstream through protein called ferroportin, regulated by the hormone hepcidin. In the bloodstream, iron gets attached to transferrin and is transported across cells. The absorption of dietary iron involves many factors like stomach acid, enzymes, and transporters. Vitamin C enhances absorption, whereas inhibitors like polyphenols can disturb it (Piskin et al. 2022). The typical Western diet provides around 7 mg of iron per 1,000 kcal, but only 1–2 mg is absorbed daily. Nonheme iron, constituting up to 90% of dietary iron, is present in the form of $Fe+3$ complexes in foods (Ramírez et al. 2019).

In contrast, heme iron, accounting for 10% of dietary iron, exhibits a higher absorption rate and is less affected by dietary factors. Both heme and nonheme iron enter the same intracellular pool after absorption and can be stored in iron storage proteins. Factors such as body iron status, dietary food types, and the use of cast iron pots and cookware can influence intestinal iron absorption. Ensuring an adequate intake of iron is essential for a healthy life (Zarjou et al. 2011). Reference Dietary Allowance (RDA) values have been established to guide nutrient intake for various age groups. For infants aged 0–6 months, an average intake (AI) for iron equivalent to the mean intake of iron in healthy, breastfed infants is recommended. For children, adolescents, and adults, RDAs vary based on age, gender, and life stage. Vegetarians, due to differences in iron absorption from plant-based sources, have specific RDAs tailored to their dietary patterns. Iron deficiency occurs when the body's iron requirement is not met, potentially leading to health problems. Meeting the recommended iron intake is essential for preventing iron deficiency and maintaining overall well-being (Sherman et al. 2018).

9.6 REGULATION OF IRON HOMEOSTASIS

Iron is a vital micronutrient, but excessive amounts may be harmful. Therefore, mammals have evolved sophisticated processes to maintain appropriate levels of iron in both individual cells and the entire body. Iron in the diet is either stored as heme or exists in several nonheme forms. The mechanism by which heme iron is absorbed is not well known. However, nonheme iron is transferred from the outer surface of the intestinal enterocyte by a protein called divalent metal-ion transporter 1 (DMT1). It is then released into the bloodstream through another protein called ferroportin 1 (FPN1). Recently assimilated iron attaches to plasma transferrin and is dispersed throughout the body to locations where it is needed, with the erythroid marrow having notably elevated iron demands. Transferrin saturated with iron attaches to transferrin receptor 1 located on the outer layer of most cells in the body. Once the complex is taken into the cell by endocytosis, iron is transported into the cytoplasm by DMT1, a protein found in the membrane of endosomes. This iron can be used for metabolic processes, retained in cytosolic ferritin, or transported out of the cell by FPN1. The iron regulatory proteins (IRPs), IRP1 and IRP2, control cellular iron concentrations. Hepcidin, a peptide produced by the liver, regulates the absorption of dietary iron and the transfer of iron from tissues to the plasma at the overall body level.

9.6.1 Hepcidin

Hepcidin may be regulated by liver-expressed HFE, HJV, and TfR2. The "hepcidin hypothesis" states that iron excess increases hepcidin expression, which lowers FPN expression and iron efflux from duodenal enterocytes, macrophages that recycle iron from senescent erythrocytes, and hepatocytes, which store most iron. Iron deficiency increases FPN expression and iron uptake (Siddique et al. 2012). Hepcidin concentrations are inversely proportional to tissue iron needs. Inadequate or excessive iron levels might have significant clinical implications. The majority of cases of iron deficiency are caused by an insufficient intake of iron in the diet, whereas iron overload is often linked to genetic problems. These illnesses encompass several types of hemochromatosis, which are marked by insufficient generation of hepcidin and therefore, higher consumption of dietary iron. Additionally, there are iron-loading anemias in which both increased absorption of iron and transfusion treatment contribute to the excess iron in the body (Wallace 2016; Sangkhae and Nemeth 2017).

9.7 IRON OVERLOAD SYNDROMES

Iron overload is when bodily iron stores surpass the usual amount, which is roughly 1 g in adult men and 300 mg in women. The most common cause of clinically relevant systemic iron overload is hereditary (idiopathic, primary) hemochromatosis, a disorder of iron metabolism that abnormally regulates dietary iron absorption and gradually accumulates stored iron. In this condition, body iron stores may reach 20–40 g. Similar symptoms are seen in other illnesses. Examples include iron overload from several blood transfusions or increased iron absorption and inefficient erythropoiesis. Ingestion of traditional home-brewed beer with high iron content causes iron overload in indigenous Sub-Saharan Africans. The extra bodily iron in this illness can reach hereditary hemochromatosis levels, with similar harmful repercussions (see African Iron Overload). Porphyria cutanea tarda and alcoholic liver disease patients can show mild iron excess (McLaren et al. 2002). In 1865, Armand Trousseau labeled hemochromatosis "case of bronze diabetes and cirrhosis". Since these individuals possessed an iron-containing liver pigment, von Recklinghausen called this ailment "hemochromatosis" in 1889. Sheldon discovered that this condition is hereditary and linked to iron metabolism in 1935. Feder et al. found the HFE mutation in 1996. Genetic abnormalities in multiple iron regulation genes produce primary iron overload syndromes, which are marked by low hepcidin levels that enhance dietary iron absorption and iron overload. Primary and secondary iron overload disorders exist (Siddique et al. 2012).

9.7.1 Hereditary Hemochromatosis

HFE-related hemochromatosis causes most genetic iron metabolism issues. Variable penetrance appears in autosomal recessive inheritance. The ailment usually appears in men in their 40s and 50s. The HFE gene mutation causes homozygous hereditary hemochromatosis. HFE, a nonclassical MHC class I protein, interacts with TfR1 via β2-microglobulin on the cell surface and its effects on hepcidin transcription and function are new. Functionally,

TBI binds cell membrane TfR1. HFE and Tf compete for TfR1 to regulate iron absorption (Roy et al. 1999). Systemic iron homeostasis is explained by duodenal crypt cell HFE and TfR1 interaction in the crypt-programming theory (Siddique et al. 2012). Plasma Tf gives crypt enterocytes iron, which they absorb in the villus. Duodenal TBI uptake was significantly reduced in Hfe–/– mice. A defective HFE protein limits enterocyte iron uptake, leaving crypt cells iron-deficient. Incorrectly upregulating iron transport proteins and increasing dietary iron absorption to correct the apparent shortfall occurs when these cells migrate to the villus (Fleming et al. 2002). Dietary iron absorption was regulated by the liver due to hepcidin, a negative regulator. Hfe–/– mice exhibit decreased hepatic hepcidin mRNA expression and elevated iron deposition, resembling human hemochromatosis (Ahmad et al. 2002). Hepcidin is crucial for iron homeostasis, as Hfe–/– mice bred with hepcidin-overexpressing transgenic mice did not experience iron overload. Inhibiting mouse enterocyte HFE expression does not affect iron metabolism. HFE appears to be more important in liver cells than intestinal crypts (Siddique et al. 2012).

Hepcidin may be regulated by liver-expressed HFE, HJV, and TfR2. The "hepcidin hypothesis" states that iron excess increases hepcidin expression, which lowers FPN expression and iron efflux from duodenal enterocytes, macrophages that recycle iron from senescent erythrocytes, and hepatocytes, which store most iron. Iron deficiency increases FPN expression and iron uptake (Siddique et al. 2012). Hepcidin may indirectly affect iron transport protein gene transcription by changing enterocytes' labile iron pool. Several HFE mutations exist. Most clinically significant mutations are C282Y and H63D. C282Y replaces HFE protein cysteine at 282 with tyrosine on the short arm of chromosome 6 (Siddique et al. 2012). At amino acid 63, the H63D mutation replaces histidine with aspartic acid. HH patients are 85–90% C282Y homozygotes and 3–5% C282Y/H63D compound heterozygotes. C282Y homozygosity affects 1 in 250 people and 1 in 200 northern Europeans (Beutler et al. 2002). Many C282Y homozygotes lack iron overload symptoms, suggesting incomplete penetrance and other genes cause HH.43 H63D is 10–20% more prevalent among Europeans than C282Y. Only 0.5–2% of compound heterozygosity for C282/H63D suffer iron overload, hence the clinical implications of H63D without C282Y are unknown (Bacon et al. 2008). H63D homozygosity should not induce illness without alcohol or viral hepatitis (Siddique et al. 2012).

9.7.2 Secondary Hemochromatosis

Iron overload in the liver and portal cirrhosis are two of the hallmarks of secondary hemochromatosis, which can be brought on by either anemia or blood transfusions, or both. Excess iron damages organs (Siddique et al. 2012). In their 20s, homozygous Mediterranean anemia (thalassemia major) patients die of myocardial iron deposition-related heart failure without iron chelation therapy. On September 2006, Europe approved the oral iron chelator deferasirox. To some who took parenteral deferoxamine for years, this medicine is a breakthrough. Because thalassemia is rare in Germany, secondary hemochromatosis primarily affects older myelodysplastic syndrome patients. Such problems affect 4 per 100,000 people annually. Thorough consideration should identify MDS iron chelation indication. Thalassemia and MDS secondary hemochromatosis causes go beyond transfusions. Iron accumulates before transfusing erythrocytes due to high intestinal iron resorption (Gattermann et al. 2009).

The erythropoiesis-deficient erythroid disorders can cause hemochromatosis, i.e. large percentage of bone marrow erythropoietic precursor cells not enduring. Four hematological disorders cause iron overload: Congenital dyserythropoietic anemias like pyruvate kinase deficiency, chronic pernicious anemia, hereditary spherocytosis, and sickle cell anemia; acquired myelodysplastic syndrome. Thalassemia major and intermedia. A majority of secondary iron overload and poor erythropoiesis are thalassemia syndromes (Siddique et al. 2012). Myelodysplastic syndrome and thalassemia cause transfusion dependency. RBCs have 200–250 mg of elemental iron. After several transfusions, iron overload may occur.

In homozygotic thalassemia patients, excessive (alpha or beta) globin chains precipitate, causing oxidative stress and inefficient erythropoiesis. Apoptosis is enhanced in myelodysplastic syndromes, although the cause is unknown. Chronic duodenal iron absorption and compensatory erythroid hyperplasia result from ineffective erythropoiesis. For years, the mechanism of this iron uptake increase was unknown (Gattermann et al. 2009).

Other than transfusional iron excess, hepcidin downregulation and growth differentiation factor 15 (GDF15) may cause iron overload in these patients. Hypoxia reduces hepatocyte hepcidin production (Peyssonnaux et al. 2007). Soluble HJV (sHJV) competing with membrane HJV may also reduce BMP signaling and hepcidin. Hypoxia, iron shortage, and other sHJV-inducing factors may decrease hepcidin expression. In vitro, tissue hypoxia improves EPO expression, which decreases hepcidin. Iron regulatory "signals" may be GDF15 and TWSG1. Beta-thalassemia and other congenital anemia patients have high GDF15 levels, which inhibit hepcidin and induce iron overload. TWSG1 blocks BMP-dependent Smad-mediated signal transduction, overloading iron (Tanno et al. 2009). Unlike primary hemochromatosis, these cases frequently cause liver macrophage iron accumulation and anemia. Phlebotomy is intolerable for many due to anemia; therefore, chelation therapy prevents long-term consequences (Siddique et al. 2012).

9.7.3 Sideroblastic Anemia

Inefficient erythropoiesis, bone marrow ring sideroblasts (RS), and decreased mature red blood cell generation describe sideroblastic anemia (SA), a group of inherited and acquired anemias. Nucleated erythroblasts with pathologic mitochondrial matrix iron granules called RS (Abu-Zeinah et al. 2020). Low heme synthesis, iron-sulfur (Fe-S) cluster building and transport, or mitochondrial and cytosolic protein synthesis cause SA. Contrary to mitochondrial protoporphyrin IX, these processes collect iron granules. Sideroblast accumulation and red cell maturation arrest result from hemoglobin heme deficiencies. Homeostatic processes improve oxygen transport in mature red blood cells to maintain the MCHC during hemoglobin deficiency by maintaining a low mean corpuscular volume (MCV). The processes that cause microcytosis in iron-deficient people are comparable. They differ from iron-deficient red cells on a Wright-Giemsa blood smear by basophilic stippling ribosomal RNA aggregates with degenerating mitochondria and siderosomes. Erythropoietin-driven anemic hypoxia promotes marrow reticulocyte release, generating macrocytic or normocytic anemia with a broad red cell distribution" (Aivado et al. 2006). Circulating reticulocytes and macrocytic red cells contain most hemoglobin (Abu-Zeinah et al. 2020).

9.7.4 Aceruloplasminemia

Aceruloplasminemia is a genetic condition that takes the form of an autosomal recessive inheritance pattern and is brought on by a mutation in the gene that codes for the ceruloplasmin protein (Siddique et al. 2012). The hepatocytes are responsible for the production of a multicopper ferroxidase known as ceruloplasmin (CP). The concentration of CP is necessary for the mobilization of iron and the oxidation of $Fe2+$ to $Fe3+$, both of which are requirements for the release of transferrin. The accumulation of iron in a variety of organs, including the basal ganglia, liver, and pancreas, can be caused by deficiencies in the protein ceruloplasmin. The typical trinity of characteristics associated with aceruloplasminemia is the presence of diabetic mellitus, neurological symptoms, and retinal degeneration. People who have aceruloplasminemia have normal copper levels in their livers, but their iron levels and SF concentrations are equal to those of people who have hemochromatosis (McNeill et al. 2008).

9.7.5 Hemosiderosis

The condition known as hemosiderosis is characterized by an abnormally high concentration of iron deposits in the tissues, which are referred to as hemosiderin. Respiratory and renal hemosiderosis are common (Saha et al. 2021). Hemosiderosis can occur due to red blood cell disintegration and tissue iron release after direct bleeding. Damage to red blood cells in blood arteries releases iron into the blood, which accumulates in the kidneys as they filter waste. There are various types of hemosiderosis, such as transfusion-related, idiopathic, pulmonary, and transfusional diabetes (Lu et al. 1995, Lu et al. 1994, Saha et al. 2021).

Damaged organs include: In cases of idiopathic pulmonary hemosiderosis, Goodpasture's syndrome, or granulomatosis with polyangiitis, hemosiderin deposition in the lungs is a common complication of diffuse alveolar hemorrhage. In addition, mitral stenosis might result in pulmonary hemosiderosis at times. Iron overload/hemosiderosis from hemosiderin buildup (Saha BK et al. 2021). Deposition of hemosiderin causes hemochromatosis liver failure. Preferential iron deposition induces hyperpigmentation and diabetes due to skin and pancreatic beta cell transferrin receptor distribution (Lu et al. 1994). Brain bleeding from persistent subdural hemorrhage, cerebral arteriovenous malformations, and cavernous hemangiomata can deposit hemosiderin. After bruising, hemostain is gradually eliminated, but in stasis dermatitis, it may remain. Kidney hemosiderin causes rare paroxysmal nocturnal hemoglobinuria and severe hemolysis. Iron excess can cause hemosiderin buildup. Sickle cell anemia and thalassemia necessitate frequent blood transfusions due to blood loss. Even without transfusions, beta-thalassemia minor can develop liver hemosiderin deposits in non-alcoholic fatty liver disease patients (Valenti et al. 2010). Iron overdose can result from whole blood and red cell transfusions or GI absorption. Intermedia thalassemia patients who aren't transfused are generally concerned about increased gastrointestinal absorption, while thalassemia major patients usually have ferritin overload from blood transfusions. Blood has 200 mg iron. Siderosis causes light-induced hyperpigmentation, infection risk, stunted growth, and delayed sexual maturation and puberty after 50 units of transfusion or earlier in children. Annually, β-thalassemia patients should get 116–232 mg iron per kg (0.32–0.64 mg/kg/day) by red cell transfusions.

9.7.6 Iron Overload Due to Chronic Liver Disease

Overconsumption of iron may be linked to chronic viral hepatitis, specifically Hepatitis C virus infection (HCV) (Sherrington et al. 2002). HFE mutations, hepcidin dysregulation, necrotic hepatocyte iron release, and HCV's direct effect on iron homeostasis may cause iron overload in HCV (Kaito et al. 2007). ROS from HCV inhibited C/EBPa, downregulating hepcidin and hepatic iron buildup in transgenic mice. When liver macrophages release pro-inflammatory cytokines, they may activate hepatic stellate cells, leading to enhanced fibrogenesis by upregulating alpha-smooth muscle actin and procollagen α-1 (Siddique et al. 2012).

Iron deposits in hepatocytes are the first indicator of alcoholic liver disease; however, as the disease progresses, iron accumulates in macrophages as well (Kohgo et al. 2005). The toxic effects on the liver are amplified when used with alcohol. Abstinence from alcohol for 2–6 weeks considerably lowers serum iron levels. Alcohol may cause hepatic iron excess like HCV. Hepatocytes are damaged by ROS and lipid peroxidation products from alcohol and its metabolites (Harrison-Findik et al. 2006). ALD patients have considerably greater thioredoxin, an indication of oxidative stress, than healthy subjects. C/EBPa suppression may depress hepcidin expression, causing iron buildup and macrophage activation like HCV (Siddique et al. 2012).

NAFLD is the most frequent cause of chronic liver disease, ranging from benign fatty liver to non-alcoholic steatohepatitis (NASH), which can lead to cirrhosis and hepatocellular cancer. Patients with NASH often have mild to moderate iron indices and hepatic iron concentrations (Siddique et al. 2012). Iron overload, insulin resistance, and oxidative stress cause liver damage. A "multiple-hit hypotheses" may cause NASH. Hepatic fatty acids accumulate in the initial "hit", causing steatosis. Second "hit" causes steatohepatitis from simple steatosis (Day et al. 1998). Hepatic iron may increase oxidative stress and be the second cause of NASH in some patients. Multiple factors may cause NAFLD and NASH's elevated hepatic iron. NASH patients had a higher prevalence of HFE mutations, although data from groups with a low prevalence have not. Recent research suggests that NASH may boost TNF-alpha expression, which downregulates FPN and HJV (Aigner et al. 2008). NASH hepcidin's role is unclear. High insulin levels may enhance adipose tissue hepcidin expression but decrease it. We need more research to determine if NAFLD and NASH enhance or decrease hepcidin expression. Porphyria Cutanea Tarda (PCT) is an iron-dependent disorder that causes cheek and hand vesiculo-bullous eruptions. 60–70% of PCT patients may have mild iron excess (Siddique et al. 2012).

9.8 TREATMENT AND MANAGEMENT

9.8.1 Phlebotomy (Blood Removal)

Phlebotomy is the standard treatment for primary hemochromatosis. Iron toxicity can be reduced by removing red blood cells, the body's main mobilizer of iron. To return iron levels to normal, patients may need 50 to 100, 500 mL phlebotomies. Phlebotomy is often done once or twice a week (https://www.niddk.nih.gov/health-information/liver-disease/hemochromatosis/treatment). Once iron levels have adjusted, phlebotomy (usually 3–4 times a year) is necessary for life. The goal is to have a ferritin level of less than 50 µg/L. Iron elimination with phlebotomy improves insulin sensitivity, skin pigmentation, and weariness, but not cirrhosis, hypogonadism, or arthropathy. This technique frequently debilitated the patient and resulted in death. President George Washington died in 1799 after having around 1.7 L of blood removed during a bloodletting treatment for acute epiglottitis3. Several thousand years ago, phlebotomy was used to treat a variety of illnesses, but in addition to its curative effects, phlebotomy also had a prophylactic function (Assi and Baz 2014). Adams et al. reviewed the use a 16-gauge straight needle and collecting bag (Blood Pack MR6102; Baxter); the second employs a 19-gauge butterfly needle linked to an evacuated bottle via an extension set (Baxter 1A8503 and 1C8624, respectively). During the course of 15–30 minutes, blood (usually 500 mL) is extracted (Adams and Barton 2010). An expert phlebotomist can alter the needle size and the venipuncture location as needed. At the time of each therapy, the hemoglobin concentration is tested. If the reading is less than 11 g/dL, the treatment plan is changed to 500 mL every other week; lesser quantities (250–400 mL each session) are ideal for certain people with petite bodies or those whose hemoglobin levels are slowly recovered following phlebotomy.

9.8.2 Iron Chelation Therapy

Iron chelation treatment is used to minimize the development of iron overload due to its deposition in various organs such as the liver and heart following frequent transfusions. diverse iron chelators implicated in the treatment of iron overload in diverse clinical diseases have been assessed in this review utilizing more recent investigations focused on these therapeutic agents. The most significant particular US FDA-approved iron chelators are deferroxamine, deferiprone, and deferrasirox. Each of these chelators has benefits and limitations, as well as different target illnesses, amounts of deposited iron, and clinical symptoms in patients, which may influence their selection as the optimal modality.

9.8.2.1 Deferoxamine

It is a safe iron-chelating agent that has received clinical approval and demonstrates efficacy for prolonged iron chelation therapy in conditions such as beta-thalassemia and other cases of iron overload. The significant impact of DFO on lowering serum ferritin levels and reducing hepatic iron content is undeniable, contributing to increased longevity (Dou et al. 2018).

Despite its potential for oral absorption, the pharmacokinetics of oral formulations of chelators are not optimal. The ineffectiveness of intramuscular injections has also been substantiated. Consequently, oral and intramuscular routes are not recommended, and instead, continuous intravenous or subcutaneous infusion is advised. Deferoxamine interacts with ferric iron (Fe^{3+}) to generate a stable compound. The binding of DFO to iron ions creates a soluble complex that is then eliminated from the body during the chelation process. DFO's capacity to create a tight connection with iron keeps the metal from engaging in potentially damaging reactions in tissues and organs (Chaston and Richardson 2003). The chelation capabilities of deferoxamine aid in the removal of excess iron by converting it into a form that is more easily eliminated from the body. Deferoxamine enhances iron elimination through normal physiological mechanisms by binding to it. Deferoxamine reduces free iron buildup in tissues by chelating excess iron. Excessive free iron can stimulate the creation of ROS, resulting in oxidative stress and tissue damage. Deferoxamine chelation reduces these negative consequences (Blood Removal) (https://www.niddk.nih.gov/health-information/liver-disease/hemochromatosis/treatment).

9.8.2.2 Dietary Changes

Dietary adjustments are essential in the treatment of hemochromatosis, a hereditary condition characterized by excessive iron absorption. Dietary changes in hemochromatosis management aim to minimize iron consumption while also promoting general health. Here are some dietary suggestions for people with hemochromatosis. Reduce your intake of foods high in heme iron, which is more easily absorbed by the body. Heme iron may be found in red meat, chicken, and fish. While these protein sources are necessary for a well-balanced diet, persons with hemochromatosis should consume them within a limit (Milman 2021). When ingested combined, vitamin C improves the absorption of nonheme iron (found in plant-based diets). As a result, those with hemochromatosis should avoid taking vitamin C supplements with meals, particularly those high in iron. Calcium can prevent both heme and nonheme iron absorption. Calcium-rich meals, such as dairy products or fortified plant-based substitutes, can aid in iron absorption reduction (Milman 2021). Cooking using iron pots and pans can help you get more iron. It is advisable to use non-iron cookware, such as stainless steel or nonstick choices. Tea and coffee include chemicals that can limit nonheme iron absorption. Consuming these beverages between meals rather than with meals can assist to reduce their influence on iron absorption. A varied diet rich in fruits, vegetables, and whole grains aids in the maintenance of a healthy gut microbiota. This can help with digestion, vitamin absorption, and general well-being(https://www.healthline.com/nutrition/increase-iron-absorption).

9.9 HEMOCHROMATOSIS

The hereditary disorder known as hemochromatosis causes an individual to absorb more iron from their food than their body needs. Symptomatic of the condition is an abnormal surge in iron absorption in the intestines. The hereditary condition is known as systemic iron overload, which occurs when the iron-regulating hormone hepcidin levels drop or when the binding between hepcidin and ferroportin is impaired. The sole known cellular iron exporter, ferroportin, is controlled by hepcidin. Hemochromatosis (HFE) and non-HFE hemochromatosis are the two most frequent types. Non-HFE variants of hemochromatosis caused by mutations in HAMP, HJV, or TFR2 are extremely uncommon, whereas HFE is the result of homozygous mutations (C282Y mutation) in the gene that encodes the hereditary hemochromatosis protein. Another cause of hemochromatosis is a mutation in SLC40A1 (or FPN1), which encodes ferroportin and prevents hepcidin-ferroportin interaction (Brissot et al. 2018).

9.9.1 Symptoms

Hepcidin insufficiency is a hallmark of hemochromatosis, whether it is accompanied with hemoglobin E or not. This, in turn, causes an increase in the release of iron into plasma from splenic macrophages and small intestinal cells. Hepatocytes, pancreatic cells, and cardiomyocytes are the primary organs that experience iron overload when plasma iron levels are high because these cells are responsible for transporting iron into parenchymal tissues. Symptoms of hemochromatosis often don't appear until a patient is in their 30s or 40s; however, this can be much later in the life of a patient with HFE-associated hemochromatosis. Symptoms, when they do appear, may impact many bodily systems simultaneously. Chronic tiredness stands out among the symptoms. Acute or chronic monoarthritis, oligoarthritis, or polyarthritis can also cause joint discomfort; hemochromatosis is more likely to be the cause of arthritis in the ankles, second and third metacarpophalangeal joints, and the rest of the body. An early development of osteoporosis increases the risk of spontaneous fractures, especially of the vertebrae. Melanoma is the most common dermatological symptom, but other symptoms include dry skin and changes to the nails, such as whitening, flattening, and koilonychia, which are excessively thin and bend inward; they are also known as "spoon" nails. Hepatomegaly is the primary indicator of liver disease. Hemochromatosis is unique among liver diseases in that, in the absence of hepatotoxic cofactors, cirrhotic livers in patients with the disease are typically well-functioning, meaning that neither hepatocellular insufficiency nor portal hypertension is typically observed. Hepatocellular carcinoma rather than liver failure problems is a common complication in people with hemochromatosis, and this result explains why. Adrenal insufficiency and hypopituitarism are other possible complications, albeit they occur less frequently than diabetes mellitus. Problems with the heart's rhythm and heart failure are the hallmarks of cardiac symptoms. While anemia is not seen in hemochromatosis, it is present in conditions such as congenital atransferrinemia, hereditary aceruloplasminemia, and iron overload associated with divalent cation transporter 1 (DMT1). Because arthropathies are common in hemochromatosis and can happen even after iron depletion therapies have been effective, it is unlikely that this symptom is due to an excess of iron. Additional research is needed to determine if arthropathies are associated with persistently high plasma transferrin saturation levels and labile plasma iron (Crownover and Covey 2013).

9.9.2 Diagnosis

There are a number of biological markers that can point to hemochromatosis, such as high transferrin saturation and serum ferritin levels. The first biochemical symptom seen in all subtypes of hemochromatosis is an elevated transferrin saturation level (>45%). Nevertheless, there are many processes that might lead to elevated transferrin saturation, such as hemolysis and cytolysis, which are not always associated with iron excess. Additionally, in cases of ferroportin illness or hereditary aceruloplasminemia, where iron excess is obvious, normal or even low transferrin saturation might be observed. In contrast to low ferritin levels, which usually indicate an iron deficit, elevated ferritin levels (defined as

300 μg/L in males and 200 μg/L in women) require careful analysis before being attributed to an excess of iron. Consequently, significant iron overload should not be the only explanation for elevated ferritin levels; the four most common causes are metabolic syndrome, drunkenness, inflammation, and severe cytolysis. Increased ferritin levels are essential for diagnosing hemochromatosis, despite these limitations. Some measures can reveal organ-specific elevated iron levels; for instance, hyperglycemia can reveal pancreatic iron excess, and moderate hypertransaminasemia (less than three times the upper normal range) can reveal chronic hepatic excess. Hemochromatosis may be indicated by radiological abnormalities such as X-ray detectable subchondral arthropathy or chondrocalcinosis of the knees or wrists. Furthermore, hemochromatosis might be suggested by a low T2-weighted signal on liver MRI. The R2* approach outperforms signal intensity ratio for low to moderate iron overload when utilizing the increasingly common 3 Tesla MRI, whereas the latter is better appropriate for excessive iron overload. Hemochromatosis due to hepcidin insufficiency and ferroportin disease may be distinguished using iron MRI. The term "black" refers to a very iron-loaded liver in hepcidin-deficient hemochromatosis patients, while the term "white" describes a spleen that does not have any iron excess. Hemochromatosis types 1, 2A, 2B, 3, and 4 manifest clinically with splenic and liver-like features. On T2-weighted MRI, a black spleen indicates a high iron overload, whereas a gray or black liver indicates a moderate or severe iron overload, in ferroportin disease. For hemochromatosis related with heparinized food, the underlying genetic etiology can be easily identified. By detecting C282Y homozygosity, which can be done by various laboratories, this condition is virtually invariably detected in white persons. Even though C282Y/H63D compound heterozygosity can raise plasma transferrin saturation to a certain extent, it won't lead to significantly elevated ferritin levels or severe iron overload in the organs. Mild iron overload, if any, might result from compound heterozygosity in conditions like metabolic syndrome or prolonged alcoholism. A patient with severe systemic iron overload should thus have additional hereditary and/or acquired sources of iron excess investigated if C282Y heterozygosity is found (Bacon et al. 2011).

9.9.3 Treatment and Management of Hemochromatosis

Clinical improvement is observed in patients with hemochromatosis who have increased serum ferritin levels after treatment. Phlebotomy is the backbone of therapy, and there is no evidence that limiting iron intake through food helps with daily control. In addition to reducing the danger of infection with V. vulnificus and advanced liver fibrosis, avoiding raw seafood and reducing alcohol intake should be done simultaneously with phlebotomy therapy.88 There are two parts to therapy: treatment and maintenance. A serum ferritin level of 50–100 μg/L is the aim, and treatment is administered by drawing blood once a week. After that, the desired serum ferritin level is stabilized with maintenance treatment. The frequency of phlebotomy is very varied and needs to be determined on an individual basis; however, it is often performed every 3 months. Only patients with confirmed cases of iron overload disease, polycythemia vera, or porphyria cutanea tarda, as well as those with significantly increased blood ferritin levels, are now eligible for phlebotomy treatment. People whose increased ferritin levels are caused by other illnesses, such as fatty liver disease, do not have solid evidence that phlebotomy therapy is helpful (Table 9.2).

TABLE 9.2
Treatment and Management of Hemochromatosis

Treatment	Mechanism	References
Phlebotomy (Blood Removal)	It is common in primary hemochromatosis. Iron toxicity can be reduced by removing red blood cells, the body's main iron mobilizer. Patients may need 50–100 phlebotomies of 500 mL to normalize iron levels. One or two phlebotomies per week are normal.	(https://www.niddk.nih.gov/health-information/liver-disease/hemochromatosis/treatment).
Deferoxamine	Iron-binding deferoxamine boosts physiological elimination. Chelating excess iron with deferoxamine reduces tissue iron. Free iron increases ROS, causing oxidative stress and tissue damage. Deferoxamine chelation reduces them.	(https://www.niddk.nih.gov/health-information/liver-disease/hemochromatosis/treatment).
Diet adjustments	For hemochromatosis, a hereditary disease that causes excessive iron absorption, diet adjustments are needed. Diets promote hemochromatosis health by reducing iron consumption. Vitamin C improves nonheme iron absorption. Calcium blocks heme and nonheme iron absorption. A varied diet of fruits, vegetables, and whole grains helps gut flora.	Milman (2021)
Synbiotics (S. boulardii, B. lactis, and Bacillus plantarum. Kefir, kimchi, sauerkraut, and yogurt)	Prevent hemochromatosis and reduce the body's sorption of iron. With the use of probiotics and dietary changes, like consuming more fiber and reducing iron-rich meals.	(Botta et al. (2021)

When phlebotomy fails or is not an option for treating hemochromatosis, iron chelation is an option for individuals with acquired iron overload, such as in beta-thalassemia. Deferasirox, an iron chelator, is useful in treating acquired and HFE-related iron overload. It is taken daily by mouth as a tablet. On the other hand, primary iron overload patients cannot afford to take it frequently. For cases of secondary iron overload in which venesection is not an option, it is covered by the Pharmaceutical Benefits Scheme. In addition to normal therapy, proton pump inhibitors have been demonstrated to decrease iron absorption in hereditary hemochromatosis patients, extending the period between phlebotomies. One possible treatment for hemochromatosis is the use of hepcidin analogs, as this condition is thought to be caused by either low hepcidin levels or a lack of hepcidin activity. This strategy seems to work better for maintenance treatment so far since the medications in question do not reduce iron storage in the liver. Because of their high cost and parenteral administration, these medicines will have a hard time competing with phlebotomy therapy. Doctors treat neonatal hemochromatosis in newborns with exchange transfusions—removing blood and replacing it with donor blood—and IV immunoglobulin—a solution of antibodies from healthy people. These treatments do not always work to reverse severe liver damage, and a liver transplant may be needed. Often the newborn's mother or father can serve as a living liver donor. Only a small part of the adult donor liver is needed for transplantation into a newborn (Golfeyz, Lewis, and Weisberg 2018; Kowdley et al. 2019; Crawford et al. 2023).

9.9.4 The Role of Synbiotics in Treating Hemochromatosis

When taken on a daily basis, probiotics—which consist of live bacteria and yeasts—provide several health advantages. The majority of these "good" bacteria live in the digestive tract and play an important role in maintaining healthy immunological and digestive systems. Research suggests that some types of probiotics can alleviate hemochromatosis symptoms by reducing inflammation in the body. Probiotics are known to have anti-inflammatory effects, but they also help keep iron levels in check. There is some evidence that probiotics can improve outcomes for people with hemochromatosis by reducing iron absorption in the stomach and, by extension, total body iron levels. Although there is a wide variety of probiotics to choose from, not all of them work equally well in alleviating the symptoms of hemochromatosis (Figure 9.3).

Bacillus plantarum, Bifidobacterium lactis, and Saccharomyces boulardii are three of the best probiotic strains for hemochromatosis. People with hemochromatosis may benefit from taking probiotics since they lower the

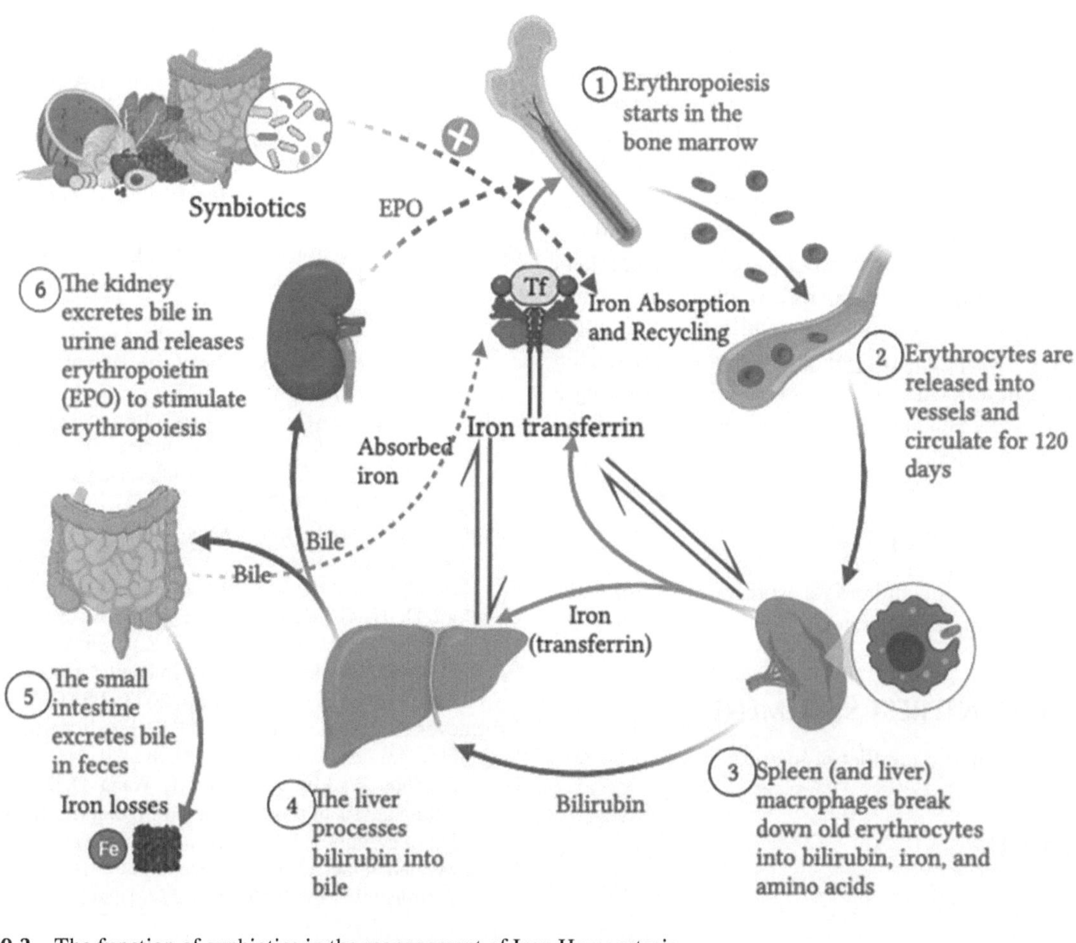

FIGURE 9.3 The function of synbiotics in the management of Iron Homeostasis.

body's iron absorption, according to research. Symptom management can be enhanced with the use of probiotics and dietary adjustments, such as limiting iron-rich foods and boosting fiber consumption. Although probiotics can alleviate some of the symptoms of hemochromatosis, they should not be considered a replacement for conventional medical care. Never begin a new treatment regimen without first discussing it with your doctor. Hemochromatosis therapy plans that include probiotics are easy to implement. Yogurt, kefir, sauerkraut, and kimchi are some foods that are rich in probiotics and may be eaten every day (Botta et al. 2021).

9.10 CONCLUSION

Autosomal recessive inheritance of a C282Y mutation in the HFE protein, affecting both alleles of the relevant gene, is the most prevalent cause of hemochromatosis. Reduced expression of the iron-regulating protein, hepcidin, causes an abnormal increase in intestinal iron absorption, which is a hallmark of the condition. Iron poisoning of the liver and other organs could result from its gradual accumulation in parenchymal tissues. Along with genetic testing and new MRI-based diagnostic tools, the hallmark biochemical abnormalities of elevated blood ferritin and transferrin saturation can identify the disease. Clinical manifestations of progressive iron overload include severe fibrosis, cirrhosis, and hepatocellular cancer. In people with hereditary hemochromatosis, the penetrance of both elevated iron indices and clinically severe illness is mysteriously incomplete. Whatever the case may be, faster detection and more public understanding of the condition have reduced the frequency of severe clinical manifestations. People with hereditary (HFE) hemochromatosis are already at a higher risk of liver damage, but being overweight and drinking excessively can make their condition worse. Researchers are currently looking at the possibility of altering genes that might affect how the disease manifests in the body. The first-line therapy is still phlebotomy, which, if started early, results in a normal life expectancy. Incorporating a healthy, balanced diet into the continuous therapy of the condition is suggested.

ACKNOWLEDGMENT

I am thankful to all the authors for working with full dedication in completing this chapter.

COMPETING INTEREST STATEMENT

The authors declare no conflict of interest.

DISCLAIMER

None.

REFERENCES

Abbaspour N, Hurrell R, and Kelishadi R. Review on iron and its importance for human health. *J Res Med Sci.* 2014 Feb;*19*(2):164–74. 24778671; PMC3999603.

Abu-Zeinah G, and DeSancho M. T. Understanding sideroblastic anemia: an overview of genetics, epidemiology, pathophysiology and current therapeutic options. *J Blood Med.* 2020, *11*:305–18.

Adams PC, and Barton JC. How I treat hemochromatosis. *Blood.* 2010; *116*(3):317–25.

Ahmad K. A, Ahmann J. R, Migas M. C, Waheed A, Britton R. S, Bacon B. R, Sly W. S, and Fleming R. E. Decreased liver hepcidin expression in the Hfe knockout mouse. *Blood Cells Mole Dis.* 2002 Nov 1;*29*(3):361–6.

Aigner E, Theurl I, Theurl M, Lederer D, Haufe H, Dietze O, Strasser M, Datz C, and Weiss G. Pathways underlying iron accumulation in human nonalcoholic fatty liver disease. *Am J Clin Nutr.* 2008 May 1;*87*(5):1374–83.

Aisen P, Enns C, and Wessling-Resnick M. Chemistry and biology of eukaryotic iron metabolism. *Int J Biochem Cell Biol.* 2001;*33*:940–59.

Aivado M, Gattermann N, Rong A, Giagounidis A. A, Prall W. C, Czibere A, Hildebrandt B, Haas R, and Bottomley S. S. X-linked sideroblastic anemia associated with a novel ALAS2 mutation and unfortunate skewed X-chromosome inactivation patterns. *Blood Cells Mole Dis.* 2006 July 1;*37*(1):40–5.

Assi T. B., and E. Baz. Current applications of therapeutic phlebotomy. *Blood Transfus.* 2014. *12* Suppl 1 (Suppl 1):s75–83.

Bacon B. R, and Britton R. S. Clinical penetrance of hereditary hemochromatosis. *N Eng J Med.* 2008 Jan 17;*358*(3):291–2.

Bacon B. R., Adams P. C, Kowdley K. V, Powell L. W, and Tavill A. S. Diagnosis and management of hemochromatosis: 2011 practice guideline by the American Association for the Study of Liver Diseases. *Hepatology.* 2011;*54*(1):328–43.

Beutler E, Felitti V. J, Koziol J. A, Ho N. J, and Gelbart T. Penetrance of 845G→ A (C282Y) HFE hereditary haemochromatosis mutation in the USA. *The Lancet.* 2002 Jan 19;*359*(9302):211–8.

Botta A, Nicole G. Barra, and Nhat Hung L, et al. Iron reshapes the gut microbiome and host metabolism. *J Lipid Atheroscler.* 2021;*10*(2):160–83.

Brissot P, Antonello P, Paul C. A., Barbara de G, Christine E. M, and Olivier L. Haemochromatosis. *Nat Rev Dis Primers.* 2018;*4*(1):18016.

Camaschella C, Nai A, and Silvestri L. Iron metabolism and iron disorders revisited in the hepcidin era. *Haematol.* 2020 Jan 31;*105*(2):260–72. doi: 10.3324/haematol.2019.232124. 31949017; PMC7012465.

Chaston T, and Des R. Iron Chelators for the treatment of iron overload disease: relationship between structure, redox activity, and toxicity. *Am J Hematol.* 2003;*73*:200–10.

Crawford D. H. G., Ramm G. A., Bridle K. R., Nicoll A. J., Delatycki M. B., and Olynyk. J. K. Clinical practice guidelines on hemochromatosis: Asian Pacific Association for the Study of the Liver. *Hepatol Int.* 2023;.*17*(3):522–41.

Crownover B. K., and Covey C. J. 2013. Hereditary hemochromatosis. *Am Fam Physician 87* (3):183–90.

Dang D, Zhou W, Lun Z. J, Mu X, Wang D. X, and Wu H. Meta-analysis of probiotics and/or prebiotics for the prevention of eczema. *J Int Med Res.* 2013 Oct;*41*(5):1426–36.

Day C. P, and James O. F. Steatohepatitis: a tale of two "hits"? *Gastroenterology.* 1998 Apr 1;*114*(4):842–5.

DeLoughery T. G. Safety of oral and intravenous iron. *Acta Haematol.* 2019;*142*(1):8–12

Dou H, Yuanhan Q, Guoli C, and Yanjun Z. Effectiveness and safety of deferasirox in thalassemia with iron overload: a meta-analysis. *Acta Haematol.* 2018;*141*(1):32–42.

Fleming R. E, and Sly W. S. Mechanisms of iron accumulation in hereditary hemochromatosis. *Annu Rev Physiol.* 2002 Mar;*64*(1):663–80.

Gafter-Gvili A, Schechter A, and Rozen-Zvi B. Iron deficiency anemia in chronic kidney disease. *Acta Haematol.* 2019;*142*(1):44–50.

Gattermann N. The treatment of secondary hemochromatosis. *Deutsches Ärzteblatt International.* 2009 July;*106*(30):499.

Gibson G. R, Probert H. M, Van Loo J, Rastall R. A, and Roberfroid M. B. Dietary modulation of the human colonic microbiota: updating the concept of prebiotics. Nutr Res Rev. 2004 Dec;*17*(2):259–75.

Golfeyz S., Lewis S., and Weisberg. I. S. 2018. Hemochromatosis: pathophysiology, evaluation, and management of hepatic iron overload with a focus on MRI. *Expert Rev Gastroenterol Hepatol 12*(8):767–78.

Gómez-Ramírez S, Bisbe E, Shander A, Spahn D. R, and Muñoz M. Management of perioperative iron deficiency anemia. *Acta Haematol.* 2019;*142*(1):21–29.

Goswami T, Rolfs A, and Hediger M. A. Iron transport: Emerging roles in health and disease. *Biochem Cell Biol.* 2002;*80*(5):679–89. doi: 10.1139/o02-159. 12440707.

Harrison-Findik D. D, Schafer D, Klein E, Timchenko N. A, Kulaksiz H, Clemens D, Fein E, Andriopoulos B, Pantopoulos K, and Gollan J. Alcohol metabolism-mediated oxidative stress down-regulates hepcidin transcription and leads to increased duodenal iron transporter expression. *J Biol Chem.* 2006 Aug 11;*281*(32):22974–82.

Hoppe M, Gramatkovski² E, Onning G, Björklund M, Larsson N, and Hulthén. L. 2015. IMPROVED IRON ABSORPTION BY CONSUMPTION OF PROBIOTICS.

Fuad A. S, Amran N. A, Nasruddin N. S, Burhanudin N. A, Dashper S, and Arzmi M. H. The mechanisms of probiotics, prebiotics, synbiotics, and postbiotics in oral cancer management. *Probiotics & Antimicro. Prot. 15*(5): 1298–1311.

https://casadesante.com/blogs/probiotics/best-probiotic-for-hemochromatosis.

https://www.healthline.com/nutrition/increase-iron-absorption.

https://www.niddk.nih.gov/health-information/liver-disease/hemochromatosis/treatment.

Huo C, Li G, Hu Y, and Sun H. The impacts of iron overload and ferroptosis on intestinal mucosal homeostasis and inflammation. Int. J. Mol. Sci. 2022;*23*(22):14195.

Jenkins T. A, Nguyen J. C, Polglaze K. E, and Bertrand P. P. Influence of tryptophan and serotonin on mood and cognition with a possible role of the gut-brain axis. *Nutrients.* 2016 Jan 20;*8*(1):56. doi: 10.3390/nu8010056. 26805875; PMC4728667.

Johnston B. C, Supina A. L, and Vohra S. Probiotics for pediatric antibiotic-associated diarrhea: a meta-analysis of randomized placebo-controlled trials. *CMAJ.* 2006 Aug 15;*175*(4):377–83.

Kaito M. Molecular mechanism of iron metabolism and overload in chronic hepatitis C. *J Gastroenterol.* 2007 Jan;*42*(1):96–9.

Kane S. F, Roberts C, Paulus R. Hereditary hemochromatosis: rapid evidence review. *Am Fam Physician.* 2021 Sep;*104*(2):263–70.

Kohgo Y, Ohtake T, Ikuta K, Suzuki Y, Hosoki Y, Saito H, Kato J. Iron accumulation in alcoholic liver diseases. *Alcoholism: Clinical and experimental research.* 2005 Nov;*29*:189S–93S.

Kowdley K. V, Brown K. E, Ahn J, and Sundaram V. ACG clinical guideline: hereditary hemochromatosis. *Am J Gastroenterol.* 2019;*114*(8):1202–1218.

Lieu P. T, Heiskala M, Peterson P. A, and Yang Y. The roles of iron in health and disease. *Mol Aspects Med.* 2001 Feb–Apr;*22*(1–2):1–87. doi: 10.1016/s0098-2997(00)00006-6. 11207374.

Lu J. P, and Hayashi K. Selective iron deposition in pancreatic islet B cells of transfusional iron-overloaded autopsy cases. *Pathol Int.* 1994 Mar;*44*(3):194–9.

Lu J. P, and Hayashi K. Transferrin receptor distribution and iron deposition in the hepatic fobufe of iron-overloaded rats. *Pathol Int.* 1995 Mar;*45*(3):202–6.

Manigandan T, Mangaiyarkarasi S. P, Hemalatha R, Hemalatha V. T, and Murali N. P. Probiotics, prebiotics and synbiotics: A review. *Biomed Pharmacol J.* 2012;*5*(2):295.

Markowiak P, and Śliżewska K. Effects of probiotics, prebiotics, and synbiotics on human health. *Nutrients.* 2017 Sep 15;*9*(9):1021.

Markowiak-Kopeć P, and K. Śliżewska. The effect of probiotics on the production of short-chain fatty acids by human intestinal microbiome. *Nutrients.* 2020;*12*(4): 1107.

McLaren G. D. Hereditary hemochromatosis and other iron-overload disorders. *Manual Clin Hematol.* 2002; *15*(6): 261–76.

McNeill A, Pandolfo M, Kuhn J, Shang H, and Miyajima H. The neurological presentation of ceruloplasmin gene mutations. *Euro Neurol.* 2008 July 30;*60*(4):200–5.

Milman, N. T. Managing genetic hemochromatosis: An overview of dietary measures, which may reduce intestinal iron absorption in persons with iron overload. *Gastroenterology Res.* 2021;*14*(2):66–80.

Muir A, and Hopfer U. Regional specificity of iron uptake by small intestinal brush-boarder membranes from normal and iron deficient mice. 1985; *248*(3 Pt 1): G376-9.

Osterholm, E. A., and M. K. Georgieff. Chronic inflammation and iron metabolism. *J Pediatr.* 2015;*166*(6):1351–7e1.

Pandey K. R, Naik S. R, and Vakil B. V. Probiotics, prebiotics and synbiotics-a review. *J Food Sci and Tech.* 2015 Dec;*52*:7577–87.

Papanikolaou G, and Pantopoulos K. Iron metabolism and toxicity. *Toxicol Appl Pharmacol.* 2005 Jan 15;*202*(2):199–211. doi: 10.1016/j.taap.2004.06.021. 15629195.

Pérez-Conesa D, López G, Abellán P, and Ros G. Bioavailability of calcium, magnesium and phosphorus in rats fed probiotic, prebiotic and synbiotic powder follow-up infant formulas and their effect on physiological and nutritional parameters. *J Sci Food Agri.* 2006 Nov;*86*(14):2327–36.

Peyssonnaux C, Zinkernagel A. S, Schuepbach R. A, Rankin E, Vaulont S, Haase V. H, Nizet V, and Johnson R. S. Regulation of iron homeostasis by the hypoxia-inducible transcription factors (HIFs). *J Clin Invest.* 2007 July 2;*117*(7):1926–32.

Piskin E, Cianciosi D, Gulec S, Tomas M, and Capanoglu E. Iron absorption: factors, limitations, and improvement methods. *ACS Omega.* 2022 June 10;*7*(24):20441–20456. doi: 10.1021/acsomega.2c01833. 35755397; PMC9219084.

Pantopoulos K. (2008). Function of the hemochromatosis protein HFE: Lessons from animal models. *World Journal of Gastroenterology*, *14*(45), 6893–6901. https://doi.org/10.3748/wjg.14.6893

Rodgers G. M, and Gilreath J. A. The role of intravenous iron in the treatment of anemia associated with cancer and chemotherapy. *Acta Haematol.* 2019;*142*(1):13–20.

Roy C. N, Penny D. M, Feder J. N, and Enns C. A. The hereditary hemochromatosis protein, HFE, specifically regulates transferrin-mediated iron uptake in HeLa cells. *J Biol Chem.* 1999 Mar 26;*274*(13):9022–8.

Saha B. K. Idiopathic pulmonary hemosiderosis: a state of the art review. *Respir Med.* 2021 Jan 1;*176*:106234.

Sangkhae, V., and E. Nemeth. Regulation of the iron homeostatic hormone hepcidin. *Adv Nutr.* 2017;*8*(1):126–36.

Santa, K, Watanabe K, Kumazawa Y, and Nagaoka I. Phytochemicals and vitamin D for a healthy life and prevention of diseases. *Int J Mol Sci.* 2023;*24*(15):12167.

Sekhon B. S, and Jairath S. Prebiotics, probiotics and synbiotics: An overview. *J Pharm Educ Res.* 2010 Dec 1;*1*(2).

Puig1* S, Lucia Ramos-Alonso1, Antonia Maria Romero1 and Maria Teresa Martinez-Pastor2* DOI: 10.1039/C7MT00116A.

Seyoum, Y, Baye K, and Humblot C. 2021. Iron homeostasis in host and gut bacteria - a complex interrelationship. *Gut Microbes 13*(1):1874855.

Sherman, H. G., Jovanovic, C., Stolnik, S., Baronian, K., Downard, A. J., and Rawson, F. J. (New perspectives on iron uptake in eukaryotes. *Front Mol Biosci.*2018;*5*, Article 97. https://doi.org/10.3389/fmolb.2018.00097

Sherrington C. A, and Olynyk J. K. Iron as a cofactor in chronic hepatitis C infection. *Liver.* 2002 June 1;*22*(3):187–9.

Siddique A, and Kowdley K. V. The iron overload syndromes. *Aliment Pharm Ther.* 2012 Apr;*35*(8):876–93.

Socha P, Stolarczyk M, and Socha J. Wpływ probiotyków i prebiotyków na gospodarke lipidowa. *Pediatr. Współcz. Gastroenterol. Hepatol. Zyw. Dziecka.* 2002;*4*:85–8.

Soyano A, Gómez M. Participación del hierro en la inmunidad y su relación con las infecciones [Role of iron in immunity and its relation with infections]. *Arch Latinoam Nutr.* 1999 Sep;*49*(3 Suppl 2):40S–46S. Spanish. 10971835.

Tanno T, Porayette P, Sripichai O, Noh S. J, Byrnes C, Bhupatiraju A, Lee Y. T, Goodnough J. B, Harandi O, Ganz T, Paulson R. F. Identification of TWSG1 as a second novel erythroid regulator of hepcidin expression in murine and human cells. *Blood.* 2009 July 2;*114*(1):181–6.

Valenti L, Canavesi E, Galmozzi E, Dongiovanni P, Rametta R, Maggioni P, Maggioni M, Fracanzani A. L, and Fargion S. Beta-globin mutations are associated with parenchymal siderosis and fibrosis in patients with non-alcoholic fatty liver disease. *J Hepatol.* 2010 Nov 1;*53*(5):927–33.

Wallace D. F. The regulation of iron absorption and homeostasis. *Clin Biochem Rev.* 2016; *37*(2):51–62.

You S., Ma Y, and Yan B, et al. The promotion mechanism of prebiotics for probiotics: A review. *Front Nutr.* 2022;*9*:1000517.

Zakrzewska Z, Zawartka A, and Schab M., et al. 2022. Prebiotics, probiotics, and postbiotics in the prevention and treatment of Anemia. *Microorganisms 10*(7): 1330.

Zarjou, A., Balla, J., Balla, G., Agarwal, A. (2011). Iron metabolism and oxidative stress. In: Miyata, T., Eckardt, K. U., Nangaku, M. (eds.), *Studies on Renal Disorders. Oxidative Stress in Applied Basic Research and Clinical Practice.* Humana Press. https://doi.org/10.1007/978-1-60761-857-7_11

Zhang M. M, Cheng J. Q, Lu Y. R, Yi Z. H, Yang P, and Wu X. T. Use of pre-, pro- and synbiotics in patients with acute pancreatitis: A meta-analysis. *WJG.* 2010 Aug 8;*16*(31):3970.

10 Correlation between Synbiotic Supplements and Lipid Metabolism

A Novel Strategy to Counter-Attack Metabolic Disorders

Alamgir Khan, Arshad Farid, Fazal Haq, Sohail Ahmad, Amin Ullah, Muhammad Muzammal, and Muhammad Ajmal Khan

10.1 INTRODUCTION

Lipid metabolism covers the production, breakdown, digestion, absorption, and transportation of lipids, including phospholipids, glycolipids, sphingolipids, cholesterol, and prostaglandins, among others. Lipids are organic compounds characterized by their insolubility and solubility in water organic solvents, respectively. Lipids primarily consist of fatty acid (FA) esters, with occasional inclusion of phosphate or alcohol group molecules. They serve as energy reservoirs in animals and play various roles including regulating body temperature and constituting essential components of cell membranes. They also act as chemical couriers (Ratnayake & Galli, 2009; Tocher, 2003).

To maintain the optimal functioning of bodily systems, the human body relies on various beneficial lipid fats. Balancing the levels of lipids in the bloodstream is a critical aspect of overall health. Irregular lipid levels can lead to the accumulation of fat depositions in artery walls, resulting in complications within the blood vessels. Increased lipid adherence to the inner walls of blood vessels can cause the development of various atherosclerotic disorders, i.e. stroke or heart attack (Natesan & Kim, 2021).

Numerous factors influence lipid metabolism, including age, gender, prolonged consumption of diets high in cholesterol, and calories, genetic predisposition, apolipoprotein irregularities, mental exertion, physical inactivity, and psychological stress, among others. Notably, imbalances in cholesterol, triacylglycerol, or free FA (FFA) ratio in the blood or peripheral tissues are key indicators of lipid metabolic disorders. Disruptions in lipid metabolism have been established as the primary causal factor behind a range of illnesses including cardiovascular diseases, obesity, nonalcoholic fatty liver disease, hypertension, and/or atherosclerosis. As a result, investigating the maintenance of lipid metabolism equilibrium holds significant importance in the context of preventing and treating metabolic disorders (Hou et al., 2019).

10.2 LIPID METABOLISM AND METABOLIC DISORDERS

Metabolic diseases, stemming from the absence of proper chemical reactions within our bodies, have a detrimental impact on our quality of life. Enzymes crucial for lipid metabolism may exhibit malfunction or insufficient production (Lattimer & Haub, 2010).

Obesity has become a prevalent metabolic disorder expressed by an unnecessary accumulation of fats in the body. It elevates susceptibility to other ailments and complications, including cardiac defects, diabetes, and various types of cancer (Arslan, 2014; Song et al., 2019). Disturbances in intestinal microbiota can also trigger the amount of fat in the liver, contributing to obesity and other metabolic disorders. Remarkably, approximately part of heart disease is linked to metabolism. Obesity serves a major role for cardiometabolic factors, i.e. raised glucose levels, high blood pressure, and atherogenic dyslipidemia (Grundy 2009).

As per information from the Mayo Clinic, some metabolic diseases can be detected through newborn screening tests, the majority of cases are diagnosed later in adulthood, often after the manifestation of symptoms (Dibaise et al., 2008). For instance, the population of microbes in human digestive system, which plays a significant role in helpful metabolic processes, is substantial. In contrast, metabolic diseases related to obesity stem from pathophysiological interactions leading to adverse metabolic activities (Hur & Lee, 2015). Depending on a child's perspective and developmental progress, these conditions can sometimes be identified in childhood (Denisenko et al., 2020). Healthcare professionals and researchers have yet to pinpoint ideal treatment for the metabolic syndromes (Metbd).

Metabolic diseases often started by commence with obesity and progress through a range of other conditions, including type I and II diabetes, various types of cancer, vaginal atrophy, testosterone replacement, nonalcoholic steatohepatitis, hypoactive sexual desire disorder, hypothyroidism, and infertility. Recently, insulin resistance

DOI: 10.1201/9781032702438-10

(IR) related to lipid metabolism has appeared as a worldwide health problem, necessitating increased research and diagnostic efforts (Pischon et al., 2008; Monnerie et al., 2020). Diseases linked to obesity are often a consequence of excessive consumption of saturated fat lipids (Cena & Calder, 2020; Novgorodtseva et al., 2011).

Furthermore, kwonlic syndrome and other chronic cardiac disorders have been linked to elevated levels of "lipoxin A4" lipids, according to several readings (Dogan et al., 2019). The National Institute of Neurological Diseases and Stroke reports that the buildup of superfluous fats can result in a number of health issues, such as brain and spleen diseases and tissue damage (Kim and Natesan, 2021).

In humans and other animals, FAs have a variety of uses, but their main job is as essential parts of lipids. These FAs, which have two to thirty-six carbon atoms, can be classified as saturated or unsaturated carboxylic acids. Polyunsaturated FAs (PUFAs) have a methyl end, sometimes referred to as the omega end, and a carboxylic acid group at one end. The first unsaturation site in omega-3 and omega-6 FAs, respectively, is after the third and sixth carbon atoms from the omega end. Only dietary sources can provide some necessary polyunsaturated FAs, such as linoleic and alpha-linolenic acid, which our bodies are unable to produce on their own. Omega-3 can be obtained via fish oils, which are rich in docosahexaenoic and eicosapentaenoic acids (22:6n3). On the other hand, flora contains the majority of the omega-6 PUFA linoleic acid (Tortosa et al., 2017).

The pathophysiology of several metabolic syndromes (MetS), which frequently present in the presence of abdominal obesity, is mostly triggered by IR. The importance of lipids—in particular, FAs—as potent signaling molecules that control insulin and inflammatory pathways has been highlighted by recent studies. Uncertain inflammation can arise when the body's molecular processes controlling glucose transport are interfered with by n-3 PUFA deficiency. Oxidative stress in MetS emerges concurrently with the needless production of FFAs. A thorough understanding of the molecular processes that FAs and their metabolites play in the pathophysiology of MetS may lead to the development of innovative MetS diagnostic techniques as well as focused treatment approaches.

Recent research has shown that a number of pathogenic events cascade into one another to cause the development of IR. Lipids are essential for initiating inflammation (IR) and for MetS development afterward (Lee et al., 2020; Grgurevic et al., 2020). It is widely known that not all lipids are created equal and that consuming too much saturated fat leads to obesity and other related disorders (Cena & Calder, 2020). According to recent research, IR in people with obesity and type 2 diabetes may be linked to elevated levels of FFAs in general and saturated FAs in particular (Jimenez et al., 2017). Lack of PUFAs can cause inflammation and upset the glucose-insulin balance (Kytikova et al., 2019).

Conversely, numerous research studies have established a clear link between alterations in lipids and with MetS (Reddy et al., 2019). Changes in FA metabolism disturb the production of lipid mediators accountable for immune-metabolic balance (Headland & Norling, 2015). Recent investigations have further clarified the importance of these compounds, causative to chronic low-grade inflammatory state observed in MetS (Kwon, 2020; Denisenko et al., 2020).

10.3 TARGETING LIPID METABOLISM TO COMBAT METABOLIC DISORDERS

The pursuit of innovative methods to tackle these intricate issues has demonstrated that relying solely on conventional treatments and interventions may not be adequate. Novel medicines that address the underlying causes of metabolic dysfunction need to be investigated in order to effectively treat these illnesses. Metabolic illnesses are frequently intimately linked to disruptions in lipid metabolism. Triglycerides (TGs) and other lipids at elevated levels may be the catalyst for the onset of MetS, inflammation, and IR. This connection emphasizes how crucial it is to target lipid metabolism as the main area for intervention, with synbiotics emerging as innovative practitioners in this regard.

10.3.1 Synbiotics

Synbiotics are dietary supplements that combine probiotics and prebiotics in a synergistic formulation. These synbiotics encompass together substrates and beneficial microorganisms, which may have crucial effects within the intestinal tract (GiT). They exert positive influence by enhancing the existence and growing of live microbes in the GiT. Several researches have demonstrated that the practice of synbiotics can lead to improvements in various MtS, and also the functionality of the gut microorganisms (Ghazalpour et al., 2016) (Figure 10.1).

10.4 CORRELATION BETWEEN SYNBIOTICS AND LIPID METABOLISM: A NOVEL THERAPEUTIC STRATEGY TO COUNTER METABOLIC DISORDERS

The primary question that comes to mind is this: what role do synbiotics play in this intricate puzzle? Because of their special impact on the gut microbiota, synbiotics provide a multimodal approach to address anomalies in lipid metabolism. By promoting the development of beneficial gut bacteria, they restore microbial equilibrium, which has a cascading effect on the balance of lipids. Hepatic lipogenesis, bile acid metabolism, and lipid absorption are just a few of the numerous facets of lipid metabolism that are impacted by this complex relationship. The synergistic link between lipid metabolism and metabolic illnesses seems to be a promising avenue in the study of metabolic disorders. The optimal dosages, formulations, and individual reactions are the focus of this field of study, which

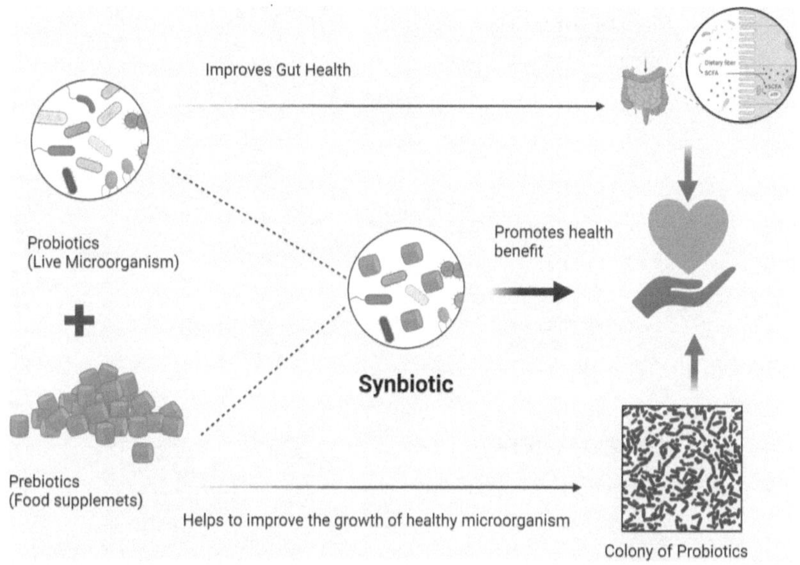

FIGURE 10.1 Schematic representation of synbiotics.

is always evolving. Rethinking the prevention and treatment of metabolic illnesses is being fueled by the encouraging relationship found between lipid metabolism and synbiotics.

We will go deeper into this intricate link in the parts that follow, looking at the mechanics, supporting evidence, and potential uses of synbiotics as a cutting-edge therapeutic strategy to treat metabolic diseases (Figure 10.2).

Here are some helpful examples in this regard.

10.4.1 Microbiome Restoration

It has been found that adding synbiotics to a diet helps some beneficial bacteria, like Lactobacillus and Bifidobacterium species. It has been demonstrated that these microorganisms contribute to improved gut health and lipid metabolism.

Probiotic restoration is directly associated with improved lipid metabolism. Notably, LDL cholesterol levels are decreased in synbiotic users, indicating a positive impact on cardiovascular health.

10.4.2 Inflammation Reduction

Chronic inflammation is a key marker of metabolic illnesses and is closely linked to issues with lipid metabolism. The use of synbiotics reduces intestinal inflammation.

There is a connection between reduced inflammation and better lipid profiles. TGs, which are known to be harmful for heart disease, are decreased, whereas HDL cholesterol, also known as "good cholesterol," increases.

10.4.3 Enhanced Nutrient Absorption

Particular probiotics in the synbiotic formulation improve the bioavailability of the dietary lipids. This impact is assumed to be caused by the probiotics' ability to transform complex lipids into forms that are easier to absorb. Better meal absorption leads to improved lipid metabolism.

10.4.4 Combination Therapies

Combination of synbiotics with standard drugs prescribed for metabolic disorders has astounding results. The combined therapy works better than any one of the medications alone to improve lipid profiles. A significant increase in HDL cholesterol—often considered a protective factor against cardiovascular disease—and a rapid decrease in LDL cholesterol and TGs are observed in the synbiotic-medication combination group.

The synergistic effect of this revolutionary technique not only shows that metabolic disorders might be better managed, but it also opens up new avenues for optimizing treatment strategies. The quality of life for people with these conditions may be enhanced by this combination therapeutic approach.

10.4.5 Effects on Triglycerides

High levels of TGs can cause cardiac irregularities and a characteristic that characterizes metabolic disorders. TGs are demonstrated to have dropped with synbiotics treatment, which implies that synbiotics may improve cardiovascular health and may be a targeted approach to reducing this significant biomarker.

10.4.6 Pediatric Metabolic Health

Children who are at risk of developing metabolic illnesses may benefit from taking synbiotics as a preventative measure to reduce the disease's progression. The children lipid profiles improve as a result of the synbiotic supplementation, and it also improves their growth and development.

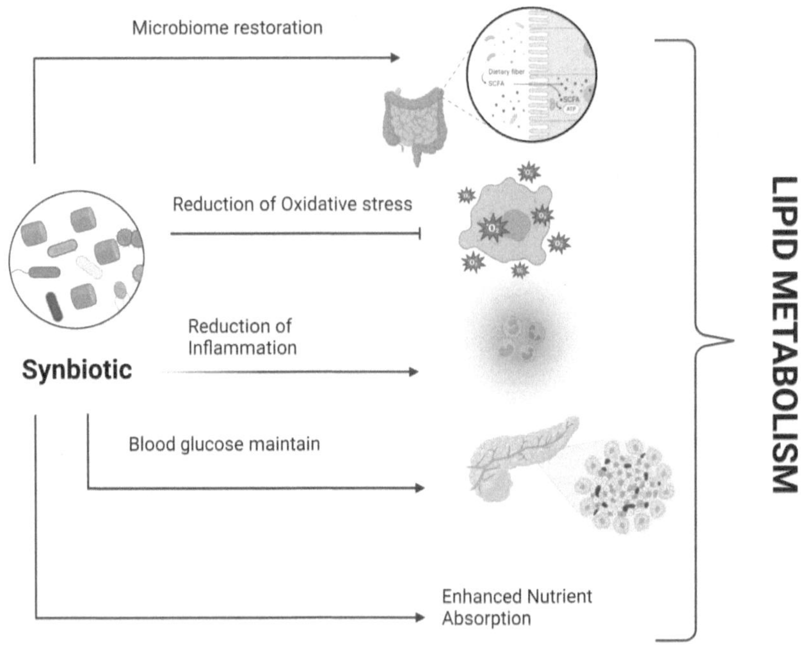

FIGURE 10.2 Effects of synbiotics on lipid metabolism through different pathways.

10.4.7 In Vivo Applications of Some Specific Synbiotics

10.4.7.1 Applications of Synbiotics in Lipid Metabolism in Humans

The application of synbiotics as functional food ingredients is an expanding field of study, with relatively few human trials investigating their effects on lipid metabolism. After three weeks of daily supplementation of a milk product consisting of *L. acidophilus* and fructo-oligosaccharides, in comparison to a control milk which was fermented by the traditional yogurt. There was a development in LDL: HDL cholesterol, which was a sign of improved cardiovascular health (Schaafsma et al., 1998) (Table 10.1).

A study by Kiessling et al. showed that after six weeks of drinking a milk product composed of *B. longum*, *L. acidophilus* as well as 1% OFS added, the total cholesterol levels of hypercholesterolemic women increased. Remarkably, neither TAG nor LDL-C levels were impacted by this alteration (Kiessling et al., 2002).

Another study reported a decrease in total cholesterol and LDL cholesterol in men and women, having high cholesterol after 10 weeks of supplementation of *L. gasseri* with inulin (Ooi et al., 2010). Notably, despite Ooi and his colleagues consuming 8.2 g less fructan daily, comparable decreases in LDL-C were recorded. The use of a varied Lactobacillus strain, a longer intervention period (3 vs. 12 weeks), and the inclusion of contributors who are hyperlipidemic may all contribute to similar findings.

A smoothie composed of *L. acidophilus* and inulin significantly reduced TAG levels and cholesterol in a trial including type II diabetic women by 26% and 37%, respectively (Moroti et al., 2012).

The majority of synbiotic research has mainly examined how they affect the structure of the gut microbiota. In a study involving healthy volunteers, Bifidobacterium sp. was administered for a period of twelve days. The participants were divided into two groups - one group received a fermented milk product containing 18 g of inulin daily, while the other group received no inulin (Bouhnik et al., 1996). According to the study's findings, giving probiotics—fermented milk products—significantly increased the amount of Bifidobacteria in the intestines. It's interesting to note that adding 18 g of inulin did not raise the proportion

TABLE 10.1
Synbiotic Impacts on Human Fasting Lipid Levels (Jackson & Lovegrove, 2012)

Synbiotic	Probiotic Strain	Change Observed
125 ml fermented milk product with 9 g OFS	L. acidophilus (DN 112.053/112.096)	4% reduction in TC, 5% reduction in LDL Cholesterol,
300g fermented milk product with 3 g OFS	*L. acidophilus* 145 and *B. longum 913*	24% increase in HDL Cholesterol
Fermented milk product (300 g) with1%OFS (~3 g)	L. acidophilus 145	10% increase in TC, 25% increase in HDL Cholesterol
Capsule-containing probiotic with 0.8 g inulin	*L. gasseri* and *B. longum*	8% decrease in TC, 9% Decrease in LDL Cholesterol
Shake (200 ml) with 2 g inulin	L. acidophilus B. Bifidum	26% decrease in TC, 37% decrease in TAG

any further. The patients treated with fermented milk product and inulin maintained their Bifidobacteria population compared to those who received only fermented milk product 2 weeks after the supplementation completion period, according to an assessment of gut microbiota composition (Grill et al., 1995).

A supplement containing *B. lactis* and Bifidum, coupled with a prebiotic containing inulin, was found to have boosted the overall number p of *B. lactis* and Bifidum, in a trial with aged people. Three weeks or more after the study's conclusion, at least one of these Bifidobacteria could still be found in fecal samples (Bartosch et al., 2005). This suggests that synbiotics might have further advantages, particularly for people whose gut microbiota is out of balance.

Additionally, eating a synbiotic including Bifidobacterium longum, Lactobacillus acidophilus, and OFS (0.5 g) for thirty days enhanced the metabolic activity of gut microorganisms significantly, according to a study done on healthy persons. According to Ndagijimana et al. (2009), there was a rise in a particular metabolite that positively connected with the quantity of Bifidobacteria in fecal samples. Although a high Bifidobacteria population in the gut is good for gut health in general, further research is still needed to determine how the synbiotic product affects the lipid profile during fasting.

10.4.7.2 Effects of Synbiotic Supplement (*Lactobacillus rhamnosus* KY3 & Cellobiose) on the Lipid Metabolism in Rats

A fermentative bacterium called Lactobacillus rhamnosus KY-3 is used in the commercial synthesis of L-lactic acid. Using a rat model, the effects of L. rhamnosus KY-3 synbiotics in conjunction with cellobiose on lipid metabolism were studied. For a period of 13 days, the rats were fed a diet that included 20% casein (C) with *Lactobacillus rhamnosus* KY3, Cellobiose, or a mixture of *Lactobacillus rhamnosus* KY3 and Cellobiose. The findings demonstrated that, as compared to rats on Casein, KY3 and Cellobiose, rats on KY3 and Cellobiose had significantly lower serum concentrations of total cholesterol, total lipids, phospholipids, and triacylglycerol.

Additionally, there was a notable increase in the weight of the cecal contents as well as the amounts of short-chain FAs (SCFA) in the cecum. Furthermore, when KY3 and Cellobiose were given concurrently, the dry weight of voided fecal matter increased additively. There were no appreciable variations in the amount of fecal bile acids excreted between the study's groups.

These results provide credence to the theory that lowering serum cholesterol levels may be facilitated by encouraging cecal fermentation. All things considered, these findings point to a beneficial effect on lipid metabolism from the concurrent administration of KY3 and Cellobiose (Umeki et al., 2004).

10.4.7.3 Role of Synbiotic in Glucose and Lipid Metabolism in Females Having Gestational Diabetes Mellitus

Glucose intolerance initially identified during pregnancy is the hallmark of gestational diabetes mellitus (GDM), which affects about 12.8% of pregnancies globally (Wan & Ma, 2022). Pregnancy-related concerns for women with GDM include eclampsia, shoulder dystocia, and cesarean sections. Furthermore, according to Homayouni et al. (2020), they have a higher chance of acquiring cardiovascular diseases, pancreatic cancer, and type 2 diabetes after giving birth. The developing fetus needs a lot of energy to grow throughout gestation, and about 80% of this energy comes from glucose. Placental blood vessels carry the fetus's blood glucose, which causes the fetal pancreas to secrete insulin and release insulin-like growth factors. These factors are important for organ development and for storing fat and glycogen to prevent glycemic imbalances in the newborn after birth (Mirabelli et al., 2021). Persistently high blood sugar levels in GDM may cause fetal insulin to increase over time, changing the hypothalamic response to glucose and perhaps causing IR and long-term mediobasal hypothalamus gliosis (Chandrasekaran et al., 2022). The increased risk of congenital abnormalities, neonatal hypoglycemia, obesity, cardiometabolic diseases, respiratory disorders, autism, and possibly neonatal mortality later in the newborn's life is a concern raised by this situation (Lowe et al., 2019). The health of women and their children is seriously endangered by GDM.

Studies have indicated a connection between the onset of GDM and a disturbance in gut microbiota (Wang et al., 2020). In late pregnancy, there is an increase in the Firmicutes: Bacteroidetes, and GDM is linked to decreased alpha diversity in the gut microbiota throughout mid- and late gestation (Davidson et al., 2021). IR, increased blood glucose, and fat mass formation are all associated with these pertaining to composition of gut microbiota (Liu et al., 2019). In addition, mothers of GDM who experience changes in the composition of their gut microbiota may pass on to their children long-term health consequences (Mahdizade et al., 2022).

Researchers have investigated a range of interventions, such as dietary modifications, exercise, combined diet and exercise programs, dietary supplements, and pharmaceutical management, in an effort to mitigate the adverse effects and reduce the risk factors associated with GDM (Rasmussen et al., 2020). Nonetheless, these interventions' supporting data have typically been assessed as having low to intermediate quality. In an effort to find new, safe, and effective population-level therapeutic approaches, recent research has identified indigestible foods known to promote and activate gut flora as synbiotics (Masulli et al., 2020). Research has shown that taking supplements containing synbiotics can help pregnant women by reducing IR and enhancing their lipid metabolism (Kunasegaran et al., 2021).

A comprehensive literature search covering the period from January 1, 2012 to November 1, 2022 was conducted using online databases, including the Cochrane Library, Web of Science, PubMed, and EBSCO. Eleven RCTs, or randomized controlled trials, in all were looked at.

The trial results showed that when probiotics and synbiotics were compared to a placebo, there were statistically significant improvements in HOMA-IR, FSI, TC, and FPG compared to several other parameters. In conclusion, there is evidence that in pregnant women having GDM, probiotics, and synbiotics may regulate glucose as well as lipid metabolism. According to Mu et al. (2023), this suggests that using specific probiotic supplements may be a good way to manage and prevent GDM.

10.4.7.4 Diet-Induced Obesity Can Be Prevented in Adulthood by Early Life Synbiotics

The metabolic status of adults is intricately connected to their gut microbiome. This symbiotic relationship between the host and the microbiome commences at birth, and disruptions in the early life microbiome can have enduring health consequences. We set out to investigate how interventions that positively influence the microbiome during early life can impact metabolic health in adulthood (Table 10.2).

Obesity is a multifaceted illness with broad health consequences (WHO Fact sheet, 2016). It is frequently associated with abnormalities in the management of glucose and fat, which increases the likelihood of developing illnesses like type 2 diabetes, cardiovascular disease, and fatty liver disease (Wilson et al., 2005). There is a direct correlation between person's metabolic condition and their gut microbiota, independent of dietary and environmental influences (Tremaroli et al., 2012). Throughout the early years of life, the gut microbiota develops dynamically under the influence of a variety of internal and external stimuli, with diet playing a critical role (Wopereis et al., 2014). Nowadays, it is widely accepted that an early postnatal diet has a significant and enduring influence on metabolic health (Adkins & Ozanne, 2011); this idea is frequently referred to as "nutritional programming." For example, compared to their formula-fed counterparts, breastfed individuals had a higher prevalence of beneficial Bifidobacteria and lower risk of glucose intolerance and obesity as well as elevated cholesterol levels in adulthood (Nauta et al., 2013). Antibiotic exposure during infancy can interfere with gut microbiota's maturation, decreasing the number of Bifidobacterium and increasing the risk of obesity in later life (Azad et al., 2014). These findings highlight the possibility of purposefully modifying the gut microbiota during infancy to reduce the likelihood of obesity as well as metabolic diseases in later life.

Up until postnatal (PN) day 42, postnatal meals were supplemented with synbiotics and prebiotics. For dietary programming, a reliable rodent model was created. After that, the mice were fed with Western-style diet (WSD) that was heavy in fat for eight weeks.

Throughout the study, changes in body weight and composition were closely observed as well as alterations in composition of gut microbiota at PN21, PN42, and PN98. In addition, various markers were assessed, related to glucose regulation, lipid metabolism, and conducted transcriptomic analyses of six target tissues during adulthood (PN98).

It was observed that early life synbiotic interventions provided protective effects in mice against excessive fat accumulation induced by a WSD, and this effect was consistent across two independent animal facilities in Europe. These interventions led to improved insulin sensitivity and a reduction in dyslipidemia in adulthood. The most significant alterations in gene expression were observed in the ileum. Additionally, an enhanced abundance of Bifidobacterium was observed in both early life and adulthood (Mischke et al., 2018).

TABLE 10.2
Findings of the Meta-Analysis on Effects of Synbiotics on Glucose and Lipid Metabolism in Females with Gestational Diabetes Mellitus (Mu et al., 2023)

Parameters	Significant Improvement
HOMA-1R	YES
FPG (mg/dL)	YES
QUICKI	NO
FSI (mg/dL)	YES
HDL cholesterol (mg/dL)	NO
LDL cholesterol (mg/dL)	NO
TC (mg/dL)	YES
GWG (kg)	NO
TG (mg/dL)	NO

10.4.7.5 Promotion of Glucose and Lipid Metabolism in Adulthood by Early Life Synbiotics

In order to ascertain if improved metabolic characteristics were also associated with protection against obesity, the HOMA-IR index was evaluated as a proxy for IR. The findings suggested that the SYN group had improved insulin sensitivity since they showed a tendency toward lower HOMA-IR in comparison to the CTRL group. While the levels of fasting glucose did not have any difference between the groups, the SYN group's lower insulin levels relative to the CTRL group were the main cause of this impact. TG plasma levels were comparable across all WSD-challenged groups, while total plasma cholesterol significantly decreased in the SYN group when compared to the CTRL group, matching levels in the REF group. In addition, higher beta-hydroxybutyrate plasma levels were found in the SYN group as compared to the CTRL group, suggesting more FA oxidation. This rise may be linked to enhanced glucose metabolism and protection against obesity.

Reductions in liver weight and hepatic TG content were similarly linked to improvements in adult plasma parameters brought about by early life synbiotic treatment. These findings suggest that improvements in metabolism, particularly glucose and lipid homeostasis indices, are associated with the preventive effect of synbiotic supplementation against obesity.

10.4.7.6 Alteration of Cholesterol Metabolism in Ileum in Adulthood by Early Life Synbiotics

In comparison to the CTRL group, six relevant tissues were harvested on PN98 and subjected to microarray analysis in order to explore the possible molecular mechanisms behind the effects of synbiotics in early life retained in the long run. These tissues included the duodenum, jejunum, ileum, colon, liver, and white adipose tissue. Comparing SYN vs. CTRL revealed differential regulation ($q \leq 0.05$) of 144 genes in the ileum. Of these genes, the SYN group showed comparatively lower expression of 57% of them than the CTRL group did. On the other hand in a comparison between synbiotic vs control group, no tissues showed differentially expressed genes after FDR adjustment, indicating that the most substantial effect on ileal gene expression in adults comes from early life synbiotic supplementation.

Ingenuity pathway analysis (IPA) was performed on differentially expressed genes ($q \leq 0.05$) to uncover regulated biological processes and canonical pathways in the ileum for the SYN vs. CTRL comparison. In comparison to the CTRL group, "lipid metabolism" was shown to be among the most tightly controlled biological processes in the ileum of adult mice that had received early life synbiotic supplements. The four most strongly regulated canonical pathways—"Superpathway of cholesterol biosynthesis"; "LPS/IL-1 mediated inhibition of RXR," which is linked to the regulation of lipid, cholesterol, and xenobiotic metabolism; "Zymosterol Biosynthesis," which aids in the biosynthesis of cholesterol; and "LXR/RXR activation," which is also connected to the metabolism of lipids and cholesterol—corroborated this. This suggests that after early life synbiotic supplementation, lipid and cholesterol metabolism are the most highly controlled processes in adult mice.

Focus was placed on gene sets associated with cholesterol metabolism and fate, including biosynthesis, esterification, transport, distribution, and control, in order to look into this more. Interestingly, in the comparison of synbiotic vs control group, 6 of the 31 genes that were chosen showed a substantial degree of regulation ($q \leq 0.05$), with the remaining genes displaying a similar trend of regulation. In comparison to the CTRL group, adult mice receiving early life synbiotic supplementation showed upregulation of gene sets linked to cholesterol biosynthesis. On the other hand, the SYN group exhibited down-regulation of genes associated with cholesterol storage, distribution, and excretion, compared to the control group. In conclusion, compared to CTRL animals receiving a WSD, early life synbiotic supplementation resulted in the expression of genes involved in intestinal cholesterol synthesis and uptake in adult mice's ileal cells.

Collectively, these findings provided an insight into the role of early life synbiotics in development of gut microbiota and the potential of synbiotics to improve cholesterol metabolism in adult life (Mischke et al., 2018).

10.5 THE WAY FORWARD

There are several key areas that need more research and potential therapeutic applications as we continue to investigate the fascinating science of synbiotics and their potential to revolutionize the treatment of metabolic disorders by regulating lipid metabolism:

10.5.1 Personalized Approaches

Individual differences exist in the degree to which synbiotics can regulate lipid metabolism. Subsequent research ought to focus on customized approaches, tailoring synbiotic therapies to an individual's distinct genetic composition, metabolic characteristics, and gut microbiome composition. People with metabolic illnesses may benefit and get the greatest outcomes with this tailored strategy.

10.5.2 Dietary Incorporation

It makes sense to look at the synbiotic supplements and dietary modifications together. A synergistic effect that enhances the therapeutic effects on lipid metabolism may result from combining a synbiotic regimen with a diet rich in gut-healthy foods, such as fermented foods and fiber. Customized diet plans may prove to be an essential part in treating metabolic diseases.

10.5.3 Long-Term Results

Longer follow-up periods are required to assess the long-term effects of synbiotic therapy, notwithstanding the positive short-term results of previous trials. It's critical to investigate if synbiotics can prevent the progression of metabolic illnesses as well as how their benefits change over time.

10.5.4 Mechanistic Perspectives

Understanding the intricate processes by which synbiotics influence lipid metabolism is crucial. Further studies should explore the molecular mechanisms and metabolic pathways underlying these effects. This expanded understanding could aid in the development of more concentrated and effective synbiotic formulations.

10.5.5 Clinical Recommendations

As the evidence for treating metabolic disorders with synbiotics increases, clinical recommendations need to be defined. Medical professionals would find it easier to prescribe synbiotics to patients with metabolic disorders if they followed these recommendations, which contain details on dosages, duration of administration, and potential interactions with other drugs.

10.5.6 Regulatory Approvals

Synbiotics cannot be included into conventional medical procedures without regulatory approval. Establishing a system that will guarantee the safe and effective use of synbiotics as a therapeutic strategy will require collaboration between regulatory bodies, healthcare facilities, and researchers.

10.5.7 Patient Awareness

It is imperative to educate patients about the potential benefits of synbiotics and how they impact lipid metabolism regulation. Enabling individuals with metabolic diseases to make informed decisions about their health, including dietary and supplement choices, may lead to better outcomes.

In summary, "The way forward" in the domains of synbiotics and lipid metabolism offers a plethora of prospects for enhancing the management of metabolic disorders. The process includes more research, customized approaches, long-term assessments, and the application of findings to therapeutic practice. As we continue along this path, the potential to improve metabolic health and the lives of those with metabolic disorders offers hope for a healthier future.

REFERENCES

Ashique, S., Afzal, O., Hussain, A., Zeyaullah, M., Altamimi, M. A., Mishra, N., ... & Anand, K. It's all about plant derived natural phytoconstituents and phytonanomedicine to control skin cancer. *Journal of Drug Delivery Science and Technology*, 2023, 84, 104495.

Ashique, S., Faruk, A., Ahmad, F. J., Khan, T., & Mishra, N. It is all about probiotics to control cervical cancer. *Probiotics and Antimicrobial Proteins*, 2023, 1–14, doi: 10.1007/s12602-023-10183-2

Ashique, S., Garg, A., Bhatt, S., Sirohi, E., Fatima, N., Bajwa, N., ... & Mishra, N. (2023). Synbiotics in cervical cancer. In *Synbiotics for the Management of Cancer* (pp. 135–155). Singapore: Springer Nature Singapore.

Ashique, S., Mishra, N., Garg, A., Sibuh, B. Z., Taneja, P., Rai, G., ... & Gupta, P. K. (2023). Recent updates on correlation between reactive oxygen species and synbiotics for effective management of ulcerative colitis. *Frontiers in Nutrition*, *10*, 1126579.

Azad, M. B., Bridgman, S. L., Becker, A. B., & Kozyrskyj, A. L. (2014). Infant antibiotic exposure and the development of childhood overweight and central adiposity. *International journal of Obesity*, *38*(10), 1290–1298.

Bartosch, S., Woodmansey, E. J., Paterson, J. C., McMurdo, M. E., & Macfarlane, G. T. (2005). Microbiological effects of consuming a synbiotic containing Bifidobacterium bifidum, Bifidobacterium lactis, and oligofructose in elderly persons, determined by real-time polymerase chain reaction and counting of viable bacteria. *Clinical Infectious Diseases*, *40*(1), 28–37.

Bouhnik, Y., Flourie, B., Andrieux, C., Bisetti, N., Briet, F., & Rambaud, J. C. (1996). Effects of Bifidobacterium sp fermented milk ingested with or without inulin on colonic bifidobacteria and enzymatic activities in healthy humans. *European Journal of Clinical Nutrition*, *50*(4), 269–273.

Cena, H., & Calder, P. C. (2020). Defining a healthy diet: evidence for the role of contemporary dietary patterns in health and disease. *Nutrients*, *12*(2), 334.

Cena, H., & Calder, P. C. (2020). Defining a healthy diet: evidence for the role of contemporary dietary patterns in health and disease. *Nutrients*, *12*(2), 334.

Davidson, S. J., Barrett, H. L., Price, S. A., Callaway, L. K., & Nitert, M. D. (2021). Probiotics for preventing gestational diabetes. *Cochrane Database of Systematic Reviews*, (4), CD009951.

Denisenko, Y. K., Kytikova, O. Y., Novgorodtseva, T. P., Antonyuk, M. V., Gvozdenko, T. A., & Kantur, T. A. (2020). Lipid-induced mechanisms of metabolic syndrome. *Journal of Obesity*, *2020*, 5762395.

DiBaise, J. K., Zhang, H., Crowell, M. D., Krajmalnik-Brown, R., Decker, G. A., & Rittmann, B. E. (2008, April). Gut microbiota and its possible relationship with obesity. *Mayo Clinic Proceedings*, *83*(4), 460–469.

Doğan, E. S. K., Doğan, B., Fentoğlu, Ö., & Kırzıoğlu, F. Y. (2019). The role of serum lipoxin A4 levels in the association between periodontal disease and metabolic syndrome. *Journal of Periodontal & Implant Science*, *49*(2), 105–113.

Ghazalpour, A., Cespedes, I., Bennett, B. J., & Allayee, H. (2016). Expanding role of gut microbiota in lipid metabolism. *Current Opinion in Lipidology*, *27*(2), 141.

Grill, J. P., Manginot-Dürr, C., Schneider, F., & Ballongue, J. (1995). Bifidobacteria and probiotic effects: action of Bifidobacterium species on conjugated bile salts. *Current Microbiology*, *31*, 23–27.

Headland, S. E., & Norling, L. V. (2015, May). The resolution of inflammation: principles and challenges. *Seminars in Immunology*, 27(3), 149–160.

Homayouni, A., Bagheri, N., Mohammad-Alizadeh-Charandabi, S., Kashani, N., Mobaraki-Asl, N., Mirghafurvand, M., ... & Pourjafar, H. (2020). Prevention of gestational diabetes mellitus (GDM) and probiotics: mechanism of action: a review. *Current Diabetes Reviews*, *16*(6), 538–545.

Hou, C., Zhang, W., Li, J., Du, L., Lv, O., Zhao, S., & Li, J. (2019). Beneficial effects of pomegranate on lipid metabolism in metabolic disorders. *Molecular Nutrition & Food Research*, *63*(16), 1800773.

Hur, K. Y., & Lee, M. S. (2015). Gut microbiota and metabolic disorders. *Diabetes & Metabolism Journal*, *39*(3), 198–203.

Jackson, K. G., & Lovegrove, J. A. (2012). Impact of probiotics, prebiotics and synbiotics on lipid metabolism in humans. *Nutrition and Aging*, *1*(3–4), 181–200.

Kiessling, G., Schneider, J., & Jahreis, G. (2002). Long-term consumption of fermented dairy products over 6 months increases HDL cholesterol. *European Journal of Clinical Nutrition*, *56*(9), 843–849.

Kunasegaran, T., Balasubramaniam, V. R., Arasoo, V. J. T., Palanisamy, U. D., & Ramadas, A. (2021). The modulation of gut microbiota composition in the pathophysiology of gestational diabetes mellitus: a systematic review. *Biology*, *10*(10), 1027.

Kwon, Y. (2020). Immuno-resolving ability of resolvins, protectins, and maresins derived from omega-3 fatty acids in metabolic syndrome. *Molecular Nutrition & Food Research*, *64*(4), 1900824.

Kytikova, O. Y., Novgorodtseva, T. P., Antonyuk, M. V., & Gvozdenko, T. A. (2019). Plasmalogenes in the pathophysiology and therapy of age-specific diseases. *Advances in Gerontology = Uspekhi Gerontologii*, *32*(6), 948–958.

Lattimer, J. M., & Haub, M. D. (2010). Effects of dietary fiber and its components on metabolic health. *Nutrients*, *2*(12), 1266–1289.

Lee, M. K., Han, K., Kim, M. K., Koh, E. S., Kim, E. S., Nam, G. E., & Kwon, H. S. (2020). Changes in metabolic syndrome and its components and the risk of type 2 diabetes: a nationwide cohort study. Scientific Reports, *10*(1), 2313.

Liu, H., Pan, L. L., Lv, S., Yang, Q., Zhang, H., Chen, W., ... & Sun, J. (2019). Alterations of gut microbiota and blood lipidome in gestational diabetes mellitus with hyperlipidemia. Frontiers in Physiology, 10, 1015.

Lowe Jr, W. L., Scholtens, D. M., Kuang, A., Linder, B., Lawrence, J. M., Lebenthal, Y., ... & Metzger, B. E. (2019). Hyperglycemia and adverse pregnancy outcome follow-up study (HAPO FUS): maternal gestational diabetes mellitus and childhood glucose metabolism. Diabetes Care, *42*(3), 372–380.

Mahdizade Ari, M., Teymouri, S., Fazlalian, T., Asadollahi, P., Afifirad, R., Sabaghan, M., ... & Darbandi, A. (2022). The effect of probiotics on gestational diabetes and its complications in pregnant mother and newborn: a systematic review and meta-analysis during 2010-2020. *Journal of Clinical Laboratory Analysis*, *36*(4), e24326.

Masulli, M., Vitacolonna, E., Fraticelli, F., Della Pepa, G., Mannucci, E., & Monami, M. (2020). Effects of probiotic supplementation during pregnancy on metabolic outcomes: a systematic review and meta-analysis of randomized controlled trials. Diabetes Research and Clinical Practice, 162, 108111.

Mirabelli, M., Chiefari, E., Tocci, V., Greco, E., Foti, D., & Brunetti, A. (2021). Gestational diabetes: implications for fetal growth, intervention timing, and treatment options. *Current Opinion in Pharmacology*, *60*, 1–10.

Monnerie, S., Comte, B., Ziegler, D., Morais, J. A., Pujos-Guillot, E., & Gaudreau, P. (2020). Metabolomic and lipidomic signatures of metabolic syndrome and its physiological components in adults: a systematic review. Scientific Reports, *10*(1), 669.

Monnerie, S., Comte, B., Ziegler, D., Morais, J. A., Pujos-Guillot, E., & Gaudreau, P. (2020). Metabolomic and lipidomic signatures of metabolic syndrome and its physiological components in adults: a systematic review. Scientific Reports, *10*(1), 669.

Moroti, C., Souza Magri, L. F., de Rezende Costa, M., Cavallini, D. C., & Sivieri, K. (2012). Effect of the consumption of a new symbiotic shake on glycemia and cholesterol levels in elderly people with type 2 diabetes mellitus. *Lipids in Health and Disease*, *11*, 1–8.

Mu, J., Guo, X., Zhou, Y., & Cao, G. (2023). The effects of probiotics/synbiotics on glucose and lipid metabolism in women with gestational diabetes mellitus: A meta-analysis of randomized controlled trials. Nutrients, 15(6), 1375.

Natesan, V., & Kim, S. J. (2021). Lipid metabolism, disorders and therapeutic drugs-review. *Biomolecules & Therapeutics*, *29*(6), 596.

Natesan, V., & Kim, S. J. (2021). Lipid metabolism, disorders and therapeutic drugs-review. *Biomolecules & Therapeutics*, *29*(6), 596.

Nauta, A. J., Ben Amor, K., Knol, J., Garssen, J., & Van der Beek, E. M. (2013). Relevance of pre-and postnatal nutrition to development and interplay between the microbiota and metabolic and immune systems. *The American Journal of Clinical Nutrition*, *98*(2), 586S–593S.

Ndagijimana, M., Laghi, L., Vitali, B., Placucci, G., Brigidi, P., & Guerzoni, M. E. (2009). Effect of a synbiotic food consumption on human gut metabolic profiles evaluated by 1H nuclear magnetic resonance spectroscopy. *International Journal of Food Microbiology*, *134*(1–2), 147–153.

Novgorodtseva, T. P., Karaman, Y. K., Zhukova, N. V., Lobanova, E. G., Antonyuk, M. V., & Kantur, T. A. (2011). Composition of fatty acids in plasma and erythrocytes and eicosanoids level in patients with metabolic syndrome. *Lipids in Health and Disease*, *10*, 1–5.

Obesity, W. H. O. (2016). overweight. Fact sheet N 311. Updated January 2015. *Dostupno na: https://www. who. int/mediacentre/factsheets/fs311/en/Pristupljeno, 24.*

Ooi, L. G., Ahmad, R., Yuen, K. H., & Liong, M. T. (2010). Lactobacillus acidophilus CHO-220 and inulin reduced plasma total cholesterol and low-density lipoprotein cholesterol via alteration of lipid transporters. *Journal of Dairy Science*, *93*(11), 5048–5058.

Pischon, T., Nöthlings, U., & Boeing, H. (2008). Obesity and cancer: symposium on 'Diet and cancer'. *Proceedings of the Nutrition Society*, *67*(2), 128–145.

Rasmussen, L., Poulsen, C. W., Kampmann, U., Smedegaard, S. B., Ovesen, P. G., & Fuglsang, J. (2020). Diet and healthy lifestyle in the management of gestational diabetes mellitus. *Nutrients*, *12*(10), 3050.

Reddy, P., Lent-Schochet, D., Ramakrishnan, N., McLaughlin, M., & Jialal, I. (2019). Metabolic syndrome is an inflammatory disorder: a conspiracy between adipose tissue and phagocytes. *Clinica Chimica Acta*, *496*, 35–44.

Schaafsma, G., Meuling, W. J. A., Van Dokkum, W., & Bouley, C. (1998). Effects of a milk product, fermented by Lactobacillus acidophilus and with fructo-oligosaccharides added, on blood lipids in male volunteers. *European Journal of Clinical Nutrition*, *52*(6), 436–440.

Solomon, M., & Muro, S. (2017). Lysosomal enzyme replacement therapies: historical development, clinical outcomes, and future perspectives. *Advanced Drug Delivery Reviews*, *118*, 109–134.

Tarry-Adkins, J. L., & Ozanne, S. E. (2011). Mechanisms of early life programming: current knowledge and future directions. *The American Journal of Clinical Nutrition*, *94*(suppl_6), 1765S–1771S.

Tocher, D. R. (2003). Metabolism and functions of lipids and fatty acids in teleost fish. *Reviews in Fisheries Science*, *11*(2), 107–184.

Tortosa-Caparrós, E., Navas-Carrillo, D., Marín, F., & Orenes-Piñero, E. (2017). Anti-inflammatory effects of omega 3 and omega 6 polyunsaturated fatty acids in cardiovascular disease and metabolic syndrome. *Critical Reviews in Food Science and Nutrition*, *57*(16), 3421–3429.

Tremaroli, V., & Bäckhed, F. (2012). Functional interactions between the gut microbiota and host metabolism. *Nature*, *489*(7415), 242–249.

Umeki, M., Oue, K., MOc HIZUKI, S., Shirai, Y., & Sakai, K. (2004). Effect of Lactobacillus rhamnosus KY-3 and cellobiose as synbiotics on lipid metabolism in rats. *Journal of Nutritional Science and Vitaminology*, *50*(5), 330–334.

Vázquez-Jiménez, J. G., Roura-Guiberna, A., Jiménez-Mena, L. R., & Olivares-Reyes, J. A. (2017). Role of free fatty acids on insulin resistance. Gaceta medica de Mexico, *153*, 773–783.

Wan, J., & Ma, J. (2022). Efficacy of dietary supplements targeting gut microbiota in the prevention and treatment of gestational diabetes mellitus. *Frontiers in Microbiology*, *13*,

Wang, X., Liu, H., Li, Y., Huang, S., Zhang, L., Cao, C., ... & Qi, H. (2020). Altered gut bacterial and metabolic signatures and their interaction in gestational diabetes mellitus. Gut Microbes, *12*(1), 1840765.

Wilson, P. W., D'Agostino, R. B., Parise, H., Sullivan, L., & Meigs, J. B. (2005). Metabolic syndrome as a precursor of cardiovascular disease and type 2 diabetes mellitus. *Circulation*, *112*(20), 3066–3072.

Wopereis, H., Oozeer, R., Knipping, K., Belzer, C., & Knol, J. (2014). The first thousand days-intestinal microbiology of early life: establishing a symbiosis. *Pediatric Allergy and Immunology*, *25*(5), 428–438.

11 Probiotics, Prebiotics, and Postbiotics on Metabolic Diseases Targeting Gut Microbiota

Priyanka Ray, Mohammad Abdul Faseeh, Debojyoti Adak, and Himanshu Sharma

11.1 INTRODUCTION

Metabolic disorders have become worldwide epidemics and pose a major danger to public health, including obesity, cardiovascular disease, and type 2 diabetes. Sedentary behavior and poor dietary choices are two lifestyle factors that are often linked to chronic disorders (Li et al., 2021). However, new research has shown how crucial the gut microbiota is to the development and progression of metabolic diseases (Lanthier and Delzenne, 2022). The gut microbiota, a complex community of billions of bacteria that reside in the human digestive tract, has a substantial influence on inflammation, energy balance, food metabolism, and overall metabolic homeostasis (Bourebaba et al., 2022). Recent studies have shown that dysbiosis—an imbalance in the composition and activity of the gut microbiota—is strongly associated with metabolic diseases (Oh et al., 2022). Dysbiosis has been linked to the development of several illnesses, including increased inflammation, insulin resistance, altered lipid metabolism, and impaired appetite control (Ojeda et al., 2016). Because of this, therapies that target the gut microbiota, such as probiotics, prebiotics, and postbiotics, have generated a lot of attention as practical ways to lower the prevalence of metabolic illnesses (Xavier-Santos et al., 2020). Żółkiewicz et al. (2020) define probiotics as live bacteria that, when administered in enough amounts, benefit the host's health. According to Vallianou et al. (2020), they could positively affect the composition and function of the gut microbiota, which might reduce inflammation and improve metabolic parameters. Prebiotics are inactive food components that particularly enhance the growth and activity of beneficial gut flora, aiding in the restoration of a balanced microbiota (Huang et al., 2022). By strengthening the intestinal barrier and altering the immune system, postbiotics may enhance metabolic health (Kaur et al., 2021). This chapter summarizes and analyzes the current state of research on probiotics, prebiotics, and postbiotics in the context of metabolic diseases, with a focus on their effects on the gut microbiota and associated processes (Park et al., 2022). The study aims to explore the potential of these medicines in mitigating metabolic disorders by restoring the balance of gut microbiota, reducing inflammation, and improving metabolic parameters (Huang et al., 2022). Additionally, it will assess the safety, efficacy, and potential future directions of these medicines, offering insights into their potential value in the treatment and prevention of metabolic disorders (Cuevas-Sierra et al., 2015).

11.2 GUT MICROBIOTA AND METABOLIC DISEASES

The gastrointestinal tract is home to a complex collection of microorganisms called the gut microbiota, which are mostly bacteria (Arora and Bäckhed, 2016). With hundreds of species, it creates a dynamic ecosystem with a special makeup and purpose (Shi et al., 2022). Numerous variables impact the gut microbiota, such as genetics, age, nutrition, and environmental exposures (Hernández-Ceballos et al., 2021). Its many roles include the manufacture of beneficial chemicals, the fermentation of dietary fibers, and the control of immunological responses (D'Aversa et al., 2013).

11.2.1 Gut Microbiota and Metabolic Diseases

According to Cani and Delzenne (2009), the gut microbiota is a fascinating and intricately balanced colony of bacteria that inhabit the human digestive system. A diverse community of bacteria, viruses, fungi, and other microbes make up the digestive system (Pascale et al., 2018). The gut microbiota, which is made up of billions of different microorganisms, is crucial to maintaining human health since it performs several immunological, metabolic, and digestive processes (Fan and Pedersen, 2021). Gálvez-Ontiveros et al. (2020) state that a person's genetics, diet, lifestyle, and exposure to the environment all affect the composition of their gut microbiota. The gut microbiome is critical to metabolic health because of its functions in nutrition metabolism, energy regulation, and the synthesis of bioactive compounds. Numerous metabolic processes in the host are impacted, including immune responses, energy balance regulation, and the uptake and use of nutrients. According to Wang et al. (2020), this microbial community produces a dynamic, ever-evolving ecosystem that responds to external stimuli like as food changes and medication interactions.

DOI: 10.1201/9781032702438-11

11.2.2 Gut Microbiota Dysbiosis and Metabolic Disorders

A disruption in the balance and composition of the gut microbiota, known as dysbiosis, has emerged as a critical factor in the development of various metabolic disorders (Erejuwa et al., 2014). Dysbiosis can occur due to factors like poor diet, overuse of antibiotics, stress, and sedentary lifestyle, leading to an imbalance in beneficial and harmful microbes. This microbial imbalance can promote inflammation, oxidative stress, and metabolic disturbances, which are central to the pathogenesis of metabolic diseases (Burcelin et al., 2015). Dysbiosis is associated with conditions such as obesity, type 2 diabetes, and cardiovascular diseases (Carding et al., 2015). In obese individuals, for instance, there is often a shift in the gut microbiota composition, characterized by a decrease in beneficial bacteria and an increase in potentially harmful microbes (Fukuda and Ohno, 2014). This imbalance can contribute to chronic inflammation and insulin resistance, key drivers of metabolic disorders (Dutta et al., 2019).

11.2.3 The Gut–Brain Axis in Metabolic Health

Through the gut–brain axis, the central nervous system and the gastrointestinal tract can communicate with one another in both ways (Grasset and Burcelin, 2019). This intricate web of impulses and data may allow the stomach and brain to interact with one another. According to Heijboer et al. (2006), the gut–brain axis controls appetite, energy balance, and metabolic processes in connection to metabolic health. The gut microbiota is a crucial intermediary in this communication network. The gut–brain axis can be impacted by it through several mechanisms, such as neurotransmitter production and gut hormone control. According to Moser et al. (2022), microbial signals have the capability to influence hunger and satiety, hence modifying food choices and the total energy equilibrium. Unbalances in gut microbiota can upset the gut–brain axis, which can lead to abnormalities in appetite regulation and metabolic diseases (Wachsmuth et al., 2022). Research in this area, according to Mishra et al. (2021), may help to clarify how gut microbiota-targeting treatments, such as probiotics and prebiotics, may affect metabolic health by reestablishing the homeostasis of the gut–brain axis and improving hunger control. Understanding this intricate interplay is crucial for managing metabolic diseases.

11.3 PROBIOTICS: GUARDIANS OF GUT HEALTH

When consumed in adequate proportions, probiotics, often known as "guardians of gut health," are live bacteria that offer several health benefits. They have a critical role in maintaining and sustaining healthy, strong gut flora. Derived from the Greek terms "pro" (meaning "for") and "bios" (meaning "life"), the term "probiotics" emphasizes how these microbes help to improve life via the gastrointestinal system (Zhou and Hong, 2023).

11.3.1 Definition and Classification of Probiotics

These beneficial bacteria, also referred to as "good bacteria," are an integral part of the gut microbiota and support the maintenance of a balanced and healthy gut environment. Probiotics can be found in nutritional supplements as well as naturally occurring in some fermented foods such as kefir, sauerkraut, and yogurt (Simmering and Blaut, 2001). Though there are numerous varieties of probiotics, lactobacilli and bifidobacteria are the most often used types. Because different probiotic strains may have distinct modes of action and health effects, it is important to consider the specific strains used in various products and research (Nerlich and Koteyko, 2008).

11.3.2 Mechanisms of Probiotic Action

Probiotics influence the gut microbiota and its interactions with the host, which is one of the main ways in which they promote health (Oelschlaeger, 2010). Probiotics function through many pathways. Figure 11.1 shows the schematic depiction of the prebiotics' mode of action. By battling bad bacteria for resources and adherence sites, probiotics aid in the maintenance of a balanced gut microbiota and stop pathogenic microorganisms from growing out of control. In addition to their potential benefits for gut health and the host's metabolism, probiotics can also create bioactive substances such as short-chain fatty acids (SCFAs) and antimicrobial peptides. By affecting the host's immunological responses and assisting in the reduction of inflammation, probiotics interact with the gut-associated lymphoid tissue. Intestinal leakage of toxic compounds into the circulation is a phenomenon commonly linked to inflammatory and metabolic illnesses. Probiotics may fortify the intestinal barrier and prevent this from happening.

11.3.3 Probiotic Strains and Their Metabolic Effects

Probiotics may affect metabolism differently depending on the specific strains used. A number of probiotic strains have shown promise in lowering metabolic disorders including obesity and type 2 diabetes, according to Østlie et al. (2003). For example, certain strains of lactobacilli and bifidobacteria have been associated with improved insulin sensitivity, reduced inflammation, and improved weight control. Probiotics may affect the host's metabolism via altering the composition of the gut microbiota, boosting the creation of molecules that are beneficial to metabolism, and reducing inflammation (LeBlanc et al., 2017). There is still more research to be done on how they affect metabolism, and various strains may affect different metabolic indicators differently.

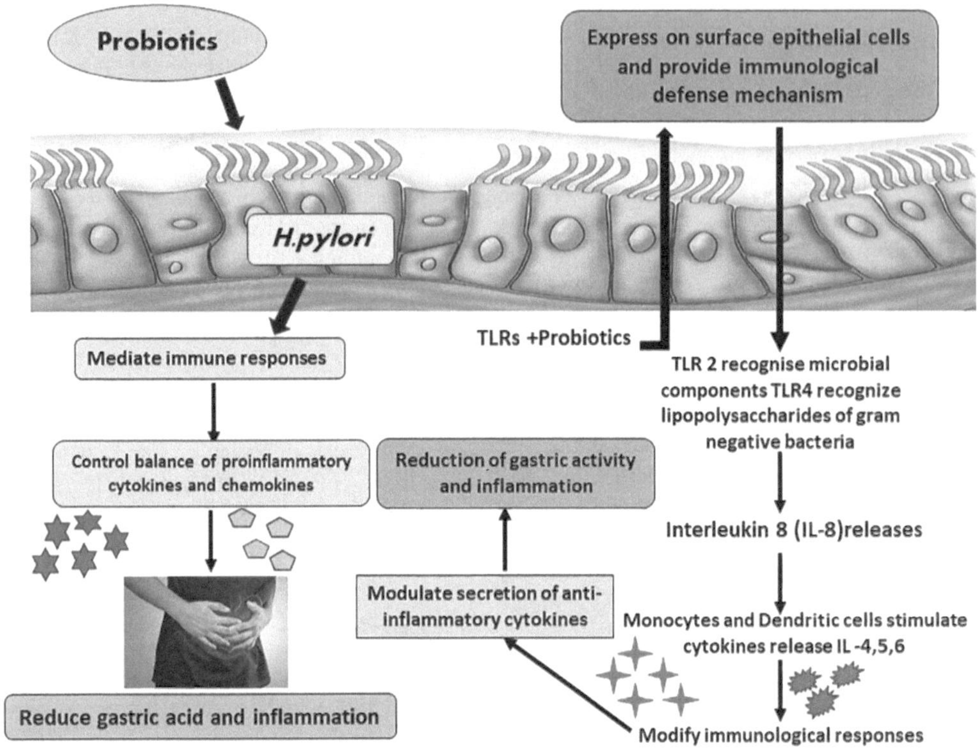

FIGURE 11.1 Mechanism of action of probiotics.

11.3.4 Clinical Applications and Evidence

There is growing interest in the potential use of probiotics to enhance metabolic health in clinical settings. Research suggests that probiotics may aid in the management of a number of illnesses, such as non-alcoholic fatty liver disease, type 2 diabetes, and obesity. While research results vary, some have shown promising effects, such as reduced body weight, improved insulin sensitivity, and decreased levels of inflammatory markers (Gogineni et al., 2013). Probiotics are often offered for sale in a range of formats, including fermented foods, powders, and tablets. Those who wish to enhance their metabolic health might take probiotics as a dietary supplement or add them to their cuisine. It's crucial to keep in mind that the ideal probiotic strains and dosage for each individual should be determined by their specific needs and health goals. Further research and clinical investigations are needed to completely understand the potential of probiotics in improving metabolic health (Aureli et al., 2011).

11.4 PREBIOTICS: FUELING BENEFICIAL BACTERIA

Since probiotics support the maintenance of a healthy and balanced digestive system, they are frequently discussed in relation to gut health. Even nevertheless, prebiotics—a less well-known hero—are subtly assisting these beneficial microbes (Appanna and Appanna, 2018). These nondigestible fibers are necessary for the growth and nutrition of probiotics, which in turn promotes gut health and overall wellness. A schematic representation of the prebiotics' method of action is presented in Figure 11.2.

11.4.1 Understanding Prebiotics

Prebiotics are dietary fibers of a kind that the body is unable to digest. Rather from being broken down, these fibers end up in the colon, where they feed the billions of bacteria that inhabit the digestive system (Bindels et al., 2015). Prebiotics are largely used to support the growth and activity of beneficial bacteria, such as Bifidobacteria and Lactobacilli. Prebiotics are found in many different foods, so it's easy to incorporate them into a balanced diet. Chicory root, a potent prebiotic with a high inulin content that may be added to a range of meals or taken as a supplement, is one of the most well-known sources. These aromatic vegetables include a kind of prebiotic fiber called fructans, which helps to support the growth of healthy bacteria. Particularly rich in Fructooligosaccharides (FOS), which nourish bacteria, are ripe bananas. A great source of inulin, asparagus, also provides several other essential nutrients and prebiotic support. Oats, barley, and whole wheat are rich in prebiotics, which support the maintenance of a diverse and balanced microbiota in the gut.

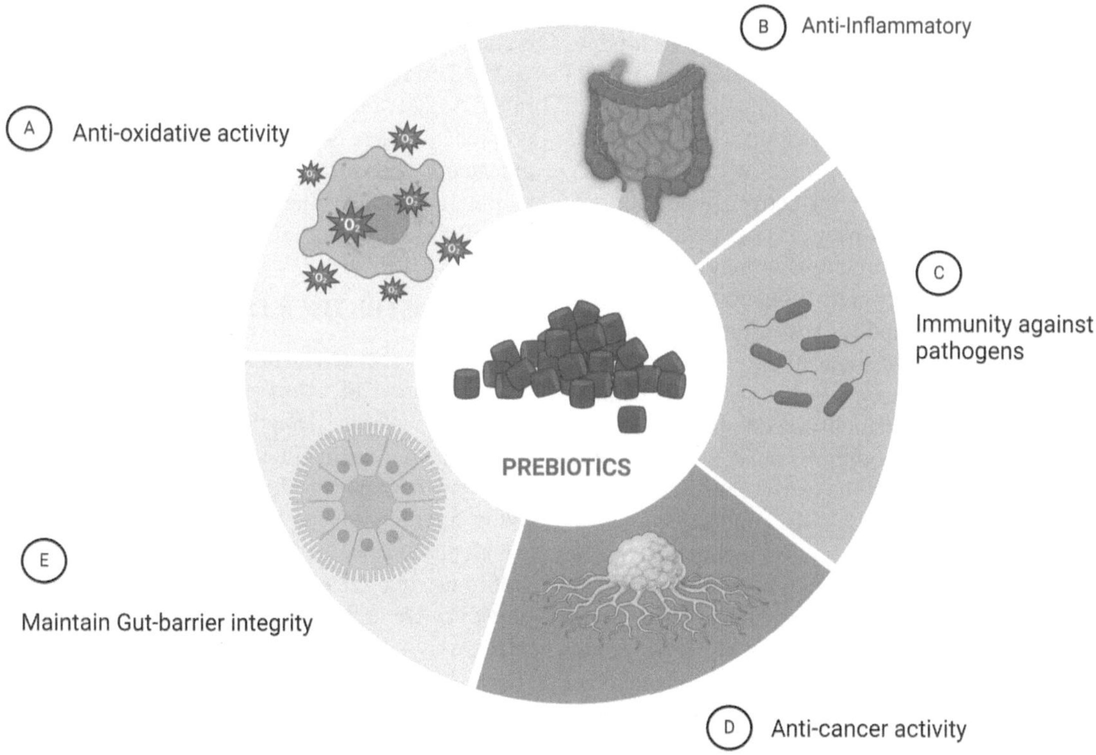

FIGURE 11.2 Mechanism of action of prebiotics.

11.4.2 Prebiotics and Gut Microbiota Modulation

The immune system and digestion are two areas of human health that are significantly impacted by the gut microbiota. Prebiotics, a type of dietary fibers that give essential energy to the thriving population of bacteria residing in our intestines instead of being digested, have gained attention in recent years (Vassileva et al., 2020). Here, we explore the dynamic relationship between prebiotics and gut microbiota change to provide insight into how these indigestible fibers sustain a stable and harmonious internal environment. The gut microbiota, which is made up of billions of different bacteria, viruses, fungi, and other microorganisms, is found in the gastrointestinal system. The complex ecosystem affects processes like immunity, metabolism, and digestion and is essential to maintaining a delicate balance that is necessary for overall health. Prebiotics are indigestible fibers that provide the beneficial bacteria in the stomach with a particular type of fuel. They are often disregarded in favor of probiotic supplements. Unlike probiotics, which are live microorganisms taken into the body, prebiotics provide these friendly bacteria—especially Bifidobacteria and Lactobacilli—with the food they need to thrive and operate (Delgado and Tamashiro, 2018). Because prebiotics have the ability to control the diversity of the gut microbiota, they are important for gut health. A diverse and well-balanced microbial population is associated with several health benefits, including improved digestion, increased immunological function, and improved absorption of nutrients (Doré and Blottière, 2015). Prebiotics stimulate the growth of specific beneficial bacterial strains, hence promoting microbial diversity. Variety is essential for resilience because a more diversified microbiota may adapt better to dietary changes, environmental changes, and other challenges. Prebiotics are necessary not just to sustain microbial variety but also to maintain the integrity of the intestinal barrier. A healthy gut barrier keeps harmful substances from the intestines from entering the bloodstream, protecting the body against inflammation and other potential health issues. Prebiotics assist in the maintenance of a robust gut barrier by controlling the production of SCFAs during fermentation. Butyrate is one of the SCFAs that have been linked to improved gut barrier function, a decreased risk of inflammatory illnesses, and overall improvements in gut health.

11.4.3 Prebiotics and Their Impact on Metabolic Health

With the growing comprehension of the complex correlation between gut health and general wellbeing, prebiotics are becoming recognized as the unsung heroes of metabolic health. The composition of the gut flora and other metabolic processes that go beyond digestion are significantly influenced by these indigestible fibers. Frequently, they are eclipsed by their probiotic equivalents. Prebiotics' impacts on metabolic health are discussed here, along with how they may help maintain a healthy metabolic profile, help control blood sugar levels, and promote weight management (Xavier-Santos et al., 2020). The gut flora is one of the many elements that contribute to a healthy weight, making it a complex process. According to research, prebiotics may help with weight management in a number of ways, such as: Increased satiety has been linked to prebiotics such oligofructose and inulin, which may lead to a decrease in total caloric consumption. Prebiotics may affect the equilibrium that aids in maintaining weight by influencing the release of gut hormones that regulate appetite, such as peptide YY (PYY) and ghrelin. A more slim body composition has been associated with certain bacteria that prebiotics support, indicating that the gut microbiota may influence the advantages associated with weight reduction. According to Nikbakht et al. (2018), prebiotics have shown encouraging results in the areas of blood sugar management and metabolic health. Insulin sensitivity, which is critical for controlling blood sugar, has been demonstrated to be enhanced by prebiotics that increase the synthesis of SCFAs. Prebiotics may affect how the body uses glucose by changing the flora in the stomach and encouraging the production of molecules that affect insulin signaling. Prebiotics may aid in preserving a healthy gut flora, which may lessen the incidence of type 2 diabetes, per a recent study. Through the gut–brain axis, prebiotics have an impact on mental health and wellbeing in addition to the physiological elements of metabolism (Barengolts, 2016). Stress reactions and mood are influenced by the gut microbiota's communication with the brain. By promoting a healthy gut flora, prebiotics may improve mental health. Prebiotics have an impact on some gut bacteria that are involved in the synthesis of neurotransmitters like serotonin, which are important for mood regulation.

11.4.4 Synergistic Effects: The Concept of Synbiotics

In the ever-evolving landscape of gut health, the symbiotic relationship between probiotics and prebiotics has given rise to a fascinating concept known as synbiotics. This dynamic duo, working in harmony, represents a holistic approach to nurturing the gut microbiota for enhanced wellbeing. We'll explore here the concept of synbiotics, unraveling the synergistic effects of combining probiotics and prebiotics to promote a balanced and thriving gut ecosystem (Barengolts et al., 2016). Synbiotics, as the name suggests, are a combination of "probiotics" and "prebiotics." While probiotics are live microorganisms that confer health benefits when consumed in adequate amounts, prebiotics are nondigestible fibers that serve as food for beneficial gut bacteria. Synbiotics, therefore, bring together these two elements to create a powerful synergy that maximizes the positive impact on gut health (Ren et al., 2019). Prebiotics act as a nourishing substrate for probiotics, promoting their survival as they travel through the digestive system. This ensures that a sufficient number of live probiotics reach the colon, where they exert their beneficial effects (De Souza Oliveira et al., 2011). Prebiotics selectively stimulate the growth and activity of specific strains of beneficial bacteria, such as Bifidobacteria and Lactobacilli. When combined with probiotics, which are often members of these bacterial groups, synbiotics create an environment conducive to the proliferation of these friendly microbes (Sharma and Padwad, 2020). The fermentation of prebiotics by probiotics results in the production of SCFAs, such as butyrate, acetate, and propionate. These SCFAs play a crucial role in maintaining gut health by nourishing colonocytes, regulating inflammation, and influencing metabolic processes (Cukkemane et al., 2020).

11.5 POSTBIOTICS DEFINED

Fermentation-related metabolic activity in probiotics results in the creation of a large class of bioactive compounds known as postbiotics. Peptides, organic acids (SCFAs), and other various metabolites are among these compounds; however, they are not the only ones. As an alternative to living microorganisms for gut health support, postbiotics are a consequence of fermentation itself. In contrast, probiotics are live microorganisms given into the body, while prebiotics are indigestible fibers that serve as food for good bacteria.

11.5.1 Production and Classification of Postbiotics

Postbiotic fermentation is closely related to the fermentation process that probiotics do. Probiotics are living microorganisms that ferment when added to a substrate. Usually, they are bacteria or yeast. As a result of these microbes' breakdown of the substrate's numerous components during fermentation, a variety of beneficial chemicals are produced as metabolic byproducts (Thorakkattu et al., 2022). Postbiotic characteristics differ across probiotic strains. A significant factor in influencing the kinds and amounts of postbiotics produced during fermentation is the selection of probiotic strains (Gibson et al., 2017). Probiotics produce a wide range of beneficial substances by breaking down the substrate's constituent parts. Postbiotic composition and concentration are dependent on the length and circumstances of the fermentation process. The postbiotic-rich mixture is collected when fermentation is finished. To extract certain postbiotic chemicals for diverse uses, the next processing stages could involve filtering, concentration, and purification. A variety of substances make up postbiotics; each has special qualities and could have health advantages (Collado et al., 2019).

11.5.2 Biological Activities of Postbiotics

A promising approach to enhancing wellbeing in the complex field of gut health is the use of postbiotics. Beyond the conventional boundaries of probiotics and prebiotics, these inert microbial metabolites, which originate from the fermentation processes of probiotics, exhibit a wide range of biological activity. Postbiotics have several biological roles that may have intricate consequences on human health (Nataraj et al., 2020). In order to control the variety and makeup of the gut microbiota, postbiotics are essential. Postbiotics provide a microbial community with balance and harmony by encouraging the growth of helpful bacteria and preventing the spread of destructive germs. Postbiotics have an impact on immune cell activity and strengthen the body's defenses through immunomodulatory actions. According to Turnbaugh et al. (2006), this may lead to a stronger immune response that is better able to fight off infections and illnesses.

11.5.3 Potential Therapeutic Applications

Within the dynamic realm of gut health, which is always growing, postbiotics have become recognized as adaptable substances with exciting therapeutic possibilities. The fermentation processes of probiotics produce these non-living microbial metabolites, which are becoming more and more well-known for their wide variety of uses outside of digestive health. These are a few possible therapeutic uses for postbiotics (Gibson and Roberfroid, 1995). Owing to their anti-inflammatory qualities, some postbiotics, especially those containing SCFAs, may be useful in the treatment of inflammatory diseases such as cancer and ulcerative colitis. According to Rastall (2010), postbiotics have the potential to alleviate symptoms of irritable bowel syndrome (IBS) by modifying the makeup of the gut microbiota and treating symptoms including abdominal discomfort and irregular bowel movements. Postbiotics have immunomodulatory effects that affect immunological responses, which can lead to infections and allergies. As a result, they may be useful partners in the fight against allergies and infections by strengthening the body's defenses. Postbiotics have the potential to improve immune system dysregulated illnesses including multiple sclerosis and rheumatoid arthritis by modulating the immune system. Diabetes type 2: Postbiotics, especially those that affect glucose metabolism, may help control blood sugar levels and insulin sensitivity, which may be beneficial for patients who have the condition. Cani and Everard (2015) have shown that the metabolic effects of some postbiotics, such as SCFAs, may have potential uses in aiding in weight control and resolving issues associated with obesity. Cholesterol Regulation: A number of postbiotics have demonstrated potential in terms of their ability to affect lipid metabolism, help control cholesterol levels, and improve cardiovascular health. Certain postbiotics may have vasodilatory effects that may promote cardiovascular health and blood pressure management. Postbiotics affect the gut–brain axis, a communication channel between the gut and the brain. The link between the two points to possible therapeutic uses for treating mood disorders including anxiety and depression. The neuroprotective potential of postbiotics is being investigated by emerging research, which may have implications for treating disorders like Parkinson's and Alzheimer's. Bioactive substances obtained from postbiotics may be used in dermatology to help treat inflammatory skin diseases including eczema, acne, and other skin problems. Postbiotics, such as bacteriocins, have the potential to be used as antimicrobial agents to help heal wounds and manage infections. According to Pandey et al. (2015), postbiotics have the potential to enhance the effectiveness of immunotherapies by altering the immune system, hence providing support for cancer therapy.

11.6 INTERPLAY BETWEEN PROBIOTICS, PREBIOTICS, AND POSTBIOTICS

The triad of probiotics, prebiotics, and postbiotics collaborates to create a robust and harmonious gut microbiota in the complex realm of gut health. In order to understand the complex interactions that support digestive health and general wellbeing, we'll examine how these three essential elements interact. In order to support probiotics' survival and function in the gut, prebiotics serve as a nutritious substrate. There are plenty of living, helpful microorganisms present because of this synergy. Metabolite Generation: Postbiotics are the byproduct of probiotics fermenting prebiotics. A dynamic ecosystem with both living and non-living components working together to promote good gut health is created by this complex interaction. It is possible to address gut health holistically by combining probiotics, prebiotics, and postbiotics.

11.6.1 The Holobiont Concept

Beyond the traditional notion of the gut as an isolated organ, Aguilar-Toalá et al. (2018) claim that the holobiont concept acknowledges the gut as a dynamic ecosystem that encompasses the host, probiotics, prebiotics, and postbiotics. This holistic approach recognizes the interconnectedness of these components and emphasizes the importance of their combined effect on health. Prebiotics provide the nourishing foundation that sustains the probiotic population, and their relationship with probiotics symbolizes symbiosis. This synergy ensures the vitality of the living collective. Prebiotics provide energy for the metabolic activities carried out by probiotics, which produce postbiotics. Probiotics, prebiotics, and postbiotics are three types of helpful bacteria that work together to support gut health. The intricate interactions of the holobiont foster harmony and balance in the stomach. A digestive symphony is produced by the harmonious interaction of every member of the live probiotic ensemble, the nutritious prebiotic support, and the sophisticated metabolic activity of postbiotics (Parvez et al., 2006). Sturdy holobionts, characterized by a diverse microbial community, offer adaptability and durability. Adaptability is essential for managing dietary changes, environmental factors, and other stressors that impact gut health.

11.6.2 Symbiotic Approaches for Metabolic Health

Combining probiotics and prebiotics improves the production of SCFA. Among the SCFAs, butyrate in particular is engaged in energy metabolism and may be useful in weight control (Corsetti and Settanni, 2007). It has been shown that probiotics and prebiotics combine to improve insulin sensitivity, a crucial factor in preserving metabolic health and averting insulin resistance. The synergistic combination of probiotics, prebiotics, and postbiotics supports metabolic resilience. Together, these three support gut flora health, metabolic functions, and overall metabolic health. Potential benefits for weight management have been linked to symbiotic approaches. The way these three components interact may have an impact on appetite regulation and fat metabolism. Symbiotic therapy may be used to treat metabolic ailments such as obesity, type 2 diabetes, and cardiovascular problems. The combined benefits of probiotics, prebiotics, and postbiotics offer a multimodal approach to preserving metabolic health, claim Taverniti and Guglielmetti (2011).

11.6.3 Case Studies and Clinical Trials

The interplay between probiotics, prebiotics, and postbiotics has gained prominence as scientists dive further into the complex realm of gut health. Beyond theoretical frameworks, we'll discuss the interactions here via the prism of case studies and clinical trials from real-world applications, which highlight the usefulness of combining the strength of these three pillars of gut health (Bordenstein and Theis, 2015). The benefits of a symbiotic intervention including probiotics, prebiotics, and postbiotics were investigated in a case study involving people with metabolic syndrome. A symbiotic supplement combining prebiotic fibers, purified postbiotic metabolites, and a carefully chosen probiotic strain was given to the participants. The symbiotic intervention showed a noteworthy enhancement in participants' insulin sensitivity, indicating a favorable effect on metabolic wellbeing. A positive change in the number of beneficial bacteria was seen in the fecal sample analysis, demonstrating the impact of the symbiotic strategy on the gut microbiota. Participants showed lower levels of inflammatory markers after the probiotic, prebiotic, and postbiotic interventions, suggesting that these treatments had anti-inflammatory effects. Round and Mazmanian (2009) conducted a randomized controlled clinical experiment to examine the impact of a synbiotic strategy on gastrointestinal resilience and the integration of functional foods.

Either the synbiotic group, which received probiotics and prebiotics together, or the control group received the same supplements. Foods high in postbiotic substances that are functional were included in all groups. Digestion comfort, including less bloating and pain, was reported to have significantly improved by the synbiotic group. Examining stool samples revealed that the synbiotic group had more diverse microbiota, highlighting the beneficial effects of prebiotics and probiotics on the richness of the gut microbiota. As evidence of the value of a comprehensive strategy, functional meals enhanced with postbiotics were included in the synbiotic intervention, which increased its overall effectiveness. Postbiotics for the treatment of inflammatory bowel disease (IBD). Sanders et al. (2019) investigated the therapeutic potential of postbiotics through a case series centered on persons with IBD. An assortment of SCFAs and other bioactive compounds obtained from probiotic fermentation were included in the postbiotic supplement given to the participants. Postbiotics may have a function in the treatment of inflammatory diseases, as evidenced by the reduction in disease activity ratings and IBD symptoms observed in some subjects. According to immunological evaluations, immune responses changed, suggesting that postbiotics might influence immune system regulation in IBD. The gut lining's health is supported by postbiotics, as seen by the improvement in biomarkers linked to gut barrier integrity. Practical insights into the effects of probiotics, prebiotics, and postbiotics interacting are offered by these case studies and clinical trials. According to Lozupone and Knight (2005), the symbiotic method demonstrates its promise in real-world circumstances, ranging from improved digestion and metabolic benefits to the therapy of inflammatory disorders. Combining these three pillars into gut health treatments is a viable way to support overall wellbeing as research progresses. Probiotics, prebiotics, and postbiotics work together to create a robust and healthy gut ecology, and this process of going from theory to implementation highlights the transformational potential of doing so (Costea et al., 2018).

11.7 METHODOLOGIES FOR ASSESSING GUT MICROBIOTA

A complex and diverse collection of bacteria living in the gastrointestinal system called the human gut microbiota is essential to preserving general health and wellbeing. Deciphering the gut microbiota's role in many facets of human physiology requires an understanding of its makeup and functioning. Our immune system, digestion, and even mental health are all impacted by these tiny residents, which are crucial to our overall health and wellbeing (Salminen et al., 2021).

11.7.1 Tools and Techniques for Gut Microbiota Analysis

Researchers examine this microbial world using a range of cutting-edge tools and techniques in an effort to understand the complex mechanisms of the gut microbiota. To further our understanding of the advancements driving our understanding of this intricate ecosystem, we will discuss some of the most advanced tools and techniques for gut microbiota research (Hemarajata and Versalovic, 2013). Researchers studying the microbiome have benefited greatly from next-generation sequencing, which has made it possible to examine microbes' genetic makeup in previously unheard-of depth. The variety and possible functions of the gut microbiota are revealed by methods such as whole-genome shotgun sequencing and 16S rRNA sequencing. Because NGS can produce enormous volumes of sequencing data and is capable of high throughput, it has become a mainstay in the investigation of gut microbiota (Hill et al., 2014). Specific DNA sequences may be quantified thanks to the potent molecular biology technique known as quantitative PCR. Quantification of the abundance of certain bacterial species or functional genes is a common use of qPCR in gut microbiota investigation. According to Lynch and Pedersen (2016), this focused method gives researchers accurate data on the relative abundance of important microbial actors, enabling them to monitor changes in response to different treatments or circumstances. Researchers can see and identify certain bacteria groups in the stomach using a technique called Fluorescence In Situ Hybridization (FISH), which is based on microscopy. FISH offers geographic information on the distribution and abundance of microorganisms in their natural habitat by employing fluorescently labeled DNA probes that attach to target sequences (Leihr, 2017). Understanding the spatial structure of the gut microbiota in respect to host tissues is made possible by this method (Bayani and Squire, 2004). Small chemicals generated by microbial metabolism are the main subject of metabolomics research. Researchers can learn more about the functional activity of the microbiota by examining the metabolites found in the gut. Metabolomics offers an overview of the metabolic activities taking place in the gut environment, which is a useful supplement to other omics techniques. Understanding how the gut microbiota affects host health and illness depends on knowing this information (Pabinger et al., 2014). Advanced bioinformatics and computational tools are needed for the processing of the massive quantity of data produced by contemporary microbiota analysis techniques. To handle, analyze, and interpret massive microbiological information, researchers employ databases and specialized tools. These resources aid in the identification of microbial species, the prediction of functional pathways, and the discovery of patterns that further our knowledge of the gut microbiota (O'Grada et al., 2014).

11.7.2 Biomarkers of Metabolic Health

Emerging research reveals the intricate relationship between gut microbiota and metabolic health, offering insights into the ways in which the microbes residing in our digestive system influence several aspects of metabolism. Biomarkers, which are measurable indicators of biological processes, are necessary to decipher this complex relationship. The interaction between metabolic health indices and their use in assessing the dynamic ecology of the gut microbiota will be examined here (Dreher, 2021). Metabolic byproducts of gut microbiological fermentation include SCFAs. Notable SCFAs with established functions in immunological regulation and energy metabolism include butyrate, propionate, and acetate. Higher levels of SCFAs are linked to better metabolic outcomes and a healthy gut microbiome. Functional analysis conducted using scenarios as a basis. Analysis of faecal samples' short-chain fatty acid (SCFAs) provides valuable insights on the fermentative activities of gut bacteria and their impact on metabolic health (Sellin, 1998). Originating from the microbial breakdown of food substances like carnitine and choline, Trimethylamine N-oxide (TMAO) has become a biomarker that connects the gut microbiota to metabolic and cardiovascular health. Insulin resistance and cardiovascular disease risk are both correlated with elevated TMAO levels. TMAO level monitoring offers insight into the role of gut bacteria in the metabolism of dietary nutrients and their consequences for metabolic health. During inflammation, neutrophils produce a protein called calprotectin. The equilibrium of the gut microbiota can be upset by intestinal inflammation, which is shown by elevated fecal calprotectin levels. Calprotectin levels can be tracked as a biomarker to evaluate gut health and its possible influence on metabolic outcomes (Ricciuto and Griffiths, 2019). Certain bacteria's outer membranes include lipopolysaccharides (LPS), and gut dysbiosis and metabolic endotoxemia are linked to elevated LPS levels in the blood. Inflammation and insulin resistance can be brought on by elevated LPS levels. The integrity of the intestinal barrier and its significance for metabolic health may be understood via measuring blood levels of LPS (Jayashree et al., 2014). The makeup of the gut microbiota may now be profiled as a biomarker for metabolic health because of developments in high-throughput sequencing methods. Obesity and metabolic syndrome have been associated with certain microbial taxa, such as the ratio of Firmicutes to Bacteroidetes. In order to evaluate the general health of the gut microbiota and its possible influence on metabolic processes, important microbial group abundance analysis is utilized as a biomarker (Bibbo et al., 2016). The systemic effects of the gut microbiota on host metabolism can be understood using biomarkers linked to glucose metabolism, such as insulin levels, HbA1c, and fasting blood glucose. The composition and function of the gut microbiota may be unbalanced, impacting metabolic health, if these indicators are dysregulated (Fallah et al., 2020).

11.8 SAFETY AND CONSIDERATIONS

In the ever-expanding landscape of gut health interventions, the triumvirate of probiotics, prebiotics, and postbiotics has emerged as a promising avenue for promoting a balanced and resilient microbiota. As individuals and healthcare professionals explore these microbial therapies, understanding their safety profiles becomes paramount (Żółkiewicz et al., 2020).

11.8.1 Safety Profiles of Probiotics, Prebiotics, and Postbiotics

We'll explore the intricacies that govern the use of probiotics, prebiotics, and postbiotics for optimum health, as well as the safety concerns related to each. Fermented foods and supplements are typical sources of probiotics, which are living bacteria that may have health advantages. Despite being widely accepted as safe, the following factors should be taken into account: Individuals may respond differently to different probiotic strains. Selecting strains for certain health objectives that have been shown to be safe and effective is essential. Probiotic administration to people with weakened immune systems should be done with caution. To evaluate each person's unique risk factors, consultation with medical specialists is crucial. In certain people, probiotics might result in moderate gastrointestinal symptoms like gas or bloating. Infections can be serious adverse effects, albeit they are uncommon, especially in those with underlying medical issues. For certain people, introducing prebiotics may result in gastrointestinal distress. Tolerance can be increased by including foods in the diet gradually. Certain prebiotics may exacerbate symptoms in people with specific gastrointestinal illnesses, such as IBS. Customizing prebiotic selections to meet specific requirements is advised. Bloating and excessive gas production might result from consuming too much prebiotics. An equilibrium gut ecology is facilitated by diversity and moderation in prebiotic sources. Postbiotics are the components generated during the breakdown of probiotics, or the metabolic byproducts of probiotic fermentation. Even though it's usually thought to be safe, there are several things to keep in mind. Individuals may respond differently to postbiotics. When introducing new foods or supplements that are high in probiotics, it is especially important to keep an eye out for any negative responses. Postbiotics' safety depends on where they come from. To reduce possible dangers, it is essential to use well-researched and quality-controlled postbiotic sources. People who suffer from certain medical issues might need to take extra care. Healthcare professionals' consultations can assist in customizing postbiotic therapies to meet the needs of each patient.

11.8.2 Potential Side Effects and Allergies

Probiotics, prebiotics, and postbiotics are components that are essential for maintaining a robust and balanced microbiota, and their study is frequently a part of the path toward gut health. It's important to be aware of any potential side effects and allergies, even though these procedures are usually well-tolerated. In order to provide people the tools they need to pursue their best possible health, we will delve into the subtleties of probiotic, prebiotic, and postbiotic allergies and side effects. Fermented foods and supplements are popular ways to ingest probiotics, living bacteria that have been shown to contribute to health. Starting probiotic supplements might cause moderate gastrointestinal symptoms in certain people, such as gas, bloating, or diarrhea. As the gut microbiome adapts, these symptoms frequently go away. Rarely, infections may result with probiotic use, especially in immunocompromised people or those with underlying medical issues. It is recommended that those with weakened immune systems seek advice from healthcare specialists. Allergy responses to substances included in probiotic supplements are possible, but rare. Those who have established sensitivities or allergies should carefully read product labels and, in case of doubt, see a physician. The addition of prebiotics to the diet may result in gas and bloating, among other minor gastrointestinal problems. Pain can be reduced by incorporating prebiotics gradually and by using a variety of prebiotic sources. Prebiotics of a particular kind may exacerbate symptoms in people with gastrointestinal diseases, such as IBS. Individual tolerances should be taken into account while selecting a probiotic.

11.8.3 Regulatory Aspects and Quality Control

Probiotics, prebiotics, and postbiotics are integral parts of the evolving landscape of gut health therapies; it is crucial to oversee their quality control and regulatory elements. It is vital to create and follow strict guidelines to ensure the safety and effectiveness of these components as their potential advantages make them more and more popular. The importance of these procedures in fostering consumer trust and wellbeing will be emphasized as we examine the legal frameworks and quality control procedures controlling probiotics, prebiotics, and postbiotics. In many parts of the world, probiotics are categorized as functional foods or nutritional supplements. Guidelines are provided for the assessment and promotion of probiotic products by regulatory organizations including the European Food Safety Authority (EFSA) and the U.S. Food and Drug Administration (FDA). But the regulatory environment is not uniform, and broad guidelines are always changing. Exact identification and recording of strains are necessary for thorough quality control. In order to enable customers and regulatory agencies to evaluate the safety and effectiveness of probiotics based on empirical data, probiotic producers are required to provide a precise description of the strains their products include. Probiotic strain viability during storage must be guaranteed. During the product's specified shelf life, quality control methods include evaluating the stability of live cultures and confirming their potency at the time of manufacturing. Food and dietary supplement safety authorities regulate prebiotics, which are often categorized as dietary fibers. Regulating bodies such as the FDA and EFSA offer recommendations for labeling, safety evaluations, and health claims; however, regulations are different around the world. Verifying the content and purity of prebiotics is part of quality control. To guarantee that prebiotic products fulfill specified requirements and are free of impurities that might jeopardize safety, manufacturers must abide by set criteria. Clinical data supporting health claims related to prebiotic products is typically required to satisfy regulatory criteria. Good research design is another way that quality control methods are used to support the stated health benefits. Regulatory definitions for postbiotics are not established because they are a relatively new category. Regulations that guarantee the safe and efficient use of postbiotics are anticipated to change as scientific knowledge of them expands. Establishing guidelines for postbiotic manufacturing, such as identifying and measuring certain metabolites or bioactive substances, is part of quality control. To ensure uniformity and safety throughout batches, rigorous testing is necessary. To determine the postbiotics' regulatory status, ongoing research and safety evaluations are essential. The safety, modes of action, and any health advantages of these substances must be established with strong scientific evidence. Protecting consumer health is fundamentally dependent on the regulatory landscape and quality control of probiotics, prebiotics, and postbiotics. International regulatory agencies need to adjust as the use of these treatments becomes more widespread in order to guarantee that standards remain current with advances in science. In order to maintain the safety, efficacy, and purity of their products, manufacturers must, in turn, put strict quality control procedures into place. For the purpose of building consumer confidence and achieving the maximum benefit of these ingredients in supporting gut health and general wellbeing, cooperation between industry players and regulators is needed.

11.9 FUTURE PERSPECTIVES AND EMERGING RESEARCH

Future research on probiotics, prebiotics, and postbiotics will be critical to gut health as our understanding of the gut microbiota expands. Due to their revolutionary potential to transform wellbeing, these dynamic components have attracted significant interest. As we explore new findings and potential advancements in the fields of probiotics, prebiotics, and postbiotics, we are taking a trip into the future with you. Probiotic, prebiotic, and postbiotic domains continue to be active research topics in the constantly changing field of gut health (Vallianou et al., 2020). Many unsolved concerns and information gaps remain despite the great progress made in comprehending their potential advantages. Here, we will explore the mysterious properties of probiotics, prebiotics, and postbiotics, emphasizing the unanswered questions that pique scientific interest. Probiotic strains and their unique health benefits are still poorly understood due to their complex interactions. Deciphering the subtle differences across strains, or why some may offer certain advantages while others might not, is a constant source of frustration. Probiotic treatments can be more effectively tailored if future studies can decipher the complex language of the microbiome. The durability of these microbes in the gut and the long-term effects of probiotic administration are topics that remain unclear. It will need substantial longitudinal studies to monitor changes in the gut microbiota over time in order to determine whether the advantages of probiotics are temporary or long-lasting. The subtleties of host–microbe interactions continue to be a challenging riddle, particularly the signaling pathways and molecular processes that underpin probiotics' communication with their hosts. Understanding the ways in which probiotics influence different physiological systems will need an understanding of these relationships. For prebiotic therapies to be as effective as possible, the ideal dosage and length of time to provide them are yet unknown. Prebiotics are meant to specifically support good gut flora, but it's still unclear how much and how long these microbes must be present in order to have long-term effects. It's difficult to anticipate how different people will react to particular prebiotics because of the inherent heterogeneity in each person's gut flora. To customize prebiotic treatments to a range of microbial environments, it is imperative to identify the elements that create this heterogeneity. The precise benefits of prebiotics on different health issues are still being researched, even though they appear to be promising in supporting gut health. In order to enable tailored therapeutic applications, research gaps remain in our understanding of how prebiotics may influence particular illnesses or situations.

11.10 CONCLUSION

In summary, the field of research on probiotics, prebiotics, and postbiotics and their impact on metabolic diseases through gut microbiota modification is a vibrant and fascinating one. Maintaining overall health and metabolic equilibrium is critical for preventing or treating metabolic disorders such as obesity, type 2 diabetes, and cardiovascular issues. These treatments present potential methods for creating a gut microbiota that is in good condition. Probiotics are live microorganisms that have been shown to have positive effects on metabolic parameters and the composition of the gut microbiota. On the other hand, prebiotics nourish and stimulate the growth of beneficial gut flora by giving them food. Probiotics and prebiotics work together to promote health by enhancing the symbiotic relationship between the host and gut microorganisms. A promising new therapy option for metabolic diseases is emerging: postbiotics, which are the metabolites of probiotic digestion. These bioactive compounds have the potential to impact the gut environment and host metabolism, which may provide a novel approach to improving metabolic health. Research on the topic is still in its early phases, but it is clear that a holistic approach that includes probiotics, prebiotics, and postbiotics and is tailored to the individual needs of each patient offers a viable treatment and prevention plan for metabolic disorders. As the intricate relationship between gut microbiota and metabolic health continues to be understood, these treatments have the potential to revolutionize medicine and offer more personalized and effective treatment strategies for metabolic disorders in the future. More investigation, long-term follow-up studies, and clinical trials are required to better understand the processes involved and identify the most effective therapies for specific metabolic illnesses.

REFERENCES

Aguilar-Toalá, J. E., Garcia-Varela, R., Garcia, H. S., Mata-Haro, V., González-Córdova, A. F., Vallejo-Cordoba, B., & Hernández-Mendoza, A. (2018). Postbiotics: an evolving term within the functional foods field. *Trends in Food Science & Technology*, *75*, 105–114.

Appanna, V. D., & Appanna, V. D. (2018). Dysbiosis, probiotics, and prebiotics: in diseases and health. *Human Microbes-The Power Within: Health, Healing and Beyond*, *2018*, 81–122.

Arora, T., & Bäckhed, F. (2016). The gut microbiota and metabolic disease: current understanding and future perspectives. *Journal of Internal Medicine*, *280*(4), 339–349.

Aureli, P., Capurso, L., Castellazzi, A. M., Clerici, M., Giovannini, M., Morelli, L., ... & Zuccotti, G. V. (2011). Probiotics and health: an evidence-based review. *Pharmacological Research*, *63*(5), 366–376.

Barengolts, E. (2016). Gut microbiota, prebiotics, probiotics, and synbiotics in management of obesity and prediabetes: review of randomized controlled trials. *Endocrine Practice*, *22*(10), 1224–1234.

Bayani, J., & Squire, J. A. (2004). Fluorescence in situ hybridization (FISH). *Current Protocols in Cell Biology*, *23*(1), 22–24.

Bibbo, S., Ianiro, G., Giorgio, V., Scaldaferri, F., Masucci, L., Gasbarrini, A., & Cammarota, G. (2016). The role of diet on gut microbiota composition. *European Review for Medical & Pharmacological Sciences*, *20*(22), 4742–4749.

Bindels, L. B., Delzenne, N. M., Cani, P. D., & Walter, J. (2015). Towards a more comprehensive concept for prebiotics. *Nature Reviews Gastroenterology & Hepatology*, *12*(5), 303–310.

Bordenstein, S. R., & Theis, K. R. (2015). Host biology in light of the microbiome: ten principles of holobionts and hologenomes. *PLoS Biology*, *13*(8), e1002226.

Bourebaba, Y., Marycz, K., Mularczyk, M., & Bourebaba, L. (2022). Postbiotics as potential new therapeutic agents for metabolic disorders management. *Biomedicine & Pharmacotherapy*, *153*, 113138.

Burcelin, R., Courtney, M., Amar, J. (2015). Gut microbiota and metabolic diseases: From pathogenesis to therapeutic perspective. In: Kochhar, S., Martin, FP. (eds) *Metabonomics and Gut Microbiota in Nutrition and Disease. Molecular and Integrative Toxicology*. Springer, London. https://doi.org/10.1007/978-1-4471-6539-2_11

Cani, P. D., & Delzenne, N. M. (2009). The role of the gut microbiota in energy metabolism and metabolic disease. *Current Pharmaceutical Design*, *15*(13), 1546–1558.

Cani, P. D., & Everard, A. (2015). Talking microbes: when gut bacteria interact with diet and host organs. *Molecular Nutrition & Food Research*, *59*(1), 3–17.

Carding, S., Verbeke, K., Vipond, D. T., Corfe, B. M., & Owen, L. J. (2015). Dysbiosis of the gut microbiota in disease. *Microbial Ecology in Health and Disease*, *26*(1), 26191.

Cook, S. I., & Sellin, J. H. (1998). Review article: short chain fatty acids in health and disease. *Alimentary Pharmacology & Therapeutics*, 12(6), 499–507. https://doi.org/10.1046/j.1365-2036.1998.00337.x

Corsetti, A., & Settanni, L. (2007). Lactic acid bacteria in sourdough fermentation. *Food Research International*, *40*(5), 539–558.

Costea, P. I., Hildebrand, F., Arumugam, M., Bäckhed, F., Blaser, M. J., Bushman, F. D., ... & Raes, J. (2018). Enterotypes in the landscape of gut microbial community composition. *Nature Microbiology*, *3*(1), 8–16.

Cuevas-Sierra, A., Ramos-Lopez, O., Riezu-Boj, J. I., Milagro, F. I., & Martinez, J. A. (2019). Diet, gut microbiota, and obesity: links with host genetics and epigenetics and potential applications. *Advances in Nutrition*, *10*(suppl_1), S17–S30.

Cukkemane, A., Kumar, P., & Sathyamoorthy, B. (2020). A metabolomics footprint approach to understanding the benefits of synbiotics in functional foods and dietary therapeutics for health, communicable and non-communicable diseases. *Food Research International*, 128, 108679.

D'Aversa, F., Tortora, A., Ianiro, G., Ponziani, F. R., Annicchiarico, B. E., & Gasbarrini, A. (2013). Gut microbiota and metabolic syndrome. *Internal and Emergency Medicine*, *8*, 11–15.

DeSouza Oliveira, R. P., Perego, P., de Oliveira, M. N., & Converti, A. (2011). Effect of inulin as prebiotic and synbiotic interactions between probiotics to improve fermented milk firmness. *Journal of Food Engineering*, *107*(1), 36–40.

Delgado, G. T. C., & Tamashiro, W. M. D. S. C. (2018). Role of prebiotics in regulation of microbiota and prevention of obesity. *Food Research International*, *113*, 183–188.

Doré, J., & Blottière, H. (2015). The influence of diet on the gut microbiota and its consequences for health. *Current Opinion in Biotechnology*, *32*, 195–199.

Dreher, M. L. (2021). A comprehensive review of almond clinical trials on weight measures, metabolic health biomarkers and outcomes, and the gut microbiota. *Nutrients*, *13*(6), 1968.

Dutta, S. K., Verma, S., Jain, V., Surapaneni, B. K., Vinayek, R., Phillips, L., & Nair, P. P. (2019). Parkinson's disease: the emerging role of gut dysbiosis, antibiotics, probiotics, and fecal microbiota transplantation. *Journal of Neurogastroenterology and Motility*, *25*(3), 363.

Erejuwa, O. O., Sulaiman, S. A., & Ab Wahab, M. S. (2014). Modulation of gut microbiota in the management of metabolic disorders: the prospects and challenges. *International Journal of Molecular Sciences*, *15*(3), 4158–4188.

Fallah, A. A., Sarmast, E., & Jafari, T. (2020). Effect of dietary anthocyanins on biomarkers of glycemic control and glucose metabolism: a systematic review and meta-analysis of randomized clinical trials. *Food Research International*, *137*, 109379.

Fan, Y., & Pedersen, O. (2021). Gut microbiota in human metabolic health and disease. *Nature Reviews Microbiology*, *19*(1), 55–71.

Fukuda, S., & Ohno, H. (2014). Gut microbiome and metabolic diseases. *Seminars in Immunopathology*, *36*(1), 103–114. https://doi.org/10.1007/s00281-013-0399-z

Gálvez-Ontiveros, Y., Páez, S., Monteagudo, C., & Rivas, A. (2020). Endocrine disruptors in food: impact on gut microbiota and metabolic diseases. *Nutrients*, *12*(4), 1158.

Gibson, G. R., Hutkins, R., Sanders, M. E., Prescott, S. L., Reimer, R. A., Salminen, S. J., Scott, K., Stanton, C., Swanson, K. S., Cani, P. D., Verbeke, K., & Reid, G. (2017). Expert consensus document: The International Scientific Association for Probiotics and Prebiotics (ISAPP) consensus statement on the definition and scope of prebiotics. *Nature Reviews. Gastroenterology & Hepatology*, *14*(8), 491–502. https://doi.org/10.1038/nrgastro.2017.75

Gibson, G. R., & Roberfroid, M. B. (1995). Dietary modulation of the human colonic microbiota: introducing the concept of prebiotics. *Journal of Nutrition, 125*(6), 1401–1412.

Gogineni, V. K., Morrow, L. E., & Malesker, M. A. (2013). Probiotics: mechanisms of action and clinical applications. *Journal of Probiotics & Health, 1*(1), 1–11.

Grasset, E., & Burcelin, R. (2019). The gut microbiota to the brain axis in the metabolic control. *Reviews in Endocrine and Metabolic Disorders, 20*(4), 427–438.

Heijboer, A. C., Pijl, H., Van den Hoek, A. M., Havekes, L. M., Romijn, J. A., & Corssmit, E. P. M. (2006). Gut-brain axis: regulation of glucose metabolism. *Journal of Neuroendocrinology, 18*(12), 883–894.

Hemarajata, P., & Versalovic, J. (2013). Effects of probiotics on gut microbiota: mechanisms of intestinal immunomodulation and neuromodulation. *Therapeutic Advances in Gastroenterology, 6*(1), 39–51.

Hernández-Ceballos, W., Cordova-Gallardo, J., & Mendez-Sanchez, N. (2021). Gut microbiota in metabolic-associated fatty liver disease and in other chronic metabolic diseases. *Journal of Clinical and Translational Hepatology, 9*(2), 227.

Hill, C., Guarner, F., Reid, G., Gibson, G. R., Merenstein, D. J., Pot, B., ... & Sanders, M. E. (2014). Expert consensus document. The International Scientific Association for Probiotics and Prebiotics consensus statement on the scope and appropriate use of the term probiotic. *Nature Reviews Gastroenterology & Hepatology, 11*(8), 506–514.

Huang, Y. H., Tain, Y. L., & Hsu, C. N. (2022). Maternal supplementation of probiotics, prebiotics or postbiotics to prevent offspring metabolic syndrome: the gap between preclinical results and clinical translation. *International Journal of Molecular Sciences, 23*(17), 10173.

Jayashree, B., Bibin, Y. S., Prabhu, D., Shanthirani, C. S., Gokulakrishnan, K., Lakshmi, B. S., ... & Balasubramanyam, M. (2014). Increased circulatory levels of lipopolysaccharide (LPS) and zonulin signify novel biomarkers of proinflammation in patients with type 2 diabetes. *Molecular and Cellular Biochemistry, 388*, 203–210.

Kaur, S., Thukral, S. K., Kaur, P., & Samota, M. K. (2021). Perturbations associated with hungry gut microbiome and postbiotic perspectives to strengthen the microbiome health. *Future Foods, 4*, 100043.

Lanthier, N., & Delzenne, N. (2022). Targeting the gut microbiome to treat metabolic dysfunction-associated fatty liver disease: ready for prime time? *Cells, 11*(17), 2718.

LeBlanc, J. G., Chain, F., Martín, R., Bermúdez-Humarán, L. G., Courau, S., & Langella, P. (2017). Beneficial effects on host energy metabolism of short-chain fatty acids and vitamins produced by commensal and probiotic bacteria. *Microbial Cell Factories, 16*(1), 1–10.

Li, H. Y., Zhou, D. D., Gan, R. Y., Huang, S. Y., Zhao, C. N., Shang, A., ... & Li, H. B. (2021). Effects and mechanisms of probiotics, prebiotics, synbiotics, and postbiotics on metabolic diseases targeting gut microbiota: a narrative review. *Nutrients, 13*(9), 3211.

Liehr, T. (2017). *Fluorescence In Situ Hybridization (FISH)*. Berlin Heidelberg: Springer.

Lozupone, C., & Knight, R. (2005). UniFrac: a new phylogenetic method for comparing microbial communities. *Applied and Environmental Microbiology, 71*(12), 8228–8235.

Lynch, S. V., & Pedersen, O. (2016). The human intestinal microbiome in health and disease. *New England Journal of Medicine, 375*(24), 2369–2379.

Mishra, S. P., Jain, S., Taraphder, S., & Yadav, H. (2021). New horizons in microbiota and metabolic health research. *The Journal of Clinical Endocrinology & Metabolism, 106*(2), e1052–e1059.

Moser, B., Milligan, M. A., & Dao, M. C. (2022). The microbiota-Gut-Brain axis: clinical applications in obesity and type 2 diabetes. *Revista de investigación clínica, 74*(6), 302–313.

Nataraj, B. H., Ali, S. A., Behare, P. V., & Yadav, H. (2020). Postbiotics-parabiotics: the new horizons in microbial biotherapy and functional foods. *Microbial Cell Factories, 19*(1), 1–22.

Nerlich, B., & Koteyko, N. (2008). Balancing food risks and food benefits: the coverage of probiotics in the UK national press. *Sociological Research Online, 13*(3), 15–28.

Nikbakht, E., Khalesi, S., Singh, I., Williams, L. T., West, N. P., & Colson, N. (2018). Effect of probiotics and synbiotics on blood glucose: a systematic review and meta-analysis of controlled trials. *European Journal of Nutrition, 57*, 95–106.

O'Grada, C. M., Morine, M. J., Morris, C., Ryan, M., Dillon, E. T., Walsh, M., ... & Roche, H. M. (2014). PBMCs reflect the immune component of the WAT transcriptome-implications as biomarkers of metabolic health in the postprandial state. *Molecular Nutrition & Food Research, 58*(4), 808–820.

Oelschlaeger, T. A. (2010). Mechanisms of probiotic actions-a review. *International Journal of Medical Microbiology, 300*(1), 57–62.

Oh, K. K., Gupta, H., Min, B. H., Ganesan, R., Sharma, S. P., Won, S. M., ... & Suk, K. T. (2022). Elucidation of prebiotics, probiotics, postbiotics, and target from gut microbiota to alleviate obesity via network pharmacology study. *Cells, 11*(18), 2903.

Ojeda, P., Bobe, A., Dolan, K., Leone, V., & Martinez, K. (2016). Nutritional modulation of gut microbiota-The impact on metabolic disease pathophysiology. *The Journal of Nutritional Biochemistry, 28*, 191–200.

Østlie, H. M., Helland, M. H., & Narvhus, J. A. (2003). Growth and metabolism of selected strains of probiotic bacteria in milk. *International Journal of Food Microbiology, 87*(1–2), 17–27.

Pabinger, S., Rödiger, S., Kriegner, A., Vierlinger, K., & Weinhäusel, A. (2014). A survey of tools for the analysis of quantitative PCR (qPCR) data. *Biomolecular Detection and Quantification, 1*(1), 23–33.

Pandey, K. R., Naik, S. R., & Vakil, B. V. (2015). Probiotics, prebiotics and synbiotics-a review. *Journal of Food Science and Technology, 52*(12), 7577–7587.

Park, M., Joung, M., Park, J. H., Ha, S. K., & Park, H. Y. (2022). Role of postbiotics in diet-induced metabolic disorders. *Nutrients, 14*(18), 3701.

Parvez, S., Malik, K. A., Kang, S. A., & Kim, H. Y. (2006). Probiotics and their fermented food products are beneficial for health. *Journal of Applied Microbiology*, *100*(6), 1171–1185.

Pascale, A., Marchesi, N., Marelli, C., Coppola, A., Luzi, L., Govoni, S., ... & Gazzaruso, C. (2018). Microbiota and metabolic diseases. *Endocrine*, *61*, 357–371.

Rastall, R. A. (2010). Functional oligosaccharides: application and manufacture. *Annual Review of Food Science and Technology*, *1*, 305–339.

Ren, H., Vahjen, W., Dadi, T., Saliu, E. M., Boroojeni, F. G., & Zentek, J. (2019). Synergistic effects of probiotics and phytobiotics on the intestinal microbiota in young broiler chicken. *Microorganisms*, *7*(12), 684.

Ricciuto, A., & Griffiths, A. M. (2019). Clinical value of fecal calprotectin. *Critical Reviews in Clinical Laboratory Sciences*, *56*(5), 307–320.

Round, J. L., & Mazmanian, S. K. (2009). The gut microbiota shapes intestinal immune responses during health and disease. *Nature Reviews Immunology*, *9*(5), 313–323.

Salminen, S., Collado, M. C., Endo, A., Hill, C., Lebeer, S., Quigley, E. M., ... & Szajewska, H. (2021). The International Scientific Association of Probiotics and Prebiotics (ISAPP) consensus statement on the definition and scope of postbiotics. *Nature Reviews Gastroenterology & Hepatology*, *18*(10), 649–667.

Sanders, M. E., Merenstein, D. J., Ouwehand, A., Reid, G., Salminen, S., Cabana, M. D., ... & Gibson, G. R. (2019). Probiotic use in at-risk populations. *Journal of the American Pharmacists Association*, *59*(6), 732–739.

Sharma, R., & Padwad, Y. (2020). Plant-polyphenols based second-generation synbiotics: emerging concepts, challenges, and opportunities. *Nutrition*, *77*, 110785.

Shi, Q., Dai, L., Zhao, Q., & Zhang, X. (2022). A review on the effect of gut microbiota on metabolic diseases. *Archives of Microbiology*, *204*(3), 192.

Simmering, R., & Blaut, M. (2001). Pro-and prebiotics-the tasty guardian angels? Applied *Microbiology and Biotechnology*, *55*, 19–28.

Taverniti, V., & Guglielmetti, S. (2011). Health-promoting properties of *Lactobacillus helveticus*. *Frontiers in Microbiology*, *2*, 1–14.

Thorakkattu, P., Khanashyam, A. C., Shah, K., Babu, K. S., Mundanat, A. S., Deliephan, A., ... & Nirmal, N. P. (2022). Postbiotics: current trends in food and pharmaceutical industry. *Foods*, *11*(19), 3094.

Turnbaugh, P. J., Ley, R. E., Mahowald, M. A., Magrini, V., Mardis, E. R., & Gordon, J. I. (2006). An obesity-associated gut microbiome with increased capacity for energy harvest. *Nature*, *444*(7122), 1027–1031.

Vallianou, N., Stratigou, T., Christodoulatos, G. S., Tsigalou, C., & Dalamaga, M. (2020). Probiotics, prebiotics, synbiotics, postbiotics, and obesity: current evidence, controversies, and perspectives. *Current Obesity Reports*, *9*, 179–192.

Vassileva, M., Flor-Peregrin, E., Malusá, E., & Vassilev, N. (2020). Towards better understanding of the interactions and efficient application of plant beneficial prebiotics, probiotics, postbiotics and synbiotics. *Frontiers in Plant Science*, *11*, 1068.

Wachsmuth, H. R., Weninger, S. N., & Duca, F. A. (2022). Role of the gut-brain axis in energy and glucose metabolism. *Experimental & Molecular Medicine*, *54*(4), 377–392.

Wang, P. X., Deng, X. R., Zhang, C. H., & Yuan, H. J. (2020). Gut microbiota and metabolic syndrome. *Chinese Medical Journal*, *133*(07), 808–816.

Xavier-Santos, D., Bedani, R., Lima, E. D., & Saad, S. M. I. (2020). Impact of probiotics and prebiotics targeting metabolic syndrome. *Journal of Functional Foods*, *64*, 103666.

Zhou, Y. L., & Hong, J. (2023). Gut microbiota: guardians of the female gut health. *Cancer Cell*, *41*(8), 1392–1394.

Żółkiewicz, J., Marzec, A., Ruszczyński, M., & Feleszko, W. (2020). Postbiotics-a step beyond pre-and probiotics. *Nutrients*, *12*(8), 2189.

12 Impact of Bacterial Metabolites on the Gut Environment to Manage Metabolic Disorders

Sohail Ahmad, Maria Faraz, Muhammad Badar, Alamgir Khan, Roomah Javed, and Arshad Farid

12.1 INTRODUCTION

Gut microbiome (GM) is a collection of various bacteria that coexist harmoniously with their host in the gastrointestinal tract. Although the significance of GM has been known for decades, the advancement in technologies like metabolomics and genomics opened the door for hidden knowledge about the microbiome (Lagier et al.., 2018). Dysbiosis of GM has been previously associated with different kinds of diseases. Besides causing diseases, GM can interact with oral drugs to modify their toxicity and effectiveness (Feng et al., 2020). The medical world is concentrating on this issue since GM not only affects how diseases develop but also has the power to change the toxicity and effectiveness of oral drugs (Vancamelbeke and Vermeire, 2017). The GM has evolved as a way to get over this spatial limitation by producing several classes of metabolites to affect both humans and other gut bacteria. In light of these developments, researchers must identify the GM's metabolites in detail to fully understand their roles. Many metabolites which include choline, bile, and short-chain fatty acids (SCFAs) were discovered using technologies like tandem mass spectrometry and liquid chromatography (Milshteyn et al., 2018). Metabolites of the GM have an impact on bacteria as well as the host they live in Perino et al. (2021). Knowing the interaction of these metabolic substances between bacteria as well as with the host stands as a significant clue in the analysis of both disease and healthy conditions.

12.2 NORMAL GUT MICROBIOTA COMPOSITION

It was previously believed that 500–1,000 species of microorganisms made up the GM (Frank et al., 2007). GM of humans is composed of almost 35,000 distinct species of bacteria (Ramakrishna, 2007). Moreover, the human gut is home to around ten million non-redundant genes. A study composed of 169 obese and 123 non-obese Dutch individuals was done to investigate GM. The study provided the concepts of high gene count (HGC) and low gene count (LGC), both of which are connected to health and disease (Le Chatelier et al., 2013). The HGC microbiome contains a significant amount of Akkermansia (Verrucomicrobia), along with Anaerotruncus coli hominis, Butyrivibrio crossotus, and Fecalibacterium sp. ratio. Large quantity of butyrate, less amount of hydrogen sulfide, augmented susceptibility of hydrogen, and the advancement of acetogenic bionetwork are very advantageous for digestive well-being (Le Chatelier et al., 2013). Highly concentrated pro-inflammatory bacteria are present in patients having LGC. These are connected with irritable bowel syndrome which affects the digestive system of the body (Swidsinski et al., 2005a; Joossens et al., 2011). LGC contains some bacteria like Staphylococcus, Anaerostipes, Dialister, etc. which are comprehensively used at gene level in the gut microbiota.

The number of the organism changes as one moves from the esophagus toward the rectum. The esophagus has almost 10^1 bacteria/gram while rectum has a huge number and is estimated to be around 10^{12} bacteria/gram (O'Hara and Shanahan, 2006). Streptococcus is an abundant genus in proximal esophagus, jejunum and duodenum (Pei et al., 2004). The general microbial landscape of the gastric flora, Helicobacter, is determined by the main species found in the stomach. In the stomach, Helicobacter pylori coexist as a commensal alongside several important species, including the most common Streptococcus, Prevotella, Rothia, and Veillonella (Blaser, 1999). When addressing gut-residing flora in connection to disease states, the term "colonic flora" is often used, especially when referring to bacterial strains derived from the metagenomic of the stool. The large intestine is home to two major phyla: Firmicutes and Bacteroidetes. Numerous illnesses are linked to the increased ratio of the following two phyla (Hollister et al., 2014). Apart from Bacteroidetes and Firmicutes species, other bacterial genera identified in the human colon include *Salmonella enterica, Campylobacter jejuni, Vibrio cholera, Bacteroides fragilis*, and Escherichia coli. However, they account for less than 0.1% of the GM, which is a very small contribution (Curtis et al., 2012; Gillespie et al., 2011). Contrary to prominent prevalence of hallmark taxa like Bacteroides, Prevotella, and Ruminococcus, healthy gut has lower prevalence of species from proteobacteria phylum (Hollister et al., 2014) (Figure 12.1)

Apart from the difference in longitudinal section, an axial difference is also found in mucosal surface and that of

DOI: 10.1201/9781032702438-12

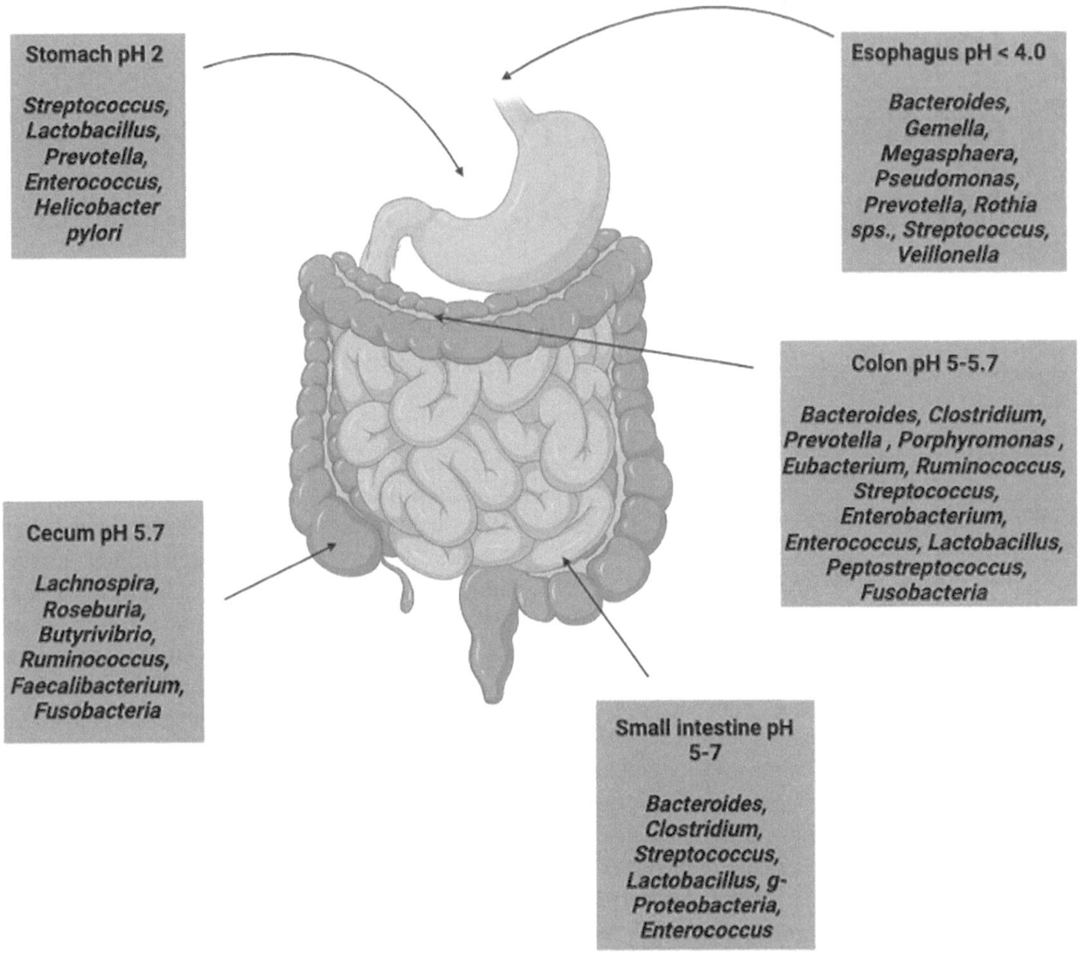

FIGURE 12.1 Gut microbiota distribution.

intestinal lumen. Although, most common luminal microbial species include *Bifidobacterium*, *Enterobacteriaceae*, *Bacteroides*, *Enterococcus*, *Streptococcus*, *Lactobacillus*, *Ruminococcus*, and *Clostridium*. The only genera related to mucus and common mucosa are *Lactobacillus*, *Clostridium*, *Akkermansia*, and *Enterococcus* (Swidsinski et al., 2005b).

12.3 CLASSIFICATION OF GUT MICROBIOTA METABOLITES

According to an estimate, there are around 22 million microbial genes related to the normal flora of the gut and approximately 10^{15} microbial cells, both of which are higher than those found in humans (Qin et al., 2010). Gut metabolites are usually of three kinds, based on their origin: the first kind of metabolites are produced as a result of gut microbes' action at the meal. Examples of such type of metabolites include indole derivatives and SCGAs while the 2nd kind of metabolites are those metabolites produced in the host body and gut microbes only modify them and examples of such metabolites are secondary bile acid and the third kind of metabolites are produced from scratch like polysaccharides A (Postler and Ghosh, 2017). A specific metabolite of the gut microbiota has numerous functions since it might affect different organs or tissues. More specifically, butyrate can impact the immune system overall as well as the intestinal barrier. Moreover, it can supply colonocytes with energy and nutrition.. The GM metabolites that have been investigated the most are bile acids, amino acid-derived metabolites, and SCFAs.

SCFAs are comprised carbon 1–6. The most prominent SCFAs generated in gut by bacteria are propionate, butyrate, and acetate. Much SCFA is produced when stomach and small intestine proteins ferment undigested branched-chain amino acids. This mechanism is also responsible for the fermentation of carbohydrates that have evaded the action of host enzymes (Russell et al., 2011). SCFAs after their production are absorbed in the large intestine by colonocytes and the process is helped by hydrogen or sodium-dependent monocarboxylate transporters (Vijay and Morris, 2014). A substantial amount of SCFAs in colonocytes act as an energy source, while rest of the SCFAs can enter the bloodstream and be absorbed by other tissues including the heart, brain, and lung (Tan et al., 2014).

Indoles, Indigos, phenols, p-cresol sulfate, amines, ammonia, nitrogen compounds, sulfides, and phenols, are some of the compounds produced from the undigested peptides and proteins of the host (Smith and Macfarlane, 1996). A significant number of researchers have focused on tryptophan and its derivatives out of all these substances. Within the gastrointestinal system, unabsorbed tryptophan is converted to different kinds of derivative substances like skatole, indole-3-propionic acid, and 3-methyl-indole (Agus et al., 2021). A protein Aryl hydrocarbon receptor (AhR) can affect the metabolism, social behavior, and immunity of the host. Different kind of gut metabolites binds to this protein and brings changes in their function (Modoux et al., 2021; Roager and Licht, 2018).

Gut-residing microbes also produce other metabolites despite those already discussed and these metabolites have important physiological functions related to the host. Certain gases, namely, carbon dioxide (CO_2), hydrogen sulfide (H_2S), nitric oxide (NO), methane (CH_4), and hydrogen (H_2), can modify the physiological state of their hosts. These gases are produced in the host through microflora present in gut of the host (Kalantar-Zadeh et al., 2019). The host's behavior may be influenced by lipids generated by gut microorganisms, such as lipopolysaccharides and conjugated fatty acids (Nicholson et al., 2012). Based on an analysis of the human gut bacterial genomes for B-vitamin biosynthesis pathways, 40%–65% of the bacteria were shown to be capable of producing vitamins, and the GM is a significant source of these substances (Magnúsdóttir et al., 2015). Even though the significance of GM metabolites has been established, a significant portion of them are yet unknown. Therefore, it has become crucial to investigate the gut microbiota for metabolites with specific functions (Wang et al., 2019). Numerous techniques, including metabolomics, functional metagenomics, and sequence-based (meta)genomics have been developed to find these compounds (Behsaz et al., 2021; Kenshole et al., 2021).

12.4 GUT MICROFLORAL MODE OF ACTION ON THEIR TARGET

Numerous host processes are regulated by the metabolites of the GM, either directly or indirectly (Figure 12.2). The host health condition is reliable on the composition of the GM's heterogeneity. Furthermore, metabolism depends on the makeup of GM. For instance, SCFAs give gut organisms energy while also preventing some gut bacteria from growing or developing and changing the makeup of genetically modified organisms (Sun and O'Riordan, 2013). A non-inflammatory secretory antibody A produced by host is modulated by SCFAs to stop pathogen invasion (Takeuchi and Ohno, 2021). Additionally, gut microbial metabolites can directly modify host processes by acting on targets within or outside of the gastrointestinal system. Moreover, SCFAs may be distributed to distant organs and tissues, where they are immediately detected by the target organs and tissues and cause significant physiological alterations in the hosts (Cait et al., 2018).

Bacterial products are taken up by one organism and exchanged with another, a process known as bacterial cross-feeding (Smith et al., 2019). Lactate is the end product of cross-feeding which is produced by bifiodiobacterium. *Eubacterium hallii* is not able to live in a pure culture of starch. Growing *Bifidobacterium adolescentis* and *E. hallii* together in a culture results in a notable decrease in lactate concentration while butyrate concentration rises (Zelezniak et al., 2015). Thus, utilizing the lactose produced by *B. adolescentis*, *E. hallii* may synthesize butyric acid. In low-nutrient environments, cross-feeding confers major benefits to bacteria and modifies antibiotic resistance in bacterial populations (Adamowicz et al., 2018).

12.5 GUT MICROBIOTA METABOLITES AND ITS FUNCTIONAL ROLE

12.5.1 Alteration of GM Composition

Proper composition of GM is thought to maintain the integrity of GIT and prevent pathogen invasion. This is done by inducing the host system to release antimicrobial substances, repressing adhesion sites for the pathogens, and enhancing nutrient uptake (Maynard et al., 2012). Changes in GM composition are known as gut dysbiosis and this condition is linked to different kinds of disorders (Wilkins et al., 2019). Many metabolites of GM, aside from the SCFAs, have a tendency to change the chemical composition and function of GM. Pathogenicity, motility, and antibiotic resistance of gut microbiota can be controlled by indole (Lee et al., 2015). The structure of bacterial membrane is disrupted by the use of bile acids, which also inhibit the growth of gut bacteria (Wahlström et al., 2016). Several important metabolites are formed in the gut microbiota. Along with that ribosomally synthesized antibiotics are also of special interest (Garcia-Gutierrez et al., 2019). In an era where there is serious concern over the overuse of antibiotics, such kind of metabolites are the spark of the hope to be an alternative for antibiotics against a vast spectrum of bacteria (Garcia-Gutierrez et al., 2019). Apart from their main duty, these metabolites have an indirect effect on the host immune system and bring certain kind of changes in their immune system (Figure 12.2). Synthesis of cecal slgA by SCFAs changes the complete setup of GM (Kim et al., 2016). Similar to this, bile acids can influence FXR, which in turn can trigger the transcription of antimicrobial molecules like interleukin (IL)-18 and inducible nitric oxide synthase. These molecules maintain the composition of gut microflora (Inagaki et al., 2006).

12.5.2 GM Metabolites as Nutrition/Nutrient Absorption Facilitators

Many vitamins, particularly vitamin B and K group vitamins, may be synthesized by gut microbes like *Bifidobacteria* (Hill, 1997). Although these vitamins have their main function to support the metabolism of bacteria,

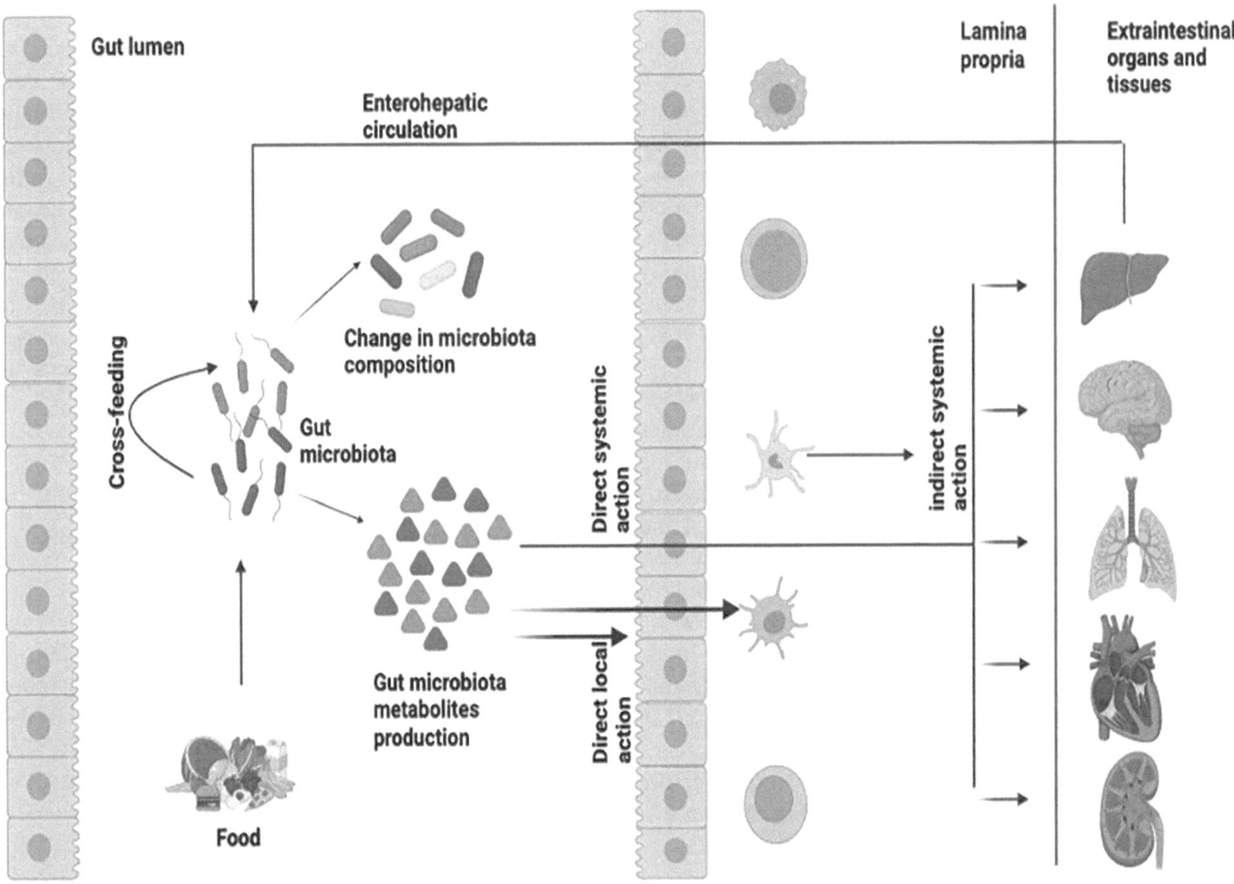

FIGURE 12.2 Interaction of GM metabolites with targets. In the lumen, some bacteria nourish over the metabolites of the other neighboring bacteria and affect the composition of GM. Immune cells and intestinal epithelia are affected by GM metabolites. Later on, these local effects may have systemic implications. Compounds produced by GM can move to other places and be reabsorbed so performs action on and in distant organs. The composition and function of GM may sometimes be transformed by the metabolites of the other gut-residing bacteria which ultimately leads to the production of new anti-bacterial compounds. The GM may circulate certain compounds via enterohepatic circulation.

they are also an additional source of vitamin supplies for mammals, maintaining their physiological and metabolic processes. SCFAs can be used as resources for lipid biosynthesis and gluconeogenesis, or they can be immediately broken down to provide energy (Feng et al., 2020). Production of amino acid metabolites by GM like valine, tryptophan, leucin, and isoleucine stands as raw material for the production of other metabolites that have a major impact on mammalian physiology (Skrypnik and Suliburska, 2018). In humans, minerals serve a variety of vital roles, including being an essential component of hemoglobin, bones, and enzymes. The bioavailability of minerals can be impacted by gut microbiota metabolites, particularly SCFAs, which alter intestinal tissue architecture and transport proteins. It also lowers the pH of the substances present in the intestinal lumen (Whisner and Castillo, 2018). Bile acids, being water-soluble and amphipathic molecules, emulsify fat-soluble vitamins and dietary lipids to aid in their absorption after they are released from the gall bladder into the duodenum (Perino et al., 2021).

12.5.3 Modulation of Host Metabolism

Maintaining an equilibrium between storing and releasing energy is essential to an organism's ability to survive and maintain health. Maintaining a positive energy balance for the long term in adults is responsible for obesity and other supplementary diseases, like colon cancer, type II diabetes, asthma, arthritis, hypercholesterolemia, and liver disease (Mokdad et al., 2003; Must et al., 1999). Contrary to that negative energy balance in the long term leads to a variety of diseases and other physiological conditions, such as reduced fertility, decreased thyroid hormone production, loss of bone mass, and decreased athletic performance (Kurpad et al., 2005; Pollock et al., 2010). Lipids and glucose are two nutrients that are essential for energy metabolism and the development of illness. The control of satiety, nutrition metabolism, non-shivering thermogenesis, insulin sensitivity, synthesis and secretion, and organ motility are all manipulated by the GM and its metabolites (Figure 12.3).

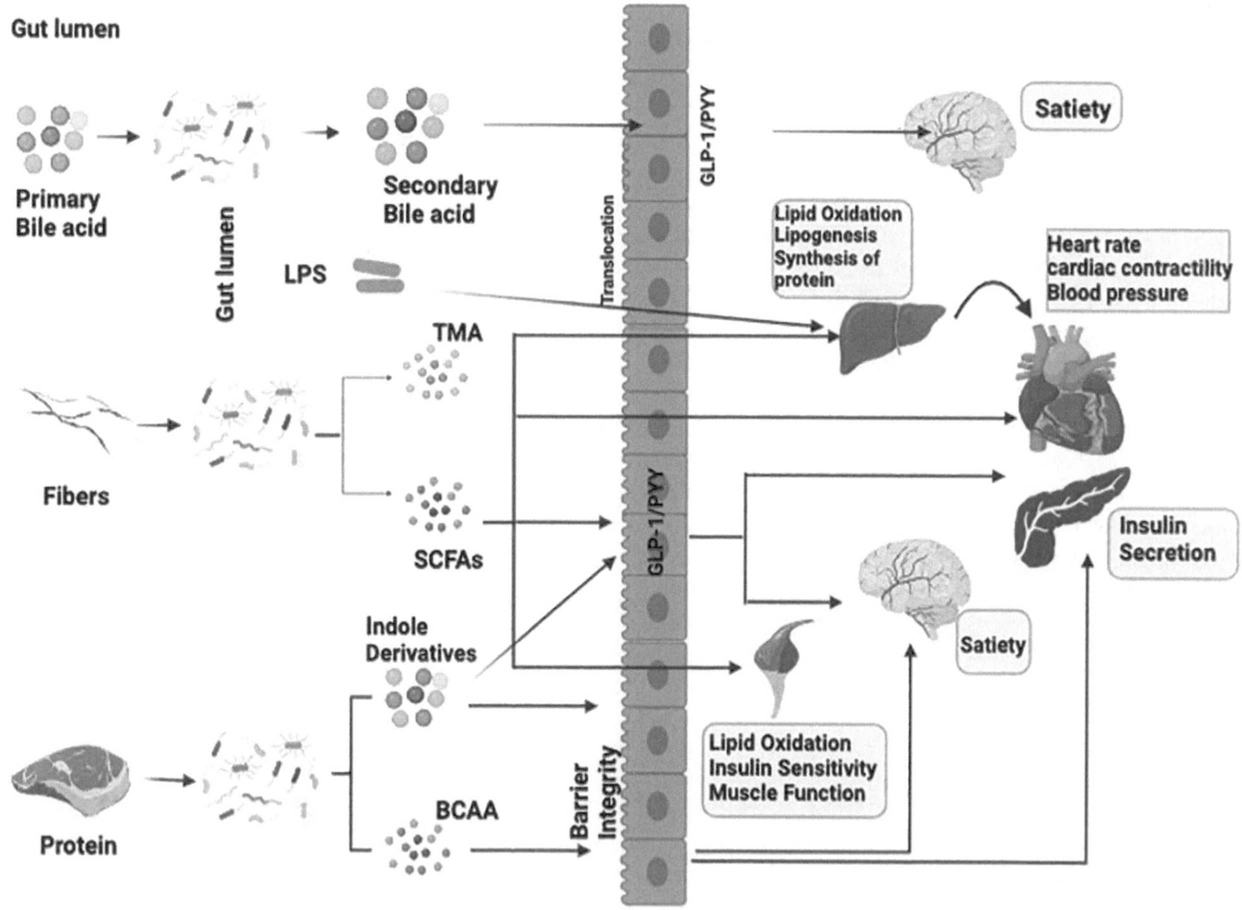

FIGURE 12.3 GM's essential metabolites in modulating host metabolism. The modulation primarily operates through the regulation of nutritional metabolism (glucose, lipids, and), satiety (via hormone production of GLP-1 and PYY), insulin formation, secretion, and sensitivity. Additionally, it extends to non-shivering thermogenesis and organ motility (including muscle and heart). The metabolites produced by the gut microbiome contribute significantly to maintaining energy balance through these mechanisms.

The ability of adipose cells to store fat is enhanced by SCFAs, particularly acetate, which can boost adipogenesis, and reduce lipolysis (Jocken et al., 2018). To a lesser extent butyrate can restore compromised thermogenesis occurred as a result of antibiotics in a cold environment by enhancing BAT thermogenesis and browning WAT (Li et al., 2019a). Type II diabetes is the result of improper functioning of insulin and β-cells. β-Cell activity and insulin secretion are positively impacted by SCFAs via GPR43 (Pingitore et al., 2017; Priyadarshini et al., 2015). SCFAs can impact skeletal muscle, which is the biggest organ, via GPR41, GPR43, and HDACs (Frampton et al., 2020). SCFAs can lower blood pressure, cardiac contractility, and heart rate while providing energy to the heart (Carley et al., 2021; Poll et al., 2021). The liver is the prime organ performing most of the carbohydrates and lipid metabolism (Den Besten et al., 2013). In obese individuals, SCFAs shift the momentum from lipogenesis toward beta-oxidation of fats by increasing energy expenditure.

The control of energy metabolism is significantly influenced by metabolites produced by the GM in addition to SCFAs. TGR5 and FXR are bile acid receptors known for their potential to enhance insulin sensitivity, increase hepatic glycogen production, and promote improved energy metabolism in brown adipose tissue, muscle, and liver, while also stimulating insulin secretion (Agus et al., 2021). Similar to SCFAs, bile acids possess the capacity to engage with enteroendocrine cells, leading to the stimulation of the release of gut hormones responsible for regulating hunger and motility (Cani et al., 2019; Perino et al., 2021). Bile acids control triglyceride metabolism, particularly lipogenesis and VLDL synthesis, whose dysbolism contributes to obesity, atherosclerosis, TIID, and other cardiovascular disorders (Jonsson and Bäckhed, 2017). GM synthesizes essential amino acids and branched-chain amino acids. The following helps in insulin production (Floyd et al., 1966; Felig et al., 1969). Reduced BCAAs can enhance body composition and glucose tolerance (Fontana et al., 2016). Many investigations have shown the critical functions of BCAAs in controlling insulin resistance, hepatocyte proliferation, protein synthesis, glucose and lipid metabolism, and BAT thermogenesis (Tajiri and Shimizu, 2018). Tryptophan, LPS, TMAO, and indole-derived metabolites are a few more gut microbiota compounds that have a strong impact on the metabolism of nutrients and energy (Agus et al., 2021). Disrupted synthesis of these GM compounds is linked to diseases such as dyslipidemia, nonalcoholic fatty liver disease, atherosclerosis, TIIDs, heart failure, and obesity, (Chávez-Talavera et al., 2017; Đanić et al., 2018).

12.5.4 Influencing the Nervous System

Connection between the gut and central nervous system (CNS) has been known for decades. CNS also controls, blood flow, nociception, immunological response, and digestive juice production of the gut (Silva et al., 2020). Furthermore, GM's composition and functions can be further influenced by brain-to-gut signaling through the intestinal immune system (Silva et al., 2020). Instead, a rising corpus of research reveals that the metabolites of the GM greatly influence brain function (Figure 12.4), and thus influence the onset of neurological and psychological conditions such as autism, major depressive disorder, Alzheimer's disease, multiple sclerosis, anxiety disorder, and Parkinson's disease (Fung et al., 2017). BBB is a constituent of the neurovascular unit, which consists of microglia, neurons, extracellular matrix, astrocytes, brain microvascular endothelial cells, and pericytes. To protect the brain from direct interaction of drugs or their components and also prevent it from pathogens and injuries BBB acts as a protective cover. Brain damage, autoimmune disorders, and infections can alter the BBB's integrity, increasing the brain's susceptibility to harmful substances in the bloodstream (Grab et al., 2005). SCFAs play a significant role in maintaining BBB coherence. It has also been confirmed through the administration of sodium butyrate in traumatic brain injury which inhibits or stops BBB breakdown (Li et al., 2016). The BBB can be crossed by SCFAs through monocarboxylate transporters which are sodium- or H+-dependent. SCFAs directly control behavior, learning, memory, and the development of disease in the brain (Dalile et al., 2019).

Immune cells like astrocytes, CD8+T, mast cells, microglia, perivascular macrophages, and CD4+T are present in the CNS and may cause inflammation in the brain (Fung et al., 2017).

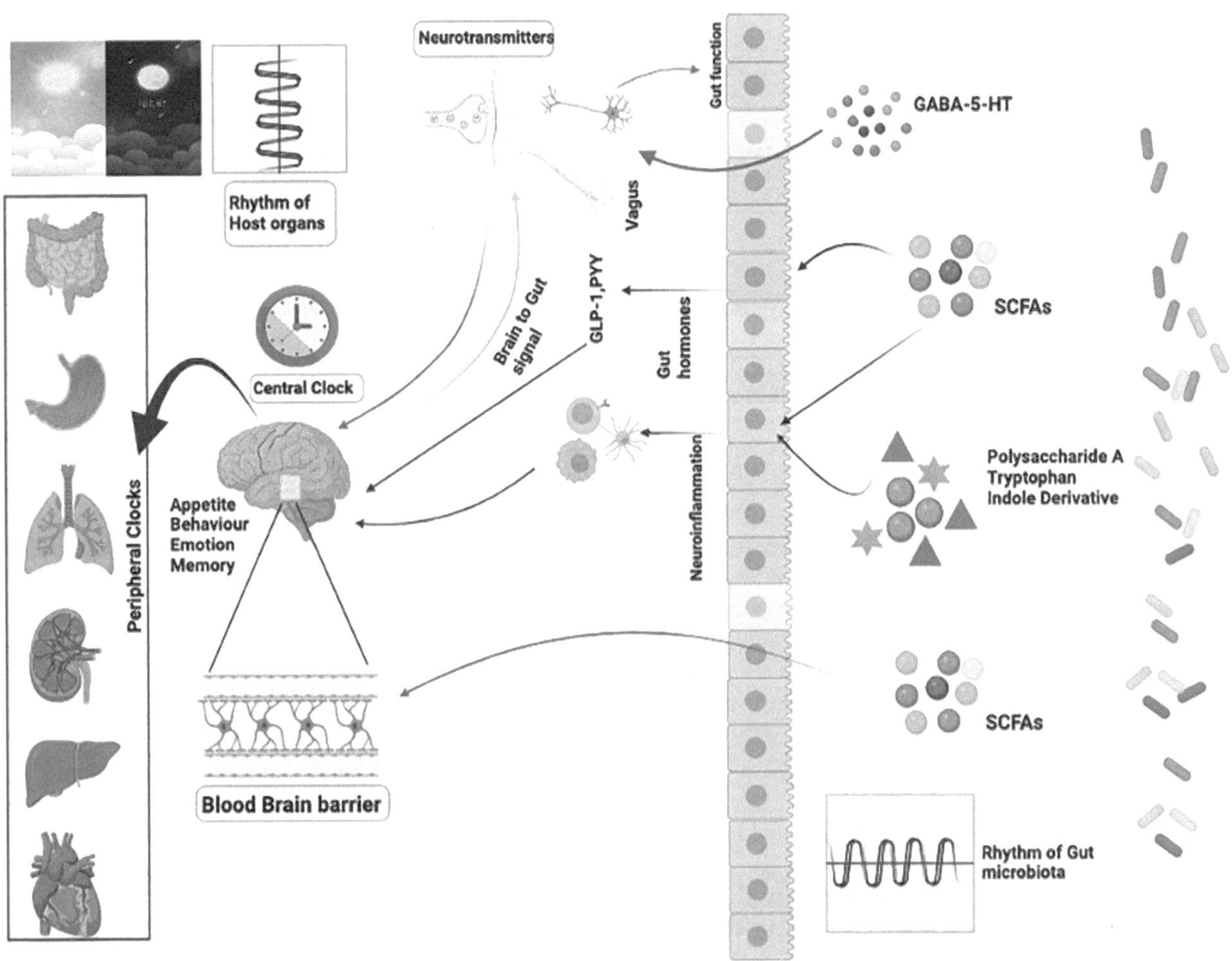

FIGURE 12.4 Circadian rhythm modulation. The gut microbiome produces metabolites that can regulate a variety of brain functions, including mood and hunger regulation, blood-brain barrier function, neural impulse transmission, and cerebral inflammation. On the other hand, the production of digestive juice and the motility of the stomach may be controlled by the brain. The gut microbiota produces compounds that exhibit day-night rhythms. These rhythms can be transmitted to the central and peripheral clocks, so modifying the systemic activity of the hosts. In a similar vein, the gut microbiota and peripheral organs can receive light and dark cues from the central clock, allowing the microbiota to synchronize with the host clock.

Usually, the production of cytokines by the immune cells does not have a significant effect on CNS. Conversely, persistent systemic inflammation may result in notable behavioral changes and cognitive impairments (Perry et al., 2003, 2007). Axonal damage and experimental autoimmune encephalomyelitis in mice were reduced by SCFA treatment, which also enhanced Treg differentiation by blocking the c-Jun NH2- terminal kinase 1 and p38 pathway (Haghikia et al., 2015). Similarly, a Toll-like receptor (TLR)-2 dependent mechanism shields wild-type mice against inflammation and CNS demyelination when a gut bacterial product called polysaccharide A is administered (Ochoa-Reparaz et al., 2010). The most prevalent type of brain cells are called astrocytes and they produce cytokines and present antigens to influence neural inflammatory responses (Dong and Benveniste, 2001). GM metabolites including tryptophan and indole derivatives affect animal multiple sclerosis by triggering AhR (Rothhammer et al., 2016).

One of the main drivers of feeding behavior is the experience of hunger and fullness. Metabolites of the GM can either stimulate a variety of metabolic diseases or protect the host metabolic health by influencing hunger. Enteroendocrine cells in the colon may be stimulated by gut microbiota metabolites to produce peripheral hormones (insulin, ghrelin, and leptin), neurotransmitter 5-HT, and anorexigenic hormones, i.e. GLP-1, cholecystokinin, PYY (Han et al., 2021). The release of GLP-1, PYY, insulin, and leptin can result from SCFAs binding to GRP43 (Lerche et al., 2008; Song et al., 2019). In the brain, anorexigenic hormones activate Proopiomelanocortin, which may cross the blood-brain barrier. Furthermore, certain metabolites of the GM, including GABA, can act as neurotransmitters to control hunger. The fact is corroborated by the observation that distraction of the signaling pathways of GABA reduced the appetite associated with hunger, decreased the hyperphagia produced by neuropeptide Y, and inhibited postweaning feeding (Kim et al., 2015; Xu et al., 2018). Additionally, the GM is able to synthesize protein sequences that are the same as peptides that regulate appetite, such as caseinolytic protease, which mimics the actions of alpha-melanocyte-stimulating hormone and causes anorexic effects (Sharon et al., 2016).

12.5.5 Transitions in the Circadian Rhythm

Humans have progressed to fit into a circadian cycle of around 24 hours, which corresponds to the light and dark cycle of the earth. Circadian cycle has a great influence on gastrointestinal motility, sleep-wake cycles, hormone production, behavior, molecular fluctuations of genes, and all the metabolites (Pearson et al., 2020; Segers and Depoortere, 2021). The central circadian clock is located in the hypothalamic suprachiasmatic nucleus. It gathers cues of light and darkness from the environment and synchronizes this information with peripheral clocks in various tissues, ensuring a consistent rhythm (Frazier and Chang, 2020). A number of lifestyle factors, such as working shifts, traveling, getting too little sleep, being exposed to artificial light at night, and when and what kind of food is consumed, can cause disruptions in circadian rhythms. Many diseases, including cancer, heart disease, neurological diseases, gastrointestinal problems, metabolic diseases, sleep and mental health issues, and metabolic diseases are linked to disruption of circadian rhythms (Lopez et al., 2021; Sancar and Van Gelder, 2021).

It has been observed recently that GM can control or have an impact on both the central and peripheral circadian clocks (Figure 12.4). Similar to mammal circadian rhythm, the gut microbiota exhibits both functional and compositional oscillation. The host transcriptome oscillations can be influenced by these oscillations, which ultimately impact medication hepatotoxicity and liver detoxification (Thaiss et al., 2016). GM influences both contact-dependent and contact-independent mechanisms of host circadian rhythms (Bishehsari et al., 2020). Direct contact between gastrointestinal cells and gut bacteria is necessary for the contact-dependent processes to function, and pattern recognition receptors like TLRs and NOD-like receptors must then be activated (Bishehsari et al., 2020). Majority of the small molecular GM metabolites like SCFAs and bile function as mediators are required for contact-independent pathways (Frazier and Chang, 2020). For instance, there is a clear diurnal fluctuation in butyrate and propionate levels, which disappears with a high-fat diet (Leone et al., 2015). Important hepatic circadian genes, such as Per2 and Bmall, have their oscillations of expression dramatically altered by treatment with SCFAs in both murine and hepatic-derived organoids (Leone et al., 2015). Quite the reverse; the rhythmicity of fecal SCFA levels was eliminated upon deletion of Bmall, indicating that the hosts' circadian rhythm can control the rhythmicity of the gut microbiota (Segers et al., 2019).

Numerous activities of metabolites produced by GM, like immune response and energy metabolism regulation, are inextricably linked to their profound impact on circadian rhythm. For a comprehensive knowledge of the gut microbiota metabolites functions, it is crucial to comprehend the connections between various functions via the interconnection of these metabolites. For instance, the gut microbiota synchronizes the daily oscillations in histone acetylation via programming the diurnal oscillations of a SCFAs receptor, HDAC3 (Kuang et al., 2019). Furthermore, obesity and lipid transporter gene Cd36 rhythmic transcription were produced by HDAC3 oscillations and high-fat diets. The study demonstrated the close connections between the various roles of gut microbiota metabolites (Selmer and Andrei., 2001).

12.5.6 Impacting the Systemic Immune Response

Additionally, to regulate intestinal immunity, the GM can impact the innate and adaptive immune responses in several extraintestinal organs by interacting with a wide range of immune cells, including B cells, T cells, and macrophages.

SCFAs increase acetyl-CoA and regulate metabolic sensors in spleen B cells to enhance antibody synthesis (Kim et al., 2016). Reduced SCFA synthesis was associated with abnormalities in pathogen-specific antibody responses and homeostasis, which increased susceptibility to infections. However, SCFA consumption can compensate for this immunological deficit (Kim et al., 2016). In the lungs, the defense against allergies and asthma is provided by gut microbiota metabolites, primarily SCFAs. Antibiotic therapy exacerbates allergic lung inflammation; synthetic cannabidiols (SCFAs) reduce it by affecting T helper type 2 cells and reducing blood levels of immunoglobulin E (Cait et al., 2018; Russell et al., 2012). Acetate in drinking water prevented adult asthma in the offspring of pregnant mice, and the mechanism involved is related to controlling mucosal immune responses by activating GPCRs including GPR109A and GPR41 (Trompette et al., 2014). HDAC inhibition to increase the number and capacity of Treg cells. In influenza-infected mice, butyrate prevented lung damage by controlling the CD8+ T cells metabolism specific to influenza and influencing the hematopoiesis of Ly6c-patrolling monocytes (Thorburn et al., 2015).

Examples of autoimmune cholestatic liver illnesses characterized by aberrant bile secretion and the primary conditions associated with the excessive accumulation of toxic bile acids are primary biliary cholangitis and primary sclerosing cholangitis (Dyson et al., 2020). Elevated bile acid levels in the liver can activate pro-inflammatory pathways and produce NF-κB-dependent mediators, which in turn can lead to autoimmune liver damage (Allen et al., 2011; Gujral et al., 2003). Bile acids can also directly harm biliary epithelial cells and result in the generation of IL-6 and IL-1β, both of which exacerbate inflammation (O'Brien et al., 2013). Hepatic inflammation can be diminished by obstructing the stimulation of pro-inflammatory macrophages (Deng et al., 2020).

Risks of certain cardiovascular disorders have increased due to high trimethylamine N-oxide (Peng et al., 2018). Trimethylamine N-oxide has the ability to increase monocyte linkage and diminish endothelial cells by stimulating protein kinase C (Ma et al., 2017). TMAO also proliferate the TNF-α which affects the heart inflammation.

Osteoporosis diminished the microstructural integrity and bone mineral density. Immunological functions are also disrupted by the metabolites present in gut microbiota (Li et al., 2019). Harmful substances enter the bloodstream due to the permeability of intestinal barrier which decreases the density of minerals in bone (Behera et al., 2020; Lu et al., 2021). These mechanisms are associated with the activation of TLR2 and TLR4 in mesenchymal stromal cells, which inhibits the differentiation of osteoblasts, and the start of the MAPK signaling and NF-κB pathways, which encourages the conversion of macrophages into osteoclasts (Wikoff et al., 2009). Renal injury, inflammation, and fibrosis can be brought on by metabolites in the kidney, which can build up and aid in the etiology and advancement of chronic kidney disease (CKD) (Vijay and Morris, 2014).

Gut microbiota metabolites not only influence other organs or tissues but are also reported to be the main cause of rheumatoid arthritis, systemic lupus erythematosus, HIV, and various inflammatory skin conditions (Salem et al., 2018; Yang and Cong, 2021). By increasing the amount of the serotonin product 5-hydroxyindole-3-acetic acid, butyrate reduces arthritis in a way that is dependent on regulatory B cells. AhR, a transcriptional marker for regulating B cell activity, may be further activated as a result (Rosser et al., 2020).

12.5.7 Affecting Drug Efficacy and Toxicity

GM affects the toxicity and effectiveness of herbal medicine like aconitine, berberine, and metformin. The gut microbiota is involved in altering the toxicity and effectiveness of medications and herbal remedies, including aconitine, berberine, and metformin (Feng et al., 2020). Drug-metabolizing enzymes are in competition with gut microbial metabolites, change the expression of drug metabolization-related enzymes, and also may interfere with the process of hepatic drug-metabolizing enzymes and in this way can affect the toxicity and effectiveness of the drugs. Microorganisms from the phyla Firmicutes, *Bacteroidetes, Actinobacteria*, and *Fusobacteria* produce *p-Cresol* are a metabolic product of tyrosine and phenylalanine (Bone et al., 1976; Selmer and Andrei, 2001). One common non-steroidal anti-inflammatory medication used to relieve fever and discomfort is acetaminophen. In clinical settings, an overdose of acetaminophen can result in severe lethal hepatotoxicity (Hodgman and Garrard, 2012). Acetaminophen's toxicity in the liver can be decreased by converting it to the inactive form acetaminophen sulfate; however, cytochrome P450 (CYP) 2E1 and CYP3A4 can convert a small amount of it into the hazardous molecule N-acetyl-p-benzoquinone imine (Laine et al., 2009, Li et al., 2021). Human cytosolic sulfotransferase 1A1, an enzyme that changes p-cresol into harmless compounds, may be in competition with acetaminophen. The liver's ability to decrease acetaminophen toxicity is compromised by this competition (Gamage et al., 2006). The membrane proteins known as drug transporters are involved in the metabolization of the drug in the body. They facilitate the movement of a diverse range of substances in and out of cells. The brain, liver, and intestine are known to express the following transporter proteins. By inhibiting the HDAC/NF-κB pathways, butyrate has the potential to decrease the expression and functionality of the drug transporter P-glycoprotein (Tolson and Wang, 2010). Nuclear receptors like constitutive androstane receptor and PXR are major regulators of xenobiotic hepatic metabolism (Tolson and Wang, 2010), CYP4501a genes in the liver and duodenum may be further regulated by the AhR modulation by tryptophan and indole derivatives (Dempsey and Cui, 2019). Additional effects on drug metabolism might be caused by altered drug transporters and metabolic enzymes.

12.5.8 Effect on Gut Motility and Intestinal Barrier

The gastrointestinal tract, which has a surface area of 200 m^2, is the part of the body that is most exposed to the external environment (Scaldaferri et al., 2012). The gut lumen and the mucosal tissues are separated by the intestinal barrier, a layer of chemical, physical, immunological, and microbiological barriers, which are essential for immune regulation and nutritional absorption. Intestinal barrier is composed of: the layer known as the inner lamina propria, which is comprised of dendritic cells, B cells, macrophages, T cells, and plasma cells that produce IgA. The outermost layer is primarily composed of beneficial gut commensal microorganisms. The mucus layer contains antimicrobial peptides and secretory immunoglobulin A (sIgA) that reinforce the mucosal barrier on the extraepithelial side. The epithelial layer is a single-cell layer consisting of various types of epithelial cells, including enteroendocrine cells, Goblet cells, absorptive enterocytes, and Paneth cells (Liu et al., 2021; Natividad and Verdu, 2013). The cells that line the inside of your body have special connections near their tops that decide what can pass through them (Wells et al., 2017). When the lining of your gut has tiny holes, it is called "leaky gut". This lets bad things like germs and toxins get into your blood and inside your gut wall (Camilleri, 2019). This can cause many health problems like diabetes, obesity, celiac disease, cancer, IBD, IBS, and others. These problems can also change how your immune system and your body's chemicals work (König et al., 2016; Meddings, 2008). The good bacteria in your gut make some substances that help your gut lining work well. One of these substances is butyrate, which can change how some genes work and help fix the holes in your gut lining (Jung et al., 2015; Sunkara et al., 2012). INF-α, IL-10, IL-1β, IL-6, IL-22, and other inflammatory cytokines are released by immune cells in the intestinal barrier to sustain the immune system's appropriate operation. On the other hand, diseases and systemic inflammation might result from overproduction of these cytokines SCFAs exhibit anti-inflammatory properties through the modulation of cytokine production and immune cell activity (Park et al., 2015). Indole and its derivatives can function as epithelial nuclear receptors, including AhR, PXR, and retinoid-related orphan receptor gamma-t ligand, thereby prompting the functions of the intestinal barrier (Park et al., 2015). For instance, indole demonstrates the ability to enhance the trans-epithelial resistance of epithelial cells, promote the synthesis of tight junction proteins in the intestines, and lower the concentrations of inflammatory cytokines like TNF-α, IL-1α, IL-1β, and IL-6. Moreover, BAR501 triggers the activation of the bile acid receptor TGR5, resulting in a transformation of macrophage phenotypes from pro-inflammatory to tissue-protective (Biagioli et al., 2017).

For digestion, absorption, and waste product release, intestinal motility must function effectively. In contrast, intestinal dysmotility can result in infections, nutritional malabsorption, diarrhea, and constipation (Di Lorenzo and Youssef, 2010; Rao, 2020). Ammonia and aromatic derivatives of amino acids are two harmful metabolites that are produced in greater quantities by bacteria during slow intestinal transit, along with protein catabolism and carbohydrate shortage (Verbeke et al., 2015). Fast transit, on the other hand, has been linked to improved intestinal health and a decrease in low-grade intestinal inflammation (Müller et al., 2018). In order to influence gastric emptying and colonic motility, Methane, LPS, SCFAs, and secondary bile acids are examples of gut microbiota metabolites that can interact with enteric neurons and smooth muscles through humoral and neuronal pathways that include GLP-1, PYY, motilin, and serotonin (Cherbut et al., 1997; Guarino et al., 2016).

It has been studied that the overall composition of gut microflora has been greatly affected by the age of the host. The colonization of microbiota differs according to the birth method (vaginal or cesarean). Soon after birth, there is a greater colonization of the microbiota, such as *Proteobacteria* which is an aerobic bacterium, are the foremost to have existed in the host intestines. These bacteria cause anaerobic species, such as Firmicutes, Actinobacteria, and Bacteroides, to colonize by lowering the oxygen levels (Del Chierico et al., 2015).

The first growth years of host life are crucial for the gut microbiota development and growth. The taxonomic diversity is initially rather modest but gradually rises (Schanche et al., 2015). Bacteroides, bifidobacteria, and the synthesis of SCFAs are considerably decreased in old people. Furthermore, it has been verified that there are more abundant facultative anaerobes, *clostridia*, *eubacteria*, and *fusobacteria* than bifidobacteria (Thompson et al., 2015). In people (ages 2–5), their gut microbiota composition is considerably far stable and includes a range of Firmicutes and Bacteroidetes species, including butyrate-producing species (Fouhy et al., 2019). The GM of pre-adolescents (7–12 years old) was also more abundant in processes that could be related to continuous growth, such as folate synthesis and vitamin B12 production (Hollister et al., 2014). The adolescent microflora, i.e. genera *Clostridium* and *Bifidobacterium* are considerably more prevalent in young people (ages 11–18), than adults. *Bacteroidetes* and *Firmicutes* predominate in the gut microbiota of healthy adults, although, species of *Actinobacteria, Proteobacteria,* and *Verrucomicrobia* are also existed in lower amounts (Reyes et al., 2010).

Aging greater than 65 has a substantial influence on the geriatric microbiota function and composition. Age-related dietary changes may be linked to a variety of physiological and behavioral changes. Reduced salivary and dental health, impaired absorption and digestion, and altered appetite as a result of medication and mental health are some of these alterations. The elderly microbiota has fewer types of microbes, which can lead to an increase in harmful pathogens and a decrease in beneficial microbes (Biagi et al., 2017). This can cause inflammation and other health problems (Mariat et al., 2009; Voreades et al., 2014).

12.5.9 Diet

The gut microflora can be influenced by food in both positive and negative ways. The effect of food on the gut microflora depends on the substances produced in the gut (Hills et al., 2019). After birth, the nutrition of the infant plays a crucial role in the growth of the gut microbiota. Genes for the breakdown of breast milk oligosaccharides are abundant in the gut microbiota of newborns, but vitamins and polysaccharide metabolism genes are more abundant in the metagenome subsequent to the intake of solid meals (Backhed et al., 2015). Furthermore, Thompson et al. (2015) found that the kind of feeding has a notable impact on the microbiota's microbial composition in newborns. Breastfed babies have an inhibition of *Proteobacteria* and *Firmicutes* and an increase of *Actinobacteria*. These bacterial species can efficiently metabolize the oligosaccharides in breast milk, which causes the immune system to synthesize more immunoglobulin G and huge quantity of SCFAs. However, the prevalence of Clostridia, Streptococci, Bacteroides, and Enterobacteria is rising in formula-fed newborns (Azad et al., 2013; Lee et al., 2015). The GM continues to grow after childhood, and food becomes the primary factor in determining how the gut microbiota is structured, shaped, and varied.

Vegetarian diets are found to have great association with improved health, and a wide range of microbiota species in the gut, with *Firmicutes* as well as *Bacteroidetes* predominating. The integrity of the mucosal barrier of the gut depends on the consumption of dietary fiber (Ray 2018). It has been demonstrated that T2DM patients who follow a high-fiber diet have better glucose management and their metabolic profile is healthier (Zhao et al., 2018). Conversely, increased amounts of fat and protein in the diet have been associated with a decrease in Firmicutes and an increase in species that are resistant to bile such as *Bacteroides*, *Bilophila*, and *Alistipes* (David et al., 2014; Forouhi et al., 2018). Notably, consuming this diet more frequently lowers immunity, increases susceptibility to infection, and raises the likelihood of metabolic disease development (Jethwani and Grover, 2019).

12.5.10 Genetics of the Host

It is commonly established that host genetic makeup influences species richness, taxonomic abundances, and variance in disease susceptibility. The microbiota of gut and the host's innate immunity genes have been connected in a variety of ways: Bacteria in the gut are identified by pattern recognition receptors and subsequently modify the microbiota makeup and associated disorders (Zoetendal et al., 2001). The microbial profiles of monozygotic twins who spent years apart exhibited a significant degree of similarity. While married couples who shared the same environment and similar eating practices did not exhibit the same level of resemblance in their microbial profiles. According to Kurilshikov et al. (2017), the phyla *Firmicutes*, *Actinobacteria*, *Tenericutes*, and *Euryarchaeota* exhibit more heritability than the extremely common Bacteroidetes phylum. Together, these studies suggested a compelling suggestion that microbiota is significantly shaped by genetic factors (Kurilshikov et al., 2017). Furthermore, it was found that GM has remarkable effect on the host genetic makeup (Chen et al., 2018). They verified that the functional categories of candidate genes and the great similarity of heritable taxa among mice, pigs, and humans were all in favor of a similar mechanism whereby host genetics influence the gut microbiota in all mammals (Chen et al., 2018).

12.5.11 Exercise

According to many studies, human exercise improved the variety of microbiota and was definitely linked with the consumption of protein and creatine kinase levels (Clarke et al., 2014). The microbiota exhibits increased diversity with physical activity. Athletes tend to have elevated levels of Firmicutes and reduced quantities of Bacteroidetes compared to non-athletes. Exercise has been demonstrated to boost the abundance of various bacterial groups, such as Lactobacillus, Bifidobacterium, and Akkermansia, while certain genera like Proteobacteria, Turicibacter, and Rikenellaceae appear to decrease in response (Hughes, 2020). Furthermore, it has been demonstrated that SCFAs synthesis, a measure of the health of the gut, and taxa that produces butyrate, including *Clostridiales*, *Roseburia*, *Lachnospiraceae*, and *Erysipelotrichaceae*, increase in response to exercise. These taxa are regulated by exercise and thus have a great effect the overall host's GM (Allen et al., 2018).

Exercise generally improves a diverse bacterial community through a combination of internal and external causes. Athletes have healthier lifestyles generally and are exposed to their surrounding biosphere, which promotes a more diverse microbiota. Furthermore, the GI tract may alter as a result of intrinsic adaptations to prolonged physical activity, including reduced blood flow, tissue hypoxia, and accelerated transit (Rosa et al., 2005).

Exercise is linked to decrease the morbidity because it reduces chronic inflammation, and athletes exhibited better metabolic markers and decreased inflammatory levels compared to controls (Clarke et al., 2014). Neuronal circuits of children at a young age are still developing, thus physical activity can protect the brain from stress-related mental illnesses including anxiety and depression in later life (Mika and Fleshner, 2016). Furthermore, exercise may be considered as a therapeutic support in the management of gastrointestinal disorders and other conditions linked to dysbiosis, such as obesity (Estaki et al., 2016).

12.5.12 Antibiotics

Using antibiotics disrupts the gut microbiota, leading to dysbiosis, and eliminates both good and harmful bacteria (Klingensmith and Coopersmith, 2016). Antibiotics change the competitive exclusion process that microbiota uses to avoid infections (Ramnani et al., 2012). The kind of antibiotic and the duration of the dosage determine the particular effects of antibiotic therapy on GM (Dethlefsen and Relman, 2010). For example, 2 years of clindamycin treatment changes the microbiota but does not allow the variety of Bacteroides to return (Jernberg et al., 2007). Furthermore, Actinobacteria species decrease when clarithromycin is used to treat Helicobacter pylori infections, and ciprofloxacin has been demonstrated to cause a decrease in Ruminococcus species (Jakobsson et al., 2010). Treatment with vancomycin results in rise of *Proteobacteria* species but a reduction in Bacteroidetes, *Fuminococcus*, and Faecalibacterium (Isaac et al., 2016).

12.5.13 Smoking

Another factor affecting the GM composition is smoking (Biedermann et al., 2013). The fecal microbiota of healthy people quitting smoking showed notable alterations as well, with decrease in Bacteroidetes and Proteobacteria and an increase in the relative abundance of Firmicutes and Actinobacteria. Furthermore, studies have revealed that the smokers' and nonsmokers' oral gut microbiota differs significantly (Biedermann et al., 2014). Specifically, there is a drop in Gemella species and an increase in Porphyromonas and Neisseria proliferation in the oral cavity of smokers. On the other hand, no noticeable differences have been found between smokers' and nonsmokers' lungs (Morris et al., 2013).

12.6 RELATIONSHIPS OF GUT MICROBIOTA WITH DISEASES

The interaction between the microbiota and the host is intricate and could be disrupted and have negative consequences on both. The resulting dysbiosis (change in the makeup of microorganisms) might be detrimental and linked to the emergence of the many illnesses listed below.

12.6.1 Gastrointestinal and Hepatic Diseases

12.6.1.1 Irritable Bowel Syndrome (IBS)

IBS is an illness marked by several symptoms, including altered bowel habits, flatulence, and abdominal discomfort. The onset of syndrome symptoms may be related to increased fermentation and gas generation. According to studies, patients with IBS have higher concentrations of SCFAs, and they may also stimulate serotonin release from the intestinal mucosa, hence encouraging digestion (Kadooka et al., 2010). Around 10%–15% of the population suffers from IBS worldwide (Gupta et al., 2016). Research has shown a strong correlation between brain and gut health (Jeffery et al., 2012).

Several studies have proved the involvement of GM in IBS. Qualitative and quantitative changes in the GM lead to IBS (Bennet et al., 2015). Additionally, it is thought that the pathophysiology of IBS includes microbial dysbiosis in the gut, which promotes pathogenic bacterial attachment with intestinal wall (Ghoshal et al., 2012). The individuals encountering IBS have been reported to have high concentrations of firmicutes, particularly *Clostridium*, *Ruminococcus*, and *Dorea*, and lower concentrations of Bacteroides fragilis, *B. vulgates*, *R. callidus*, and *Ruminococcus albus* (Jeffery et al., 2012).

12.6.1.2 Inflammatory Bowel Disease (IBD)

IBD originates from stimulation of the immune system and causes inflammation in the gastrointestinal tract which persists over time (Lane et al., 2017). A variety of hereditary and environmental factors are responsible for inflammatory bowel disease (IBD). These factors include stress, sleep habits, the use of antibiotics, cleanliness, food, and smoking. Host genome is greatly influenced by gut microbiota composition. There are two main types of IBD, i.e. ulcerative colitis and Crohn's disease (Schirmer et al., 2018).

Colon and rectum are significantly affected by ulcerative colitis and are marked by a chronic large bowel inflammation while Crohn's disease is not limited to a specific area but affects the whole GI tract (Kudelka et al., 2016). It has been established by several studies that diets and microbiota in those at risk for IBD are directly correlated (Dolan and Chang, 2017). Conversely, nutrition containing a higher number of fruits and vegetables produces extra SCFAs thereby lowering the chances of contracting CD (Lane et al., 2017). It is believed that individuals with IBD develop weakened mucus layer in their intestinal tracts, which allows entry of luminal bacteria into intra-epithelial cells and triggers the events of inflammatory and proliferative procedures (Parekh et al., 2015). Intestinal dysbiosis can affect the digestive system by initiating several problems in the body (Lane et al., 2017). Different types of IBD can also make some changes in the bacterial gut (Sokol et al., 2009; Zhu et al., 2018) and form the disease more dangerous and severe (Lane et al., 2017).

12.6.2 Hepatic Sickness

Fatty liver disease can cause inflammation and scarring. It occurs due to several reasons such as overeating, excessive alcohol consumption, or metabolic issues. Nonalcoholic fatty liver disease causes hepatocellular carcinoma and liver cirrhosis. Alterations in gut flora increase the rate of such disease (Betrapally et al., 2016). The pathophysiology of nonalcoholic fatty liver disease may be caused due to several reasons. Fatty liver diseases reduce the levels of Firmicutes and Bacteroides. Increased levels of SCFA and a decrease in ratio of Bacteroidetes to Firmicutes cause elevated energy collection, leading to liver's gluconeogenesis and lipogenesis processes. Furthermore, dysbiosis reduces the production of butyrate, which activates lipoprotein lipase and causes the liver to accumulate triglycerides (Leung et al., 2016).

By raising intestinal penetrability and lipopolysaccharide (LPS) entry levels, ethanol may contribute to hepatic injury. Another process involves the gut microbiota's catalysis of choline to produce poisonous methylamines. These toxic compounds are absorbed by the liver, which intensifies inflammation (Pevsner-Fischer et al., 2016). Increased liquor consumption exerts over overburden of Gram-negative bacteria, thereby increasing gut permeability and availability of pro-inflammatory chemicals including bacterial toxins and LPS to the liver as well as bacterial metabolites (Betrapally et al., 2016).

12.6.3 Metabolic Diseases

12.6.3.1 Obesity

Obesity is defined as the increase of the body mass index (BMI) from 30 kg/m^2. A buildup of extra fats in the tissues causes obesity (Pasco et al., 2014). Approximately 2 billion people worldwide suffer from obesity, a condition that leads to several metabolic disorders referred to as metabolic syndrome. These metabolic disorders are characterized by osteoarthritis, diabetes, insulin resistance, hyperlipidemia, malignancy, and hepatic steatosis (Kang et al., 2010). Different factors like behavior, genetics, and environmental factors contribute to cause obesity. Furthermore, the development and progression of obesity are significantly influenced by gut bacteria (Villanueva-Millan et al., 2015). The GM ferments the food in obese people and absorbs energy from it. Obese individuals have higher levels of Firmicutes to Bacteroides/Prevotella, which promotes the genes of microbiota responsible for the breakdown of polysaccharides and raises SCFA levels (Andoh et al., 2016). Moreover, it has been noted that as compared to lean individuals obese people have higher concentrations of some bacteria. These bacteria are Campylobacter, Staphylococcus, Bacteroides, Dialister, Porphyromonas, Ruminococcus, and Parabacteroides (Le Chatelier et al., 2013). Conversely, there was a small percentage of *Methanobrevibacter*, *Coprococcus*, *Akker-mansia*, *Bifidobacterium*, *Faecalibacterium*, and *Lactobacillus*.

12.6.3.2 Diabetes

Type 1 diabetes (T1D) results from a compromised immune system. In T1D the patients are unable to produce pancreatic B cells and these pancreatic B cells are responsible for the production of insulin. TID is usually conferred in childhood and careful observation of these individuals has shown a certain chain in the GM which indicates their role in the immune modulation and ultimately affecting T1D (Clemente et al., 2012). TID patients have been reported to have high concentrations of Bacteroidetes (butyrate and lactate-producing bacteria) (Knip and Siljander, 2016).

The condition in which the human body is unable to properly metabolize glucose even in the presence of a sufficient amount of insulin is known as type diabetes. This condition is marked by the diminished presence of insulin receptors or body shows insulin resistance. According to Muscogiuri et al. (2016), the GI tract microflora composition and the risk of type 2 diabetes have been greatly affected by both host genetics and lifestyle variables. When compared to healthy persons, the microbiota of diabetic people revealed increased growth of certain taxa, including Proteobacteria, Bacteroidetes, and Firmicutes (Qin et al., 2012). Lipopolysaccharides that are isolated from Gram-negative bacteria's outer membranes may elevate the metabolic endotoxemia by encouraging the pro-inflammatory cytokines secretion. Numerous investigations indicated a high fat intake might alter the composition of GI tract microbiota and boost the LPS level in the bloodstream (Harte et al., 2012). In other words, the bacteria in the gut make some chemicals called SCFAs from the food we eat. Some of the chemicals affect the effects of sugars and energy on our body (Zhu et al., 2018).

12.6.3.3 Cardiovascular Diseases (CVD)

Diabetes and heavy weight are the main causes of cardiovascular disease (Garcia-Rios et al., 2017). Western diet contains meat and eggs having a chemical "trimethylamine" which can make this disease more severe and aggressive (Estruch et al., 2018). Trimethylamine destruct the blood vessels and habituate the arteries by passing into the liver and convert into TMAO (Zhu et al., 2016). Trimethylamine-N-oxide also affects the effects of liver cholesterol and bile acids (Griffin et al., 2015). They also cause inflammation in the people having atherosclerosis (Karlsson et al., 2012, 2013).

12.7 CONCLUSION

Environmental factors are the things around the host and the GM that affect them, such as temperature, moisture, soil, sunlight, and other living things. A pool of unique metabolites is produced from the genes produced by the GM which significantly changes the GM microbiota itself activities and also the activities of the host. Targeting these metabolites is essential to precision medicine, and this may be done with dynamic integrative biomarkers or diagnostic microbial biomarkers. Even though there are many known gut microbiota compounds, rigorous research to identify more metabolites is necessary to develop novel medications for the treatment of disease. Numerous factors, such as drugs, host genetics, diet, lifestyle choices, and age can impact the overall makeup of GM. It also has an impact on host metabolism, physiology, and immune system development. Differences in the gut microbiota's makeup and activity directly affect human health and are a major contributor to a wide range of diseases. Treatment for these illnesses involves effective strategies to counterbalance these detrimental fluctuations.

REFERENCES

Adamowicz EM, Flynn J, Hunter RC, Harcombe WR (2018). Cross-feeding modulates antibiotic tolerance in bacterial communities. *ISME J* 12:2723–2735.

Agus A, Clément K, Sokol H (2021). Gut microbiota- derived metabolites as central regulators in metabolic disorders. *Gut* 70:1174–1182.

Allen JM, Mailing LJ, Niemiro GM, Moore R, Cook MD, White BA, et al. (2018). Exercise alters gut microbiota composition and function in lean and obese humans. *Med Sci Sport Exer* 50:747–757.

Allen K, Jaeschke H, Copple BL (2011). Bile acids induce inflammatory genes in hepatocytes: a novel mechanism of inflammation during obstructive cholestasis. *Am J Pathol* 178:175–186.

Andoh A, Nishida A, Takahashi K, Inatomi O, Imaeda H, Bamba S, et al. (2016). Comparison of the gut microbial community between obese and lean peoples using 16S gene sequencing in a Japanese population. *J Clin Biochem Nutr* 59(1):65–70.

Azad M, Konya T, Maughan H, Guttman D, Field C, Chari S, et al. (2013). Gut microbiota of healthy Canadian infants: profiles by mode of delivery and infant diet at 4 months. *CMAJ* 185:385–394.

Backhed F, Roswall J, Peng Y, Feng Q, Jia H, Kovatcheva P, et al. (2015). Dynamics and stabilization of the human gut microbiome during the first year of life. *Cell Host Microbe* 17:690–703.

Behera J, Ison J, Tyagi SC, Tyagi N (2020). The role of gut microbiota in bone homeostasis. *Bone* 135:115317.

Behsaz B, Bode E, Gurevich A, Shi YN, Grundmann F, Acharya D, et al. (2021). Integrating genomics and metabolomics for scalable non-ribosomal peptide discovery. *Nat Commun* 12:3225.

Bennet S, Ohman L, Simren M (2015). Gut microbiota as potential orchestrators of irritable bowel syndrome. *Gut Liver* 9:318–931.

Betrapally N, Gillevet P, Bajaj J (2016). Changes in the intestinal microbiome and alcoholic and nonalcoholic liver diseases: causes or effects? *Gastroenterol* 150:1745–1770.

Biagi E, Rampelli S, Turroni S, Quercia S, Candela M, Brigidi P (2017). The gut microbiota of centenarians: signatures of longevity in the gut microbiota profile. *Mech Age Dev* 165:180–184.

Biagioli M, Carino A, Cipriani S, Francisci D, Marchianò S, Scarpelli P, et al. (2017). The bile acid receptor GPBAR1 regulates the M1/M2 phenotype of intestinal macrophages and activation of GPBAR1 rescues mice from murine colitis. *J Immunol* 199:718–733.

Biedermann, L., Brülisauer, K., Zeitz, J., Frei, P., Scharl, M., Vavricka, S. R., Fried, M., Loessner, M. J., Rogler, G., & Schuppler, M. (2014). (2014). Smoking cessation alters intestinal microbiota: insights from quantitative investigations on human fecal samples using FISH. *Inflam Bowel Dis* 20:1496–1501.

Biedermann, L., Zeitz, J., Mwinyi, J., Sutter-Minder, E., Rehman, A., Ott, S. J., Steurer-Stey, C., Frei, A., Frei, P., Scharl, M., Loessner, M. J., Vavricka, S. R., Fried, M., Schreiber, S., Schuppler, M., & Rogler, G. (2013).Smoking cessation induces profound changes in the composition of the intestinal microbiota in humans. *PLOS One* 8:59–63.

Bishehsari F, Voigt RM, Keshavarzian A (2020). Circadian rhythms and the gut microbiota: from the metabolic syndrome to cancer. *Nat Rev Endocrinol* 16:731–739.

Blaser MJ (1999). Hypothesis: the changing relationships of Helicobacter pylori and humans: implications for health and disease. *J Infect Dis* 179(6):1523–1530.

Bone E, Tamm A, Hill M (1976). The production of urinary phenols by gut bacteria and their possible role in the causation of large bowel cancer. *Am J Clin Nutr* 29:1448–1454.

Cait A, Hughes MR, Antignano F, Cait J, Dimitriu PA, Maas KR, et al. (2018). Microbiome-driven allergic lung inflammation is ameliorated by short-chain fatty acids. *Mucosal Immunol* 11:785–795.

Camilleri M (2019). Leaky gut: mechanisms, measurement and clinical implications in humans. *Gut* 68:1516–1526.

Cani PD, Van Hul M, Lefort C, Depommier C, Rastelli M, Everard A (2019). Microbial regulation of organismal energy homeostasis. *Nat Metab* 1:34–46.

Carley AN, Maurya SK, Fasano M, Wang Y, Selzman CH, Drakos SG, et al. (2021). Short-chain fatty acids outpace ketone oxidation in the failing heart. *Circulation* 143:1797–1808.

Chávez-Talavera O, Tailleux A, Lefebvre P, Staels B (2017). Bile acid control of metabolism and inflammation in obesity, type 2 diabetes, dyslipidemia, and nonalcoholic fatty liver disease. *Gastroenterol* 152:1679–1694.

Chen C, Huang X, Fang S, Yang H, He M, Zhao Y, Huang L (2018). Contribution of host genetics to the variation of microbial composition of cecum lumen and feces in pigs. *Front Microbiol* 9:2626–2639.

Cherbut C, Aube AC, Blottiere HM, Galmiche JP (1997). Effects of short-chain fatty acids on gastrointestinal motility. *Scand J Gastroenterol Suppl* 222:58–61.

Clarke SF, Murphy EF, O'Sullivan O, et al. (2014). Exercise and associated dietary extremes impact on gut microbial diversity. *Gut* 63(12):1913–1920.

Clemente J, Ursell L, Parfrey L, Knight R (2012). The impact of the gut microbiota on human health: an integrative view. *Cell* 148(6):1258–1270.

Curtis H, Blaser MJ, Dirk G, Kota KC, Rob K, Liu B, et al. (2012). Structure, function and diversity of the healthy human microbiome. *Nature (London)* 486(7402):207–214.

Dalile B, Van Oudenhove L, Vervliet B, Verbeke K (2019). The role of short-chain fatty acids in microbiota-gut-brain communication. *Nat Rev Gastroenterol Hepatol* 16:461–478.

Đanić M, Stanimirov B, Pavlović N, Goločorbin-Kon S, Al-Salami H, Stankov K, et al. (2018). Pharmacological applications of bile acids and their derivatives in the treatment of metabolic syndrome. *Front Pharmacol* 9:1382.

David L, Maurice C, Carmody R, Gootenberg D, Button J, Wolfe B, et al. (2014). Diet rapidly and reproducibly alters the human gut microbiome. *Nature* 505:559–563.

Del Chierico F, Vernocchi P, Petrucca A, Paci P, Fuentes S, Pratic G, et al. (2015). Phylogenetic and metabolic tracking of gut microbiota during perinatal development. *PLoS One* 10:137–247.

Dempsey JL, Cui JY (2019). Microbiome is a functional modifier of P450 drug metabolism. *Curr Pharmacol Rep* 5:481–490.

den Besten G, Lange K, Havinga R, van Dijk TH, Gerding A, van Eunen K, et al. (2013). Gut-derived short-chain fatty acids are vividly assimilated into host carbohydrates and lipids. *Am J Physiol Gastrointest Liver Physiol* 305:G900–G910.

Deng MJ, Qu F, Chen L, Liu C, Zhang M, Ren FZ, et al. (2020). SCFAs alleviated steatosis and inflammation in mice with NASH induced by MCD. *J Endocrinol* 245:425–437.

Dethlefsen L, Relman DA (2010). Incomplete recovery and individualized responses of the human distal gut micro- biota to repeated antibiotic perturbation. *Proc Natl Acad Sci USA* 108:4554–4561.

Di Lorenzo C, Youssef NN (2010). Diagnosis and management of intestinal motility disorders. *Semin Pediatr Surg* 19:50–58.

Dolan K, Chang E (2017). Diet, gut microbes, and the pathogenesis of inflammatory bowel diseases. *Mol Nutr Food Res, 61(1):* 61–80.

Dong Y, Benveniste EN (2001). Immune function of astrocytes. *Glia* 36:180–190.

Dyson JK, Blain A, Shirley MD, Hudson M, Rushton S, Jones DE (2020). Geo-epidemiology and environmental co-variate mapping of primary biliary cholangitis and primary sclerosing cholangitis. *JHEP Rep* 3:100202.

Estaki M, Pither J, Baumeister P, Little JP, Gill SK, Ghosh S, et al. (2016). Cardiorespiratory fitness as a predictor of intestinal microbial diversity and distinct metagenomic functions. *FASEB J* 30(1):1027–1035.

Estruch R, Ros E, Salas-Salvado J, Covas M, Corella D, Aros F, et al. (2018). Primary prevention of cardiovascular disease with a mediterranean diet supplemented with extra-virgin olive oil or nuts. *N Engl J Med* 378:34–50.

Felig P, Marliss E, Cahill Jr GF (1969). Plasma amino acid levels and insulin secretion in obesity. *N Engl J Med* 281:811–816.

Feng WW, Liu J, Ao H, Yue SJ, Peng C (2020). Targeting gut microbiota for precision medicine: focusing on the efficacy and toxicity of drugs. *Theranostics* 10:11278–11301.

Floyd JC, Fajans SS, Conn JW, Knopf RF, Rull J (1966). Stimulation of insulin secretion by amino acids. *J Clin Invest* 45:1487–1502.

Fontana L, Cummings NE, Apelo SI, Neuman JC, Kasza I, Schmidt BA et al.. (2016). Decreased consumption of branched-chain amino acids improves metabolic health. *Cell Rep* 16:520–530.

Forouhi N, Krauss R, Taubes G, Willett W (2018). Dietary fat and cardiometabolic health: evidence, controversies, and consensus for guidelines. *BMJ* 361:21–39.

Fouhy F, Watkins C, Hill C, O'Shea C, Nagle B, Dempsey E, et al. (2019). Micro- biome memory of perinatal factors that affect the gut microbiota four years after birth. *Nat Commun* 10:151–167.

Frampton J, Murphy KG, Frost G, Chambers ES (2020). Short-chain fatty acids as potential regulators of skeletal muscle metabolism and function. *Nat Metab* 2:840–848.

Frank DN, St. Amand AL, Feldman RA, Boedeker EC, Harpaz N, Pace NR (2007). Molecular-phylogenetic characterization of microbial community imbalances in human inflammatory bowel diseases. *Proceedings of the National Academy of Sciences* 104(34):13780–13785.

Frazier K, Chang EB (2020). Intersection of the gut microbiome and circadian rhythms in metabolism. *Trends Endocrinol Metab* 31:25–36.

Fung TC, Olson CA, Hsiao EY (2017). Interactions between the microbiota, immune and nervous systems in health and disease. *Nat Neurosci* 20:145–155.

Gamage N, Barnett A, Hempel N, Duggleby RG, Windmill KF, Martin JL et al. (2006). Human sulfotransferases and their role in chemical metabolism. *Toxicol Sci* 90:5–22.

Garcia-Gutierrez E, Mayer MJ, Cotter PD, Narbad A (2019). Gut microbiota as a source of novel antimicrobials. *Gut Microbes* 10:1–21.

Garcia-Rios A, Torres-Pena J, Perez-Jimenez F, Perez-Martinez P (2017). Gut microbiota: a new marker of cardiovascular disease. *Curr Pharm Des* 23(22):3233–3238.

Ghoshal U, Shukla R, Ghoshal U, Gwee K, Ng S, Quigley E (2012). The gut microbiota and irritable bowel syndrome friend or foe? *Int J Inflam* 2012:151–185.

Gillespie JJ, Wattam AR, Cammer, SA, Gabbard JL, Shukla MP, Dalay O, et al. (2011). PATRIC: the comprehensive bacterial bioinformatics resource with a focus on human pathogenic species. *Infec Immun* 79(11):4286–4298.

Grab DJ, Perides G, Dumler JS, Kim KJ, Park J, Kim YV et al. (2005). Borrelia burgdorferi, host-derived proteases, and the blood-brain barrier. *Infect Immun* 7:1014–1022.

Griffin J, Wang X, Stanley E (2015). Does our gut microbiome predict cardiovascular risk? A review of the evidence from metabolomics. *Circ Cardiovasc Genet* 8:187–191.

Guarino MP, Cicala M, Putignani L, Severi C (2016). Gastrointestinal neuromuscular apparatus: An underestimated target of gut microbiota. *World J Gastroenterol* 22:9871–9879.

Gujral JS, Farhood A, Bajt ML, Jaeschke H (2003). Neutrophils aggravate acute liver injury during obstructive cholestasis in bile duct-ligated mice. *Hepatology (Baltimore, Md.)*, *38*(2), 355–363. https://doi.org/10.1053/jhep.2003.50341

Gupta S, Allen-Vercoe E, Petrof E (2016). Fecal microbiota transplantation in perspective. *Ther Adv Gastroenterol* 9(2):229–239.

Haghikia A, Jörg S, Duscha A, Berg J, Manzel A, Waschbisch A, et al. (2015). Dietary fatty acids directly impact central nervous system autoimmunity via the small intestine. *Immunity*, 43:817–829.

Han H, Yi B, Zhong RQ, Wang MY, Zhang SF, Ma J, et al. (2021). From gut microbiota to host appetite: gut microbiota-derived metabolites as key regulators. *Microbiome* 9:1–6.

Harte A, Varma M, Tripathi G, McGee K, Al-Daghri N, Al-Attas O, et al. (2012). High fat intake leads to acute postprandial exposure to circulating endotoxin in type 2 diabetic subjects. *Diabetes Care* 35:375–382.

Hill MJ (1997). Intestinal flora and endogenous vitamin synthesis. *Eur J Cancer Prev* 6:S43–S45.

Hills R, Pontefract B, Mishcon H, Black C, Sutton S, Theberge C (2019). Gut microbiome profound implications for diet and disease. *Nutrition* 11:1613–1653.

Hodgman MJ, Garrard AR (2012). A review of acetaminophen poisoning. *Crit Care Clin* 28:499–516.

Hollister EB, Gao C, Versalovic J (2014). Compositional and functional features of the gastrointestinal microbiome and their effects on human health. *Gastroenterol* 146(6):1449–1458.

Hughes RL (2020). A review of the role of the gut microbiome in personalized sports nutrition. *Front Nutr* 6:191–218.

Inagaki T, Moschetta A, Lee YK, Peng L, Zhao G, Downes M, et al. (2006). Regulation of antibacterial defense in the small intestine by the nuclear bile acid receptor. *Proc Natl Acad Sci U S A* 103:3920–3925.

Isaac S, Scher J, Djukovic A, Jiménez N, Littman D, Abramson S, Pamer E, Ubeda C (2016). Short-and long-term effects of oral vancomycin on the human intestinal microbiota. *J Antimicrob Chem* 72(1):128–136.

Jakobsson H, Jernberg C, Andersson A, Sjolund-Karlsson M, Jansson J, Engstrand L (2010). Short-term antibiotic treatment has differing long-term impacts on the human throat and gut microbiome. *PLOS ONE* 5(3):983–996.

Jeffery I, O'Toole P, Öhman L, Claesson M, Deane J, Quigley E, Simrén M (2012). An irritable bowel syndrome subtype defined by species-specific alterations in faecal microbiota. *Gut* 61:997–1006.

Jernberg C, Lo¨fmark S, Edlund C, Jansson J (2007). Long-term ecological impacts of antibiotic administration on the human intestinal microbiota. *ISME J* 1(1):56–66.

Jethwani P, Grover K (2019). Gut microbiota in health and diseases-a review. *Int J Curr Microbiol Appl Sci* 8(8):1586–1599.

Jocken JW, González Hernández MA, Hoebers NT, van der Beek CM, Essers YP, Blaak EE, et al. (2018). Short-chain fatty acids differentially affect intracellular lipolysis in a human white adipocyte model. *Front Endocrinol* 8:372.

Jonsson AL, Bäckhed F (2017). Role of gut microbiota in atherosclerosis. *Nat Rev Cardiol* 14:79–87.

Joossens M, Huys G, Cnockaert M, De Preter V, Verbeke K, Rutgeerts P, et al. (2011). Dysbiosis of the faecal microbiota in patients with Crohn's disease and their unaffected relatives. *Gut* 60(5):631–637.

Jung TH, Park JH, Jeon WM, Han KS (2015). Butyrate modulates bacterial adherence on LS174T human colorectal cells by stimulating mucin secretion and MAPK signaling pathway. *Nutr Res Pract* 9:343–349.

Kadooka Y, Sato M, Imaizumi K, Ogawa A, Ikuyama K, Akai Y, et al. (2010). Regulation of abdominal adiposity by probiotics (*Lactobacillus gasseri* SBT2055) in adults with obese tendencies in a randomized controlled trial. *Eur J Clin Nutr* 64:636–643.

Kalantar-Zadeh K, Berean KJ, Burgell RE, Muir JG, Gibson PR (2019). Intestinal gases: influence on gut [44] disorders and the role of dietary manipulations. *Nat Rev Gastroenterol Hepatol* 16:733–747.

Kang S, Denman S, Morrison M, Yu Z, Dore J, Leclerc M, et al. (2010). Dysbiosis of fecal microbiota in Crohn's disease patients as revealed by a custom phylogenetic microarray. *Inflamm Bowel Dis* 16:2034–2042.

Karlsson F, Tremaroli V, Nielsen J, Backhed F (2013). Assessing the human gut microbiota in metabolic diseases. *Diabetes* 62(10):3341–3349.

Karlsson FH, Fåk F, Nookaew I, Tremaroli V, Fagerberg B, Petranovic D, et al. (2012). Symptomatic atherosclerosis is associated with an altered gut metagenome. *Nat Commun* 3(1):1245.

Kenshole E, Herisse M, Michael M, Pidot SJ (2021). Natural product discovery through microbial genome mining. *Curr Opin Chem Biol* 60:47–54.

Kim ER, Wu Z, Sun H, Xu Y,Mangieri LR, Xu Y, et al. (2015). Hypothalamic non-AgRP, non-POMC GABAergic neurons are required for postweaning feeding and NPY hyperphagia. *J Neurosci* 35:10440–10450.

Kim M, Qie Y, Park J, Kim CH (2016). Gut microbial metabolites fuel host antibody responses. *Cell Host Microbe* 20:202–214.

Klingensmith N, Coopersmith C (2016). The gut as the motor of multiple organ dysfunction in critical illness. *Crit Care Clin* 32(2):203–212.

Knip M, Siljander H (2016). The role of the intestinal microbiota in type 1 diabetes mellitus. *Nat Rev Endocrinol* 12:154–167.

Kö nig J, Wells J, Cani PD, García-Ródenas CL, MacDonald T, Mercenier A, et al. (2016). Human intestinal barrier function in health and disease. *Clin Transl Gastroenterol* 7:e196.

Kuang Z, Wang Y, Li Y, Ye C, Ruhn KA, Behrendt CL, et al. (2019). The intestinal microbiota programs diurnal rhythms in host metabolism through histone deacetylase 3. *Science*, 365:1428–1434.

Kudelka M, Hinrichs B, Darby T, Moreno C, Nishio H, Cutler C, et al. (2016). Cosmc is an X-linked inflammatory bowel disease risk gene that spa- tially regulates gut microbiota and contributes to sex- specific risk. *Proc Natl Acad Sci USA* 113:14787–14792.

Kurilshikov A, Wijmenga C, Fu JY, Zhernakova A (2017). Host genetics and gut microbiome: challenges and perspectives. *Trend Immunol* 38:633–647.

Kurpad AV, Muthayya S, Vaz M (2005). Consequences of inadequate food energy and negative energy balance in humans. *Public Health Nutr* 8:1053–1076.

Lagier JC, Dubourg G, Million M, Cadoret F, Bilen M, Fenollar F, et al. (2018). Culturing the human microbiota and culturomics. *Nat Rev Microbiol* 16:540–550.

Laine JE, Auriola S, Pasanen M, Juvonen RO (2009). Acetaminophen bioactivation by human cytochrome P450 enzymes and animal microsomes. *Xenobiotica* 39:11–21.

Lane E, Zisman T, Suskind D (2017). The microbiota in inflammatory bowel disease: current and therapeutic insights. *J Inflamm Res* 10:63–73.

Le Chatelier E, Nielsen T, Qin J, Prifti E, Hildebrand F, Falony G, et al. (2013). Richness of human gut microbiome correlates with metabolic markers. *Nature* 500(7464):541–546.

Lee JH, Wood TK, Lee J (2015). Roles of indole as an interspecies and interkingdom signaling molecule. *Trends Microbiol* 23:707–718.

Lee S, Lim J, Kim B, Cho S, Kim N, Kim O, et al. (2015). Comparison of the gut microbiota profile in breast-fed and formula-fed Korean infants using pyrosequencing. *Nutr Res Pract* 9:242–257.

Leone V, Gibbons SM, Martinez K, Hutchison AL, Huang EY, Cham CM, et al. (2015). Effects of diurnal variation of gut microbes and high-fat feeding on host circadian clock function and metabolism. *Cell Host Microbe* 17:681–689.

Lerche S, Brock B, Rungby J, Bøtker HE, Møller N, Rodell A, et al. (2008). Glucagon-like peptide-1 inhibits blood-brain glucose transfer in humans. *Diabetes* 57:325–331.

Leung C, Rivera L, Furness J, Angus P (2016). The role of the gut microbiota in NAFLD. *Nat Rev Gastroenterol Hepatol* 13:412–425.

Li B, Li L, Li M, Lam SM, Wang G, Wu Y, et al. (2019a). Microbiota depletion impairs thermogenesis of brown adipose tissue and browning of white adipose tissue. *Cell Rep* 26: 2720–2737.

Li HX, Sun J, Wang FY, Ding GQ, Chen WQ, Fang RC, et al. (2016). Sodium butyrate exerts neuroprotective effects by restoring the blood-brain barrier in traumatic brain injury mice. *Brain Res* 1642:70–78.

Li J, Chiew AL, Isbister GK, Duffull SB (2021). Sulfate conjugation may be the key to hepatotoxicity in paracetamol overdose. *Br J Clin Pharmacol* 87:2392–2396.

Li LS, Rao ST, Cheng YZ, Zhuo XY, Deng CH, Xu NN, et al. (2019b). Microbial osteoporosis: The interplay between the gut microbiota and bones via host metabolism and immunity. *Microbiologyopen* 8:e00810.

Li X, Geng J, Zhao J, Ni Q, Zhao C, Zheng Y, et al. (2019c). Trimethylamine N-oxide exacerbates cardiac fibrosis via activating the NLRP3 inflammasome. *Front Physiol* 10:866.

Liu W, Luo X,T ang J, Mo Q, Zhong H, Zhang H, et al. (2021). A bridge for short-chain fatty acids to affect inflammatory bowel disease, type 1 diabetes, and non- alcoholic fatty liver disease positively: by changing gut barrier. *Eur J Nutr* 60:2317–2330.

Lopez DE, Lashinger LM, Weinstock GM, Bray MS (2021). Circadian rhythms and the gut microbiome synchronize the host's metabolic response to diet. *Cell Metab* 33:873–887.

Lu LY, Chen XX, Liu Y, Yu XJ (2021). Gut microbiota and bone metabolism. *FASEB J* 35:e21740.

Ma G, Pan B, Chen Y, Guo C, Zhao M, Zheng L, Chen B (2017). Trimethylamine N-oxide in atherogenesis: impairing endothelial self-repair capacity and enhancing monocyte adhesion. *Biosci Rep* 37:BSR20160244.

Magnúsdóttir S, Ravcheev D, de Crécy-Lagard V, Thiele I (2015). Systematic genome assessment of B-vitamin biosynthesis suggests co-operation among gut microbes. *Front Genet* 6:148.

Mariat D, Firmesse O, Levenez F, Guimaraes V, Sokol H, Dore, et al. (2009). The Firmicutes/Bacteroidetes ratio of the human microbiota changes with age. *BMC Microbiol* 9:123–137.

Maynard CL, Elson CO, Hatton RD, Weaver CT (2012). Reciprocal interactions of the intestinal microbiota and immune system. *Nature* 489:231–241.

Meddings J (2008). The significance of the gut barrier in disease. *Gut* 57:438–440.

Mika A, Fleshner M (2016). Early-life exercise may promote lasting brain and metabolic health through gut bacterial metabolites. *Immunol Cell Biol* 94:151–157.

Milshteyn A, Colosimo DA, Brady SF (2018). Accessing bioactive natural products from the human microbiome. *Cell Host Microbe* 23:725–736.

Modoux M, Rolhion N, Mani S, Sokol H (2021). Tryptophan metabolism as a pharmacological target. *Trends Pharmacol Sci* 42:60–73.

Mokdad AH, Ford ES, Bowman BA, Dietz WH, Vinicor F, Bales VS, et al. (2003). Prevalence of obesity, diabetes, and obesity-related health risk factors. *JAMA* 289:76–79.

Morris A, Beck J, Schloss P, Campbell TB, Crothers K, Curtis JL, et al. (2013). Comparison of the respiratory microbiome in healthy nonsmokers and smokers. *Am J Res Crit Care Med* 187:1067–1075.

Mü ller M, Canfora EE, Blaak EE (2018). Gastrointestinal transit time, glucose homeostasis and metabolic health: modulation by dietary fibers. *Nutrients* 10:275.

Muscogiuri G, Balercia G, Barrea L, Cignarelli A, Giorgino F, Holst J, et al. (2016). Gut A key player in the pathogenesis of type 2 diabetes? *Crit Rev Food Sci Nutr* 58(8):1294–1309.

Must A, Spadano J, Coakley EH, Field AE, Colditz G, Dietz WH (1999). The disease burden associated with overweight and obesity. *JAMA* 282:1523–1529.

Natividad JM, Verdu EF (2013). Modulation of intestinal barrier by intestinal microbiota: pathological and therapeutic implications. *Pharmacol Res* 69:42–51.

Nicholson JK, Holmes E, Kinross J, Burcelin R, Gibson G, Jia W, Pettersson S (2012). Host-gut microbiota metabolic interactions. *Science* 336:1262–1267.

O'Brien KM, Allen KM, Rockwell CE, Towery K, Luyendyk JP, Copple BL (2013). IL-17A synergistically enhances bile acid-induced inflammation during obstructive cholestasis. *Am J Pathol* 183:1498–1507.

O'Hara AM, Shanahan F (2006). The gut flora as a forgotten organ. *EMBO Reports* 7(7):688–693.

Ochoa-Reparaz J, Mielcarz DW, Wang Y, Begum-Haque S, Dasgupta S, Kasper DL, et al. (2010). A polysaccharide from the human commensal Bacteroides fragilis protects against CNS demyelinating disease. *Mucosal Immunol* 3:487–495.

Parekh P, Balart L, Johnson D (2015). The influence of the gut microbiome on obesity, metabolic syndrome and gas- trointestinal disease. *Clin Trans Gastroent* 6(6):e91.

Park J, Kim M, Kang SG, Jannasch AH, Cooper B, Patterson J, et al. (2015). Short-chain fatty acids induce both effector and regulatory T cells by suppression of histone deacetylases and regulation of the mTOR-S6K pathway. *Mucosal Immunol* 8:80–93.

Pasco JA, Holloway K, Dobbin A, Kotowicz M, Williams L, Brennan S (2014). Body mass index and measures of body fat for defining obesity and underweight: a cross-sectional, population-based study. *BMC Obes* 1:9–16.

Pearson JA, Wong FS, Wen L (2020). Crosstalk between circadian rhythms and the microbiota. *Immunol* 161:278–290.

Pei Z, Bini EJ, Yang L, Zhou M, Francois F, Blaser MJ (2004). Bacterial biota in the human distal esophagus. *Proc Nat Acad Sci* 101(12):4250–4255.

Peng J, Xiao X, Hu M, Zhang X (2018). Interaction between gut microbiome and cardiovascular disease. *Life Sci* 214:153–157.

Perino A, Demagny H, Velazquez-Villegas L, Schoonjans K (2021). Molecular physiology of bile acid signaling in health, disease, and aging. *Physiol Rev* 101:683–731.

Perry VH, Cunningham C, Holmes C (2007). Systemic infections and inflammation affect chronic neurodegeneration. *Nat Rev Immunol* 7:161–167.

Perry VH, Newman TA, Cunningham C (2003). The impact of systemic infection on the progression of neurodegenerative disease. *Nat Rev Neurosci* 4:103–112.

Pevsner-Fischer M, Tuganbaev T, Meijer M, Zhang S, Zeng Z, Chen M, et al. (2016). Role of the microbiome in non- gastrointestinal cancers. *World J Clin Oncol* 7:200–213.

Pingitore A, Chambers ES, Hill T, Maldonado IR, Liu B, Bewick G, et al. (2017). The diet-derived short chain fatty acid propionate improves beta-cell function in humans and stimulates insulin secretion from human islets in vitro. *Diabetes Obes Metab* 19:257–265.

Poll BG, Xu J, Jun S, Sanchez J, Zaidman NA, He X, et al. (2021). Acetate, a short-chain fatty acid, acutely lowers heart rate and cardiac contractility along with blood pressure. *J Pharmacol Exp Ther* 377:39–50.

Pollock N, Grogan C, Perry M, Pedlar C, Cooke K, Morrissey D, et al. (2010). Bone-mineral density and other features of the female athlete triad in elite endurance runners: a longitudinal and cross-sectional observational study. *Int J Sport Nutr Exerc Metab* 20:418–426.

Postler TS, Ghosh S (2017). Understanding the holobiont: how microbial metabolites affect human health and shape the immune system. *Cell Metab* 26:110–130.

Priyadarshini M, Villa SR, Fuller M, Wicksteed B, Mackay CR, Alquier T, et al. (2015). An acetate-specific GPCR, FFAR2, regulates insulin secretion. *Mol Endocrinol* 29:1055–1066.

Qin J, Li R, Raes J, Arumugam M, Burgdorf KS, Manichanh C, et al. (2010). A human gut microbial gene catalogue established by metagenomic sequencing. *Nature* 464:59–65.

Qin J, Li Y, Cai Z, Li S, Zhu J, Zhang F, et al. (2012). A metagenome-wide association study of gut microbiota in type 2 diabetes. *Nature* 490:55–60.

Ramakrishna BS (2007). The normal bacterial flora of the human intestine and its regulation. *J Clin Gastroenterol* 41:S2–S6.

Ramnani P, Chitarrari R, Tuohy K, Grant J, Hotchkiss S, Philp K, Campbell R, Gill C, Rowland I (2012). In vitro fer- mentation and prebiotic potential of novel low molecular weight polysaccharides derived from agar and alginate seaweeds. *Anaerobe* 18(1):1–6.

Rao M (2020). An increasingly complex view of intestinal motility. *Nat Rev Gastroenterol Hepatol* 17:72–73.

Ray K (2018). Gut microbiota filling up on fibre for a healthy gut. *Nat Rev Gastroenterol Hepatol* 15(2):67.

Reyes, A., Haynes, M., Hanson, N., Angly, F. E., Heath, A. C., Rohwer, F., & Gordon, J. I. (2010). Viruses in the faecal microbiota of monozygotic twins and their mothers. *Nature* 466:334–338.

Roager HM, Licht TR (2018). Microbial tryptophan catabolites in health and disease. *Nat Commun* 9:3294.

Rosa EF, Silva AC, Ihara SS, Mora OA, Aboulafia J, Nouail-hetas VL (2005). Habitual exercise program protects murine intestinal, skeletal, and cardiac muscles against aging. *J Appl Physiol* 99(4):1569–1575.

Rosser EC, Piper CJ, Matei DE, Blair PA, Rendeiro AF, Orford M, et al. (2020). Microbiota-derived metabolites suppress arthritis by amplifying aryl-hydrocarbon receptor activation in regulatory B cells. *Cell Metab*, 31:837–851.

Rothhammer V, Mascanfroni ID, Bunse L, Takenaka MC, Kenison JE, Mayo L, et al. (2016). Type I interferons and microbial metabolites of tryptophan modulate astrocyte activity and central nervous system inflammation via the aryl hydrocarbon receptor. *Nat Med* 22:586–597.

Russell SL, Gold MJ, Hartmann M, Willing BP, Thorson L, Wlodarska M, et al. (2012). Early life antibiotic-driven changes in microbiota enhance susceptibility to allergic asthma. *EMBO Rep* 13:440–447.

Russell WR, Gratz SW, Duncan SH, Holtrop G, Ince J, Scobbie L, et al. (2011). High-protein, reduced- carbohydrate weight-loss diets promote metabolite profiles likely to be detrimental to colonic health. *Am J Clin Nutr* 93:1062–1072.

Salem I, Ramser A, Isham N, Ghannoum MA (2018). The gut microbiome as a major regulator of the gut-skin axis. *Front Microbiol* 9:1459.

Sancar A, Van Gelder RN (2021). Clocks, cancer, and chronochemotherapy. *Science*, 371:eabb0738.

Scaldaferri F, Pizzoferrato M, Gerardi V, Lopetuso L, Gasbarrini A (2012). The gut barrier: new acquisitions and therapeutic approaches. *J Clin Gastroenterol* 46:S12–S17.

Schanche M, Avershina E, Dotterud C, Øien T, Storrø O, Johnsen R, Rudi K (2015). High-resolution analyses of overlap in the microbiota between mothers and their children. *Curr Microbiol* 71:283–290.

Schirmer M, Franzosa E, Lloyd-Price J, McIver R, Schwager T, Poon A, et al. (2018). Dynamics of metatranscription in the inflammatory bowel disease gut microbiome. *Nat Microbiol* 3:337–346.

Segers A, Depoortere I (2021). Circadian clocks in the digestive system. *Nat Rev Gastroenterol Hepatol* 18:239–251.

Segers A, Desmet L, Thijs T, Verbeke K, Tack J, Depoortere I (2019). The circadian clock regulates the diurnal levels of microbial short-chain fatty acids and their rhythmic effects on colon contractility in mice. *Acta Physiol* 225:e13193.

Selmer T, Andrei PI (2001). P-Hydroxyphenylacetate decarboxylase from Clostridium difficile: A novel glycyl radical enzyme catalysing the formation of p- cresol. *Eur J Biochem* 268:1363–1372.

Sharon G, Sampson TR, Geschwind DH, Mazmanian SK (2016). The central nervous system and the gut microbiome. *Cell* 167:915–932.

Silva YP, Bernardi A, Frozza RL (2020). The role of short-chain fatty acids from gut microbiota in gut-brain communication. *Front Endocrinol* 11:25.

Skrypnik K, Suliburska J (2018). Association between the gut microbiota and mineral metabolism. *J Sci Food Agric* 98:2449–2460.

Smith EA, Macfarlane GT (1996). Enumeration of human colonic bacteria producing phenolic and indolic compounds: effects of pH, carbohydrate availability and retention time on dissimilatory aromatic amino acid metabolism. *J Appl Bacteriol* 81:288–302.

Smith NW, Shorten PR, Altermann E, Roy NC, McNabb WC (2019). The classification and evolution of bacterial cross-feeding. *Front Ecol Evol* 7:153.

Song Y, Koehler JA, Baggio LL, Powers AC, Sandoval DA, Drucker DJ (2019). Gut-proglucagon-derived peptides are essential for regulating glucose homeostasis in mice. *Cell Metab* 30:976–986.

Sun Y, O'Riordan MX (2013). Regulation of bacterial pathogenesis by intestinal short-chain fatty acids. *Adv Appl Microbiol* 85:93–118.

Sunkara LT, Jiang W, Zhang G (2012). Modulation of antimicrobial host defense peptide gene expression by free fatty acids. *PLoS One* 7:e49558.

Swidsinski A, Loening-Baucke V, Lochs H, Hale LP (2005a). Spatial organization of bacterial flora in normal and inflamed intestine: a fluorescence in situ hybridization study in mice. *World J Gastroenterol* 11(8):1131.

Swidsinski A, Weber J, Loening-Baucke V, Hale LP, Lochs H (2005b). Spatial organization and composition of the mucosal flora in patients with inflammatory bowel disease. *J Clin Microbiol* 43(7):3380–3389.

Tajiri K, Shimizu Y (2018). Branched-chain amino acids in liver diseases. *Transl Gastroenterol Hepatol* 3:47.

Takeuchi T, Ohno H (2021). Reciprocal regulation of IgA and the gut microbiota: a key mutualism in the intestine. *Int Immunol* 33(12):781–786.

Tan J, McKenzie C, Potamitis M, Thorburn AN, Mackay CR, Macia L (2014). The role of short-chain fatty acids in health and disease. *Adv Immunol* 121:91–119.

Thaiss C A, Levy M, Korem T, Dohnalová L, Shapiro H, Jaitin DA, et al. (2016). Microbiota diurnal rhythmicity programs host transcriptome oscillations. *Cell* 167:1495–1510.

Thompson A, Monteagudo-Mera A, Cadenas M, Lampl M, Azcarate-Peril M, Mcgavin MJ, Eckstein T (2015). Milk- and solid-feeding practices and daycare attendance are associated with differences in bacterial diversity, pre- dominant communities, and metabolic and immune func-tion of the infant gut microbiome. *Front Cell Infect Microbiol* 5:3–14.

Thorburn A N, McKenzie CI, Shen SJ, Stanley D, Macia L, Mason LJ, et al. (2015). Evidence that asthma is a developmental origin disease influenced by maternal diet and bacterial metabolites. *Nat Commun* 6:7320.

Tolson A H, Wang H (2010). Regulation of drug- metabolizing enzymes by xenobiotic receptors: PXR and CAR. *Adv Drug Deliv Rev* 62:1238–1249.

Trompette A, Gollwitzer ES, Yadava K, Sichelstiel AK, Sprenger N, Ngom-Bru C, et al. (2014). Gut microbiota metabolism of dietary fiber influences allergic airway disease and hematopoiesis. *Nat Med* 20:159–166.

Vancamelbeke M, Vermeire S (2017). The intestinal barrier: a fundamental role in health and disease. *Expert Rev Gastroenterol Hepatol* 11:821–834.

Verbeke KA, Boobis AR, Chiodini A, Edwards CA, Franck A, Kleerebezem M, et al. (2015). Ton microbial fermentation metabolites as markers for health benefits of prebiotics. *Nutr Res Rev* 28:42–66.

Vijay N, Morris ME (2014). Role of monocarboxylate transporters in drug delivery to the brain. *Curr Pharm Des* 20:1487–1498.

Villanueva-Millan M, Perez-Matute P, Oteo J (2015). Gut microbiota a key player in health and disease. A review focused on obesity. *J Physiol Biochem* 71:509–525.

Voreades N, Kozil A, Weir T (2014). Diet and the development of the human intestinal microbiome. *Front Microbiol* 5:1–9.

Wahlstr öm A, Sayin SI, Marschall HU, Bäckhed F (2016). Intestinal crosstalk between bile acids and microbiota and its impact on host metabolism. *Cell Metab* 24:41–50.

Wang L, Ravichandran V, Yin Y, Yin J, Zhang Y (2019). Natural products from mammalian gut microbiota. *Trends Biotechnol* 37:492–504.

Wells JM, Brummer RJ, Derrien M, MacDonald TT, Troost F, Cani PD, et al. (2017). Homeostasis of the gut barrier and potential biomarkers. *Am J Physiol Gastrointest Liver Physiol* 312:G171–G193.

Whisner CM, Castillo LF (2018). Prebiotics, bone and mineral metabolism. *Calcif Tissue Int* 102:443–479.

Wikoff WR, Anfora AT, Liu J, Schultz PG, Lesley SA, Peters EC, et al. (2009). Metabolomics analysis reveals large effects of gut microflora on mammalian blood metabolites. *Proc Natl Acad Sci U S A* 106:3698–3703.

Wilkins LJ, Monga M, Miller AW (2019). Defining dysbiosis for a cluster of chronic diseases. *Sci Rep* 9:12918.

Xu J, Bartolome CL, Low CS, Yi X, Chien CH, Wang P, et al. (2018). Genetic identification of leptin neural circuits in energy and glucose homeostases. *Nature* 556:505–509.

Yang W, Cong Y (2021). Gut microbiota-derived metabolites in the regulation of host immune responses and immune-related inflammatory diseases. *Cell Mol Immunol* 18:866–877.

Zelezniak A, Andrejev S, Ponomarova O, Mende DR, Bork P, Patil KR (2015). Metabolic dependencies drive species co-occurrence in diverse microbial communities. *Proc Natl Acad Sci U S A* 112:6449–6454.

Zhao L, Zhang F, Ding X, Wu G, Lam Y, Wang X, et al. (2018). Gut bacteria selectively promoted by dietary fibers alleviate type 2 diabetes. *Science* 359:1151–1156.

Zhu W, Gregory J, Org E, Buffa J, Gupta N, Wang Z, et al. (2016). Gut microbial metabolite TMAO enhances platelet hyper-reactivity and thrombosis risk. *Cell* 165:111–124.

Zhu W, Winter M, Byndloss M, Spiga L, Duerkop B, Hughes E, et al. (2018). Precision editing of the gut microbiota ameliorates colitis. *Nature* 553:208–211.

Zoetendal EG, Akkermans AD, Akkermans-van Vliet WM, de Visser JA, De Vos WM (2001). The host genotype affects the bacterial community in the human gastrointestinal tract. *Microb Ecol Health Dis* 13:129–134.

13 The Potential Role of Prebiotics, Probiotics, and Synbiotics in Cancer Prevention and Therapy

Phool Chandra, Himanshu Sharma, and Neetu Sachan

13.1 INTRODUCTION

Cancer, a complex and heterogeneous group of diseases, continues to take a significant toll on global health [1]. As our understanding of the intricate interplay between the human microbiome and various physiological processes deepens, a compelling avenue for novel therapeutic interventions emerges. This chapter aims to unravel the potential role of prebiotics, probiotics, and synbiotics in the prevention and treatment of cancer, exploring the dynamic relationship between these bioactive compounds and the human microbiome [2]. The human microbiome, an ecosystem of diverse microorganisms inhabiting various body niches, has emerged as a crucial determinant of health and disease [3]. Recent research illuminates the bidirectional relationship between the microbiome and cancer, highlighting the potential for microbiome modulation as a strategy to influence cancer initiation, progression, and response to therapy. Traditional approaches to cancer prevention and therapy have predominantly focused on genetic and environmental factors [4]. However, the microbiome introduces a paradigm shift, emphasizing the significance of microbial communities in modulating systemic health. This shift prompts a reevaluation of conventional strategies and opens new avenues for interventions that target the microbiome to complement existing therapies. Prebiotics, non-digestible fibers that selectively nourish beneficial microbes, and probiotics, live microorganisms conferring health benefits, have gained attention for their potential in shaping the microbiome [5]. Synbiotics, the synergistic combination of prebiotics and probiotics, offer a comprehensive approach to microbiome modulation [6]. Understanding the unique contributions of each and their combined effects forms the crux of this exploration. This chapter aims to provide a comprehensive overview of the current understanding of the microbiome's role in cancer, the potential of prebiotics, probiotics, and synbiotics in cancer prevention and therapy, and the underlying mechanisms driving their effects [7]. By synthesizing existing knowledge, we seek to elucidate the promise and challenges of microbiome-focused interventions in the dynamic landscape of cancer care. As we embark on this exploration, the integration of microbiome-centric approaches into mainstream oncology holds the promise of enhancing therapeutic outcomes and ushering in a new era in cancer research and treatment (see Figure 13.1) [8].

13.1.1 Microbiome and Its Impact on Health

The human microbiome, an intricate and dynamic community of microorganisms residing predominantly in the gastrointestinal tract, has emerged as a critical player in maintaining health and influencing various physiological processes [9]. Comprising bacteria, viruses, fungi, and archaea, this ecosystem forms a symbiotic relationship with the host, collectively referred to as the microbiota [10]. The genetic material of these microorganisms, known as the microbiome, significantly exceeds the human genome, contributing an extensive repertoire of functional genes that play a pivotal role in human biology [11]. The microbiome's impact extends far beyond its historical association with digestion. Recent research has illuminated its profound influence on the immune system, metabolism, and even neurological functions. Microbes within the gut actively participate in the breakdown of complex carbohydrates, the synthesis of essential vitamins, and the metabolism of dietary compounds, contributing to overall nutrient absorption and energy regulation [12]. Moreover, the microbiome serves as a critical player in the development and education of the immune system. It plays a crucial role in training immune cells to distinguish between harmless and harmful entities, contributing to the body's defense mechanisms against pathogens [13]. Additionally, the microbiome acts as a barrier, preventing the colonization of pathogenic microorganisms by competing for resources and producing antimicrobial substances. Alterations in the composition and function of the microbiome, termed dysbiosis, have been implicated in a range of diseases, including inflammatory bowel diseases, metabolic disorders, and autoimmune conditions. Moreover, emerging research highlights the intricate interplay between the microbiome and cancer, with microbial communities influencing the risk, progression, and response to cancer therapy. In summary, the microbiome stands as a complex and integral component of human health, with its influence reaching far beyond the confines of the digestive system [14]. Understanding this intricate interplay provides a foundation for exploring novel therapeutic strategies centered around microbiome modulation, presenting unprecedented opportunities for improving health and preventing disease (see Figure 13.2) [15].

DOI: 10.1201/9781032702438-13

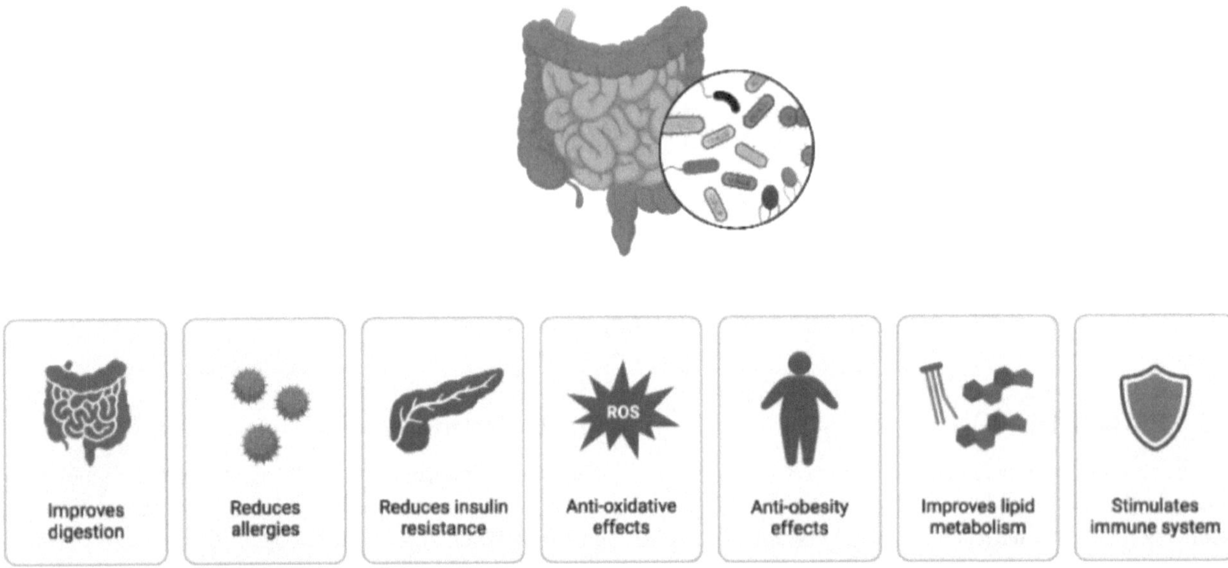

FIGURE 13.1 Microbes, and probiotics, live microorganisms conferring health benefits.

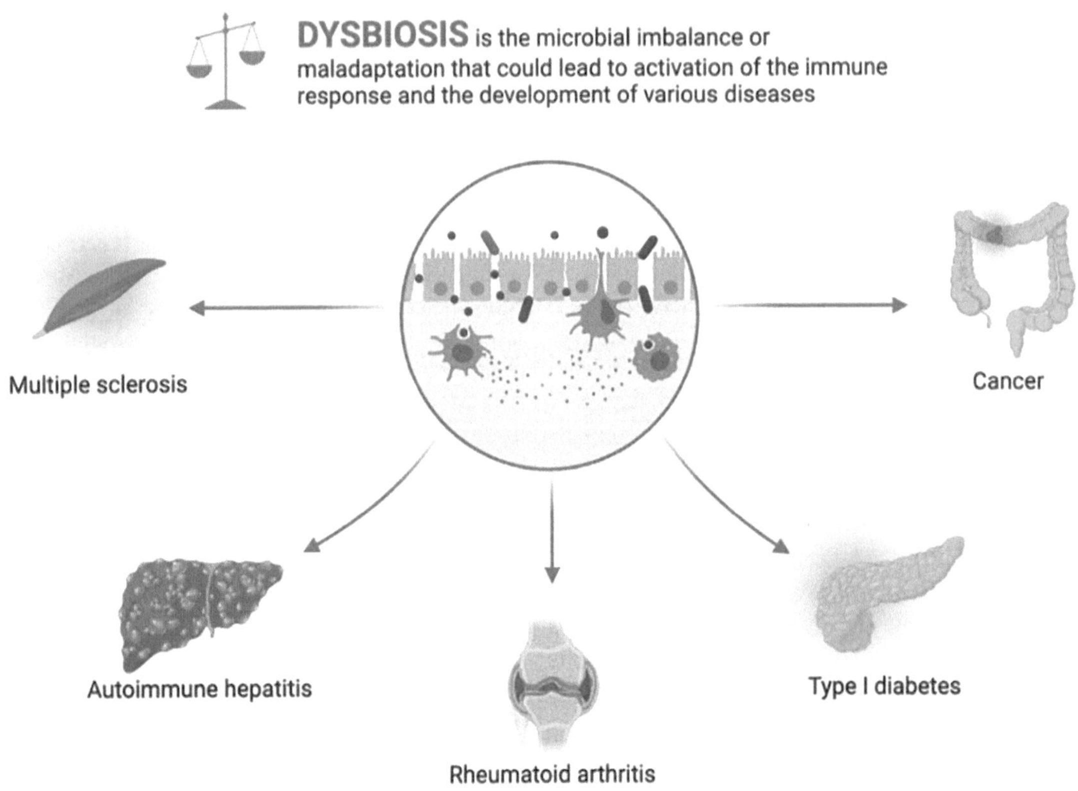

FIGURE 13.2 Background on the microbiome and its impact on health.

13.1.2 Overview of the Current Landscape of Cancer Prevention and Therapy

The current landscape of cancer prevention and therapy is marked by significant advancements in understanding the molecular basis of cancer, innovative treatment modalities, and a growing emphasis on personalized medicine [16]. While traditional approaches such as surgery, chemotherapy, and radiation therapy remain cornerstones, the evolving understanding of cancer as a complex and heterogeneous group of diseases has led to a paradigm shift in strategies. Advances in genomic profiling have paved the way for precision medicine, tailoring treatment approaches based on the specific genetic alterations present in an individual's cancer cells [17]. Targeted therapies, designed to interfere with specific molecules involved in cancer growth and progression, have shown remarkable efficacy in certain cancer types, minimizing damage to healthy cells and reducing side effects. Harnessing the body's immune system to recognize and attack cancer cells has revolutionized cancer treatment. Immunotherapeutic approaches, such as immune checkpoint inhibitors and CAR-T cell therapies, have demonstrated unprecedented success in various cancers, offering durable responses and improved outcomes for some patients [18]. Beyond therapeutic interventions, there is a growing emphasis on comprehensive cancer prevention strategies. Lifestyle modifications, including healthy dietary practices, regular physical activity, and avoidance of tobacco, contribute significantly to reducing the risk of cancer [19]. Additionally, screening and early detection programs aim to identify cancers at an early, more treatable stage. Despite these advancements, challenges persist. Resistance to treatment, side effects, and the high cost of some therapies underscore the need for continued research and innovation. Moreover, the recognition of the microbiome's role in cancer development has opened new avenues for exploration, presenting opportunities to enhance therapeutic efficacy and mitigate treatment-related side effects through microbiome-focused interventions. As the field of oncology continues to evolve, the integration of diverse and complementary approaches, including microbiome modulation with prebiotics, probiotics, and synbiotics, holds the potential to augment existing strategies and usher in a new era of personalized and more effective cancer prevention and therapy [20].

13.1.3 Rationale for Exploring Prebiotics, Probiotics, and Synbiotics in Cancer Research

The exploration of prebiotics, probiotics, and synbiotics in cancer research is rooted in a profound understanding of the intricate interplay between the human microbiome and cancer development [21]. The microbiome, a dynamic community of microorganisms inhabiting various body sites, has emerged as a key modulator of systemic health, influencing processes ranging from immune function to metabolism. As this connection becomes clearer, there is a compelling rationale for investigating how manipulating the microbiome through prebiotics, probiotics, and synbiotics may hold therapeutic potential in the realm of cancer. Microbiome and tumorigenesis scientific evidence underscores the association between alterations in the gut microbiota and the initiation and progression of various cancers [22]. Dysbiosis, characterized by an imbalance in the composition and function of the microbiome, has been implicated in creating a microenvironment conducive to tumorigenesis. This recognition forms the foundation for exploring interventions that can restore or maintain a healthy microbiome to counteract cancer-related processes [23]. Immunomodulation and anti-inflammatory effects of prebiotics, probiotics, and synbiotics have been shown to modulate the immune system, enhancing its ability to recognize and eliminate aberrant cells, including cancer cells. Moreover, these interventions exhibit anti-inflammatory effects, contributing to a microenvironment less favorable for cancer development [24]. The microbiome's influence on systemic inflammation and immune surveillance positions prebiotics, probiotics, and synbiotics as potential agents to bolster the body's natural defenses against cancer. Prebiotics, probiotics, and synbiotics have shown promise in ameliorating treatment-related side effects, improving the efficacy of chemotherapy, and mitigating the impact of radiation therapy on the gut [8]. This supportive role in conventional therapies adds another layer of significance to their exploration of the cancer research landscape. In conclusion, the rationale for investigating prebiotics, probiotics, and synbiotics in cancer research lies in their potential to influence the microbiome, modulate immune responses, and enhance the body's ability to prevent and combat cancer. These interventions represent a holistic and innovative approach that may reshape the landscape of cancer prevention and therapy, offering new avenues for therapeutic intervention and improved patient outcomes [25].

13.2 THE MICROBIOME-CANCER CONNECTION

The connection between the microbiome and cancer is an area of active research, and scientists are exploring how the trillions of microbes living in and on the human body may influence the development and progression of cancer [26]. The microbiome refers to the diverse community of microorganisms, including bacteria, viruses, fungi, and archaea, that inhabit various body sites, such as the gut, skin, mouth, and other mucosal surfaces. Certain microbes can promote inflammation, which is a known factor in the development of cancer. Chronic inflammation can create an environment that encourages the growth of cancer cells. The microbiome plays a crucial role in regulating the immune system [27]. A balanced and diverse microbiome helps maintain immune system health. Disruptions in the balance of the microbiome (dysbiosis) can affect the immune response, potentially contributing to the development of cancer. The microbiome is involved in the metabolism of various compounds, including dietary components. Some microbes can produce or modify metabolites that may influence the risk of cancer. For example, the metabolism of certain foods can produce substances that either promote or inhibit cancer growth. Some microbes may directly interact with host cells, influencing their behavior [28]. This interaction can affect cellular processes and potentially contribute to the development of cancer. The microbiome may influence the response to cancer treatments, including chemotherapy and immunotherapy. Specific microbial populations in the gut, for example, can impact how the body responds to certain drugs. Reduced diversity in the microbiome has been associated with certain types of cancer. A diverse microbiome is generally considered healthier, and alterations in microbial diversity may be linked to an increased risk of cancer [29]. The majority of research in this field has focused on the gut microbiome, given its significant influence on the immune system and overall health. However, other microbiomes, such as those in the oral cavity and skin, are also being investigated for their potential roles in cancer. It's important to note that while there is growing evidence of a microbiome-cancer connection, the field is complex, and more research is needed to fully understand the mechanisms and implications of these interactions. Additionally, individual responses to the microbiome and its influence on cancer can vary, making personalized approaches to treatment and prevention a promising area of investigation [30].

13.2.1 Understanding the Role of the Microbiome in Cancer Development

The intricate relationship between the human microbiome and cancer development is a burgeoning area of research that has unveiled the multifaceted influence of microbial communities on various aspects of tumorigenesis [31]. The microbiome, primarily residing in the gastrointestinal tract, comprises trillions of microorganisms collectively contributing to the complex landscape of the body's microbial ecosystem. Dysbiosis, characterized by alterations in the composition and function of the microbiome, has been implicated in creating a microenvironment conducive to the initiation and progression of cancer. Specific shifts in microbial populations have been associated with increased inflammation, compromised immune surveillance, and alterations in metabolic processes, all of which can contribute to the hallmarks of cancer [32]. One of the key mechanisms through which the microbiome impacts cancer development is by modulating the immune system. The gut microbiota actively communicates with immune cells, influencing their maturation, activation, and response to potential threats, including cancer cells. Dysbiosis can disrupt this delicate balance, leading to immune dysfunction and a compromised ability to recognize and eliminate aberrant cells. Microbial communities play a crucial role in shaping the inflammatory milieu within the body [33]. Chronic inflammation is a well-established driver of cancer, promoting genetic mutations and creating a microenvironment favorable for tumor growth. Dysbiosis can contribute to sustained inflammation, fostering conditions conducive to the initiation and progression of cancer. The microbiome significantly contributes to the host's metabolism, influencing the processing of dietary components and the production of bioactive metabolites [34]. Dysbiosis can disrupt these metabolic interactions, potentially promoting conditions favorable to cancer development through alterations in nutrient availability and utilization. Understanding the role of the microbiome in cancer development is a nuanced exploration of the dynamic interactions between microbial communities and the host. This comprehension not only sheds light on the mechanisms underpinning cancer initiation but also provides a foundation for developing targeted interventions that aim to modulate the microbiome to prevent or treat cancer effectively [30]. As research progresses, unraveling the complexities of this relationship holds great promise for innovative approaches in the ongoing battle against cancer [35].

13.2.2 Mechanisms Linking Gut Microbiota to Tumorigenesis

The intricate mechanisms linking the gut microbiota to tumorigenesis underscore the dynamic interplay between microbial communities and the complex processes that drive the initiation and progression of cancer [36]. Understanding these mechanisms provides crucial insights into potential therapeutic interventions aimed at modulating the microbiome to prevent or treat cancer. The gut microbiota is involved in the metabolism of dietary compounds, producing bioactive metabolites that can influence host cell function. Some metabolites, such as SCFAs, have anti-inflammatory properties and can contribute to maintaining gut homeostasis [37]. However, dysbiosis may lead to the production of genotoxic metabolites, promoting DNA damage and mutations that contribute to tumorigenesis. Dysbiosis can induce chronic inflammation in the gut, creating a pro-tumorigenic environment. Inflammatory responses trigger the release of reactive oxygen species and pro-inflammatory cytokines, which, over time, can damage cellular DNA and create conditions favorable for the survival and proliferation of cancer cells [38]. Moreover, dysbiosis can compromise the immune system's ability to detect and eliminate transformed cells, contributing to tumor development. Gut microbiota actively communicates with host cells by influencing signaling pathways crucial for cellular homeostasis. Dysbiosis may lead to aberrant signaling, disrupting regulatory mechanisms that control cell proliferation, apoptosis, and DNA repair [39]. These disruptions can drive uncontrolled cell growth, a hallmark of cancer. The microbiome significantly influences host metabolism, including the metabolism of nutrients critical for cellular function. Dysbiosis can alter nutrient availability and utilization, impacting host cell energetics. These metabolic changes can provide a supportive environment for cancer cells to thrive and proliferate. Microbial communities within the gut can influence the systemic environment, affecting distant organs, including tumor sites [40]. Dysbiosis-induced changes in the tumor microenvironment can influence angiogenesis, immune cell infiltration, and extracellular matrix remodeling, all of which contribute to tumor growth and metastasis. In conclusion, the mechanisms linking gut microbiota to tumorigenesis are diverse and multifaceted, involving genotoxicity, inflammation, immune dysregulation, alterations in host signaling, and modulation of host metabolism. Recognizing these intricate interactions provides a foundation for developing targeted interventions that aim to restore a healthy microbiome and disrupt the pro-tumorigenic processes, potentially offering novel avenues for cancer prevention and therapy [41].

13.2.3 Implications Strategies for Cancer Prevention

The insights gained from understanding the intricate relationship between gut microbiota and tumorigenesis carry profound implications for developing effective cancer prevention strategies [42]. Recognizing the role of the microbiome in influencing cancer development opens new avenues for interventions that target microbial modulation, presenting novel opportunities to reduce cancer risk and enhance overall health. Dietary interventions and prebiotics given the influence of the microbiome on the metabolism of dietary interventions play a pivotal role in cancer prevention [43]. Prebiotics, non-digestible fibers that selectively nourish beneficial gut bacteria, promote a balanced microbial ecosystem. Incorporating prebiotic-rich foods into the diet, such as fruits, vegetables, and whole grains, may contribute to maintaining a healthy gut microbiota and reducing the risk of dysbiosis-associated tumorigenesis [44]. Probiotics, live microorganisms conferring health benefits, have shown promise in modulating the gut microbiota and promoting a favorable environment for cancer prevention. Consumption of probiotic-rich foods or supplements may enhance the abundance of beneficial bacteria, supporting immune function and suppressing inflammation, thereby contributing to the prevention of cancer development [45]. Adopting a healthy lifestyle that includes regular physical activity, avoidance of tobacco, and moderation in alcohol consumption contributes to a balanced gut microbiota and reduces the risk of dysbiosis. Physical exercise has been associated with a more diverse and beneficial gut microbiome, reinforcing the importance of holistic lifestyle approaches in cancer prevention. The widespread use of antibiotics can disrupt the delicate balance of the gut microbiota, potentially promoting dysbiosis. Antibiotic stewardship, including judicious use and consideration of alternative treatments when appropriate, is crucial to preserving the integrity of the microbiome and reducing the risk of antibiotic-induced disturbances linked to cancer susceptibility [46]. Recognizing the individual variability in microbiome composition, personalized approaches to cancer prevention may emerge. Understanding a person's unique microbiome profile could inform tailored interventions, optimizing strategies to restore or maintain a healthy microbial balance based on individual needs and susceptibilities. In conclusion, leveraging the insights into the role of gut microbiota in cancer development informs a multifaceted approach to cancer prevention. Integrating dietary interventions, probiotics, lifestyle modifications, antibiotic stewardship, and personalized microbiome-based strategies holds the potential to reshape cancer prevention initiatives, providing more effective and targeted approaches for reducing the global burden of cancer [47].

13.3 PREBIOTICS: NOURISHING THE MICROBIAL ALLIES

Prebiotics, non-digestible fibers that selectively promote the growth and activity of beneficial microorganisms, constitute a pivotal component in microbiome modulation for health promotion and disease prevention, including in the context of cancer. Prebiotics encompass a diverse group of compounds, predominantly oligosaccharides, that resist digestion in the upper gastrointestinal tract and reach the colon intact. Common prebiotics include inulin, fructooligosaccharides, and galactooligosaccharides [48]. These compounds serve as substrates for beneficial bacteria, promoting their proliferation and metabolic activity. Prebiotics play a crucial role in shaping the composition and functionality of the gut microbiota. By selectively nourishing beneficial bacteria, such as Bifidobacteria and Lactobacilli, prebiotics foster a microbial ecosystem associated with health and resilience. This modulation contributes to the maintenance of a diverse and balanced microbiome, creating an environment less conducive to dysbiosis-linked pathologies, including cancer. The role of prebiotics in cancer prevention lies in their ability to create a microbiome environment that opposes tumorigenesis. Through the production of SCFAs, a byproduct of microbial fermentation of prebiotics, the gut environment becomes more acidic, inhibiting the growth of potential pathogens and promoting the health of colonocytes. Moreover, SCFAs exert anti-inflammatory effects, contributing to a milieu that discourages pro-tumorigenic processes. Prebiotics are abundantly found in various plant-based foods. Chicory root, Jerusalem artichokes, garlic, onions, leeks, bananas, and whole grains are rich sources of prebiotic fibers. Including a diverse range of these foods in the diet ensures a regular supply of prebiotics, supporting the growth of beneficial bacteria in the gut. Combining prebiotics with probiotics creates synergistic formulations known as synbiotics [49]. This approach aims to enhance the survival and activity of probiotic strains by providing them with a tailored substrate for growth. Synbiotics, therefore, offer a comprehensive strategy for microbiome modulation, potentially amplifying their impact on cancer prevention and overall health. In summary, prebiotics stand as nutritional allies in nurturing a healthy gut microbiome [50]. Their potential in cancer prevention is rooted in the modulation of microbial communities and the promotion of an environment that is less conducive to cancer development. As research advances, the incorporation of prebiotics into dietary strategies may prove to be a valuable and accessible approach in the broader context of cancer prevention and holistic health [51].

13.3.1 Definition and Types of Prebiotics

Prebiotics, a category of non-digestible fibers, are defined by their ability to selectively nourish beneficial microorganisms in the gut, fostering the growth and activity of specific bacteria associated with health and well-being [52]. These compounds resist digestion in the upper gastrointestinal tract, reaching the colon intact, where they serve as substrates for fermentation by beneficial bacteria. A fructan, inulin is naturally found in a variety of plants, including chicory root, garlic, onions, and Jerusalem artichokes. Its complex structure allows it to escape digestion in the small intestine, reaching the colon to stimulate the growth of beneficial bacteria. FOS are short-chain fructans naturally present in foods like bananas, onions, and asparagus

[53]. They consist of short chains of fructose molecules and act as prebiotics by promoting the proliferation of beneficial bacteria in the colon. GOS are oligosaccharides composed of galactose units and are found in foods such as legumes, lentils, and certain dairy products. They serve as substrates for the fermentation activity of beneficial gut bacteria. Although not a traditional prebiotic, resistant starch functions similarly by resisting digestion in the small intestine [54]. Found in foods like green bananas, raw potatoes, and legumes, resistant starch reaches the colon intact, where it undergoes fermentation by beneficial microbes. Found in fruits, especially apples and citrus fruits, pectin is a soluble fiber that acts as a prebiotic by promoting the growth of beneficial bacteria in the colon. These diverse types of prebiotics contribute to the enrichment of the gut microbiota, fostering a balanced and diverse microbial ecosystem associated with improved health outcomes. As our understanding of the microbiome advances, the incorporation of a variety of prebiotics through a diverse and balanced diet remains a key strategy for promoting gut health and potentially mitigating the risk of dysbiosis-associated conditions, including cancer [55].

13.3.2 Gut Microbiome in Cancer

The gut microbiome, a complex community of microorganisms inhabiting the gastrointestinal tract, has emerged as a crucial player in cancer development, progression, and treatment response [28]. The intricate interplay between the gut microbiota and the host's immune system, metabolism, and inflammatory processes significantly influences the dynamics of cancer-related pathways. Research has unveiled distinct differences in the composition and diversity of the gut microbiome between individuals with cancer and those without, indicating the potential role of microbial signatures as biomarkers for cancer risk and diagnosis. The gut microbiota, particularly in the context of CRC, has been extensively studied [56]. Certain microbial imbalances and the presence of specific bacterial strains have been associated with an increased risk of CRC and other gastrointestinal cancers. Mechanistically, the gut microbiome can impact cancer through various pathways. Chronic inflammation induced by dysbiosis may contribute to the initiation and progression of cancer [32]. Additionally, the microbiome can influence the metabolism of dietary components, producing bioactive metabolites that may either promote or inhibit tumorigenesis. In cancer therapy, the gut microbiome has been recognized for its role in modulating the efficacy of treatments such as immunotherapy [57]. Specific microbial communities are associated with enhanced or diminished responses to cancer immunotherapy, highlighting the potential for microbiome-based interventions to improve treatment outcomes. As our understanding of the gut microbiome's intricate relationship with cancer deepens, there is growing optimism for leveraging this knowledge to develop innovative strategies for cancer prevention, early detection, and personalized treatment approaches. However, challenges such as the complexity of microbial interactions, individual variability, and the translation of findings into clinical applications underscore the need for continued research in this dynamic field [58].

13.3.3 Composition and Function of the Gut Microbiome

The gut microbiome, a diverse community of microorganisms inhabiting the gastrointestinal tract, is integral to human health, influencing various physiological functions [59]. Comprising bacteria, viruses, fungi, and archaea, the gut microbiota's composition is highly individualized, and shaped by factors like genetics, diet, and environmental exposures [60]. The predominant bacterial phyla in the gut include Firmicutes, Bacteroidetes, Actinobacteria, and Proteobacteria. Within these phyla, numerous genera, such as Bacteroides, Prevotella, and Faecalibacterium, contribute to the microbial balance [61]. Firmicutes and Bacteroidetes are involved in breaking down complex carbohydrates, while Actinobacteria, including Bifidobacterium, ferment dietary fibers and produce beneficial metabolites. Proteobacteria, when in overabundance, can indicate dysbiosis [62]. Microbes ferment non-digestible dietary fibers, producing SCFAs like butyrate, which is vital for gut health. Vitamin synthesis certain gut bacteria contribute to the synthesis of vitamins, including B and K, essential for various physiological processes. The gut microbiome plays a pivotal role in the development and maturation of the immune system, particularly in early life. It contributes to immune tolerance, distinguishing between harmless and harmful antigens, and acts as a barrier against pathogens. The gut microbiota competes with potential pathogens, preventing their overgrowth by occupying resources and adhesion sites. Some gut microbes produce antimicrobial compounds, like bacteriocins, inhibiting the growth of pathogenic bacteria [63]. The gut microbiome influences the extraction of energy from ingested food, impacting host metabolism and energy storage. Microbial metabolites can affect host appetite and satiety, contributing to the regulation of body weight [64]. Understanding the gut microbiome's composition and function is crucial for unraveling its role in health and addressing conditions associated with microbial dysregulation, such as inflammatory bowel diseases and metabolic disorders. Ongoing research continues to shed light on the intricate interplay between the gut microbiota and human physiology [65].

13.3.4 Influence of Prebiotics on the Gut Microbiota

Prebiotics exert a profound influence on the gut microbiota, shaping its composition and functionality in ways that contribute to overall health [66]. The unique properties of prebiotics as non-digestible fibers that selectively nourish beneficial microorganisms enable them to play a crucial role in modulating the intricate ecosystem of the gastrointestinal tract [67]. Prebiotics act as a fuel source for specific beneficial bacteria, such as Bifidobacteria and Lactobacilli. By providing these microbes with a substrate for fermentation, prebiotics selectively stimulate their growth and metabolic activity in the colon [3]. This selective promotion of beneficial bacteria contributes to a microbiota profile associated with health and disease resistance. The fermentation of prebiotics by gut bacteria produces SCFAs, including acetate, propionate, and butyrate. SCFAs serve as energy sources for colonocytes and play a crucial role in maintaining the integrity of the gut barrier. Additionally, they contribute to the regulation of inflammation and immune responses, creating an environment less favorable for pathogenic bacteria and potential carcinogenesis [68]. A diet rich in diverse prebiotics supports the growth of a wide array of beneficial bacteria, fostering microbial diversity within the gut. Increased microbial diversity is associated with improved resilience and responsiveness to environmental challenges, further contributing to gut health. Prebiotic fermentation produces acids that lower the pH of the colon [69]. This acidification inhibits the growth of potentially harmful bacteria while promoting the proliferation of acid-loving beneficial bacteria, creating an environment less conducive to dysbiosis and inflammation. In summary, the influence of prebiotics on the gut microbiota is a dynamic and multifaceted process. By selectively nourishing beneficial bacteria, promoting SCFA production, enhancing microbial diversity, and modulating gut pH, prebiotics contribute to the maintenance of a balanced and resilient gut microbiota. This modulation not only supports digestive health but also holds implications for broader aspects of well-being, including the potential prevention of dysbiosis-associated conditions such as cancer [70].

13.3.5 Prebiotics as Potential Agents for Cancer Prevention

The role of prebiotics in cancer prevention is grounded in their capacity to modulate the gut microbiota, influencing factors associated with tumorigenesis [71]. As non-digestible fibers, prebiotics selectively nourish beneficial bacteria, fostering an environment that holds promise for reducing the risk of cancer development. SCFAs the fermentation of prebiotics by gut bacteria results in the production of SCFAs, particularly butyrate, propionate, and acetate. These SCFAs play a pivotal role in maintaining gut health by providing an energy source for colonocytes, promoting a healthy gut barrier, and exhibiting anti-inflammatory effects [72]. These mechanisms collectively create an environment less conducive to the initiation and progression of cancer. Chronic inflammation is a recognized contributor to cancer development, and prebiotics, through the production of SCFAs, help mitigate inflammatory processes [73]. By dampening pro-inflammatory responses, prebiotics contribute to an anti-inflammatory milieu that may reduce the risk of inflammation-driven carcinogenesis. Prebiotics influence the immune system by promoting the growth of beneficial bacteria associated with enhanced immune function. A balanced and responsive immune system is critical for detecting and eliminating aberrant cells, contributing to the body's defense against cancer [74]. Dysbiosis, an imbalance in the gut microbiota, has been linked to various cancers. Prebiotics, by selectively supporting the growth of beneficial bacteria, contribute to microbial balance. This balance may create an environment less favorable for the proliferation of potentially harmful microbes associated with cancer development. Prebiotics contribute to an acidic environment in the colon through the production of SCFAs [18]. This acidification inhibits the growth of pathogenic bacteria while favoring the growth of beneficial bacteria, further promoting a gut environment that may protect against cancer initiation. Incorporating prebiotics into the diet through sources such as chicory root, garlic, onions, bananas, and whole grains holds potential as a holistic and accessible strategy for promoting gut health and reducing the risk of cancer. As research continues to unveil the intricate connections between gut microbiota and cancer, prebiotics emerge as promising agents for inclusion in comprehensive cancer prevention approaches [75].

13.3.6 Gut Microbiome and Gastrointestinal Cancers

The gut microbiome, a complex community of microorganisms residing in the gastrointestinal tract, has emerged as a key player in influencing various aspects of human health, including the development and progression of GI cancers [31]. Comprising bacteria, viruses, fungi, and archaea, the gut microbiota plays a pivotal role in maintaining intestinal homeostasis and modulating the immune system [28]. Recent research has unveiled intricate connections between alterations in the gut microbiome and the onset of GI cancers, with CRC being a primary focus [76]. Dysbiosis, an imbalance in the gut microbiota, has been associated with increased susceptibility to GI cancers. Changes in microbial diversity, abundance, and function have been observed in individuals with colorectal, gastric, esophageal, and liver cancers. Dysbiosis can lead to the production of pro-inflammatory molecules, contributing to chronic inflammation a known driver of cancer development [77]. In CRC, specific microbial signatures have been identified. Reduced levels of beneficial bacteria, such as Bifidobacterium and Lactobacillus, and an overabundance of potentially pathogenic bacteria like Fusobacterium and Enterococcus, are associated with increased CRC risk. Microbial dysregulation may influence the progression of precancerous lesions to invasive cancer. The mechanisms through which the gut microbiome influences GI cancers are multifaceted. Chronic inflammation induced by dysbiosis can promote the survival and proliferation of cancer cells. Microbial metabolites, such as short-chain fatty acids and secondary bile acids, can impact cellular processes and modulate the host immune response, further influencing cancer development [78]. The gut microbiome's influence extends to cancer treatment outcomes. Recent studies suggest that the composition of the gut microbiota can affect the efficacy of chemotherapy and immunotherapy. Microbial modulation through interventions like fecal microbiota transplantation (FMT) or probiotics may enhance treatment responses. As the understanding of the gut microbiome's role in GI cancers deepens, there is potential for developing microbiome-based diagnostics and interventions. Integrating microbiome information into personalized treatment plans holds promise for improving therapeutic outcomes. However, challenges such as the complexity of microbial interactions and individual variability need to be addressed for effective translation into clinical practice [79].

13.4 PROBIOTICS: HARNESSING THE POWER OF BENEFICIAL MICROORGANISMS

Probiotics, live microorganisms that confer health benefits when administered in adequate amounts, represent a compelling frontier in promoting gut health and potentially mitigating the risk of cancer [80]. The power of probiotics lies in their ability to modulate the composition and function of the gut microbiota, influencing various physiological processes that extend beyond digestive health. Probiotics encompass a diverse array of bacteria, with Lactobacillus and Bifidobacterium species being the most commonly used [81]. These beneficial microorganisms can be found in fermented foods like yogurt, kefir, sauerkraut, and supplement form. Each strain of probiotic may confer unique health benefits, emphasizing the importance of strain specificity in harnessing their therapeutic potential. Probiotics interact with the immune system, influencing the balance between pro-inflammatory and anti-inflammatory responses [82]. By enhancing the activity of immune cells and promoting the production of anti-inflammatory cytokines, probiotics contribute to an immune profile associated with cancer prevention and overall health [83]. Certain probiotic strains demonstrate the ability to inhibit processes associated with carcinogenesis. This includes the production of antimicrobial substances that suppress the growth of potentially harmful bacteria, as well as the modulation of metabolic pathways involved in the formation of carcinogenic compounds. Probiotics play a key role in maintaining the balance of the gastrointestinal tract. They contribute to the integrity of the gut barrier, preventing the translocation of harmful substances into the bloodstream [84]. This barrier function is crucial in reducing inflammation and protecting against conditions linked to cancer development. Beyond prevention, probiotics show promise in cancer therapy. They may help mitigate treatment-related side effects, such as gastrointestinal toxicity associated with chemotherapy and radiation therapy. Additionally, by modulating the gut microbiota, probiotics could potentially enhance the efficacy of certain cancer treatments [85].

13.4.1 Immunomodulatory Effects of Probiotics

The immunomodulatory effects of probiotics highlight their pivotal role in shaping the intricate interplay between the gut microbiota and the immune system [86]. This capacity to modulate immune responses constitutes a fundamental aspect of probiotic functionality, offering potential benefits not only for gastrointestinal health but also for broader systemic immune function and disease prevention. Probiotics exert profound influences on various immune cell populations, including macrophages, dendritic cells, and T lymphocytes [87]. These microorganisms communicate with immune cells, enhancing their activity and promoting a balanced immune response. Probiotics can stimulate the production of cytokines, signaling molecules that coordinate immune responses, contributing to the regulation of inflammation and immune homeostasis. Phagocytosis, the process by which immune cells engulf and eliminate pathogens, is a critical defense mechanism. Probiotics have been shown to enhance phagocytic activity, bolstering the immune system's ability to recognize and clear potential threats [88]. This heightened phagocytic capacity contributes to the overall resilience of the immune system. Probiotics play a crucial role in fortifying mucosal immunity, which is particularly significant in the context of the gut [89]. By promoting the production of immunoglobulins, such as IgA, probiotics contribute to the defense of mucosal surfaces against invading pathogens. This reinforcement of mucosal immunity is vital for preventing infections and maintaining gut health. Chronic inflammation is implicated in various diseases, including cancer. Probiotics exhibit anti-inflammatory effects by downregulating the production of pro-inflammatory cytokines [90]. This modulation of the inflammatory milieu contributes to an environment less conducive to chronic inflammation, potentially reducing the risk of inflammation-driven carcinogenesis. Probiotics engage in a form of immune system training, influencing the maturation and education of immune cells. This training enhances the immune system's ability to distinguish between harmful pathogens and harmless antigens, contributing to a well-regulated and responsive immune defense [91]. Understanding the immunomodulatory effects of probiotics illuminates their potential to support immune health and prevent diseases associated with immune dysregulation, including certain cancers [92].

13.4.2 Inhibition of Carcinogenic Processes by Probiotics

Probiotics, the beneficial microorganisms inhabiting the gut, demonstrate a remarkable ability to inhibit various processes associated with carcinogenesis. Through intricate interactions with the host and the gut microbiota, probiotics contribute to a microenvironment that opposes the initiation and progression of cancer [93]. Probiotics produce antimicrobial substances, such as bacteriocins and organic acids, which create an inhospitable environment for potential carcinogenic bacteria. By inhibiting the growth of harmful microorganisms, probiotics contribute to the maintenance of a balanced and protective microbial ecosystem in the gut. Certain probiotic strains have been shown to modulate metabolic pathways, influencing the production of metabolites associated with cancer development [94]. For instance, probiotics may reduce the conversion of carcinogenic compounds into active carcinogens, thereby mitigating the risk of cancer initiation. Probiotics participate in the detoxification of carcinogens by enhancing the expression of enzymes involved in the breakdown and elimination of harmful substances [95]. This detoxification process contributes to reducing the burden of potential carcinogens in the gut and systemic circulation. A compromised gut barrier allows the translocation of harmful substances, potentially contributing to inflammation and carcinogenesis. Probiotics play a crucial role in enhancing the integrity of the gut barrier, preventing the leakage of toxins and pathogenic bacteria into the bloodstream. This barrier function is pivotal in reducing the risk of inflammation-driven cancers [96]. Probiotics exert immunomodulatory effects that contribute to the surveillance and elimination of cancer cells. By enhancing immune responses, probiotics assist in the recognition and removal of abnormal cells, reducing the likelihood of tumorigenesis. Chronic inflammation is a hallmark of cancer development, and probiotics have demonstrated anti-inflammatory effects by modulating the production of inflammatory cytokines. This regulation of inflammatory responses creates an environment less conducive to the promotion and progression of cancer [97].

13.4.3 Probiotics in Cancer Therapy: Current Evidence and Challenges

The exploration of probiotics in cancer therapy represents a burgeoning area of research, reflecting the evolving understanding of the gut microbiome's impact on overall health, including cancer [98]. While there is promising evidence regarding the potential benefits of probiotics in cancer treatment, challenges and complexities persist. Modulation of treatment-related side effects probiotics show promise in alleviating treatment-related side effects, particularly those associated with conventional cancer therapies such as chemotherapy and radiation. Studies suggest that certain probiotic strains can mitigate gastrointestinal symptoms, including nausea, diarrhea, and mucositis, enhancing the overall quality of life for cancer patients undergoing treatment [99]. The immunomodulatory effects of probiotics have implications for cancer therapy. By enhancing immune responses, probiotics may complement immunotherapeutic approaches. However, the complexity of the immune system and the need for a nuanced understanding of specific cancer types and treatments present challenges in optimizing probiotic interventions [100]. The efficacy of probiotics is highly dependent on strain specificity. Different strains may exert varying effects, and identifying the most beneficial strains for specific cancers remains a challenge. Precision in selecting probiotic strains tailored to individual patient profiles and cancer types is crucial for optimizing therapeutic outcomes. The gut microbiome's composition varies among individuals, contributing to the challenge of developing universal probiotic interventions. Personalized approaches that consider the unique microbial landscape of each patient are essential for harnessing the full potential of probiotics in cancer therapy [101]. Standardizing probiotic formulations for therapeutic use presents challenges due to the multitude of available strains and their diverse effects. Regulatory frameworks for probiotic products also vary globally, necessitating a cohesive and evidence-based approach to ensure the safety and efficacy of probiotics in cancer therapy [102].

13.5 SYNBIOTICS: OPTIMIZING SYNERGY FOR ENHANCED IMPACT

Synbiotics represent a dynamic approach to microbiome modulation by combining prebiotics and probiotics, aiming to maximize the synergistic effects of these two components for enhanced impact on gut health and overall well-being [103]. Synbiotics are formulations that incorporate both prebiotics and probiotics. Prebiotics, typically non-digestible fibers, serve as substrates for the growth and activity of beneficial bacteria. Probiotics, live microorganisms conferring health benefits, are introduced alongside prebiotics to enhance their survival, growth, and beneficial effects in the gut [10]. The combination of prebiotics and probiotics creates a synergistic relationship, where prebiotics selectively nourish and stimulate the growth of probiotic microorganisms. This synergistic interaction fosters the establishment and maintenance of a balanced and diverse microbial ecosystem in the gut, promoting the overall health of the host. Prebiotics act as a source of energy and sustenance for probiotics, enhancing their survival through the digestive tract and promoting their colonization in the gut. This combination ensures that a sufficient population of viable probiotics reaches the colon, where their beneficial effects are most pronounced. Synbiotics play a role in modulating the composition of the gut microbiota [104]. The selective stimulation of specific beneficial bacteria by prebiotics, coupled with the introduction of probiotics, contributes to a microbiome profile associated with improved gut health, immune function, and other systemic benefits. The synergistic effects of synbiotics have implications for cancer prevention and therapy. By promoting a balanced and resilient gut microbiota, synbiotics may contribute to reducing the risk of dysbiosis-associated conditions, including certain cancers [50]. In cancer therapy, synbiotics may enhance the efficacy of treatments and mitigate treatment-related side effects. Like other microbiome-based interventions, the effectiveness of synbiotics may vary among individuals due to the personalized nature of the gut microbiome. Tailoring synbiotic formulations to individual microbiome profiles represents a direction for future research, ensuring precision and efficacy in promoting gut health. In summary, synbiotics harness the synergistic potential of prebiotics and probiotics to optimize their impact on gut health and overall well-being. As our understanding of the gut microbiome advances, the strategic use of synbiotics holds promise for personalized interventions, offering a holistic approach to support health and potentially play a role in the prevention and management of various health conditions, including cancer [20].

13.5.1 Definition and Rationale for Synbiotics

Synbiotics, a term derived from the fusion of "probiotics" and "prebiotics," refers to formulations that combine live beneficial microorganisms (probiotics) with selectively fermentable substrates (prebiotics). The rationale behind synbiotics lies in the synergistic relationship between these two components, aiming to optimize their combined effects on the gut microbiota and, consequently, host health [55]. Synbiotics are formulations designed to maximize the symbiotic interactions between probiotics and prebiotics. Probiotics are live microorganisms that confer health benefits when consumed in adequate amounts, while prebiotics are non-digestible fibers that selectively nourish beneficial gut bacteria. The combination of these two components creates a synergistic effect, enhancing the survival, growth, and activity of probiotics in the gut [105]. The rationale for synbiotics stems from the recognition that probiotics and prebiotics exert complementary effects on the gut microbiota. Prebiotics serve as a fuel source for probiotics, promoting their colonization and activity in the gastrointestinal tract. This synergistic interaction fosters a more robust and balanced microbial ecosystem, with potential benefits for gut health, immune function, and overall well-being. The strategic combination of probiotics and prebiotics in synbiotics offers a comprehensive approach to microbiome modulation, addressing both the need for beneficial microorganisms and the substrates necessary for their optimal function [106].

13.5.2 Synergistic Effects of Combining Prebiotics and Probiotics

The synergistic effects of combining prebiotics and probiotics in synbiotics create a powerful alliance that extends beyond the individual benefits of each component. This strategic combination capitalizes on their complementary mechanisms, optimizing the impact on the gut microbiota and overall health [107]. Prebiotics, non-digestible fibers, serve as a nutritional source for probiotics, enhancing their survival through the digestive tract and promoting their colonization in the gut. This synergy ensures that a sufficient population of viable probiotics reaches the colon, where they can exert their beneficial effects on the host. Prebiotics selectively nourish specific beneficial bacteria, acting as a substrate for their fermentation. When combined with probiotics, this creates a synergistic environment where the growth and activity of these beneficial microbes are further promoted [3]. The selective stimulation fosters a balanced and diverse microbial ecosystem associated with improved gut health. The combination of prebiotics and probiotics influences the overall microbial composition of the gut. Prebiotics create an environment conducive to the growth of beneficial bacteria, and probiotics contribute to the introduction of specific strains. This combined modulation supports a microbiome profile associated with enhanced resilience and resistance to dysbiosis. The synergistic effects of synbiotics contribute to improved metabolic activity within the gut. Fermentation of prebiotics by probiotics produces SCFAs, known for their various health benefits [108]. SCFAs not only serve as an energy source for colonocytes but also exhibit anti-inflammatory and regulatory effects, contributing to overall gut and systemic health. The collective impact of synbiotics extends beyond the gut, with potential benefits for immune function, nutrient absorption, and even mental health [109].

13.5.3 Potential Applications of Synbiotics in Cancer Prevention and Therapy

Synbiotics, a combination of probiotics and prebiotics, have emerged as a promising avenue in cancer prevention and therapy due to their potential to modulate the gut microbiota and enhance overall health [2]. Probiotics, beneficial microorganisms, play a crucial role in maintaining gut microbial balance, while prebiotics provide the necessary nutrients for their growth. In cancer prevention, synbiotics may contribute to a healthy gut microbiome, which has been linked to reduced inflammation and improved immune function. Chronic inflammation is a known contributor to cancer development, and synbiotics could help mitigate this risk by promoting an anti-inflammatory environment in the gut [110]. Moreover, certain probiotic strains have demonstrated the ability to produce bioactive compounds with anti-cancer properties, further supporting their preventive potential. In cancer therapy, synbiotics hold promise as adjuncts to traditional treatments. They may enhance the efficacy of immunotherapy by modulating the immune response and promoting a favorable microenvironment for immune cells. Additionally, synbiotics could help alleviate treatment-related side effects, such as gastrointestinal issues and compromised immune function, by supporting gut health. Research suggests that the gut microbiota can influence the response to chemotherapy and other cancer treatments [111]. Synbiotics may optimize the microbial composition, potentially improving treatment outcomes and reducing complications. However, further studies are needed to elucidate specific mechanisms, identify optimal formulations, and determine the ideal timing for synbiotic interventions in cancer prevention and therapy. Overall, the potential applications of synbiotics in cancer care highlight the intricate connection between gut health and systemic well-being, paving the way for innovative approaches in the fight against cancer [112].

13.6 IMMUNE MODULATION BY MICROBIOME INTERVENTIONS

The interaction between the microbiome and the immune system has garnered increasing attention, paving the way for innovative strategies in immune modulation [113]. Microbiome interventions, which include probiotics, prebiotics, and FMT, hold promise in influencing immune responses and maintaining overall immune homeostasis. Probiotics, live microorganisms with health benefits, have been shown to modulate immune function [29]. Certain strains can enhance the activity of immune cells, regulate inflammation, and contribute to the development of a balanced immune system. These interventions are particularly relevant in conditions associated with immune dysregulation, such as autoimmune diseases and allergies. Prebiotics, non-digestible fibers that stimulate the growth of beneficial bacteria, indirectly influence immune function by shaping the composition of the gut microbiota [114]. A diverse and balanced microbiome is associated with a more robust and responsive immune system. By promoting the growth of beneficial bacteria, prebiotics contribute to a healthier microbial community that, in turn, supports immune modulation. FMT, the transfer of fecal material from a healthy donor to a recipient, is another microbiome intervention that can impact immune function. This approach has shown promise in the treatment of certain infections and conditions related to immune dysregulation. The transplanted microbiota from a healthy donor can potentially restore microbial diversity and improve immune responses in the recipient. Understanding the intricate relationship between the microbiome and the immune system opens avenues for therapeutic interventions [115]. Harnessing microbiome-based strategies for immune modulation could have implications for a range of conditions, from autoimmune disorders to infectious diseases. However, it is essential to conduct further research to unravel the specific mechanisms involved and optimize these interventions for clinical applications (see Figure 13.3) [116].

13.6.1 Anti-Inflammatory Effects on the Tumor Microenvironment

Various interventions demonstrate anti-inflammatory effects on the tumor microenvironment. Probiotics modulate gut microbiota, reducing systemic inflammation and potentially inhibiting tumor-promoting pathways. NSAIDs suppress inflammatory mediators and hinder tumor-associated angiogenesis [117]. Omega-3 fatty acids produce anti-inflammatory lipid mediators, attenuating pro-inflammatory signals. Curcumin inhibits NF-κB, suppressing inflammatory responses and potentially hindering tumor progression. Corticosteroids reduce inflammation in the tumor microenvironment. Anti-inflammatory cytokines (e.g., IL-10) promote an immunosuppressive microenvironment, potentially inhibiting tumor growth. Exercise contributes to systemic inflammation reduction and immune system modulation, potentially improving anti-tumor immune responses (Table 13.1) [118].

13.6.2 Metabolic Influences on Cancer Development and Progression

Metabolism plays a crucial role in cancer development and progression, influencing various cellular processes that contribute to the hallmarks of cancer [126]. Dysregulation of metabolic pathways can promote tumor growth, survival, and metastasis. One key aspect is altered glucose metabolism, known as the Warburg effect, where cancer cells preferentially utilize glycolysis even in the presence of oxygen [127]. This metabolic shift provides energy rapidly but less efficiently than oxidative phosphorylation. Elevated glucose consumption not only fuels tumor growth but also contributes to an acidic microenvironment, fostering invasion, and immune evasion. Beyond glucose, changes in lipid metabolism are also implicated in cancer. Enhanced lipid synthesis supports the high demands for membrane production in rapidly dividing cancer cells. Lipids act as signaling molecules, influencing pathways related to cell proliferation and survival [128]. Amino acid metabolism is vital for protein synthesis and sustaining cancer cell proliferation. Tumor cells often exhibit increased uptake of certain amino acids, such as glutamine, to meet their energetic and biosynthetic needs. Moreover, the tumor microenvironment influences metabolic adaptations. Hypoxia, a common feature in solid tumors, triggers responses that enhance angiogenesis and alter metabolism to support survival in low-oxygen conditions [129].

13.7 CLINICAL IMPLICATIONS AND CHALLENGES

Clinical implications of understanding metabolic influences on cancer involve developing targeted therapies to disrupt specific metabolic pathways, potentially enhancing treatment efficacy [130]. Challenges include tumor heterogeneity, requiring personalized approaches, and the risk of normal tissue toxicity with systemic metabolic interventions. Precision medicine, considering individual tumor metabolic profiles, is crucial. Moreover, optimizing drug delivery to the tumor microenvironment poses a challenge. Despite hurdles, integrating metabolic insights into clinical practice holds promise for more effective cancer treatments,

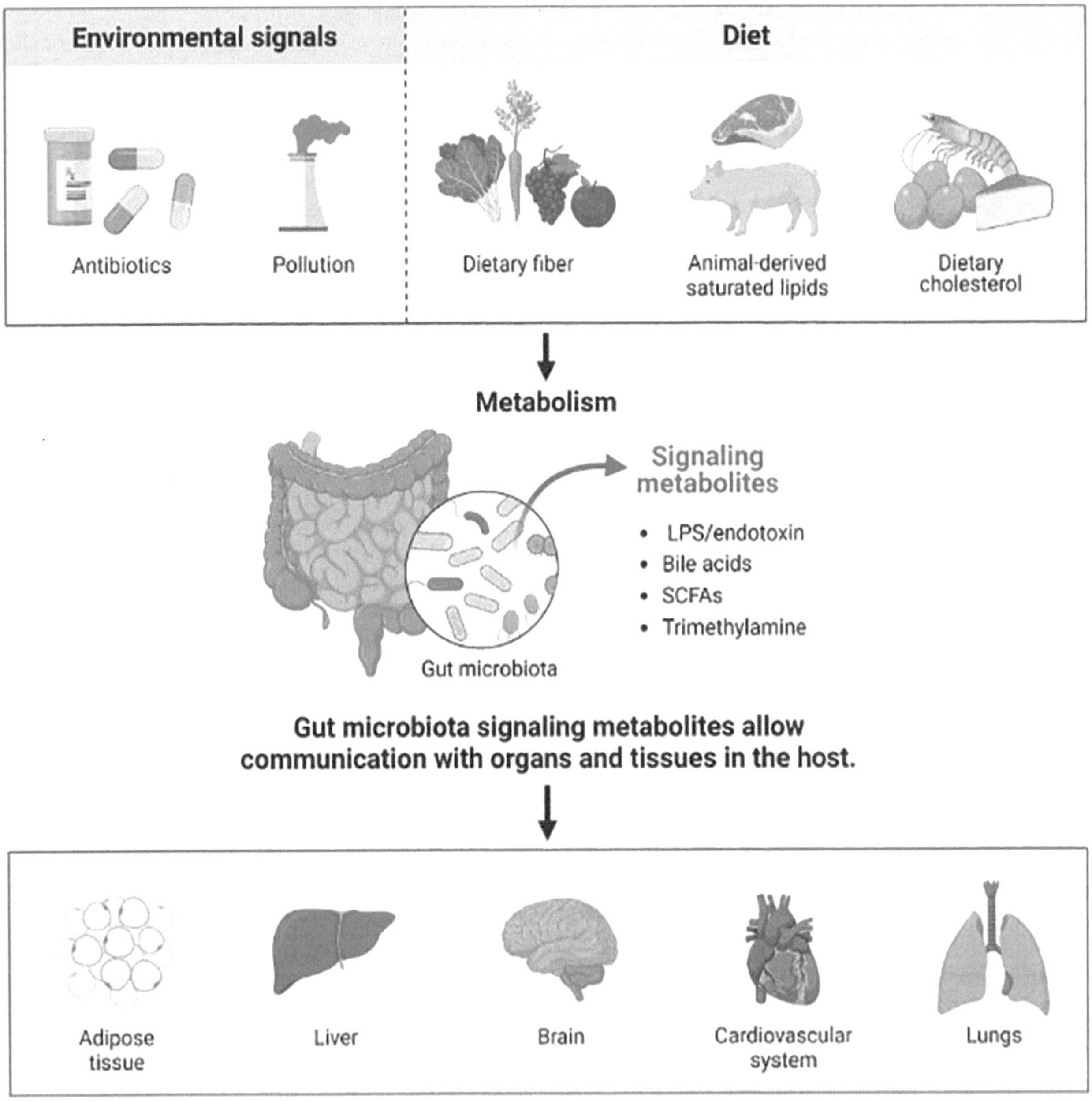

FIGURE 13.3 Role of gut microbiota in autoimmune diseases.

emphasizing the need for ongoing research, innovative technologies, and collaborative efforts to translate metabolic discoveries into tangible clinical benefits [131].

13.7.1 Overview of Clinical Studies Investigating Microbiome-Based Interventions

Clinical studies investigating microbiome-based interventions have surged in recent years, reflecting a growing recognition of the microbiome's impact on health [132]. These studies encompass a range of conditions, from gastrointestinal disorders to neurological diseases. Researchers explore the therapeutic potential of probiotics, prebiotics, FMT, and dietary interventions. Preliminary findings suggest microbiome modulation can influence disease outcomes by restoring microbial balance, modulating immune responses, and producing bioactive compounds. Challenges include standardization of interventions, establishing optimal dosages, and elucidating long-term effects. Despite complexities, these studies signify a transformative era in healthcare, with microbiome research holding promise for innovative and personalized therapeutic strategies (Table 13.2) [133].

13.7.2 Challenges and Limitations in Translating Research Findings to Clinical Practice

Translating research findings into clinical practice faces several challenges and limitations, hindering the seamless integration of innovative interventions. Heterogeneity in study populations clinical trials often involves diverse

TABLE 13.1
Potential Anti-Inflammatory Effects on the Tumor Microenvironment

Anti-Inflammatory Intervention	Mechanism of Action	Potential Impact on Tumor Microenvironment	References
Probiotics	Modulation of gut microbiota, reduction of systemic inflammation	Alleviation of chronic inflammation, potential inhibition of tumor-promoting pathways	[119]
NSAIDs	Inhibition of COX enzymes, reduction of prostaglandin synthesis	Suppression of inflammatory mediators, hindrance of tumor-associated angiogenesis	[120]
Omega-3 fatty acids	Production of anti-inflammatory lipid mediators	Attenuation of pro-inflammatory signals, potential inhibition of tumor growth	[121]
Curcumin	Inhibition of NF-κB, modulation of cytokine expression	Suppression of inflammatory responses, potential hindrance of tumor progression	[122]
Corticosteroids	Suppression of immune responses and inflammation	Reduction of inflammation in the tumor microenvironment, alleviation of symptoms	[123]
Anti-inflammatory cytokines	Administration of anti-inflammatory cytokines (e.g., IL-10)	Promotion of an immunosuppressive microenvironment, potential inhibition of tumor growth	[124]
Exercise	Systemic reduction of inflammation, immune system modulation	Attenuation of chronic inflammation, potential improvement of anti-tumor immune responses	[125]

TABLE 13.2
Overview of Clinical Studies Investigating Microbiome-based Interventions

Intervention Type	Conditions Studied	Key Findings	Challenges and Considerations	References
Probiotics	Gastrointestinal disorders, immune modulation	Improved gut microbial balance, symptom relief	Strain-specific effects, dose standardization, long-term impacts	[134]
Prebiotics	Metabolic disorders, gastrointestinal health	Promotion of beneficial bacteria, metabolic improvements	Individual response variations, optimal dosage determination	[65]
FMT	Clostridium difficile infection, Inflammatory bowel disease	Microbial community restoration, disease remission	Donor selection and screening, long-term safety and efficacy	[135]
Dietary interventions	Obesity, metabolic syndrome	Altered microbial composition, weight management	Dietary heterogeneity, individual response variability	[76]
Microbial modulation therapies	Various conditions	Targeted manipulation of specific microbial functions	Standardization of therapeutic approaches, ethical considerations	[76]

patient populations, leading to variations in treatment responses [136]. Tailoring interventions for specific subgroups can be challenging. Lack of standardization variability in study designs, endpoints, and assessment methods complicates the establishment of standardized protocols. Consistent methodologies are essential for comparing and combining results across studies [137]. Long-term effects and safety concerns may have immediate effects, but long-term safety and efficacy remain uncertain. A comprehensive understanding of potential adverse events is crucial before widespread clinical implementation. Ensuring patient safety and adherence to ethical standards poses regulatory challenges. Issues like informed consent, patient autonomy, and the responsible use of emerging technologies require careful consideration. Determining the optimal dosage and duration of interventions is challenging. The "one-size-fits-all" approach may not be suitable for microbiome-based therapies, considering individual variations in response [34]. The microbiome's dynamic nature and individual variability make it challenging to identify consistent patterns. Understanding how interventions impact diverse microbial profiles is critical for personalized treatment. Incorporating new interventions into existing clinical practices poses challenges. Resistance to change, lack of awareness, and the need for updated guidelines can slow down adoption [138]. Patient compliance with microbiome-based interventions, which may involve lifestyle changes or specific dietary habits, can be a hurdle. Non-adherence affects the reliability of outcomes. Implementing new interventions may be resource-intensive, and financial constraints can impede the widespread adoption of innovative therapies, especially in resource-limited settings. Successful integration requires collaboration between researchers, clinicians, and other healthcare professionals. Bridging gaps between disciplines is crucial for effective translation [139].

13.8 ETHICAL AND SAFETY CONSIDERATIONS

13.8.1 Ethical Issues in Microbiome Research and Applications

Microbiome research and its applications raise several ethical considerations that warrant careful attention. These issues revolve around informed consent, privacy and data security, representation and diversity, therapeutic interventions, commercialization, environmental impact, and community engagement [140]. The complexity and long-term nature of microbiome research present challenges in obtaining truly informed consent from participants. Researchers must communicate effectively about the intricacies of microbiome data and the potential implications of participation. Microbiome data is inherently personal, offering insights into an individual's health and lifestyle [141]. Protecting participant privacy and ensuring data security against unauthorized access are crucial ethical concerns, given the sensitivity of this information. Achieving diversity in participant populations is essential to ensure that microbiome research findings are applicable across different groups. Failing to include diverse populations may lead to biased results and hinder the generalizability of research outcomes. The development of microbiome-based therapies, such as FMT, introduces ethical considerations regarding safety, potential risks, and equitable access [142]. Rigorous testing, clear communication of side effects, and addressing access disparities are crucial for responsible therapeutic applications. Commercial interests in microbiome-related products and services raise ethical questions regarding intellectual property, profit motives, and conflicts of interest. Balancing these interests with ethical research conduct is essential to prevent undue influence on scientific endeavors. Manipulating the microbiome, whether through interventions or environmental changes, may have ecological consequences [143]. Ethical considerations extend to understanding and mitigating any potential negative impacts on the environment. Ethical microbiome research necessitates meaningful community engagement. Researchers should treat communities as partners, involving them in decision-making processes, addressing concerns, and ensuring that research aligns with community values and benefits the broader population. Navigating these ethical challenges requires a multidisciplinary approach involving researchers, ethicists, policymakers, and community representatives. Establishing clear ethical guidelines, prioritizing participant welfare, and fostering transparency are essential for the responsible advancement of microbiome research and its applications [144].

13.8.2 Safety Concerns and Risk Mitigation Strategies

Microbiome-based interventions introduce safety concerns that require vigilant risk mitigation. Key considerations include unknown long-term effects, ecological disruption, inadvertent introduction of pathogens, immunological responses, and individual variability. Conduct rigorous preclinical studies to assess safety, using animal models and *in vitro* experiments to identify potential adverse effects before human trials. Implement robust monitoring during and after clinical trials to promptly identify any unexpected adverse events and ensure participant safety [145]. Enhance informed consent processes, ensuring participants fully comprehend potential risks, uncertainties, and the importance of long-term follow-up [146]. Consider individual variability in responses, tailoring interventions based on factors such as genetics and baseline microbiome composition. Strengthen regulatory oversight for microbiome-based products, establishing clear guidelines to ensure safety and efficacy. Assess potential ecological impacts of microbiome interventions to minimize unintended effects on microbial ecosystems. Encourage ongoing research and collaboration between researchers, clinicians, and regulatory bodies to stay informed about emerging safety considerations and continuously improve safety protocols. By proactively addressing these concerns through these risk mitigation strategies, the development and application of microbiome interventions can proceed responsibly, minimizing potential risks and ensuring the safety of individuals and ecosystems [147].

13.9 FUTURE PROSPECTS

The potential role of prebiotics, probiotics, and synbiotics in cancer prevention and therapy holds significant promise, representing a burgeoning area of research with compelling prospects [148]. These interventions target the gut microbiome, a dynamic ecosystem linked to immune regulation, inflammation, and metabolic processes, all of which are pivotal in cancer development and progression. Prebiotics, non-digestible fibers that promote the growth of beneficial bacteria, have shown promise in fostering a healthy gut microbiota [149]. By providing a nourishing environment for beneficial microbes, prebiotics may contribute to an anti-inflammatory milieu and enhance the body's defense against cancer. Future research may delve deeper into identifying specific prebiotic compounds and their optimal combinations to maximize anti-cancer effects. Probiotics, live microorganisms with proven health benefits, demonstrate potential in cancer prevention and therapy by modulating the gut microbiota. Certain strains exhibit anti-inflammatory properties and may even produce bioactive compounds with direct anti-cancer effects [150]. The future lies in refining our understanding of strain-specific activities, dosage considerations, and personalized approaches based on individual microbiome profiles. Synbiotics, a combination of prebiotics and probiotics, present a synergistic approach. By delivering both the beneficial microorganisms and the substrates necessary for their growth, synbiotics aim to optimize the therapeutic potential. This involves uncovering the precise interactions between prebiotics and probiotics, tailoring synbiotic formulations for specific cancer types, and exploring their potential as adjuvants to conventional cancer therapies [151]. As we advance, research may focus on the intricate crosstalk between the gut microbiome and the immune system, elucidating how these interventions impact systemic anti-cancer immune responses. Additionally, clinical trials assessing the efficacy of prebiotics, probiotics, and synbiotics in various cancer types will contribute crucial evidence for their integration into cancer prevention and treatment protocols. Challenges, including the need for standardized formulations, understanding individual variability in responses, and addressing concerns regarding safety in immunocompromised patients, warrant careful consideration. However, the evolving landscape of microbiome research suggests that harnessing the potential of prebiotics, probiotics, and synbiotics could offer innovative, complementary strategies in the comprehensive approach to cancer prevention and therapy in the future [152].

13.10 CONCLUSION

In conclusion, the potential role of prebiotics, probiotics, and synbiotics in cancer prevention and therapy presents a compelling frontier in biomedical research with broad-reaching implications. The gut microbiome's influence on immune modulation, inflammation, and metabolic processes underscores the significance of these interventions in the context of cancer, a disease intricately linked to these physiological factors. Prebiotics, by fostering a supportive environment for beneficial bacteria, and probiotics, with their direct and indirect anti-cancer properties, offer avenues for personalized and targeted interventions. The combination of prebiotics and probiotics in synbiotics represents a synergistic approach, potentially amplifying therapeutic benefits. The interventions lie in unraveling the complexities of microbiome–host interactions and optimizing formulations for specific cancer types. As we look ahead, understanding the interplay between the gut microbiome and the immune system will be paramount. Advances in this field may lead to the development of tailored interventions that enhance systemic anti-cancer immune responses. Clinical trials exploring the efficacy of these interventions across diverse cancer types will provide critical insights, shaping their integration into comprehensive cancer prevention and treatment strategies. However, challenges such as the need for standardized formulations, consideration of individual variability, and addressing safety concerns must be navigated. As the field evolves, the potential benefits of incorporating prebiotics, probiotics, and synbiotics into cancer care highlight a paradigm shift toward holistic, microbiome-informed approaches. The dynamic nature of microbiome research offers optimism for innovative, personalized strategies that may complement existing cancer therapies, providing new avenues to enhance patient outcomes in the future.

ACKNOWLEDGMENT

The authors are thankful to the Principal, Department of Pharmacy, Teerthanker Mahaveer University, Moradabad, Uttar Pradesh for providing the necessary facilities and support.

LIST OF ABBREVIATIONS

DNA	Deoxyribonucleic acid
SCFAs	Short-chain fatty acids
CRC	Colorectal cancer
GI	Gastrointestinal
FMT	Fecal microbiota transplantation
NSAIDs	Non-steroidal anti-inflammatory drugs

REFERENCES

1. Xavier-Santos, D., Padilha, M., Fabiano, G. A., Vinderola, G., Gomes Cruz, A., Sivieri, K., & Costa Antunes, A. E. (2022). Evidences and perspectives of the use of probiotics, prebiotics, synbiotics, and postbiotics as adjuvants for prevention and treatment of COVID-19: A bibliometric analysis and systematic review. *Trends in Food Science and Technology, 120*, 174–192. https://www.sciencedirect.com/science/article/pii/S0924224421006907. https://doi.org/10.1016/j.tifs.2021.12.033
2. Ashique, S., Garg, A., Bhatt, S., Sirohi, E., Fatima, N., Bajwa, N., Dua, K., & Mishra, N. (2023, March 26). Synbiotics in cervical cancer. In *Synbiotics for the Management of Cancer* (pp. 135–155). Springer Nature. https://doi.org/10.1007/978-981-19-7550-9_6
3. Ashique, S., Faruk, A., Ahmad, F. J., Khan, T., & Mishra, N. (2023, October 25). It is all about probiotics to control cervical cancer. *Probiotics and Antimicrobial Proteins*, 1–4. https://doi.org/10.1007/s12602-023-10183-2
4. Zepeda-Hernández, A., Garcia-Amezquita, L. E., Requena, T., & García-Cayuela, T. (2021). Probiotics, prebiotics, and synbiotics added to dairy products: Uses and applications to manage type 2 diabetes. *Food Research International, 142*, 110208. https://www.sciencedirect.com/science/article/pii/S0963996921001071. https://doi.org/10.1016/j.foodres.2021.110208
5. Keulers, L., Dehghani, A., Knippels, L., Garssen, J., Papadopoulos, N., Folkerts, G., Braber, S., & van Bergenhenegouwen, J. (2022). Probiotics, prebiotics, and synbiotics to prevent or combat air pollution consequences: The gut-lung axis. *Environmental Pollution, 302*, 119066. https://www.sciencedirect.com/science/article/pii/S0269749122002809. https://doi.org/10.1016/j.envpol.2022.119066
6. Wong, W. Y., Chan, B. D., Leung, T. W., Chen, M., & Tai, W. C. S. (2022). Beneficial and anti-inflammatory effects of formulated prebiotics, probiotics, and synbiotics in normal and acute colitis mice. *Journal of Functional Foods, 88*, 104871. https://www.sciencedirect.com/science/article/pii/S175646462100520X. https://doi.org/10.1016/j.jff.2021.104871
7. Rani, K., Kaur, G., & Ali, S. A. (2023). Probiotic-prebiotic therapeutic potential: A new horizon of microbial biotherapy to reduce female reproductive complications.

PharmaNutrition, *24*, 100342. https://www.sciencedirect.com/science/article/pii/S2213434423000142. https://doi.org/10.1016/j.phanu.2023.100342

8. Dangi, P., Chaudhary, N., Chaudhary, V., Virdi, A. S., Kajla, P., Khanna, P., Jha, S. K., Jha, N. K., Alkhanani, M. F., Singh, V., & Haque, S. (2023). Nanotechnology impacting probiotics and prebiotics: A paradigm shift in nutraceuticals technology. *International Journal of Food Microbiology*, *388*, 110083. https://www.sciencedirect.com/science/article/pii/S0168160522005578. https://doi.org/10.1016/j.ijfoodmicro.2022.110083
9. Gadallah, S. H., Eissa, S., Ghanem, H. M., Ahmed, E. K., Hasanin, A. H., El Mahdy, M. M., & Matboli, M. (2021). Probiotic-prebiotic-synbiotic modulation of (YAP1, LATS1 and NF2 mRNAs/miR-1205/lncRNA SRD5A3-AS1) panel in NASH animal model. *Biomedicine and Pharmacotherapy*, *140*, 111781. https://www.sciencedirect.com/science/article/pii/S0753332221005631. https://doi.org/10.1016/j.biopha.2021.111781
10. Khursheed, R., Gulati, M., Wadhwa, S., Vishwas, S., Sharma, D. S., Corrie, L., Alam, A., Alnasser, S. M., Aba Alkhayl, F. F., Parveen, Z., Nammi, S., Chellappan, D. K., Gupta, G., Zacconi, F., Steel, A., Adams, J., Jha, N. K., Dua, K., & Singh, S. K. (2022). Multifaceted role of Synbiotics as nutraceuticals, therapeutics and carrier for drug delivery. *Chemico-Biological Interactions*, *368*, 110223. https://www.sciencedirect.com/science/article/pii/S0009279722004288. https://doi.org/10.1016/j.cbi.2022.110223
11. Gu, Q., Yin, Y., Yan, X., Liu, X., Liu, F., & McClements, D. J. (2022). Encapsulation of multiple probiotics, synbiotics, or nutrabiotics for improved health effects: A review. *Advances in Colloid and Interface Science*, *309*, 102781. https://www.sciencedirect.com/science/article/pii/S000186862200183X. https://doi.org/10.1016/j.cis.2022.102781
12. Kumari, R., Singh, A., Yadav, A. N., Mishra, S., Sachan, A., & Sachan, S. G. (2020). Chapter 11. Probiotics, prebiotics, and Synbiotics: Current status and future uses for human health. In A. A. Rastegari, A. N. Yadav, & N. Yadav (Eds.). *New and Future Developments in Microbial Biotechnology and Bioengineering: Trends of Microbial Biotechnology for Sustainable Agriculture and Biomedicine Systems: Perspectives for Human Health* (pp. 173–190). Elsevier. https://www.sciencedirect.com/science/article/pii/B9780128205280000120
13. Barengolts, E. (2016). Gut microbiota, prebiotics, probiotics, and synbiotics in management of obesity and prediabetes: Review of randomized controlled trials. *Endocrine Practice*, *22*(10), 1224–1234. https://www.sciencedirect.com/science/article/pii/S1530891X20355701. https://doi.org/10.4158/EP151157.RA
14. Chenhuichen, C., Cabello-Olmo, M., Barajas, M., Izquierdo, M., Ramírez-Vélez, R., Zambom-Ferraresi, F., & Martínez-Velilla, N. (2022). Impact of probiotics and prebiotics in the modulation of the major events of the aging process: A systematic review of randomized controlled trials. *Experimental Gerontology*, *164*, 111809. https://www.sciencedirect.com/science/article/pii/S0531556522001176. https://doi.org/10.1016/j.exger.2022.111809
15. Lefkovitz, A. L., & Zarowitz, B. J. (2013). It's a microscopic world after all: Prebiotics, probiotics, and synbiotics. *Geriatric Nursing*, *34*(4), 323–325. https://www.sciencedirect.com/science/article/pii/S0197457213002024. https://doi.org/10.1016/j.gerinurse.2013.06.007
16. Jampílek, J., Kráľová, K., & Chapter, B. V. (2022). Chapter 13: Probiotics and prebiotics in the prevention and management of human cancers (colon cancer, stomach cancer, breast cancer, and cervix cancer. In M. K. Dwivedi, N. Amaresan, A. Sankaranarayanan & E. Kemp (Eds.). *Probiotics in the Prevention and Management of Human Diseases: A Scientific Perspective* (pp. 187–212). Academic Press. https://www.sciencedirect.com/science/article/pii/B978012823733500009X
17. Riasatian, M., Mazloomi, S. M., Ahmadi, A., Derakhshan, Z., & Rajabi, S. (2023). Benefits of fermented synbiotic soymilk containing Lactobacillus acidophilus, Bifidobacterium lactis, and inulin towards lead toxicity alleviation. *Heliyon*, *9*(6), e17518. https://www.sciencedirect.com/science/article/pii/S2405844023047266. https://doi.org/10.1016/j.heliyon.2023.e17518
18. Ambalam, P., Raman, M., Purama, R. K., & Doble, M. (2016). Probiotics, prebiotics and colorectal cancer prevention. *Best Practice and Research. Clinical Gastroenterology*, *30*(1), 119–131. https://www.sciencedirect.com/science/article/pii/S1521691816000135. https://doi.org/10.1016/j.bpg.2016.02.009
19. Manzoor, S., Wani, S. M., Ahmad Mir, S., & Rizwan, D. (2022). Role of probiotics and prebiotics in mitigation of different diseases. *Nutrition*, *96*, 111602. https://www.sciencedirect.com/science/article/pii/S0899900722000156. https://doi.org/10.1016/j.nut.2022.111602
20. Voss, G. B., Machado, D., Barbosa, J. C., Campos, D. A., Gomes, A. M., & Pintado, M. (2022). Chapter 9: Interplay between probiotics and prebiotics for human nutrition and health. In E. Leite de Souza, J. L. de Brito Alves & V. Fusco (Eds.). *Probiotics for Human Nutrition in Health and Disease* (pp. 231–254). Academic Press. https://www.sciencedirect.com/science/article/pii/B9780323899086000273.
21. Włodarczyk, M., & Śliżewska, K. (2021). Obesity as the 21st century's major disease: The role of probiotics and prebiotics in prevention and treatment. *Food Bioscience*, *42*, 101115. https://www.sciencedirect.com/science/article/pii/S2212429221002406. https://doi.org/10.1016/j.fbio.2021.101115
22. Cunningham, M., Azcarate-Peril, M. A., Barnard, A., Benoit, V., Grimaldi, R., Guyonnet, D., Holscher, H. D., Hunter, K., Manurung, S., Obis, D., Petrova, M. I., Steinert, R. E., Swanson, K. S., van Sinderen, D., Vulevic, J., & Gibson, G. R. (2021). Shaping the future of probiotics and prebiotics. *Trends in Microbiology*, *29*(8), 667–685. https://www.sciencedirect.com/science/article/pii/S0966842X21000056. https://doi.org/10.1016/j.tim.2021.01.003
23. Geier, M. S., Butler, R. N., & Howarth, G. S. (2007). Inflammatory bowel disease: Current insights into pathogenesis and new therapeutic options; probiotics, prebiotics and synbiotics. *International Journal of Food Microbiology*, *115*(1), 1–11. https://www.sciencedirect.com/science/article/pii/S0168160506005101. https://doi.org/10.1016/j.ijfoodmicro.2006.10.006
24. O'Connor, L. E., Gahche, J. J., Herrick, K. A., Davis, C. D., Potischman, N., & Vargas, A. J. (2021). Nonfood prebiotic, probiotic, and synbiotic use has increased in US adults and children from 1999 to 2018. *Gastroenterology*, *161*(2), 476–486.e3. https://www.sciencedirect.com/science/article/pii/S0016508521006612. https://doi.org/10.1053/j.gastro.2021.04.037
25. Ghavami, A., Khorvash, F., Khalesi, S., Heidari, Z., & Askari, G. (2021). The effects of synbiotic supplementation on oxidative stress and clinical symptoms in women with

migraine: A double-blind, placebo-controlled, randomized trial. *Journal of Functional Foods*, *86*, 104738. https://doi.org/10.1016/j.jff.2021.104738

26. Parke, E. C., & Plutynski, A. (2023). Going big by going small: Trade-offs in microbiome explanations of cancer. *Studies in History and Philosophy of Science*, *97*, 101–110. https://www.sciencedirect.com/science/article/pii/S0039368122001844. https://doi.org/10.1016/j.shpsa.2022.12.007
27. Yi, J., Xiang, J., & Tang, J. (2023). Exploring the microbiome: Uncovering the link with lung cancer and implications for diagnosis and treatment. *Chinese Medical Journal Pulmonary and Critical Care Medicine*, *1*(3), 161–170. https://www.sciencedirect.com/science/article/pii/S2772558823000427. https://doi.org/10.1016/j.pccm.2023.08.003
28. Pandey, P., & Khan, F. (2023). Gut microbiome in cancer immunotherapy: Current trends, translational challenges and future possibilities. *Biochimica et Biophysica Acta. General Subjects*, *1867*(9), 130401. https://www.sciencedirect.com/science/article/pii/S0304416523000995. https://doi.org/10.1016/j.bbagen.2023.130401
29. Pacheco-Yanes, J., Reynolds, E., Li, J., & Mariño, E. (2023). Microbiome-targeted interventions for the control of oral-gut dysbiosis and chronic systemic inflammation. *Trends in Molecular Medicine*, *29*(11), 912–925. https://www.sciencedirect.com/science/article/pii/S1471491423001910. https://doi.org/10.1016/j.molmed.2023.08.006
30. Bahuguna, A., & Dubey, S. K. (2023). Relevance of tumor microbiome in cancer incidence, prognosis, and its clinical implications in therapeutics. *Biochimica et Biophysica Acta. Reviews on Cancer*, *1878*(5), 188956. https://www.sciencedirect.com/science/article/pii/S0304419X23001051. https://doi.org/10.1016/j.bbcan.2023.188956
31. Vora, K. B., & Parikh, A. (2023). Gastrointestinal cancers and the link to the microbiome. *Advances in Oncology*, *3*(1), 191–196. https://www.sciencedirect.com/science/article/pii/S2666853X23000139. https://doi.org/10.1016/j.yao.2023.01.013
32. Kaune, T., Griesmann, H., Theuerkorn, K., Hämmerle, M., Laumen, H., Krug, S., Plumeier, I., Kahl, S., Junca, H., Gustavo Dos Anjos Borges, L., Michl, P., Pieper, D. H., & Rosendahl, J. (2023). Gender-specific changes of the gut microbiome correlate with tumor development in murine models of pancreatic cancer [Internet]. *iScience*, *26*(6), 106841. https://www.sciencedirect.com/science/article/pii/S2589004223009185. https://doi.org/10.1016/j.isci.2023.106841
33. Meng, Y. F., Fan, Z. Y., Zhou, B., & Zhan, H. X. (2023). Role of the intratumoral microbiome in tumor progression and therapeutics implications. *Biochimica et Biophysica Acta. Reviews on Cancer*, *1878*(6), 189014. https://www.sciencedirect.com/science/article/pii/S0304419X23001634. https://doi.org/10.1016/j.bbcan.2023.189014
34. Burkett, W. C., Clontz, A. D., Keku, T. O., & Bae-Jump, V. (2023). The interplay of obesity, microbiome dynamics, and innovative anti-obesity strategies in the context of endometrial cancer progression and therapeutic approaches. *Biochimica et Biophysica Acta. Reviews on Cancer*, *1878*(6), 189000. https://www.sciencedirect.com/science/article/pii/S0304419X2300149X. https://doi.org/10.1016/j.bbcan.2023.189000
35. Villemin, C., Six, A., Neville, B. A., Lawley, T. D., Robinson, M. J., & Bakdash, G. (2023). The heightened importance of the microbiome in cancer immunotherapy. *Trends in Immunology*, *44*(1), 44–59. https://www.sciencedirect.com/science/article/pii/S147149062200237X. https://doi.org/10.1016/j.it.2022.11.002
36. Yue, Y., Zhang, H., Deng, P., Tan, M., Chen, C., Tang, B., Li, J., Chen, F., Zhao, Q., Li, L., Hao, R., Wang, H., Luo, Y., Tian, L., Xie, J., Chen, M., Yu, Z., Zhou, Z., & Pi, H. (2023). Environmental cadmium exposure facilitates mammary tumorigenesis via reprogramming gut microbiota-mediated glutamine metabolism in MMTV-Erbb2 mice. *Science of the Total Environment*, *897*, 165348. https://www.sciencedirect.com/science/article/pii/S0048969723039712. https://doi.org/10.1016/j.scitotenv.2023.165348
37. Bai, X., Fu, R., Liu, Y., Deng, J., Fei, Q., Duan, Z., Zhu, C., & Fan, D. (2023). Ginsenoside Rk3 modulates gut microbiota and regulates immune response of group 3 innate lymphoid cells to against colorectal tumorigenesis. *Journal of Pharmaceutical Analysis*. https://www.sciencedirect.com/science/article/pii/S2095177923002472.
38. Yang, J., Wei, H., Lin, Y., Chu, E. S. H., Zhou, Y., Gou, H., Guo, S., Lau, H. C. H., Cheung, A. H. K., Chen, H., To, K. F., Sung, J. J. Y., Wang, Y., & Yu, J. (2023). High soluble fiber promotes colorectal tumorigenesis through modulating gut microbiota and metabolites in mice. *Gastroenterology*. https://www.sciencedirect.com/science/article/pii/S0016508523051399. https://doi.org/10.1053/j.gastro.2023.10.012
39. Ashique, S., De Rubis, G., Sirohi, E., Mishra, N., Rihan, M., Garg, A., Reyes, R. J., Manandhar, B., Bhatt, S., Jha, N. K., Singh, T. G., Gupta, G., Singh, S. K., Chellappan, D. K., Paudel, K. R., Hansbro, P. M., Oliver, B. G., & Dua, K. (2022, October 23). Short chain fatty acids: Fundamental mediators of the gut-lung axis and their involvement in pulmonary diseases. *Chemico-Biological Interactions*, *368*, 110231. https://doi.org/10.1016/j.cbi.2022.110231
40. Guo, C., Guo, D., Fang, L., Sang, T., Wu, J., Guo, C., Wang, Y., Wang, Y., Chen, C., Chen, J., Chen, R., & Wang, X. (2021). Ganoderma lucidum polysaccharide modulates gut microbiota and immune cell function to inhibit inflammation and tumorigenesis in colon. *Carbohydrate Polymers*, *267*, 118231. https://www.sciencedirect.com/science/article/pii/S0144861721006184. https://doi.org/10.1016/j.carbpol.2021.118231
41. Xu, J. Y., Liu, M. T., Tao, T., Zhu, X., & Fei, F. Q. (2021). The role of gut microbiota in tumorigenesis and treatment. *Biomedicine and Pharmacotherapy*, *138*, 111444. https://www.sciencedirect.com/science/article/pii/S0753332221002298. https://doi.org/10.1016/j.biopha.2021.111444
42. Baig, M. H., Adil, M., Khan, R., Dhadi, S., Ahmad, K., Rabbani, G., Bashir, T., Imran, M. A., Husain, F. M., Lee, E. J., Kamal, M. A., & Choi, I. (2019). Enzyme targeting strategies for prevention and treatment of cancer: Implications for cancer therapy. *Seminars in Cancer Biology*, *56*, 1–11. https://www.sciencedirect.com/science/article/pii/S1044579X17301013. https://doi.org/10.1016/j.semcancer.2017.12.003
43. Seibert, T. M., Garraway, I. P., Plym, A., Mahal, B. A., Giri, V., Jacobs, M. F., Cheng, H. H., Loeb, S., Helfand, B. T., Eeles, R. A., & Morgan, T. M. (2023). Genetic risk prediction for prostate cancer: Implications for early detection and prevention. *European Urology*, *83*(3), 241–248. https://www.sciencedirect.com/science/article/pii/S0302283822028706. https://doi.org/10.1016/j.eururo.2022.12.021
44. Iloki Assanga, S. B., Lewis Luján, L. M., McCarty, M. F., & DiNicolantonio, J. J. (2023). Nutraceutical and dietary resources for breast cancer prevention - Highlighting

strategies for suppressing breast aromatase expression. *PharmaNutrition*, *23*, 100327. https://www.sciencedirect.com/science/article/pii/S2213434422000408. https://doi.org/10.1016/j.phanu.2022.100327
45. Wu, Y. P., Parsons, B., Jo, Y., Chipman, J., Haaland, B., Nagelhout, E. S., Carrington, J., Wankier, A. P., Brady, H., & Grossman, D. (2022). Outdoor activities and sunburn among urban and rural families in a Western region of the US: Implications for skin cancer prevention. *Preventive Medicine Reports*, *29*, 101914. https://www.sciencedirect.com/science/article/pii/S2211335522002212. https://doi.org/10.1016/j.pmedr.2022.101914
46. Stroud, A. M., & Coleman, M. F. (2023). Bariatric surgery in the prevention of obesity-associated cancers: Mechanistic implications. *Surgery for Obesity and Related Diseases*, *19*(7), 772–780. https://www.sciencedirect.com/science/article/pii/S1550728923000928. https://doi.org/10.1016/j.soard.2023.02.016
47. Gilpatrick, T., Long, S., Mousavi, S., Samghabadi, P., & Vohra, P. (2023). Age and race-based differences in anal cytology: Implications for screening and prevention of anal cancer disparities: A single institutional study. *Journal of the American Society of Cytopathology*, *12*(5), S20. https://www.sciencedirect.com/science/article/pii/S2213294523000959. https://doi.org/10.1016/j.jasc.2023.07.033
48. Cosme, F., Inês, A., & Vilela, A. (2022). Consumer's acceptability and health consciousness of probiotic and prebiotic of non-dairy products. *Food Research International*, *151*, 110842. https://www.sciencedirect.com/science/article/pii/S0963996921007420. https://doi.org/10.1016/j.foodres.2021.110842
49. Guergoletto, K. B., Farinazzo, F. S., Mauro, C. S. I., Fernandes, M. T. C., Alves, G., Prudencio, S. H. & Garcia, S. (2019). Chapter 8: Nondairy probiotic and prebiotic beverages: Applications, nutrients, benefits, and challenges. In A. M. Grumezescu & A. M. Holban (Eds.). *Nutrients in Beverages* (pp. 277–314). Academic Press. https://www.sciencedirect.com/science/article/pii/B9780128168424000083.
50. Chaturvedi, S., Khartad, A., & Chakraborty, S. (2021). The potential of non-dairy synbiotic instant beverage powder: Review on a new generation of healthy ready-to-reconstitute drinks. *Food Bioscience*, *42*, 101195. https://www.sciencedirect.com/science/article/pii/S2212429221003205. https://doi.org/10.1016/j.fbio.2021.101195.
51. Commane, D., Hughes, R., Shortt, C., & Rowland, I. (2005). The potential mechanisms involved in the anticarcinogenic action of probiotics. *Mutation Research*, *591*(1–2), 276–289. https://www.sciencedirect.com/science/article/pii/S0027510705002769. https://doi.org/10.1016/j.mrfmmm.2005.02.027.
52. Ángeles Stegmayer, M., Sirini, N., Frizzo, L. S., Fernández-López, J., Pérez Álvarez, J. Á., Rosmini, M. R., & Soto, L. P.(2024) Chapter 7: Enrichment of foods with prebiotics. In J. M. Lorenzo (Ed.). *Strategies to Improve the Quality of Foods: A Volume in Developments in Food Quality and Safety* (pp. 171–201). Academic Press. https://www.sciencedirect.com/science/article/pii/B9780443153464000070.
53. Iemsam-arng, J., Surassmo, S., Mahatnirunkul, T., Weizman, K., Kaweeteerawat, C. R., Panya, A., Warin, C., Chomtong, T., & Sukjarernchaikul, P. (2024). Exploring the prebiotic potential of fermented glutinous rice filtrate: In vitro skin bacterial balance and biological activities. *In Industrial Crops and Products*, 207, 117742. Elsevier. https://www.sciencedirect.com/science/article/pii/S0926669023015078
54. Turati, F., Concina, F., Bertuccio, P., Fiori, F., Parpinel, M., Garavello, W., Crispo, A., Libra, M., Negri, E., Serraino, D., & La Vecchia, C. (2023). Prebiotics and the risk of upper digestive tract and stomach cancers: The PrebiotiCa study. *Journal of the Academy of Nutrition and Dietetics*, *123*(12), 1772–1780. https://www.sciencedirect.com/science/article/pii/S2212267223012753. https://doi.org/10.1016/j.jand.2023.07.008.
55. Fagnant, H. S., Isidean, S. D., Wilson, L., Bukhari, A. S., Allen, J. T., Agans, R. T., Lee, D. M., Hatch-McChesney, A., Whitney, C. C., Sullo, E., Porter, C. K., & Karl, J. P. (2023). Orally ingested probiotic, prebiotic, and synbiotic interventions as countermeasures for gastrointestinal tract infections in nonelderly adults: A systematic review and meta-analysis. *Advances in Nutrition*, *14*(3), 539–554. https://www.sciencedirect.com/science/article/pii/S2161831323001357. https://doi.org/10.1016/j.advnut.2023.02.002.
56. Kim, C. G., Koh, J. Y., Shin, S. J., Shin, J. H., Hong, M., Chung, H. C., Rha, S. Y., Kim, H. S., Lee, C. K., Lee, J. H., Han, Y., Kim, H., Che, X., Yun, U. J., Kim, H., Kim, J. H., Lee, S. Y., Park, S. K., Park, S., … Jung, M. (2023). Prior antibiotic administration disrupts anti-PD-1 responses in advanced gastric cancer by altering the gut microbiome and systemic immune response. *Cell Reports. Medicine*, *4*(11), 101251. https://www.sciencedirect.com/science/article/pii/S2666379123004287. https://doi.org/10.1016/j.xcrm.2023.101251
57. Nandi, S. K., Basu, S., Bhattacharjya, A., Dey Ghosh, R., Bose, C. K., Mukhopadhyay, S., & Bhattacharya, R. (2022). Interplay of gut microbiome, fatty acids, and the endocannabinoid system in regulating development, progression, immunomodulation, and chemoresistance of cancer. *Nutrition*, *103–104*, 111787. https://www.sciencedirect.com/science/article/pii/S0899900722002003. https://doi.org/10.1016/j.nut.2022.111787
58. Xu, M., Qiu, X., Chen, Q., Yang, T., Xu, J., Chen, L., Shuai, L., Xu, Z., Cheng, X., Zhang, Y., & Cao, Z. (2023). Changes of gut microbiome and metabolome in the AOM/DSS mouse model of colorectal cancer with FLASH radiation. *Radiation Medicine and Protection*, *4*(1), 1–10. https://www.sciencedirect.com/science/article/pii/S2666555723000047. https://doi.org/10.1016/j.radmp.2023.02.001
59. Fan, S., Zhang, Z., Zhao, Y., Daglia, M., Zhang, J., Zhu, Y., Bai, J., Zhu, L., & Xiao, X. (2023). Recent advances in targeted manipulation of the gut microbiome by prebiotics: From taxonomic composition to metabolic function. *Current Opinion in Food Science*, *49*, 100959. https://www.sciencedirect.com/science/article/pii/S2214799322001618. https://doi.org/10.1016/j.cofs.2022.100959
60. Leibovitzh, H., Lee, S. H., Xue, M., Raygoza Garay, J. A., Hernandez-Rocha, C., Madsen, K. L., Meddings, J. B., Guttman, D. S., Espin-Garcia, O., Smith, M. I., Goethel, A., Griffiths, A. M., Moayyedi, P., Steinhart, A. H., Panaccione, R., Huynh, H. Q., Jacobson, K., Aumais, G., Mack, D. R., … Croitoru, K. (2022). Altered gut microbiome composition and function are associated with gut barrier dysfunction in healthy relatives of patients with Crohn's disease. *Gastroenterology*, *163*(5), 1364–1376.e10. https://www.sciencedirect.com/science/article/pii/S0016508522007764. https://doi.org/10.1053/j.gastro.2022.07.004.

61. Tan, S., Ge, W., Wang, J., Liu, W., Zhao, Y., Shen, W., & Li, L. (2020). Zearalenone-induced aberration in the composition of the gut microbiome and function impacts the ovary reserve. *Chemosphere*, *244*, 125493. https://www.sciencedirect.com/science/article/pii/S004565351932733X. https://doi.org/10.1016/j.chemosphere.2019.125493.
62. Altamirano, Á., Saa, P. A., & Garrido, D. (2020). Inferring composition and function of the human gut microbiome in time and space: A review of genome-scale metabolic modelling tools. *Computational and Structural Biotechnology Journal*, *18*, 3897–3904. https://www.sciencedirect.com/science/article/pii/S200103702030502X. https://doi.org/10.1016/j.csbj.2020.11.035
63. Sharpton, S. R., Ajmera, V., & Loomba, R. (2019). Emerging role of the gut microbiome in nonalcoholic fatty liver disease: From composition to function. *Clinical Gastroenterology and Hepatology*, *17*(2), 296–306. https://www.sciencedirect.com/science/article/pii/S1542356518309443. https://doi.org/10.1016/j.cgh.2018.08.065
64. Raygoza Garay, J. A., Turpin, W., Lee, S. H., Smith, M. I., Goethel, A., Griffiths, A. M., Moayyedi, P., Espin-Garcia, O., Abreu, M., Aumais, G. L., Bernstein, C. N., Biron, I. A., Cino, M., Deslandres, C., Dotan, I., El-Matary, W., Feagan, B., Guttman, D. S., Huynh, H., … Croitoru, K. (2023). Gut microbiome composition is associated with future onset of Crohn's disease in healthy first-degree relatives. *Gastroenterology*, *165*(3), 670–681. https://www.sciencedirect.com/science/article/pii/S0016508523008053. https://doi.org/10.1053/j.gastro.2023.05.032
65. Borrego-Ruiz, A., & Borrego, J. J. (2024). An updated overview on the relationship between human gut microbiome dysbiosis and psychiatric and psychological disorders. *Progress in Neuro-Psychopharmacology and Biological Psychiatry*, *128*, 110861. https://www.sciencedirect.com/science/article/pii/S0278584623001471. https://doi.org/10.1016/j.pnpbp.2023.110861
66. Pyle, S. (2022). 2.23-Human gut microbiota and the influence of probiotics, prebiotics, and micronutrients. In M. Glibetic (Eds.), Comprehensive Gut Microbiota (pp. 271–288). Elsevier. https://www.sciencedirect.com/science/article/pii/B9780128192658000760.
67. Zhou, L., Han, F., Lu, K., Qiao, Y., & Li, E. (2023). Comparative study on prebiotic effects of different types of prebiotics in an in vitro fermentation by gut microbiota of shrimp (litopenaeus vannamei). *Aquaculture*, *574*, 739687. https://www.sciencedirect.com/science/article/pii/S0044848623004611. https://doi.org/10.1016/j.aquaculture.2023.739687
68. Sajnaga, E., Socała, K., Kalwasińska, A., Wlaź, P., Waśko, A., Jach, M. E., Tomczyk, M., & Wiater, A. (2023). Response of murine gut microbiota to a prebiotic based on oligosaccharides derived via hydrolysis of fungal α-(1→3)-d-glucan: Preclinical trial study on mice. *Food Chemistry*, *417*, 135928. https://www.sciencedirect.com/science/article/pii/S0308814623005459. https://doi.org/10.1016/j.foodchem.2023.135928
69. Huang, K. C., Lee, J. W., Hu, Y. F., Ballantyne, R., & Liu, C. H. (2023). Effects of Aspergillus-meal prebiotic diet on the growth performance, health status and gut microbiota of Asian seabass, Lates calcarifer. *Fish and Shellfish Immunology*, *136*, 108696. https://www.sciencedirect.com/science/article/pii/S1050464823001821. https://doi.org/10.1016/j.fsi.2023.108696
70. Gibbons, S. M., Gurry, T., Lampe, J. W., Chakrabarti, A., Dam, V., Everard, A., Goas, A., Gross, G., Kleerebezem, M., Lane, J., Maukonen, J., Penna, A. L. B., Pot, B., Valdes, A. M., Walton, G., Weiss, A., Zanzer, Y. C., Venlet, N. V., & Miani, M. (2022). Perspective: Leveraging the gut microbiota to predict personalized responses to dietary, prebiotic, and probiotic interventions. *Advances in Nutrition*, *13*(5), 1450–1461. https://www.sciencedirect.com/science/article/pii/S2161831323000212. https://doi.org/10.1093/advances/nmac075
71. Khemiri, S., Khelifi, N., Messaoud, C., & Smaali, I. (2023). Bioprospecting of microalgae for a potential use as enzyme inhibitors, anti-ageing and prebiotic agents. *Biocatalysis and Agricultural Biotechnology*, *51*, 102759. https://www.sciencedirect.com/science/article/pii/S1878818123001603. https://doi.org/10.1016/j.bcab.2023.102759
72. Wen, Y., Wen, P., Hu, T. G., Linhardt, R. J., Zong, M. H., Wu, H., & Chen, Z. Y. (2020). Encapsulation of phycocyanin by prebiotics and polysaccharides-based electrospun fibers and improved colon cancer prevention effects. *International Journal of Biological Macromolecules*, *149*, 672–681. https://www.sciencedirect.com/science/article/pii/S0141813019344861. https://doi.org/10.1016/j.ijbiomac.2020.01.189
73. Jampílek, J., Kráľová, K., & Chapter, B. V. (2022). Chapter 13: Probiotics and prebiotics in the prevention and management of human cancers (colon cancer, stomach cancer, breast cancer, and cervix cancer. In M. K. Dwivedi, N. Amaresan, A. Sankaranarayanan & E. Kemp (Eds.). *Probiotics in the Prevention and Management of Human Diseases: A Scientific Perspective* (pp. 187–212). Academic Press. https://www.sciencedirect.com/science/article/pii/B978012823733500009X
74. Ávila, P. F., de Mello, A. H. F., Forte, M. B. S., de Almeida Costa, F. A., & Goldbeck, R. (2023). Fractionation of functional oligosaccharides produced from sugarcane straw using serial nanofiltration membranes and their influence on prebiotic potential. *Food Research International*, *172*, 113175. https://www.sciencedirect.com/science/article/pii/S0963996923007202. https://doi.org/10.1016/j.foodres.2023.113175
75. Zhao, C., Chen, N., & Ashaolu, T. J. (2023). Prebiotic and modulatory evidence of lactoferrin on gut health and function. *Journal of Functional Foods*, *108*, 105741. https://www.sciencedirect.com/science/article/pii/S1756464623003419. https://doi.org/10.1016/j.jff.2023.105741
76. Crowder, S. L., Jim, H. S. L., Hogue, S., Carson, T. L., & Byrd, D. A. (2023). Gut microbiome and cancer implications: Potential opportunities for fermented foods. *Biochimica et Biophysica Acta. Reviews on Cancer*, *1878*(3), 188897. https://www.sciencedirect.com/science/article/pii/S0304419X2300046X. https://doi.org/10.1016/j.bbcan.2023.188897
77. Ramai, D., Salati, M., Pomati, G., Amoroso, C., Facciorusso, A., Botticelli, A., & Ghidini, M. (2022). Antibiotics, the microbiome and gastrointestinal cancers: A causal interference? *Current Opinion in Pharmacology*, *67*, 102315. https://www.sciencedirect.com/science/article/pii/S1471489222001424. https://doi.org/10.1016/j.coph.2022.102315
78. Griggs, J. L., Chi, L., Hanley, N. M., Kohan, M., Herbin-Davis, K., Thomas, D. J., Lu, K., Fry, R. C., & Bradham, K. D. (2022). Bioaccessibility of arsenic from contaminated soils and alteration of the gut microbiome in an

in vitro gastrointestinal model. *Environmental Pollution*, *309*, 119753. https://www.sciencedirect.com/science/article/pii/S0269749122009678. https://doi.org/10.1016/j.envpol.2022.119753
79. Liu, Y., Lau, H. C. H., Cheng, W. Y., & Yu, J. (2023). Gut microbiome in colorectal cancer: Clinical diagnosis and treatment. *Genomics Proteomics Bioinformatics*, *21*(1), 84–96. https://www.sciencedirect.com/science/article/pii/S1672022922000869. https://doi.org/10.1016/j.gpb.2022.07.002
80. Zhang, T., Shang, C., Du, T., Zhuo, J., Wang, C., Li, B., Xu, J., Fan, M., Wang, J., & Zhang, W. (2023). *Cytoprotection of probiotics by nanoencapsulation for advanced functions. Trends in Food Science and Technology, 142,* 104227. https://www.sciencedirect.com/science/article/pii/S0924224423003424. https://doi.org/10.1016/j.tifs.2023.104227
81. Salavati Schmitz, S. (2022). Modifying the gut microbiota - An update on the evidence for dietary interventions, probiotics, and fecal microbiota transplantation in chronic gastrointestinal diseases of dogs and cats. *Advances in Small Animal Care*, *3*(1), 95–107. https://www.sciencedirect.com/science/article/pii/S2666450X22000104. https://doi.org/10.1016/j.yasa.2022.05.010
82. Schmitz, S. S. (2021). Value of probiotics in canine and feline gastroenterology. *Veterinary Clinics of North America. Small Animal Practice*, *51*(1), 171–217. https://www.sciencedirect.com/science/article/pii/S019556162030111X. https://doi.org/10.1016/j.cvsm.2020.09.011
83. Zhu, Y., Michelle Luo, T., Jobin, C., & Young, H. A. (2011). Gut microbiota and probiotics in colon tumorigenesis. *Cancer Letters*, *309*(2), 119–127. https://www.sciencedirect.com/science/article/pii/S0304383511003405. https://doi.org/10.1016/j.canlet.2011.06.004
84. Fiocchi, A., Burks, W., Bahna, S. L., Bielory, L., Boyle, R. J., Cocco, R., Dreborg, S., Goodman, R., Kuitunen, M., Haahtela, T., Heine, R. G., Lack, G., Osborn, D. A., Sampson, H., Tannock, G. W., Lee, B. W., & WAO Special Committee on Food Allergy and Nutrition. (2012). Clinical use of probiotics in pediatric allergy (cuppa): A world allergy organization position paper. *World Allergy Organization Journal*, *5*(11), 148–167. https://www.sciencedirect.com/science/article/pii/S1939455119303965. https://doi.org/10.1097/WOX.0b013e3182784ee0
85. Lowe, J. R., Briggs, A. M., Whittle, S., & Stephenson, M. D. (2020). A systematic review of the effects of probiotic administration in inflammatory arthritis. *Complementary Therapies in Clinical Practice*, *40*, 101207. https://www.sciencedirect.com/science/article/pii/S1744388119309454. https://doi.org/10.1016/j.ctcp.2020.101207
86. Elkholy, S. E., Maher, S. A., Abd el-Hamid, N. R., Elsayed, H. A., Hassan, W. A., Abdelmaogood, A. K. K., Hussein, S. M., Jaremko, M., Alshawwa, S. Z., Alharbi, H. M., & Imbaby, S. (2023). The immunomodulatory effects of probiotics and azithromycin in dextran sodium sulfate-induced ulcerative colitis in rats via TLR4-NF-κB and p38-MAPK pathway. *Biomedicine and Pharmacotherapy*, *165*, 115005. https://www.sciencedirect.com/science/article/pii/S0753332223007953. https://doi.org/10.1016/j.biopha.2023.115005
87. Yin, C., Li, Y., Li, J., Fan, X., Yao, F., Shi, D., Cheng, Y., Liu, M., Lu, Q., & Gao, H. (2022). Gastrointestinal digestion, probiotic fermentation behaviors and immunomodulatory effects of polysaccharides from *Sanghuangporus vaninii*. *International Journal of Biological Macromolecules*, *223*(A), 606–617. https://www.sciencedirect.com/science/article/pii/S0141813022025557. https://doi.org/10.1016/j.ijbiomac.2022.11.012
88. Mahooti, M., Miri, S. M., Abdolalipour, E., & Ghaemi, A. (2020). The immunomodulatory effects of probiotics on respiratory viral infections: A hint for COVID-19 treatment? *Microbial Pathogenesis*, *148*, 104452. https://www.sciencedirect.com/science/article/pii/S0882401020308184. https://doi.org/10.1016/j.micpath.2020.104452
89. Wen, J., Ma, L., Xu, Y., wu, J., Yu, Y., Peng, J., Tang, D., Zou, B., & Li, L. (2020) Effects of probiotic litchi juice on immunomodulatory function and gut microbiota in mice. *Food Research International*, *137*, 109433. https://www.sciencedirect.com/science/article/pii/S0963996920304580. https://doi.org/10.1016/j.foodres.2020.109433
90. Awais, M. M., Jamal, M. A., Akhtar, M., Hameed, M. R., Anwar, M. I., & Ullah, M. I. (2019). Immunomodulatory and ameliorative effects of Lactobacillus and Saccharomyces based probiotics on pathological effects of eimeriasis in broilers. *Microbial Pathogenesis*, *126*, 101–108. https://www.sciencedirect.com/science/article/pii/S0882401018310982. https://doi.org/10.1016/j.micpath.2018.10.038
91. Patel, A. R., Shah, N. P., & Prajapati, J. B. (2014). Immunomodulatory effects of probiotics in the treatment of HIV infection. *Biomedicine and Preventive Nutrition*, *4*(1), 81–84. https://www.sciencedirect.com/science/article/pii/S2210523913000275. https://doi.org/10.1016/j.bionut.2013.04.003
92. Chen, Y. C., Wu, Y. J., & Hu, C. Y. (2019). Monosaccharide composition influence and immunomodulatory effects of probiotic exopolysaccharides. *International Journal of Biological Macromolecules*, *133*, 575–582. https://www.sciencedirect.com/science/article/pii/S0141813019319622. https://doi.org/10.1016/j.ijbiomac.2019.04.109
93. Roldán-Pérez, S., Gómez Rodríguez, S. L., Sepúlveda-Valencia, J. U., Ruiz Villadiego, O. S., Márquez Fernández, M. E., Montoya Campuzano, O. I., & Durango-Zuleta, M. M. (2023). Assessment of probiotic properties of lactic acid bacteria isolated from an artisanal Colombian cheese. *Heliyon*, *9*(11), e21558. https://www.sciencedirect.com/science/article/pii/S2405844023087662. https://doi.org/10.1016/j.heliyon.2023.e21558
94. Naseem, Z., Mir, S. A., Wani, S. M., Rouf, M. A., Bashir, I., & Zehra, A. (2023). Probiotic-fortified fruit juices: Health benefits, challenges, and future perspective. *Nutrition*, *115*, 112154. https://www.sciencedirect.com/science/article/pii/S089990072300182X. https://doi.org/10.1016/j.nut.2023.112154
95. Chang, S., Guo, Q., Du, G., Tang, J., Liu, B., Shao, K., & Zhao, X. (2023). Probiotic-loaded edible films made from proteins, polysaccharides, and prebiotics as a quality factor for minimally processed fruits and vegetables: A review. *International Journal of Biological Macromolecules*, 253(5), 127226. https://www.sciencedirect.com/science/article/pii/S0141813023041235. https://doi.org/10.1016/j.ijbiomac.2023.127226
96. Jan, T., Negi, R., Sharma, B., Kour, D., Kumar, S., Rai, A. K., Rustagi, S., Singh, S., Sheikh, M. A., Kumar, K., Ahmed, N., & Yadav, A. N. (2023). Diversity, distribution and role of probiotics for human health: Current research and future challenges. *Biocatalysis and Agricultural Biotechnology*, *53*, 102889. https://www.sciencedirect.com/science/article/pii/S1878818123002906. https://doi.org/10.1016/j.bcab.2023.102889

97. Zhao, J., Zhao, F., Yuan, J., Liu, H., & Wang, Y. (2023). Gut microbiota metabolites, redox status, and the related regulatory effects of probiotics. *Heliyon, 9*(11), e21431. https://www.sciencedirect.com/science/article/pii/S2405844023086395. https://doi.org/10.1016/j.heliyon.2023.e21431
98. Xu, X., Zhang, M., Liu, X., Chai, M., Diao, L., Ma, L., Nie, S., Xu, M., Wang, Y., Mo, F., & Liu, M. (2023). Probiotics formulation and cancer nanovaccines show synergistic effect in immunotherapy and prevention of colon cancer [Internet]. *iScience, 26*(7), 107167. https://www.sciencedirect.com/science/article/pii/S2589004223012440. https://doi.org/10.1016/j.isci.2023.107167
99. Ma, T., Shen, X., Shi, X., Sakandar, H. A., Quan, K., Li, Y., Jin, H., Kwok, L., Zhang, H., & Sun, Z. (2023). Targeting gut microbiota and metabolism as the major probiotic mechanism - An evidence-based review. *Trends in Food Science and Technology, 138*, 178–198. https://www.sciencedirect.com/science/article/pii/S0924224423001851. https://doi.org/10.1016/j.tifs.2023.06.013
100. Han, M., Lei, W., Liang, J., Li, H., Hou, M., & Gao, Z. (2024). The single-cell modification strategies for probiotics delivery in inflammatory bowel disease: A review. *Carbohydrate Polymers, 324*, 121472. https://www.sciencedirect.com/science/article/pii/S0144861723009372. https://doi.org/10.1016/j.carbpol.2023.121472
101. Chen, Z., Cai, Z., Zhuang, P., Li, F., Cui, W., & Li, Z. (2023). Living probiotic biomaterials for osteoporosis therapy. *Biomedical Technology, 1*, 52–64. https://www.sciencedirect.com/science/article/pii/S2949723X22000095. https://doi.org/10.1016/j.bmt.2022.11.007
102. Silva, D. R., de Sardi, J. C. O., Pitangui, Nd. S., Roque, S. M., da Silva, A. C. B., & Rosalen, P. L. (2020). Probiotics as an alternative antimicrobial therapy: Current reality and future directions. *Journal of Functional Foods, 73*, 104080. https://www.sciencedirect.com/science/article/pii/S1756464620303042. https://doi.org/10.1016/j.jff.2020.104080
103. Watanabe, A., Teragaki, Y., Kitaura, Y., & Tochio, T. (2023). The synergistic synbiotic potential of 1-kestose and Bifidobacterium longum in the mouse gut. *Journal of Functional Foods, 101*, 105403. https://www.sciencedirect.com/science/article/pii/S1756464623000038. https://doi.org/10.1016/j.jff.2023.105403
104. Sun, R., Niu, Y., Li, M., Liu, Y., Wang, K., Gao, Z., Wang, Z., Yue, T., & Yuan, Y. (2023). Emerging trends in pectin functional processing and its fortification for Synbiotics: A review. *Trends in Food Science and Technology, 134*, 80–97. https://www.sciencedirect.com/science/article/pii/S0924224423000791. https://doi.org/10.1016/j.tifs.2023.03.004
105. Dawood, M. A. O., Abo-Al-Ela, H. G., & Hasan, M. T. (2020). Modulation of transcriptomic profile in aquatic animals: Probiotics, prebiotics and Synbiotics scenarios. *Fish and Shellfish Immunology, 97*, 268–282. https://www.sciencedirect.com/science/article/pii/S1050464819311830. https://doi.org/10.1016/j.fsi.2019.12.054
106. Malik, J. K., Raina, R., Ahmad, A. H., Kalpana, S., Prakash, A., & Gupta, R. C. (2021). Chapter 66. Synbiotics: Safety and toxicity considerations. In R. C. Gupta, R. Lall, & A. B. T. N. Srivastava (Eds.). *Nutraceuticals* (Second Edition, pp. 1107–1123). Academic Press. https://www.sciencedirect.com/science/article/pii/B9780128210383000665.
107. Chen, Q., Fan, J., Lin, L., & Zhao, M. (2023). Combination of *Lycium barbarum* L. and *Laminaria japonica* polysaccharides as a highly efficient prebiotic: Optimal screening and complementary regulation of gut probiotics and their metabolites. *International Journal of Biological Macromolecules, 246*, 125534. https://www.sciencedirect.com/science/article/pii/S0141813023024285. https://doi.org/10.1016/j.ijbiomac.2023.125534
108. del Valle, J. C., Bonadero, M. C., & Fernández-Gimenez, A. V. (2023). Saccharomyces cerevisiae as probiotic, prebiotic, synbiotic, postbiotics and parabiotics in aquaculture: An overview. *Aquaculture, 569*, 739342. https://www.sciencedirect.com/science/article/pii/S0044848623001151. https://doi.org/10.1016/j.aquaculture.2023.739342
109. Sáez-Orviz, S., Rendueles, M., & Díaz, M. (2023). Impact of adding prebiotics and probiotics on the characteristics of edible films and coatings- a review. *Food Research International, 164*, 112381. https://www.sciencedirect.com/science/article/pii/S0963996922014399. https://doi.org/10.1016/j.foodres.2022.112381
110. Kim, A. J., Hong, D. S., & George, G. C. (2022). Dietary influences on symptomatic and non-symptomatic toxicities during cancer treatment: A narrative review. *Cancer Treatment Reviews, 108*, 102408. https://www.sciencedirect.com/science/article/pii/S030573722200072X. https://doi.org/10.1016/j.ctrv.2022.102408
111. Kushkevych, I., & Jampílek, J. (2022). Chapter 4: Effect of intestinal microbiome, antibiotics, and probiotics in the prevention and management of ulcerative colitis. In M. K. Dwivedi, N. Amaresan, A. Sankaranarayanan, & E. Kemp (Eds.). *Probiotics in the Prevention and Management of Human Diseases: A Scientific Perspective* (pp. 59–92). Academic Press. https://www.sciencedirect.com/science/article/pii/B9780128237335000167.
112. Harandi, F. N., Khorasani, A. C., Shojaosadati, S. A., & Hashemi-Najafabadi, S. (2022). Surface modification of electrospun wound dressing material by Fe2O3 nanoparticles incorporating *Lactobacillus* strains for enhanced antimicrobial and antibiofilm activity. *Surfaces and Interfaces, 28*, 101592. https://www.sciencedirect.com/science/article/pii/S2468023021006647. https://doi.org/10.1016/j.surfin.2021.101592
113. Hitch, T. C. A., Hall, L. J., Walsh, S. K., Leventhal, G. E., Slack, E., de Wouters, T., Walter, J., & Clavel, T. (2022). Microbiome-based interventions to modulate gut ecology and the immune system. *Mucosal Immunology, 15*(6), 1095–1113. https://www.sciencedirect.com/science/article/pii/S1933021922017391. https://doi.org/10.1038/s41385-022-00564-1
114. Wang, Z., Zhong, J., Meng, X., Gao, J., Li, H., Sun, J., Li, X., & Chen, H. (2021). The gut microbiome-immune axis as a target for nutrition-mediated modulation of food allergy. *Trends in Food Science and Technology, 114*, 116–132. https://www.sciencedirect.com/science/article/pii/S0924224421003435. https://doi.org/10.1016/j.tifs.2021.05.021
115. Taboun, Z. S., & Sadeghi, J. (2023). The bidirectional relationship between opioids and the gut microbiome: Implications for opioid tolerance and clinical interventions. *International Immunopharmacology, 125*(A), 111142. https://www.sciencedirect.com/science/article/pii/S1567576923014686. https://doi.org/10.1016/j.intimp.2023.111142
116. Morshed, S. M., & Lee, T. H. (2023). The role of the microbiome on fish mucosal immunity under changing environments. *Fish and Shellfish Immunology, 139*, 108877. https://www.sciencedirect.com/science/article/pii/S1050464823003637. https://doi.org/10.1016/j.fsi.2023.108877

117. Wolff, C., Zoschke, C., Kalangi, S. K., Reddanna, P., & Schäfer-Korting, M. (2019). Tumor microenvironment determines drug efficacy in vitro - Apoptotic and anti-inflammatory effects of 15-lipoxygenase metabolite, 13–HpOTrE. *European Journal of Pharmaceutics and Biopharmaceutics*, *142*, 1–7. https://www.sciencedirect.com/science/article/pii/S0939641119300785. https://doi.org/10.1016/j.ejpb.2019.06.003
118. Tu, J., He, Y., Zhang, H., Wang, J., Li, Z., & Sun, H. (2023). Anti-tumor effect of *Crocus sativus* petals polysaccharides by reconstructing tumor microenvironment. *International Journal of Biological Macromolecules*, *248*, 125878. https://www.sciencedirect.com/science/article/pii/S0141813023027733. https://doi.org/10.1016/j.ijbiomac.2023.125878
119. Sun, X., Zhou, L., Wang, Y., Deng, G., Cao, X., Ke, B., Wu, X., Gu, Y., Cheng, H., Xu, Q., Du, Q., Chen, H., & Sun, Y. (2023). Single-cell analyses reveal cannabidiol rewires tumor microenvironment via inhibiting alternative activation of macrophage and synergizes with anti-PD-1 in colon cancer. *Journal of Pharmaceutical Analysis*, *13*(7), 726–744. https://www.sciencedirect.com/science/article/pii/S2095177923000746. https://doi.org/10.1016/j.jpha.2023.04.013
120. Tilsed, C. M., Principe, N., Kidman, J., Chin, W. L., Orozco Morales, M. L., Zemek, R. M., Chee, J., Islam, R., Fear, V. S., Forbes, C., Aston, W. J., Jansen, M., Chopra, A., Lassmann, T., Nowak, A. K., Fisher, S. A., Lake, R. A., & Lesterhuis, W. J. (2022). CD4+ T cells drive an inflammatory, TNF-α/IFN-rich tumor microenvironment responsive to chemotherapy. *Cell Reports*, *41*(13), 111874. https://www.sciencedirect.com/science/article/pii/S2211124722017703. https://doi.org/10.1016/j.celrep.2022.111874
121. Li, J., Wang, Q., Lu, H., Han, Y., Jiang, L., Qian, W., Zhu, M., Wang, B., Min, J., Hou, Y., Xu, S., Xiong, Z., Liu, H., Li, Y., Chen, C., Liu, Y., & Qian, P. (2022). Graphdiyne oxide nanosheets exert anti-lymphoma effect by killing cancer stem cells and remodeling tumor microenvironment. *Nano Today*, *46*, 101622. https://www.sciencedirect.com/science/article/pii/S174801322200250X. https://doi.org/10.1016/j.nantod.2022.101622
122. Zhang, L., Xu, S., Cheng, X., Wu, J., Wang, Y., Gao, W., Bao, J., & Yu, H. (2023). Inflammatory tumor microenvironment of thyroid cancer promotes cellular dedifferentiation and silencing of iodide-handling genes expression. *Pathology, Research and Practice*, *246*, 154495. https://www.sciencedirect.com/science/article/pii/S0344033823001954. https://doi.org/10.1016/j.prp.2023.154495
123. Yi, X. F., Gao, R. L., Sun, L., Wu, Z. X., Zhang, S. L., Huang, L. T., Han, C. B., & Ma, J. T. (2023). Dual antitumor immunomodulatory effects of PARP inhibitor on the tumor microenvironment: A counterbalance between anti-tumor and pro-tumor. *Biomedicine and Pharmacotherapy*, *163*, 114770. https://www.sciencedirect.com/science/article/pii/S0753332223005590. https://doi.org/10.1016/j.biopha.2023.114770
124. Pan, W., Han, J., Wei, N., Wu, H., Wang, Y., & Sun, J. (2022). LINC00702-mediated DUSP1 transcription in the prevention of bladder cancer progression: Implications in cancer cell proliferation and tumor inflammatory microenvironment. *Genomics*, *114*(4), 110428. https://www.sciencedirect.com/science/article/pii/S0888754322001732. https://doi.org/10.1016/j.ygeno.2022.110428
125. Guo, X., Sun, M., Yang, P., Meng, X., & Liu, R. (2023). Role of mast cells activation in the tumor immune microenvironment and immunotherapy of cancers. *European Journal of Pharmacology*, *960*, 176103. https://www.sciencedirect.com/science/article/pii/S0014299923006155. https://doi.org/10.1016/j.ejphar.2023.176103
126. Ashique, S., Upadhyay, A., Kumar, N., Chauhan, S., & Mishra, N. (2022, July 1). Metabolic syndromes responsible for cervical cancer and advancement of nanocarriers for efficient targeted drug delivery-A review. *Advances in Cancer Biology - Metastasis*, *4*, 100041. https://doi.org/10.1016/j.adcanc.2022.100041
127. Liu, Z., Wang, R., Wang, Y., Duan, Y., & Zhan, H. (2023). Targeting succinylation-mediated metabolic reprogramming as a potential approach for cancer therapy. *Biomedicine and Pharmacotherapy*, *168*, 115713. https://www.sciencedirect.com/science/article/pii/S0753332223015111. https://doi.org/10.1016/j.biopha.2023.115713
128. Xi, Y., Shen, Y., Chen, L., Tan, L., Shen, W., & Niu, X. (2023). Exosome-mediated metabolic reprogramming: Implications in esophageal carcinoma progression and tumor microenvironment remodeling. *Cytokine and Growth Factor Reviews*, *73*, 78–92. https://www.sciencedirect.com/science/article/pii/S1359610123000564. https://doi.org/10.1016/j.cytogfr.2023.08.010
129. Jaraíz-Rodríguez, M., del Prado, L., & Balsa, E. (2023). Metabolic remodeling in astrocytes: Paving the path to brain tumor development. *Neurobiology of Disease*, *188*, 106327. https://www.sciencedirect.com/science/article/pii/S0969996123003431. https://doi.org/10.1016/j.nbd.2023.106327
130. Mehraj, U., Mushtaq, U., Mir, M. A., Saleem, A., Macha, M. A., Lone, M. N., Hamid, A., Zargar, M. A., Ahmad, S. M., & Wani, N. A. (2022). Chemokines in triple-negative breast cancer heterogeneity: New challenges for clinical implications. *Seminars in Cancer Biology*, *86*(2), 769–783. https://www.sciencedirect.com/science/article/pii/S1044579X22000645. https://doi.org/10.1016/j.semcancer.2022.03.008
131. Nguyen, H. Q., Tran, K. L., Vuong, M. H., Tran, Q. T., & Ho, X. D. (2023). Chapter 10: Colorectal cancer heterogeneity and targeted therapy: Clinical implications, challenges, and solutions for treatment resistance. In P. K. Maurya PK, & V. Saini (Eds.). *Treatment Landscape of Targeted Therapies in Oncology: Challenges and Opportunities* (pp. 207–221). Academic Press. https://www.sciencedirect.com/science/article/pii/B9780443160349000058
132. Zhai, Z., Yu, X., Yang, B., Zhang, Y., Zhang, L., Li, X., & Sun, H. (2017). Colorectal cancer heterogeneity and targeted therapy: Clinical implications, challenges and solutions for treatment resistance. *Seminars in Cell and Developmental Biology*, *64*, 107–115. https://www.sciencedirect.com/science/article/pii/S1084952116302671. https://doi.org/10.1016/j.semcdb.2016.08.033
133. Wang, D., Zhang, Y., Li, Q., Zhang, A., Xu, J., Li, Y., Li, W., Tang, L., Yang, F., & Meng, J. (2023). N6-methyladenosine (m6A) in cancer therapeutic resistance: Potential mechanisms and clinical implications. *Biomedicine and Pharmacotherapy*, *167*, 115477. https://www.sciencedirect.com/science/article/pii/S0753332223012751. https://doi.org/10.1016/j.biopha.2023.115477
134. Zhu, G., Guo, M., Zhao, J., Zhang, H., Wang, G., & Chen, W. (2024). Environmental enrichment in combination with *Bifidobacterium breve* HNXY26M4 intervention amplifies neuroprotective benefits in a mouse model of Alzheimer's disease by modulating glutamine metabolism of the gut microbiome. *Food Science and Human Wellness*,

13(2), 982–992. https://www.sciencedirect.com/science/article/pii/S2213453023001866. https://doi.org/10.26599/FSHW.2022.9250084
135. Puig-Castellví, F., Pacheco-Tapia, R., Deslande, M., Jia, M., Andrikopoulos, P., Chechi, K., Bonnefond, A., Froguel, P., & Dumas, M. (2023). Advances in the integration of metabolomics and metagenomics for human gut microbiome and their clinical applications. *TrAC Trends in Analytical Chemistry*, *167*, 117248. https://www.sciencedirect.com/science/article/pii/S0165993623003357. https://doi.org/10.1016/j.trac.2023.117248
136. Aljumaah, M. R., Bhatia, U., Roach, J., Gunstad, J., & Azcarate Peril, M. A. (2022). The gut microbiome, mild cognitive impairment, and probiotics: A randomized clinical trial in middle-aged and older adults. *Clinical Nutrition*, *41*(11), 2565–2576. https://www.sciencedirect.com/science/article/pii/S0261561422003442. https://doi.org/10.1016/j.clnu.2022.09.012
137. Karim, M. R., Iqbal, S., Mohammad, S., Lee, J. H., Jung, D., Mathiyalagan, R., Yang, D. C., Yang, D. U., & Kang, S. C. (2023). A review on Impact of dietary interventions, drugs, and traditional herbal supplements on the gut microbiome. *Microbiological Research*, *271*, 127346. https://www.sciencedirect.com/science/article/pii/S0944501323000484. https://doi.org/10.1016/j.micres.2023.127346
138. Liu, Z., de Vries, B., Gerritsen, J., Smidt, H., & Zoetendal, E. G. (2020). Microbiome-based stratification to guide dietary interventions to improve human health. *Nutrition Research*, *82*, 1–10. https://www.sciencedirect.com/science/article/pii/S0271531720305017. https://doi.org/10.1016/j.nutres.2020.07.004
139. Carson, M. D., Westwater, C., & Novince, C. M. (2023). Adolescence and the microbiome: Implications for healthy growth and maturation. *American Journal of Pathology*, *193*(12), 1900–1909. https://www.sciencedirect.com/science/article/pii/S0002944023003073. https://doi.org/10.1016/j.ajpath.2023.07.004
140. Sguazzi, G., Mickleburgh, H. L., Ghignone, S., Voyron, S., Renò, F., Migliario, M., Sellitto, F., Lovisolo, F., Camurani, G., Ogbanga, N., Gino, S., & Procopio, N. (2022). Microbial DNA in human nucleic acid extracts: Recoverability of the microbiome in DNA extracts stored frozen long-term and its potential and ethical implications for forensic investigation. *Forensic Science International. Genetics*, *59*, 102686. https://www.sciencedirect.com/science/article/pii/S1872497322000278. https://doi.org/10.1016/j.fsigen.2022.102686
141. Dumitriu, A. (2022). HypersymbioticsTM: An artistic reflection on the ethical and environmental implications of microbiome research and new technologies. *Endeavour*, *46* (1–2), 100820. https://www.sciencedirect.com/science/article/pii/S0160932722000205. https://doi.org/10.1016/j.endeavour.2022.100820
142. Mayer, R., Hittmeir, M., & Ekelhart, A. (2024). Distance-based linkage of personal microbiome records for identification and its privacy implications. *Computers and Security*, *136*, 103538. https://www.sciencedirect.com/science/article/pii/S0167404823004480. https://doi.org/10.1016/j.cose.2023.103538
143. Steinbach, E., Masi, D., Ribeiro, A., Serradas, P., Le Roy, T., & Clément, K. (2024). Upper small intestine microbiome in obesity and related metabolic disorders: A new field of investigation. *Metabolism: Clinical and Experimental*, *150*, 155712. https://www.sciencedirect.com/science/article/pii/S0026049523003165. https://doi.org/10.1016/j.metabol.2023.155712
144. McGuinness, A. J., Stinson, L. F., Snelson, M., Loughman, A., Stringer, A., Hannan, A. J., Cowan, C. S. M., Jama, H. A., Caparros-Martin, J. A., West, M. L., Wardill, H. R., & Australasian Human Microbiome Research Network (AHMRN) Committee. (2024). From hype to hope: Considerations in conducting robust microbiome science. *Brain, Behavior, and Immunity*, *115*, 120–130. https://www.sciencedirect.com/science/article/pii/S0889159123002854. https://doi.org/10.1016/j.bbi.2023.09.022
145. Xu, X., Rothrock, M. J., Mishra, A., Kumar, G. D., & Mishra, A. (2023). Relationship of the poultry microbiome to pathogen colonization, farm management, poultry production, and foodborne illness risk assessment. *Journal of Food Protection*, *86*(11), 100169. https://www.sciencedirect.com/science/article/pii/S0362028X23068539. https://doi.org/10.1016/j.jfp.2023.100169
146. Ahmed, T., Noman, M., Gardea-Torresdey, J. L., White, J. C., & Li, B. (2023). Dynamic interplay between nano-enabled agrochemicals and the plant-associated microbiome. *Trends in Plant Science*, *28*(11), 1310–1325. https://www.sciencedirect.com/science/article/pii/S1360138523001899. https://doi.org/10.1016/j.tplants.2023.06.001
147. Yu, Z., Lu, T., & Qian, H. (2023). Pesticide interference and additional effects on plant microbiomes. *Science of the Total Environment*, *888*, 164149. https://www.sciencedirect.com/science/article/pii/S0048969723027705. https://doi.org/10.1016/j.scitotenv.2023.164149
148. Nanoscience, C., Kumar, P., Pandey, S. N., Ahmad, F., Verma, A., Sharma, H., Ashique, S., Bhattacharyya, S. P., Kumar, S., Kumar, S., Mishra, N., & Garg, A. (2023, November 8). Carbon nanotubes: A targeted drug delivery against cancer cell. *Current Nanoscience*, *9*, 1–31. https://doi.org/10.2174/0115734137271865231105070727
149. Chaudhari, A., Bharti, A., & Dwivedi, M. K. (2022). Chapter 21. Role of probiotics in the management of fungal infections. In M. K. Dwivedi, N. Amaresan, A. Sankaranarayanan, & E. Kemp (Eds.). *Probiotics in the Prevention and Management of Human Diseases: A Scientific Perspective* (pp. 305–320). Academic Press. https://www.sciencedirect.com/science/article/pii/B9780128237335000155.
150. Arunima, A., Das, J. K., & Suar, M. (2019). Chapter 10: Gut microbes in liver diseases: Dietary intervention for promoting hepatic health. In R. R. Watson, & V. R. Preedy (Eds.). *Dietary Interventions in Gastrointestinal Diseases: Foods, Nutrients, and Dietary Supplements* (pp. 117–131). Academic Press. https://www.sciencedirect.com/science/article/pii/B9780128144688000107.
151. Pal, D., Chandra, P., & Sachan, N. (2020). Chapter 15: Sesame seed in controlling human health and nutrition. In V. R. Preedy, & R. R. Watson (Eds.). *Nuts and Seeds in Health and Disease Prevention* (pp. 183–210). Academic Press. https://www.sciencedirect.com/science/article/pii/B9780128185537000152.
152. Chandra, P., Kishore, K., & Ghosh, A. K. (2015). Assessment of antisecretory, gastroprotective, and in-vitro antacid potential of Daucus carota in experimental rats. *Osong Public Health and Research Perspectives*, *6*(6), 329–335.https://www.sciencedirect.com/science/article/pii/S2210909915300023. https://doi.org/10.1016/j.phrp.2015.10.006

14 Key Regulatory Aspects of Prebiotics, Probiotics, and Synbiotics in the Management of Metabolic Disorders

Innocent Ayesiga, Shabnoor Iqbal, Yusuf Kyejjusa, Joash Okoboi, Timothy Omara, Thomas Adelina, Delafrique Deogratias, Arthur Amule Anyole, Braize Ben Kagimu, Denis Odongo, and Ivan Kahwa

14.1 INTRODUCTION TO METABOLIC DISORDERS AND GUT MICROBIOTA

14.1.1 Overview of Metabolic Disorders and Their Prevalence

A group of diseases known as metabolic disorders are characterized by irregularities in the body's metabolism, which is the set of chemical processes that occur within cells to maintain life [1]. These disorders can involve various aspects of metabolism, involving the creation of necessary molecules, the breakdown of nutrients to produce energy, and the removal of waste materials [2]. Metabolic disorders can be genetic (inherited) or acquired (developed over time), and they can affect different organs and systems in the body [3]. An overview of some common metabolic disorders is discussed in the following:

Phenylketonuria (PKU): PKU is a hereditary condition that prevents the body from correctly metabolizing the amino acid phenylalanine. This leads to its accumulation in the blood and can cause intellectual disabilities if not managed through a strict diet [4] and affects about 1 in 10,000–15,000 births worldwide. PKU is more common in certain populations, such as individuals of Northern European and Turkish descent [5].

Galactosemia: It affects the metabolism of galactose and is brought on by a lack of activity in the enzyme galactose-1-phosphate uridylyl transferase [6]. Without proper management, it can lead to liver damage and other complications. Prevalence: Approximately 1 in 30,000–60,000 births. It varies based on ethnic and geographical factors [7].

The so-called maple syrup urine disease is a heredity condition that hinders the metabolism of branched-chain amino acids [8]. It leads to a buildup of these amino acids and their byproducts, which can cause severe neurological symptoms. Prevalence: Roughly 1 in 185,000 to 1 in 250,000 births. This disorder is relatively rare [9].

Mitochondrial Disorders: A single problem or flaw in mitochondrial function, such as a shortened calcium buffer time, excessive production of free radicals, an increase in mitochondrial membrane permeability, or oxidative stress, can cause pathogenic alterations in cells [10]. Muscle wasting, neurological issues, and organ dysfunction are just a few of the signs of mitochondrial disorders. Prevalence: Mitochondrial disorders are relatively rare, with varying estimates for different subtypes. Some subtypes can be more prevalent than others, but overall prevalence is often cited as about 1 in 5,000–10,000 people [11].

Glycogen Storage Diseases: These are a collection of hereditary conditions that affect the way the body stores and uses glycogen, a form of energy storage in cells. It encompasses a collection of 19 hereditary disorders that are characterized by deposits or abnormal forms of glycogens in tissues and are brought on by a deficiency of one or more enzymes necessary for the synthesis or breakdown of glycogen. Different types of glycogen storage diseases can lead to various symptoms, including muscle weakness, liver enlargement, and low blood sugar [12]. Prevalence: The prevalence varies widely depending on the specific type of glycogen storage disease. Some types are more common than others, such as glycogen storage disease type I (around 1 in 100,000) and type II (Pompe disease, around 1 in 40,000–300,000) [13, 14].

Lysosomal Storage Disorders: These disorders result from deficiencies in enzymes that are responsible for breaking down specific substances within cells. Lysosomal storage abnormalities include conditions like Tay-Sachs disease and Gaucher's disease [15]. Prevalence: The prevalence varies depending on the specific disorder. Some examples include Gaucher's disease (1 in 40,000–60,000), Fabry disease (1 in 40,000–117,000 males), and Tay-Sachs disease (1 in 320,000–600,000 births in high-risk populations) [16].

Diabetes Mellitus: High blood sugar levels due to either inadequate insulin production (Type 1 diabetes) or insulin resistance (type 2 diabetes [T2D]) is characterized as diabetes, a common metabolic condition [17]. It can lead to various complications affecting the eyes, kidneys, nerves, and cardiovascular system [18]. Prevalence: Diabetes is quite common, and its prevalence has been steadily increasing globally. Ten percent (10%) of people aged 20–79 years worldwide suffered from diabetes in 2021 and this is projected to rise to 12.2% by 2045 [19]. About 5%–10% of all

 DOI: 10.1201/9781032702438-14

diabetes cases are type 1 diabetes, while the rest are type 2 cases.

Hyperthyroidism and Hypothyroidism: These are disorders of the thyroid gland, which plays a crucial role in regulating metabolism [20]. Hyperthyroidism involves an overactive thyroid, leading to excessive metabolism, while hypothyroidism involves an underactive thyroid and a decrease in metabolism [21]. Prevalence: Thyroid disorders are relatively common, with hypothyroidism being more prevalent. Hypothyroidism's prevalence varies by region, but it's estimated to affect around 1%–2% of the global population [22]

Porphyria: A series of uncommon hereditary diseases known as porphyria impair the heme, a substance necessary for the formation of hemoglobin [23]. This can lead to symptoms ranging from skin sensitivity to neurological disturbances. Prevalence: Porphyria is rare, with specific subtypes having different prevalence rates. One of the more prevalent kinds of porphyria is acute intermittent with a prevalence estimated at around 1 in 20,000–75,000 individuals [24].

Alkaptonuria: An uncommon hereditary condition called alkaptonuria causes an accumulation of homogentisic acid, causing dark pigmentation of tissues and joint problems [25]. Prevalence: Alkaptonuria is very rare. Its prevalence is estimated at around 1 in 250,000 to 1 in 1,000,000 individuals [26].

It's crucial to remember that any metabolic issue has its own specific causes, symptoms, and management strategies. Diagnosis and treatment often involve a multidisciplinary approach, including medical genetics, dietetics, endocrinology, and other specialties. To lessen the negative effects of these disorders on people's health and quality of life, early detection, and effective management are crucial.

14.1.2 Role of Gut Microbiota in Metabolic Health

Metabolic health is significantly influenced by the gut microbiome that interacts with the metabolic processes, influencing energy balance, nutrient utilization, inflammation, and various metabolic pathways. The complex collection of microbes, mostly bacteria, that live in the digestive system is referred to as the gut microbiota. The functions of the gut microbiota in metabolic health are as follows:

Energy Harvesting and Nutrient Metabolism: Gut microbiota helps break down complex carbohydrates and dietary fibers that human enzymes can't digest [27]. Due to the fermentation of these materials by specific bacteria, short-chain fatty acids (SCFAs) like acetate, propionate, and butyrate are created. The gut absorbs SCFAs, which have been linked to improved energy metabolism, reduced inflammation, and enhanced glucose homeostasis [28].

Regulation of Appetite and Weight: Gut microbiota can influence appetite and body weight through various mechanisms. Certain bacterial strains produce molecules that affect appetite-regulating hormones, potentially impacting satiety and food intake [29]. Dysbiosis, an imbalance in gut bacteria composition, was associated with conditions like metabolic syndrome and obesity [30].

Insulin Sensitivity and Glucose Regulation: The gut microbiota was improved insulin resistance and glucose metabolism [31]. Dysbiosis might exacerbate insulin resistance, a major risk factor for T2D [32]. Microbial metabolites like SCFAs can influence insulin signaling and glucose utilization in peripheral tissues [33].

Inflammation and Immune Response: The maintenance of healthy gut flora is essential for gut barrier integrity and preventing the translocation of harmful bacterial products into circulation [34]. Dysbiosis can lead to increased gut permeability, triggering a systemic inflammatory response that's implicated in metabolic disorders such as obesity and insulin resistance [35].

Bile Acid Metabolism: Bile acids, necessary for lipid breakdown and absorption, are metabolized by the gut bacteria [36]. Dysbiosis can alter bile acid composition and signaling, affecting lipid metabolism, and potentially contributing to conditions like alcohol-unrelated fatty liver disease [37]

Metabolism of Host-Derived Compounds: Gut bacteria can metabolize host-derived compounds, including dietary components and endogenous molecules [38]. This metabolism can produce bioactive metabolites that influence various physiological processes, including those related to metabolism and inflammation [39].

Personalized Responses: Everyone's gut microbiota composition is unique, leading to personalized responses to dietary interventions [40]. Factors such as genetics, diet, environment, and medical history all contribute to shaping an individual's gut microbiome and its impact on metabolic health [41].

Therapeutic Potential: Metabolic health may be enhanced by manipulating the makeup of the gut microbiota with probiotics, prebiotics, and fecal microbiota transplantation [42].

In conclusion, the gut microbiota exerts a substantial influence on metabolic health through its involvement in energy metabolism, appetite regulation, glucose homeostasis, inflammation, and more. Maintaining a balanced gut microbiota through a healthy diet, lifestyle, and potential interventions may offer promising strategies for preventing and managing metabolic disorders.

14.1.3 Introduction to Prebiotics, Probiotics, and Synbiotics

Prebiotics are dietary fibers that are not digested but instead influence the growth and activity of gut microbiota [43]. They help certain genera of microorganisms, particularly *Lactobacilli* and *Bifidobacteria* grow and function in the colon, serving as a source of nutrition for these advantageous bacteria, promoting their growth and preserving a balanced microbiome in the gut. Prebiotics are typically found in certain foodstuffs, fruits, veggies, whole grains, and legumes [44]. Inulin, fructooligosaccharides (FOS), and galactooligosaccharides (GOS) are typical examples of prebiotics [45].

Probiotics are live microorganisms, primarily bacteria but also some yeasts, that when ingested in sufficient quantities, confer health benefits. These microbes resemble the helpful bacteria that symbiotically exist in the human gut [46]. Probiotics can help maintain or restore a healthy balance of gut bacteria, which is important for digestion, immune function, and overall well-being. Probiotics can be found in certain fermented foods like yogurt, kefir, sauerkraut, kimchi, and in the form of dietary supplements [44].

Synbiotics refer to products that combine both prebiotics and probiotics. They are designed to provide a synergistic effect by supplying beneficial microorganisms (probiotics) with the necessary nourishment (prebiotics) to thrive and establish themselves in the gut [47]. The idea behind synbiotics is to enhance the survival and effectiveness of probiotics by providing them with a conducive environment for growth. Synbiotic products can include various combinations of probiotic strains and prebiotic fibers [48].

In summary, numerous aspects of human health, including digestion, metabolism, immunological response, and even mental health, are significantly influenced by gut microbiota. Both prebiotics and probiotics have gained attention for their potential to positively influence the gut microbiota and thus contribute to overall well-being.

14.2 PREBIOTICS: REGULATORY CONSIDERATIONS AND APPLICATIONS

14.2.1 Definition and Types of Prebiotics

Prebiotics were first defined in 1995 as, 'a nondigestible food ingredient that beneficially affects the host by selectively stimulating the growth and/or activity of one or a limited number of bacteria in the colon, and thus improves host health' [49]. The Food and Agriculture Organization (FAO) retained most of the components of this definition and defined prebiotics as non-viable food components that confer health benefit(s) on the host associated with modulation of gut microbiota [50]. Prebiotics are mostly fibers that are non-digestible food ingredients. They selectively promote the growth or activity of specific genera of microorganisms in the colon that confer wider nutritional and health benefits to the host [51, 52]. There are, however, renewed calls for a redefinition of prebiotics [53] because the word prebiotic was originally used in Chemistry to mean building block structures that predate living organisms [54, 55] and the expansion of the scope of substances with prebiotic properties [53]. The accepted criteria for any compound to be called a prebiotic include these three conditions; first resistance to the acidic pH of the stomach and unaffected by hydrolysis by mammalian enzymes, second not absorbable in the mammalian GIT, fermentable by gut microbiota and lastly has the ability to promote growth of specific gut microbes in such a way so as to benefit the host [56].

There are many different types of prebiotics but many of them are oligosaccharide carbohydrates that are resistant to digestion by the enzymes of the human alimentary canal. They may be derivatives of fructose, glucose, galactose, or non-carbohydrate oligosaccharides.

i. Fructans are non-reducing carbohydrates composed of fructosyl units and terminated by a single glucose molecule. They are natural heterogenous fructose polymers consisting of inulin and fructo-oligosaccharides or oligofructose [57]. They have a linear structure with fructose residues joined to form a chain of β (2→1) bonds. There are various natural sources of fructans such as wheat, onions, garlic asparagus, etc. They are known to have immune-modulatory effects and stimulate immune activity via the toll-like receptor (TLR) signaling [58]. In the human gut, the important prebiotic activity of fructans is the selective promotion of the growth of specific bacteria, especially the *Lactobacillus* and *Bifidobacterium* species [59]
ii. GOS have excess galactose residues with galactose joined to carbons three, four, and six. They may be α- or β-GOS although the latter are the most commercially produced and used as prebiotics. β-GOS are formed through trans-galactosylation of lactose in a reaction catalyzed by β-galactosidase [60, 61]. GOS are also known to promote the growth of *Bifidobacteria* whose presence in the gut inhibits the growth of pathogenic bacteria [61]. GOS are also known to promote the production of SCFAs, impact lipid and carbohydrate metabolism, and promote growth and differentiation of the epithelial cells of the colon [62].
iii. Starch and glucose-derived oligosaccharides include resistant starch and polydextrose. Polydextrose is a glucose-derived oligosaccharide. It is highly branched with randomly bonded glucose residues containing various forms of α and β linkages with 1→6 linkages in both forms predominates [63]. It is not hydrolyzed by the enzymes of the human alimentary canal and passes through the ileum to the colon unchanged. It is fermented to produce SCFAs, e.g., butyrate, propionate, and acetate [64, 65]. Resistant starch is fermented by bacteria to produce high levels of butyrate [63].
iv. Pectic oligosaccharides have significantly varying structures that are dependent on their source. They are formed from extensions of galacturonic acid or rhamnose and may have side chains that are composed of many different sugars [66]. They are derived through depolymerizations of pectin, a form of heteropolysaccharide made of a linear backbone of α(1→4) linked galacturonic acid which may be methylated or acetylated [67].

It is worth noting that many types of prebiotics are being discovered and this has of late included non-carbohydrate oligosaccharides, e.g., cocoa-derived flavanols, that stimulate lactic acid bacteria.

14.2.2 Mechanisms of Action in Metabolic Disorders

The mechanisms of action of prebiotics in metabolic diseases remain a subject of interest. However, they are as diverse as there are different types of prebiotics. The commonly observed property is their fermentation by bacteria to produce a variety of SCFAs with a direct effect on lipid metabolism, glucose metabolism, and immune-modulatory functions.

Fructans have been observed to have immunomodulatory and antioxidant activity [58, 68, 69]. The immunomodulatory activity of fructans stems from their alteration of the immune parameters in the gut-associated lymphoid tissue (GALT) whose main function is to distinguish between harmful and innocuous molecules therefore protect against infection [58]. It therefore helps to avoid the generation of hypersensitivity against commensal bacteria. TLR signaling is important in the generation of multiple specific immune-competent cells against antigen [70]. Fructans are demonstrated to influence TLR2 type of TLRs therefore influencing immune activity directly [71]. In addition, some findings have demonstrated the ability of oligofructose to bind on the membranes of pathogenic bacteria preventing their adsorption into the membrane of epithelial cells [72].

Fructans are also known to have the ability to scavenge reactive oxygen species and therefore act as antioxidants [69]. Reactive oxygen species consists of free radicals such as superoxide anions, hydroxyl radicals, and non-radical molecules such as hydrogen peroxide and singlet oxygen. Reactive oxygen species damage DNA, lipids, and proteins by oxidizing them resulting in cell damage [73]. Fructans have been shown to have a number of other effects on metabolism such as lipid lowering, reducing calorie intake by promoting satiety, decreasing blood glucose, and prevent constipation [74].

Galactooligosaccharides have also been shown to have a number of potential health benefits. They are formed by β-galactosidase trans-galactosylation of lactose. They are fermented in the colon to produce SCFAs [75]. They are also known to promote the growth and differentiation of colonic epithelial cells and reduce the adhesion of pathogenic bacteria to gut epithelial cells [76]. They are also known to promote the absorption of calcium, and magnesium and relieve lactose intolerance [77]. The absorption of calcium reduces the risk of osteoporosis, hypertension, and improves glucose uptake by improved insulin response [78, 79].

Resistant starch improves glucose metabolism and insulin sensitivity. It has the ability to improve postprandial glucose levels with no effect on hepatic and peripheral insulin sensitivity [80]. Although the exact mechanisms are not understood, resistant starch remains intact till the colon, where it is fermented to form SCFA. It also triggers the release of PYY and glucagon-like peptide 1, that are involved in regulation of appetite. Polydextrose a highly branched glucose polymer is known to promote satiety [81]. It reduces appetite, increases satiety, and reduces energy intake. It therefore is a potent approach to preventing obesity, diabetes, hypertension, and gastrointestinal disorders. It has been experimentally shown that a 12.5 g/kg daily dose of polydextrose decreases postprandial triglycerides in normal, obese, and hyperlipidaemic individuals [82]. It has also been shown that 56.77 g/day of polydextrose led to reduced insulin response [83].

14.2.3 Prebiotics as Dietary Supplements vs. Functional Foods

Dietary supplements refer to any mouth pill, capsule, tablet, or liquid that contains one or more dietary ingredients, e.g., vitamins, minerals, herbs, amino acids, or other botanicals intended to supplement the diet and is labeled as such [84]. Functional foods were first called so in the 1980s in Japan. They are defined as processed foods having disease-preventing and or health-promoting benefits in addition to their nutritional value [85]. They are food products that resemble traditional food but possess unique physiological abilities [86]. Functional foods include probiotics, functional drinks, dietary fibers, fruits, and vegetables [87]. Although most of the prebiotics are available as functional foods, there are a number of commercial supplements available and more are in clinical trials at different levels [88].

14.2.4 Regulatory Guidelines for Prebiotic Products

The regulatory framework for prebiotic products is contingent upon their intended use, similar to how it is for dietary supplements or drugs. If a prebiotic is meant to be used as a dietary supplement, it falls under the jurisdiction of the Food and Drug Administration's (FDA) Center for Food Safety and Applied Nutrition (CFSAN) as part of the category of "foods." Just as probiotics, prebiotics can also be subject to regulation as dietary supplements, foods, or drugs, contingent upon their intended purpose. Furthermore, factors beyond intended use can influence how these products are categorized and regulated [89–91].

In the European Union (EU), for any health statement made about a food product, there's a requirement for scientific proof to support it. This necessitates an evaluation by the European Food Safety Authority (EFSA) and approval from the European Commission (EC). When food companies wish to highlight the positive effects of their products on health and nutrition through labeling or advertising, they must adhere to the guidelines outlined in Regulation (EC) No. 1924/2006 [92, 93].

14.2.5 Clinical Evidence Supporting the Use of Prebiotics in Metabolic Disorders

Prebiotics are gaining attention due to their potential to lower the risk of specific health conditions and enhance overall well-being. Over the past few years, there has been a surge in consumer curiosity regarding the connection between diet and health, driving the need for accurate information about prebiotics. Consequently, the global market for prebiotic products has expanded because of technological advancements, the creation of novel products, and a growing population of health-conscious individuals seeking products that enhance their quality of life [93, 94].

Prebiotics have accumulated significant interest, and a growing body of research reinforces their positive impact on various diseases by influencing and engaging with gut bacteria. Frequently employed strains are sourced from the Bifidobacterium and Lactobacillus genera, and they have been extensively studied for their potential to address issues, for example lactose intolerance, diarrhea, and constipation. Additionally, they have been explored for their roles in immune regulation, cancer prevention, the preservation of a healthy gut microbiome, and the integrity of the gut lining in both animals and humans [95, 96].

Acute inflammation of the pancreas is typically a mild to moderate condition, severe acute pancreatitis poses a significant threat to life due to the systemic inflammatory response it triggers and affects the production of insulin which is important for regulating blood glucose levels [97]. According to a study conducted by Ref. [98], the inclusion of prebiotics in enteral nutrition formulas for patients with severe acute pancreatitis has the potential to improve clinical outcomes. These enhancements may include a reduction in infection rates, shorter ICU stays, and a faster recovery as indicated by inflammatory markers associated with pancreatitis.

Non-alcoholic fatty liver disease (NAFLD) is a common health issue linked to the global rise in obesity, metabolic syndrome, T2D, and hepatic encephalopathy. This condition varies in how it manifests clinically, ranging from minor disruptions in liver function tests to the development of liver cirrhosis [97]. A study by Daubioul [99] investigated the effects of prebiotics on liver enzymes in seven individuals diagnosed with non-alcoholic steatohepatitis, confirmed by biopsy. The results showed that over 8 weeks, prebiotics caused a decrease in the levels of one liver enzyme, AST while there were no significant statistical differences observed in another liver enzyme, ALT.

Fructans such as FOS are considered safe for individuals with diabetes because they have low-calorie content and can improve insulin sensitivity [100, 101]. Additionally, they alter the composition of gut microbiota, particularly the abundance of *Bifidobacterium*, which plays a role in regulating metabolic processes linked to obesity and T2D [102].

Prebiotics have been shown to offer advantages for cholesterol levels, including the reduction of total cholesterol, LDL-cholesterol, and triglycerides, which in turn lowers the risk of elevated triglyceride levels [93].

The increased production of SCFAs due to the fermentation of prebiotics has the impact of decreasing and restraining the production of fats in liver cells, a process referred to as liver lipogenesis. This is probably a result of changes in gene regulation, which subsequently results in the suppression of all liver enzymes responsible for fat synthesis. Prebiotics like GOS, xylooligosaccharides (XOS), and isomaltooligosaccharides have been reported to play a substantial role in reducing cholesterol and triglyceride levels in the blood [101].

Prebiotics, when combined with probiotics, have been linked to improved digestive, physiological, and nutritional functions in both humans and animals. This combination can have positive effects in addressing conditions such as acute gastroenteritis and osteoporosis, reducing the risk of cancer, regulating cholesterol levels, and potentially assisting in the management of anxiety [103].

Prebiotics offer various health advantages by supporting a healthy gut microbiome, stimulating beneficial bacteria growth, and being safe for dental health. They have promising applications in the food industry and research, including the development of enriched foods and further investigations into their properties and functions. As consumer awareness grows, prebiotics are poised for a successful future in the market.

14.3 PROBIOTICS: REGULATORY CONSIDERATIONS AND APPLICATIONS

14.3.1 Definition and Types of Prebiotics

It is now two decades or so since the scientific definition of probiotics was coined together with the guidelines to ensure the correct usage of the term [104]. In the simplest terms, probiotics are live microorganisms that are beneficial to the body when consumed in adequate amounts [105]. They are usually found in beauty products, foods, and dietary supplements with positive effects on gut health and overall well-being. Probiotic species are genetic subtypes of genera that constitute live bacteria and yeasts that are useful to the body when taken in sufficient quantities [105–107]

Functional features of probiotics include their ability to survive (for example, the environment in which it is, i.e., considering the route of administration, most probiotics are oral and have to pass the gastrointestinal tract. Hence, they must be able to survive pH, and enzymes and even be able to colonize new areas surviving the microbiota; they should also be able to survive the manufacturing process when you consider parameters like pH and temperature among others), delivery to the target organ, interaction with the host systems, antipathogenic properties (i.e., should not be toxin-producing strains) and generally should be safe [108,

109]. Technological features include the ability to produce mass biomass, genetic stability, longer shelf life of the finished product, resistance to preservation procedures, and no spoilage of the product [108, 109].

Probiotics are broadly categorized into two types namely:

1. Bacteria probiotics. Bacteria probiotics are known to be used in digestive health, immune system support, prevention of antibiotic-associated diarrhea, management of irritable bowel syndrome, and treatment and prevention of infectious diarrhea (rotavirus and traveler's diarrhea) [106, 110]. The most common are bacteria that belong to the following groups:
   i. Lactobacillus: One of the most well-known and widely used genera of probiotics is Lactobacillus. Lactobacillus species and strains are found in fermented dairy products like yogurt and kefir, as well as in supplements. Such beneficial bacteria as *L. acidophilus*, *L. casei*, and *L. rhamnosus* are examples of bacterial probiotics found in fermented foods [110].
   ii. *Bifidobacterium*: Another common genus of bacterial probiotics found in the human colon is *Bifidobacterium*. In fermentation and producing SCFAs, these bacteria play a key role. Many products containing Bifidobacterium can be found in yogurt and kefir as well as supplements. Typical examples include *B. bifidum* and *B. longum*.
   iii. *Streptococcus*: Particularly *Streptococcus thermophilus*, some strains of Streptococcus are used in the fermentation of yogurt and other dairy products. These products, despite not being marketed as probiotics, add to their overall probiotic content.
   iv. *Enterococcus*: Certain strains of *Enterococcus*, such as *E. faecium* and *E. faecalis*, have been studied for their probiotic potential, especially in animal health and agriculture.
   v. Lactic Acid Bacteria (LAB): LAB is a group of bacteria that includes *Lactobacillus*, *Streptococcus*, and others. They are known for their ability to produce lactic acid during fermentation and are commonly used in probiotic foods and supplements.
   vi. Other bacterial strains: There are many other bacterial strains used as probiotics, including *E. coli* Nissle 1917 (ECN) and *Bacillus coagulans*. These strains have specific applications and benefits.
   vii. Combination and multi-strain probiotics: Many probiotic supplements contain a combination of different bacterial strains to provide a broader spectrum of health benefits. These multi-strain formulations are designed to target various aspects of gut health and overall well-being.
2. Yeast probiotics
   1. While bacteria have been celebrated for their digestive benefits, yeast strains such as *Saccharomyces boulardii* and *Kluyveromyces marxianus* have emerged as unsung heroes in promoting intestinal harmony and overall well-being [105, 107]. *Saccharomyces boulardii* is the only commercialized probiotic yeast, and it is widely studied for its significant probiotic properties, such as survival capacity in the acidic environment of the gastrointestinal tract and improvements in the intestinal microbiota [107]. Other yeasts with potential probiotic features include *Kluyveromyces marxianus*, *Meyerozyma gruessi*, *Debaryomyces*, and *Candida*. Yeast probiotics have several advantages compared to bacterial probiotics, including higher natural resistance and robustness toward the aggressive environment encountered in the intestinal tract, bacteriophages, and antibiotics [105].
   2. Yeast probiotics have been used to improve gastrointestinal health, vaginal health, immune support, general gut health, treatment of Inflammatory Bowel Disease (IBD), irritable bowel syndrome (IBS), *Heliobacter pylori* infections, and treatment of traveler's diarrhea [107].
   3. Yeast probiotics include [107]
      i. *Saccharomyces boulardii*: This is perhaps the most extensively studied and recognized yeast probiotic strain. It's known for its effectiveness in treating various gastrointestinal issues, including antibiotic-associated diarrhea, *Clostridium difficile* infection, and infectious diarrhea.
      ii. *Saccharomyces cerevisiae* var. boulardii CNCM I-745: This strain is closely related to *S. boulardii* and has been used for its probiotic properties in supporting gastrointestinal health.
      iii. *Kluyveromyces marxianus*: This yeast strain has been studied for its potential to promote gut health and modulate gut microbiota. It's associated with digestive well-being.
      iv. *Candida milleri* (formerly *C. humilis*): Some research has explored the probiotic potential of *C. milleri*, particularly in improving gut health and preventing gastrointestinal infections.
      v. *Yarrowia lipolytica*: This has been investigated for its probiotic properties, including

its ability to modulate the gut microbiota and support digestive health.

vi. *Debaryomyces hansenii*: While more commonly associated with animal feed and livestock health, *D. hansenii* has been studied for its potential probiotic applications in humans, particularly in the context of gut health.

a. B. Mechanisms of action in metabolic disorders

Probiotics have the potential to serve as supportive treatments for metabolic disorders, such as obesity, metabolic syndrome, NAFLD, and T2D [111]. Nevertheless, there has been limited attention given to understanding the various and strain-specific mechanisms through which probiotics mediate their effects [111]. These primary mechanisms encompass actions like restoring and balancing disrupted gut microbial communities in both children and adults, outcompeting harmful pathogens, producing bacteriocins, influencing enzymatic activities related to bile salt metabolism and the deactivation of harmful substances, generating SCFAs and branched-chain fatty acids, which have broad effects on intestinal and peripheral tissues by interacting with receptors and improving insulin sensitivity, promoting cell adhesion and mucin production, modulating the immune system by fostering the development of T-regulatory cells, and increasing anti-inflammatory cytokines and growth factors like interleukin-10 and transforming growth factor, as well as influencing the brain-gut axis by regulating endocrine and neurological functions [111].

a. Colonization and normalization of perturbed intestinal microbial communities in children and adults. In children, probiotics play a crucial role in early gut colonization [111]. Various factors, such as genetics, delivery methods, antibiotics, and maternal health, influence this process [111]. Bacteria from the vaginal canal and breast milk have a significant impact. Probiotics have shown promise in restoring healthy gut balance, promoting intestinal development, and enhancing immunity in children. In premature infants, probiotics reduce the risk of severe necrotizing enterocolitis by controlling the immature immune system's response. Probiotics like *L. reuteri* can reduce crying spells in colicky infants. Probiotics can prevent and treat pediatric diarrhea by restoring microbial balance and inhibiting pathogen growth. However, specific mechanisms of action are not well-documented in most studies [111, 112]. In healthy adults, probiotics increase the production of beneficial SCFAs, fecal moisture, defecation frequency, and stool volume [113]. *Lactobacillus rhamnosus* PRSFL477 is well-tolerated but doesn't influence gastrointestinal symptoms [111]. Some probiotic strains, like *L. rhamnosus* CNCM I-4036, exhibit intestinal persistence. Probiotics can benefit individuals with overweight and obese, with formulations like the De Simone preparation reducing lipid concentrations, and inflammatory markers, and enhancing insulin sensitivity. On the other hand, *L. plantarum* TENSIA has shown promise in reducing BMI and blood pressure in individuals with obesity and hypertension [114]. IBD, which affects the gastrointestinal tract, sees alterations in gut microbiota as a contributing factor [114, 115]. Probiotic trials in Crohn's disease have shown limited effects on remission, but probiotics, especially De Simone formulation, and combinations of *Lactobacillus* and prebiotics, appear more effective in ulcerative colitis remission [114]. Certain butyrate-producing bacterial strains have been tested in CD patients, demonstrating increased butyrate production and improved epithelial barrier integrity [114]. For *C. difficile*-associated diarrhea, moderate-quality evidence suggests that probiotics are effective in alleviating this condition [114].

b. Competitive exclusion of pathogens and bacteriocin production. Probiotics also mediate their effects in adults through the competitive exclusion of pathogens and the production of bacteriocins [116]. Competitive exclusion involves probiotic bacteria outcompeting other bacteria for receptor sites in the intestinal tract [111]. While the specific regulatory mechanisms are not well understood, the proposed mechanisms include lowering the pH in the gut, competing for nutrients, and producing bacteriocins or bacteriocin-like substances [111]. Probiotics have been studied for their ability to reduce human pathogens such as *Salmonella typhi* and *E. coli* [116]. They achieve this by producing metabolites that interact with various cellular pathways, influencing processes like proliferation, differentiation, apoptosis, inflammation, angiogenesis, and metastasis [117]. Some probiotic strains, particularly *Lactobacilli* and *Bifidobacteria,* can produce antimicrobial peptides, i.e., bacteriocins [116]. These molecules disrupt the protonmotive force in bacterial cytoplasmic membranes, effectively inhibiting the growth of specific pathogens [117]. Bacteriocins are classified into four main types based on their structures and genetic characteristics [111]. Certain bacteriocins produced by probiotics like *L. plantarum* and *L. acidophilus* have been found to inhibit the growth of pathogens such as *Helicobacter*, *C. difficile*, rotaviruses multidrug-resistant *Shigella* species, and *E. coli* in the GIT [118].

c. Enzymatic activities and production of volatile fatty acids: *Lactobacilli* and *Bifidobacteria* possess over 20 different enzymatic activities, with β-galactosidase activity being a common one [118]. The enzyme β-glucuronidase, for example, converts glucuronidated metabolites into toxic forms, potentially causing intestinal damage. Low β-glucuronidase activity in feces has been associated with increased levels of harmful substances like carcinogens in the colon [114]. Bifidobacterium longum, when included in the diet, can alter the intestinal microbiota, reducing β-glucuronidase activity [119], [120]. This reduction is linked to inhibiting aberrant crypt formation, an early marker of malignant potential in colon carcinogenesis. Probiotics have also been investigated in the context of NAFLD. In clinical trials, probiotics, prebiotics, or synbiotics were found to reduce liver aminotransferase activity in adult patients with NAFLD, indicating potential liver health benefits [121]. Enzymatic activities were examined in a study involving 30 healthy adults consuming a fermented product containing two probiotic strains [111]. The probiotic-treated group exhibited increased enzymatic activities, including those associated with lactobacilli and probiotic strains, such as naphthol-AS-BI-phosphohydrolase and leucine arylamides, while β-glucuronidase activity decreased [122]. Furthermore, probiotics interact with bile acids in the gut, influencing bile acid metabolism and cholesterol absorption [122, 123]. Bile salt hydrolase (BSH) is an enzyme produced by many probiotics and other gut bacteria, playing a key role in the deconjugation of biliary salts. BSH-containing bacteria have been recognized for their beneficial effects, including the modulation of cholesterol levels [111]. Consequently, BSH activity is considered an important mechanism contributing to the hypocholesterolemia (cholesterol-lowering) effect attributed to probiotics [111].

On the other hand, probiotics can also impact adults through the production of volatile fatty acids (VFAs) in the gut, conferring various health benefits [124]. VFAs, such as butyrate, propionate, and acetic acid, are produced by probiotics and influence the gut environment [125]. In clinical trials, the consumption of specific probiotic strains has been linked to increased VFA production. For example, L. gasseri CECT5714 and L. coryniformis CECT5711 increased fecal butyrate, propionic, and acetic acid concentrations compared to controls. Even after the washout period, butyrate production remained elevated in the probiotic group [126, 127]. The production of VFAs, particularly butyrate, seems to depend on the specific probiotic strains used. Studies have shown that different probiotics can influence the gut microbiota differently, affecting VFA levels. For example, the synbiotic preparation B. longum, when combined with an insulin-based prebiotic, increased the production of acetate, succinate, butyrate, and isobutyrat [128, 129]. VFAs play a role in preventing diarrhea, especially in patients receiving total enteral nutrition. Probiotic yeast S. boulardii increased fecal butyrate concentrations, contributing to the reduction of diarrhea incidence during enteral nutrition [130]. Probiotics like L. plantarum 299v have been found to enhance fecal SCFA concentrations in patients with C. difficile-associated diarrhea, helping to counteract the negative effects of antibiotics. In elderly populations, probiotics like L. casei strain Shirota and L. casei Shirota have been associated with increased fecal acetic acid concentrations and reduced instances of gastroenteritis caused by norovirus [131]. Probiotic interventions in children have shown that probiotics like L. paracasei Lpc-37 or B. lactis HN019 can reduce the risk of diarrhea and increase selected SCFAs and branched-chain fatty acids concentrations. SCFAs, particularly butyrate, have been associated with promoting tolerance in infants with cow's milk allergy (CMA) when treated with extensively hydrolyzed casein formula (eHCF) and L. rhamnosus GG. Probiotics and synbiotics have demonstrated positive effects on obesity, insulin resistance syndrome, T2D, and NAFLD in adults [132, 133]. They can influence BMI, fat mass, insulin sensitivity, carbohydrate metabolism, and liver health, potentially through their impact on SCFA production. SCFAs play essential roles in various tissues, including the intestine, liver, adipose, muscle, and brain tissues [134]. They can regulate energy homeostasis and metabolism, influence satiety, affect fat accumulation, improve insulin sensitivity, and decrease inflammation. SCFAs interact with specific receptors like GPR41 and GPR43, enhancing these effects [135].

d. Cell adhesion and mucin production

Probiotics in adults exert their effects through various mechanisms, including adhesion to the intestinal mucosa and modulation of immune responses. Adhesion to the mucosa is a critical step for probiotics to colonize and interact effectively within the host's gastrointestinal tract. Some probiotic strains (especially

Lactobacillus) possess surface adhesins that facilitate attachment to the mucous layer lining the intestines [136]. This adhesion is vital for probiotics to carry out functions such as antagonizing pathogenic bacteria and regulating the immune system. Mucin, secreted by intestinal epithelial cells, plays a crucial role in the host's defense against harmful microbes. Probiotics may influence mucin production, enhancing the protective barrier of the intestinal lining. By promoting the secretion of mucin, probiotics contribute to preventing the adhesion of pathogenic bacteria and maintaining gut health [137]. To evaluate probiotics' adhesion capabilities, researchers often employ *in vitro* models like the Caco-2 cell line. These cells form a monolayer that closely resembles mature enterocytes found in the human small intestine [118]. Utilizing such models helps researchers understand how probiotics interact with and adhere to intestinal epithelial cells, providing insights into their colonization and functionality. Probiotics also have a significant impact on the host's immune system. For example, *L. rhamnosus* ATCC 7469 has been shown to influence immune responses. When exposed to pathogenic bacteria like *E. coli*, probiotics can attenuate the expression of immune-related receptors such as TLR-4 and nucleotide-binding oligomerization-domain–containing protein (NOD)-2. This immunomodulatory effect contributes to the probiotics' ability to protect against infections and promote immune health. Moreover, probiotics play a role in maintaining the integrity of the intestinal epithelial barrier [138]. Certain probiotics, notably *L. rhamnosus*, can enhance the barrier's function by promoting the phosphorylation of Akt and increasing the expression of proteins like zonula occludens-1 and occluding [139]. This reinforcement of the epithelial barrier is essential, particularly during bacterial infections, to prevent the passage of harmful pathogens into the bloodstream. Additionally, probiotics can influence gene transcription in the gut mucosa [114]. These changes in gene expression contribute to the overall health-promoting effects of probiotics in the gastrointestinal tract. In summary, probiotics in adults interact with the intestinal mucosa through adhesion mechanisms, which enable colonization and host interactions. They can also influence mucin production, modulate immune responses, maintain the epithelial barrier, and regulate gene transcription in the gut mucosa [140]. These multifaceted mechanisms collectively contribute to the beneficial effects of probiotics on gut health and overall well-being.

e. Modulation of the immune system

Probiotics also function by interacting with the gut microbiota and the host's immune system [141, 142]. They help regulate the immune response, which consists of innate and adaptive systems [143]. The innate system responds to common pathogen patterns through pattern recognition receptors (PRRs) [144], including TLRs [145]. Probiotics influence these receptors found on various cells, modulating the immune response [146]. One key role of probiotics is promoting immune balance. They induce the development of regulatory T cells (T-regs), which are vital for maintaining a balanced immune system [147]. Probiotics play a crucial part in fine-tuning the immune system by interacting with the gut microbiota and host cells, preserving intestinal harmony [112].

f. Modulation of sIgA and cytokine production

Probiotics play a crucial role in modulating the immune system through various mechanisms [111]. One key action is their ability to stimulate the production of secretory immunoglobulin A (sIgA), which enhances the gut's barrier function [112]. Probiotics interact with specific immune cells, leading to the production of cytokines and immunoglobulins, contributing to immune balance and intestinal health [112]. These beneficial effects are observed with various probiotic strains. For instance, Lactobacillus and Bifidobacterium strains have been shown to enhance the production of immunoglobulins and cytokines [148]. Probiotics like *L. Rhamnosus* and L. casei promote the activation of immune cells and increase the concentrations of key immunological substances like IL-10, enhancing the immune response. Bifidobacteria strains, such as B. longum subsp. infantis 35624, induce regulatory T cells (T-regs) and prevent excessive inflammation [145]. This immunoregulatory effect is crucial in conditions like psoriasis, IBS, and ulcerative colitis. Additionally, B. breve C50 releases soluble factors that reduce the secretion of pro-inflammatory cytokines, contributing to intestinal homeostasis. Probiotic mixtures have also shown promise in regulating the immune system [146]. They can upregulate the production of CD4+forkhead box P3 (FoxP3)+T-regs, leading to reduced inflammation in conditions like IBD, atopic dermatitis, and rheumatoid arthritis. These probiotics promote regulatory dendritic cells (DCs) and T-regs, making them a potential treatment for inflammatory immune disorders [147].

g. Interaction of probiotics with TLRs and cell cascade signaling

Probiotics interact with TLRs, a family of proteins that recognize microbial components. TLRs play a crucial role in immune responses

[111]. Different TLRs respond to specific microbial components. For example, TLR2 and TLR6 recognize bacterial surface components, and TLR9 responds to nucleic-acid-based molecules [149]. Probiotics can influence TLR expression and signaling, contributing to immune regulation. Probiotics like lactobacilli activate TLR2 and TLR6, stimulating cytokine production and immune responses. TLR2 recognizes components like peptidoglycan, found in gram-positive bacteria. Lactobacillus strains interact with gut-associated immune cells through TLR2, influencing receptor expression [114]. TLR9 activation by probiotics is anti-inflammatory, affecting the epithelial surface. It triggers intracellular signaling pathways, leading to the expression of key immune molecules. Different probiotic strains have varying effects on cytokine production, with some inducing cytokines in a TLR9-dependent manner. Probiotics can also modulate TLR gene expression, reducing the levels of certain TLRs. Additionally, they can affect immune signaling pathways, including p38 MAPK and extracellular-regulated kinase [150]. The effectiveness of probiotics in activating TLR9 signaling may depend on the dosing regimen. In intestinal diseases like NEC, probiotics like L. Rhamnosus HN001 activate TLR9, potentially attenuating the condition without reported toxicity. Probiotics can also influence the balance of Th1 and Th2 lymphocytes, reducing allergic responses and promoting immune homeostasis [151].

h. Interaction with the brain–gut axis

Social interactions among individuals can lead to similarities in their gut microbiota, even when controlling for factors like diet, genetics, and shared environments [152]. This social transmission of gut microbes might benefit both the microbes and host communities. The gut microbiota's role is increasingly recognized in influencing aspects of behavior, particularly in early childhood. Stress and pain, especially in preterm infants, can affect the gut microbiota and overall health. Autism spectrum disorder (ASD) is linked to gastrointestinal issues and gut dysbiosis [153]. Some studies suggest that certain probiotics, like B. fragilis, could improve ASD-related behaviors [112]. Additionally, maternal factors like obesity and diabetes have been associated with ASD incidence [154]. High-fat maternal diets can impact offspring behavior, but probiotics like L. reuteri may mitigate these effects [154]. Stress, whether physical or psychological, can disrupt the microbiota–gut–brain axis. Certain probiotics have shown promise in reducing symptoms of depression in human volunteers [155]. Gut bacteria produce various neuroactive compounds that can affect brain function, potentially influencing social behavior [114]. While more research is needed to fully understand these interactions, the gut microbiota's role in behavior and its consequences for both host and microbes are becoming increasingly clear [114].

14.3.2 Prebiotics as Dietary Supplements vs. Functional Foods

Probiotics by virtue of their composition can be consumed as nutraceuticals and functional foods [156, 157]. Functional foods are those whose ingredients improve the health of the consumers. In the context of probiotics, they can be in the form of ice cream, a fermented milk product but with some additives [158]. Goktas [159] found that the antioxidant potential of ice creams functionalized with rowanberry pulp had a 53.08% antioxidant activity. Even after storage for 120 days, the probiotic viability exceeded 8.24 log cfu/g and the survival rate of L. rhamnosus was preserved with rowanberry pulp addition. The author concluded that 5% rowanberry pulp can be used in the manufacturing of functional probiotic ice cream [159].

On the other hand, they can be taken as supplements if they are provided separately in capsule, powder, liquid, or pill form of different strains and doses [160, 161]. Probiotic yeasts, in particular, are promising cell factories and carriers [162]. However, the safety of probiotics in immunosuppressed individuals versus immune-competent individuals remains a concern [163].

14.3.3 Regulatory Guidelines for Prebiotic Products

In 2001, the requirements for probiotics with health claims were put forward by the Joint Food and Agriculture Organization of the United Nations/World Health Organization Expert Consultation on Evaluation of Health and Nutritional Properties of Probiotics. The guidelines are divided into labeling, stability testing, and storage guidelines.

1. Labeling recommendations
   a. The amount(s) of probiotics in any serving of the stated size of the food should be declared, usually in colony-forming units (CFUs). The stated quantity ought to reflect the total quantity of the live microorganisms at the end of the stated shelf life, and not at the time of manufacture [164].
   b. In addition, the product label should identify the genus, species, and strain for each microorganism in the product. The identification should employ a combination of phenotypic and genotypic tests as well as clinical evidence suggesting that the health benefits of probiotics claimed thereof are strain-specific [91].

c. The mechanism of the supposed probiotic effect was carried out in vitro [165, 166].
d. An explicit substantiation of the clinical health benefits of the probiotic agents, specifically with clinical trials in humans.
e. Further, assessment of the safety profiles of the probiotic strains should be conducted to establish (i) mechanisms of antimicrobial drug resistance, (ii) side effects observed in the conducted clinical trials and after consumption by the general market, (iii) the toxin production profile and (any) hemolytic potential of the species, especially where the strain in question is already known to elicit these effects, and (vi) evidence of no infectivity in animal studies [167].

2. Stability profile guidelines

   Assessment of product stability guidelines was established to guarantee that the shelf life of a probiotic product is scientifically proven. Stability tests should proceed under the same conditions as the recommended storage conditions. The storage temperature should be well-defined in the stability testing protocol. When defining storage temperatures, firms may consider the following storage conditions from the International Conference on Harmonisation.

3. Storage guidelines

   Since probiotics are live organisms and are therefore largely sensitive to variations or fluctuations in environmental conditions (temperature and humidity), it is expected that the degree to which a probiotic product is impacted by such conditions is dependent on the probiotic strains in the product, formulation matrix and dosage form, and product packaging [168, 169]. Thus, the storage and handling instructions for every probiotic product need to be availed to the consumers, considering the nature of the formulation as well as its packaging [170].

14.3.4 Clinical Evidence Supporting the Use of Probiotics in Metabolic Disorders

Probiotics are known to elicit beneficial effects in the management of metabolic disorders, and the clinical evidence supporting these therapeutic claims is briefly presented and discussed in the following:

For T2D (Table 14.1), studies have suggested that *Bifidobacterium*-based probiotics possess greater effects than other probiotic genera. These probiotics colonize the gut, altering the composition of the host's gut microbiota [171–173]. It can also be contended that food-type probiotics (such as yogurt) may elicit higher effects than other types of probiotics on glycemic control in type-2 diabetic patients, possibly by buffering stomach acid, and enhancing the colonization of the gut by the probiotics [174, 175]. These results suggest that the administration of probiotics could be leveraged as a promising adjuvant therapy for glycemia management in type-2 diabetic patients [176].

Probiotic supplementation has also been proven to be helpful in managing overweight, NAFLD, and obesity via modulating gut microbiota [196, 197]. For the available clinical trials on obesity (Table 14.2), at least five of the trials involved children and adolescents and yielded rather conflicting results. Three trials were in support of anti-obesity effects such as a decrease in weight, waist circumferences, or body mass index [198–200].

Among the major ten clinical trials conducted on obese adults, nine studies showed probiotic efficiency in reducing weight or waist circumferences as shown in Table 14.2 [201–208]. These observations show that specific strains of probiotics possess anti-obesity effects, but these may also depend on whether an individual is a child, an adult, pregnant, involved in some physical activity or is supplementing their diet with vitamins [197, 209–211]. For example, some probiotics modulate the intestinal microbiota by increasing the number of *Bifidobacterium* and *Lactobacillus* spp. These bacteria biosynthesize and release pro-healthy conjugated linoleic acid, which adjusts body weight through improving energy metabolism and lipolysis [212].

With regards to malignancies, probiotics are known to play useful roles in the chemoprevention, treatment, and reduction of the spread of cancers such as colorectal, colon, liver, breast, bladder, and cervical [217]. Table 14.3 gives a synopsis of reports on some clinical supporting interventions using probiotics. It is worth noting that clinical trials on the utilization of probiotics are limited, and almost always focused on gastrointestinal tumors with often unelucidated mechanisms of action and were reportedly followed by bacteremia after the interventions [218]. Therefore, more studies are required to validate which species of bacteria are best suited for intervention in particular cancer types [219].

14.4 SYNBIOTICS: SYNERGISTIC APPROACHES FOR METABOLIC HEALTH

14.4.1 Definition and Benefits of Synbiotics

Over time, the definitive understanding of synbiotics has drifted due to knowledge advancement. Pandey [225] initially describes synbiotics as a combination of prebiotics and probiotics that significantly affect the host's health. By 2019, the definition of synbiotics was revised by the "International Scientific Association for Probiotics and Prebiotics (ISAPP) panel," which involved professionals such as microbiologists, nutritionists, dieticians, and physiologists. The panel agreed that synbiotics are "a mixture of substrates and living microorganisms selectively utilized by the host organism to confer a health benefit to the host" [226]. The agreement was based on the enhanced action exhibited by these synbiotics to manage different conditions. Furthermore, these synbiotics have antioxidant activity through synergistic and complementary mechanisms vital in managing health conditions [227].

TABLE 14.1
Reports of Clinical Trials Supporting the Use of Probiotics in Treatment of T2D

Probiotic	Clinical Trial Results	References
L. rhamnosus, L. bulgaricus, B. breve, B. longum, S. thermophiles, L. casei, L. acidophilus,	The patients were recovered from inulin resistance as shown by a decrease in fasting and an increase in high-density lipoprotein	[177]
Ecologic®Barrier	After 12 weeks, Homeostasis model of assessment-insulin resistance was optimized and the waist-hip ratio decreased. For 6 weeks, the cardiometabolic profile improved with decrease in endotoxin, TNF-α and IL-6	[178, 179]
L. reuteri ADR-1, and L. reuteri ADR-3	In a 9-month trial, cholesterol and blood pressure levels decreased and there was improved fecal microbial composition (increased fecal *Lactobacillus* and *Bifidobacterium* loads)	[180]
Symbiter	In 8 weeks, there was improved insulin resistance (decreased HOMA-IR, HbA1c)	[181]
L. plantarum A7 and Soy milk	Optimized kidney function	[182]
Bifidobacterium, S. thermophiles, and Lactobacillus spp.	Retrieved the normal level of all the parameters associated with Insulin resistance after 9 weeks of treatments	[183]
B. infantis, L. acidophilus, L. lactis,B,. B. bifidum, longum, L. casei,	The probiotic improved fasting insulin level and hemoglobin A1c on 12 week of exposure	[184]
L. reuteri DSM 17938	In 12 weeks, the insulin sensitivity index and serum deoxycholic acid increased	[185]
Fermented milk by L. casei	Bacterial translocation was decreased, *C. leptum, Clostridium coccoides, Lactobacillus* were augmented	[186]
lactis, L. acidophilu, and B. animalis sub spp. Fermented	The insulin resistance was parameters included levels of HbA1c and fructosamine, and total cholesterol were optimized after 8 weeks	[187]
B. lactis and L. acidophilus strains in yogurt	Helped to normalized the insulin resistance and lipid profile in glycemic patients	[188]
Streptococcus thermophiles, L. acidophilus, L. rhamnosus, B. longum, B. breve, L. bulgaricus, L. casei,	The insulin resistant parameters included Fasting plasma glucose level, HOMA-IR score, LDL level, and the hs-CRP value were improved	[189, 190]
Strains of L. sporogenes	The levels of hs-CRP, FPG were decreased and serum levels of GSH level was increased after 6 weeks	[191]
Ecologic®Barrier	After 26 weeks, there was a decrease in systemic stated inflammatory response and decreased endotoxin levels which altered gut microbiota	[192]
Strains of *B. lactis* and *L. acidophilus* in yogurt	Assisted to optimized total antioxidant status and lipid profile while assisted to lowered the total cholesterol and low-density lipoproteins after 6 weeks	[193, 194]
FOS, B. bifidum, and L. acidophilus strains	Lowered the insulin resistance in 30 days	[195]

TABLE 14.2
Major Clinical Trials in Support of Probiotics as Interventions for the Management of Obesity and Overweight

Probiotic Intervention	Clinical Trial Outcomes	References
B. breve, L. acidophilus, B. longum, and L. bulgaricus L. rhamnosus	Helped to decrease body weights after 12 weeks of surgery	[213]
B. animalis subsp. lactis CECT 8145; heat-killed B. animalis subsp. lactis CECT 8145	After 16 weeks, BMI and WC decreased	[206]
B. bifidum W23, B. lactis W51, B. lactis W52, L. acidophilus W37, L. brevis W63, L. casei W56, L. salivarius W24, L. lactis W19, and L. lactis W58	For 12 weeks, there was an improved lipid profile and glucose metabolism, with decrease in visceral fat and waist circumference	[208]
vitamins E, A and C, L. casei, L. rhamnosus, S. thermophilus, L. bulgaricus, B. breve, L. acidophilus, and B. longum	BMI reduced in obese children after 8 weeks	[214]
L. casei, L. rhamnosus, S. thermophilus, B. breve, L. acidophilus, B. longum, L. bulgaricus, vitamins E, A, C	In 8 weeks, the BMI and WC reduced significantly	[211]
L. rhamnosus GG, B. lactis	Marked decrease in waist circumference were observed after pregnancy	[215]
L. rhamnosus GG, B. lactis	From the first trimester to the end of breastfeeding, there was a reduction in gestational diabetes among the pregnant participants	[216]

TABLE 14.3
Major Clinical Trials in Support of Probiotics as Interventions for Management of Obesity and Overweight

Probiotic Intervention	Clinical Trial Outcomes	References
L. casei Shirota (LcS)	Cervical cancer and human papillomavirus-associated infection were recovered 60% in 6 months	[220]
B. breve Yakult	Reduced the incidence of fever in patients after chemotherapy for 6 weeks	[221]
Shirota of *L. casei* and soy products in Yakult	The incidence was decreased in breast cancer patients of age 40 to 55 years	[222]
Lactobacillus acidophilus L1	The habitual intake of lactic acid bacteria reduced the risk of bladder cancer	[223]
Strains of Propionibacterium freudenreichii and Lactobacillus rhamnosus	Assisted to improved liver cancer and observed reduced urinary excretion of aflatoxin up to 61.5% after 5 weeks	[224]

14.4.2 Mechanisms of Synergistic Action in Metabolic Disorders

14.4.2.1 Synbiotics Mechanism of Action as Antioxidant

Nuclear factors can be activated and translocated by synbiotics, which is the mechanism behind their antioxidant properties. These generate antioxidant-related important molecules, activate the antioxidant defense enzymatic system, and detoxify the generation of free radicals and singlet oxygen [228, 229]. Additionally, recent studies on synbiotic dairy products have shown that they provide a range of important vitamins and regulators. These consist of antioxidants, water-soluble vitamins, and GSH, a crucial tripeptide that directly neutralizes singlet oxygen, hydroxyl radicals, and superoxide radicals chemically [228, 230]. More recently, a study on patients with diabetes revealed that supplementing with synbiotics reduced levels of malondialdehyde (MDA), a marker of lipid peroxidation (Weiss and Deutschman 2014), and increased levels of GSH, nitric oxide (NO), a crucial intra- and intercellular regulating molecule with a wide range of physiological effects, and total antioxidant capacity (TAC), a measure of the quantity of free radicals scavenged [231]. With a few representative instances in human and animal species, there is mounting data that suggests the antioxidant actions of synbiotics when the probiotic and prebiotic combinative effects are taken into consideration, either in a complementary or synergistic manner. It is believed that the most important probiotics engaged in synbiotic antioxidant activity are strains of Bifidobacterium and Lactobacillus [232]. Synbiotics containing both L. casei and inulin have been shown to be effective in shielding the human body from the harm that free radicals can inflict. Certain antioxidant enzyme activity and blood plasma antioxidant capacity may be enhanced by synbiotics [233].

Supplementing with synbiotics was associated with increased antioxidant resistance and antioxidant enzymes, according to two recent meta-analyses. Consuming synbiotics (and probiotics) increased TAC, GSH, SOD, and NO levels relative to the controls, but decreased MDA levels [234]. Furthermore, antioxidant parameters were measured before and after the synbiotic bread containing L. sporogenes, and inulin was consumed by patients in a clinical trial with T2D to investigate its effects. According to their findings, eating synbiotic bread considerably reduced MDA while having no effect on TAC, GSH, or chloramphenicol acetyltransferase (CAT) [235]. A study on the antioxidant effect of synbiotic supplementation in migraine-affected women found that a 12-week synbiotic supplementation of 109 CFU of 12 different probiotic kinds with FOS prebiotic decreased oxidative stress, including TAC and NO, as well as the clinical symptoms of migraine [236]. According to the results of another study, piglets' lipid oxidation process was postponed during the refrigeration phase when they were fed a diet supplemented with organic zinc and a synbiotic combination [237]. Additionally, it has been demonstrated that taking synbiotics increased the activity of antioxidant enzymes and inhibited the hepatic growth of MDA, hence strengthening the antioxidant defense system and reducing lipid peroxidation in rats' livers [238].

14.4.2.2 Synbiotics Assists to Modulate Composition of Gut Microbiota

One effective tactic for preventing metabolic illnesses has been suggested: probiotics [239]. *L. rhamnosus* LMG S-28148 and *B. lactis* LMG P-28149 combined effect could alter the makeup of the gut microbiota associated with obesity and increase the abundances of Rikenellaceae and *Akkermansia muciniphila* while decreasing those of Lactobacillaceae [240]. Furthermore, disruption of the digestive system and dysbiosis of the gut microbiota, which is characterized by reduced abundances of Bifidobacteria and Lactobacillus and increased abundances of Escherichia coli led to IBD [241]. Furthermore, the gut microbiota is caused metabolic inflammation in diabetic patients. *Lactobacillus reuteri* treatment was shown to enhance metabolic function by preventing the growth of pathogenic bacteria, such as *Yersinia enterocolitica* [242]. Additionally, by reducing the Firmicutes to Bacteroidetes ratio and the production of the angiotensin-converting enzyme (ACE) and elevating the abundances of Akkermansia and Lactobacillus, the consumption of *L. casei* may protect neonates from metabolically associated hypertension [243]. Furthermore, probiotic-fermented milk containing LR6 strain of *Lactobacillus reuteri* was ameliorated malnutrition related to protein energy and immunological function in mice [244]. In comparison to use of probiotics alone, the combination of omega-3 fatty acids and *Lactococcus*, *Lactobacillus*, *Propionibacterium*, and *Bifidobacterium* significantly reduced lipid accumulation [181]. Synbiotics were viewed as a new frontier in the prevention of obesity. Furthermore, by reducing the abundances of Ruminococcaceae and Desulfovibrionaceae, oral supplements containing a combination of *Bacillus licheniformis* and XOS could more successfully enhance lipid metabolism and body weight increase in obese rats [245]. Furthermore, combining *L. plantarum* PMO 08 with chia seeds showed a synergistic anti-obesity impact on obese mice and improved the intestinal milieu that supports the proliferation of *L. plantarum* [246].

14.4.2.2.1 Synbiotics Help to Modulate Metabolites of Gut Microbial

Some gut microbial metabolites may have an indirect effect on human metabolism via signaling pathways, such as AMPK, PPARγ, and GPR [247]. According to an *in vitro* investigation, a combination of *L. salivarius* and *B. lactis* could increase the fermentation system's synthesis of butyrate and propionate [240]. Furthermore, an experimental investigation that compared 23 bacterial strains found that *Ligilactobacillus salivarius* PI2 and *B. longum* PI10 might limit the formation of fat in adipocytes [248]. Furthermore, the strains of *B. longum* and *L. plantarum* were inhibited microbiota in gut and downregulated the expression of nuclear factor kappa B (NF-κB) and tumor necrosis factor α (TNF-α) in mice model of osteoporosis and obesity [249].

Consuming prebiotics may control the synthesis of bile acids and saturated fats (SCFAs), which in turn may affect how the body uses energy [250]. Furthermore, dietary fiber from rye and oat brans was shown to regulate tryptophan-serotonin metabolism and bile acids in addition to improving body weight, glucose metabolism, hepatic inflammation, and SCFA generation in mice in an *in vivo* investigation [251].

By upregulating the TLR2-AMPK signaling pathway, postbiotics such as Lactobacillus plantarum L-14's exopolysaccharide inhibited the differentiation of immature cells into mature adipocytes, regulated body weight and lipid profiles in mice [252]. Furthermore, by triggering the extracellular-regulated protein kinases (ERK) signaling pathway, *L. brevis* long-chain polyphosphate may enhance intestinal inflammation and barrier function [253]. Furthermore, it was found that the muramyl dipeptide derived from bacterial cell walls was an advantageous postbiotic that may reduce the insulin resistance caused by obesity by IRF4 and NOD2 [254]. Subsequent research revealed that the relationship with NOD1 and NOD2 may reduce insulin sensitivity and inflammation [255]. Furthermore, galactooligosaccharides were shown to delay the development of insulin resistance and obesity in mice by upregulation of GLP1 and downregulating the excretion of bile acid in the feces. The alteration in the composition of gut bacteria was assisted to increase in the signaling pathways of SIRT1-AMPK-PPARα and IRS1-Akt and downregulated ACE mRNA expression and improved the tetrathionate metabolism, hydrolase activity of hepatic cholesterol 7-alpha hydroxylase and bile salt [256] (Figure 14.1).

14.4.3 Designing Effective Synbiotic Combinations

A synbiotic is a mix of a prebiotic—a substance that specifically promotes the growth of a bacterium—and a probiotic—a microorganism that has been demonstrated—or believed—to have some positive effects when taken. Nowadays, a lot of probiotic supplements are sold as synbiotics. Combinations of Bifidobacterium, Lactobacillus, or Streptococcus species are commonly found in these products, together with a carbon source (e.g., lactose, lactulose, or inulin) that promotes the growth of these microorganisms. Food corporations have benefited historically from the use of probiotics in meals and beverages and from marketing geared toward digestive health. Companies such as Danone, Nestlé, and General Mills hold the highest market share for probiotics and are actively investing in research and development to broaden their range of probiotics and prebiotics [257]. These days, a lot of probiotic organisms on the market, make the claim to improve digestive health and are frequently used for symptoms like constipation or diarrhea. Probiotic sales are anticipated to rise, and these organisms may be marketed for purposes other than digestive disorders. The speed at which research is being conducted on the potential health benefits of the human microbiome suggests that next-generation probiotics should have some sort of proven health effect, derived from studies on animals or from human clinical trials. If there are no adverse health consequences, probiotic use may be justified by implied effects. Using this tactic, the startup company AOBiome markets ammonia-oxidizing bacteria that, when applied to skin, purport to lessen sweat odors [258]. In the USA, the majority of probiotics are thought to be safe (GRAS). This classification is significant for probiotics; however, it usually only applies to the microorganisms that aid in the fermentation of foods like yogurt and cheese. Other probiotics have GRAS designation based on a consensus of scientific and medical observations. Organisms that have been granted GRAS certification make it easier to manufacture and commercialize probiotics, as they reduce worries about possible health risks related to probiotic usage. But a lot of potentially helpful microorganisms [259, 260].

Prebiotics are substances that boost the effect of probiotics when used as a combination. For a pair to be referred to as a synbiotic, there must be some indication that one prebiotic specifically supports the growth of the new organism. This is because the majority of prebiotic substances now in use support the growth of numerous different bacteria that are native to the host. One method for creating synbiotics is to enrich living things with a target prebiotic in vivo and

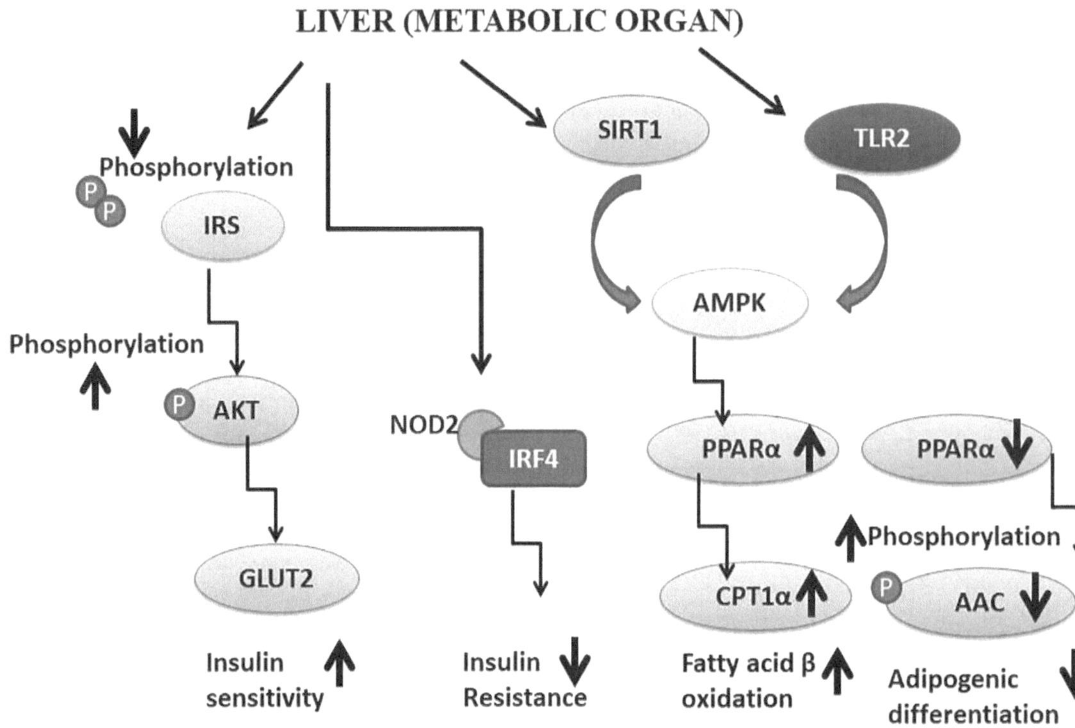

FIGURE 14.1 The mediators of different pathways crosslinked to enhance the entire metabolic system including upregulating the IRS1-Akt-GLUT2, SIRT1-AMPK-PPARα-CPR1α, TLR2-PPARγ-AMPK, and NOD-IRF4 signaling pathways.

then isolate the organisms whose numbers rise as a result of the prebiotic [261]. This strategy guarantees that the isolated organisms will be the most likely to use the target prebiotic substance even in a competitive situation. Starting with a prebiotic substance that is particular to a probiotic and unavailable to the endogenous population is an alternative strategy (e.g. a genetically produced probiotic that can break down some exotic substrate). Presumably, prebiotics can serve as a supplement for commensals that are already present in the body, even in situations where probiotics are not needed. For the treatment of inflammatory bowel illness, General Mills is developing a prebiotic formulation that enriches particular commensals [262].

Probiotics that are well-designed can utilize prebiotics that are already present in the host to create a synbiotic without having to feed the prebiotic directly. Similarly, other studies have demonstrated that two conditions must be met for an introduced Bifidobacterium probiotic to persist: (i) the source of nutrients must be endogenous; and (ii) there must be no competition from other commensal organisms for the same nutritional source [263]. The use of ammonia-oxidizing bacteria by AOBiome serves as an example of other potential components of the system, such as nitrogen, phosphorus, or iron, which may enable the development of specific prebiotics that favor respiration over fermentation. For instance, dissimilatory sulfite reduction in *Bilophila wadsworthia* is facilitated by the sulfite found in taurine [264].

The term "synbiotic" suggests that the probiotic and prebiotic work in concert. Therefore, all that is needed for the design of a synbiotic is for the probiotic to function better when a prebiotic is present than when it is not, and vice versa [265].

Subsequent studies investigating the effects of synbiotics ought to evaluate not just how the prebiotic influences the probiotic, but also how the combination of the two affects the host differently than when it is studied separately. Such data is ultimately necessary to justify the use of synbiotics, and gathering it will need significant financial contributions from the leading academic, commercial, and clinical participants in this field.

14.4.4 Regulatory Considerations for Synbiotic Products

Probiotic applications for illness prevention or treatment will need to pay attention to regulatory issues that aren't always present in the market for health foods. The following is a summary of the points Jennifer Ross of the US FDA covered in her presentation to the colloquium attendees:

1. Under the general heading of food, the FDA's Center for Food Safety and Applied Nutrition (CFSAN) regulates probiotic products, including dietary supplements. In a nutshell, a dietary supplement is a substance that is taken orally with the goal of enhancing diet (FDA). Dietary supplements and other goods classified as foods may make limited labeling claims (Dietary Supplement Health and Education Act) (CFSAN).

2. A microorganism's lengthy history of use in food may not be sufficient to support its feeding to humans for therapeutic purposes. According to the Food Drug & Cosmetic Act, United States Code (U.S.C.) Title 21, Chapter 9, an article is considered a drug if it is meant to be used in the diagnosis, cure, mitigation, treatment, or prevention of disease (CFSAN). Conventional medications are chemically manufactured, tiny molecules. According to the Public Health Service Act of 1944, 42 U.S.C. 262, any medicine that contains a virus, therapeutic serum, toxin, anti-toxin, or equivalent product is considered a biological product (CFSAN). Historically, goods containing microscopic live sources of infectious disease were considered referred to as "viruses." The term "virus" in this meaning today includes anything that contains germs like bacteria and fungi.
3. To date, the majority of probiotic-type products were under regulatory authority under CBER's Office of Vaccines Research and Review (OVRR).
4. When a license to commercialize a biological product, like an LBP, in the United States for a particular illness claim is needed, a Biologics License Application (BLA) (4) is filed. Data from many clinical studies carried out under an Investigational New Drug Application (IND) are typically included in a BLA (CFR). Therapeutic studies were often planned with the goal of evaluating a product's safety and effectiveness for a particular therapeutic indication. A population (i.e., children or adults) and a disease or condition are typically used to define a clinical indication. The contents of an IND comprise the following: (i) a cover sheet; (ii) a table of contents; (iii) an opening statement and general investigative strategy; and (iv) a description of the drug substance and drug product's composition, manufacturing method, and control tests.
5. Before formally filing an application, plans might be discussed with FDA regarding the submission of an IND. It is recommended that anyone thinking about conducting clinical research get early advice from the FDA to ascertain if the IND regulations apply in a certain circumstance. An IND is also necessary for many clinical investigations that are carried out only for research, as opposed to licensure, or marketing approval. When an IND is necessary, it may be possible to ask for a pre-IND meeting to help with regulatory compliance.

14.4.5 Clinical Evidence Supporting the Use of Synbiotics in Metabolic Disorders

Numerous literatures have demonstrated significant evidence concerning the benefits of synbiotics in managing multiple metabolic disorders. A randomized, double-blind clinical trial on the impact of synbiotics on patients with NAFLD demonstrated a significant reduction in inflammatory substrates, hepatic fibrosis, and steatosis among the affected patients [266]. Further evidence demonstrated that synbiotics have significant anti-diabetic properties among patients with Type II diabetes Mellitus, especially by reducing pro-inflammatory markers and oxidation processes [267]. Additionally, Roy and Dhaneshwar (2023) asserted that synbiotic use improved sigmoidoscopy scores among patients with IBD. Moreover, synbiotics like prebiotics and Bifidobacterium longum lowered the B-defensins and interleukins-1α among patients with ulcerative colitis. Therefore, utilizing some of these synbiotics can offer weighty benefits in managing patients with metabolic disorders.

14.5 SAFETY AND QUALITY CONTROL OF PREBIOTIC, PROBIOTIC, AND SYNBIOTIC PRODUCTS

14.5.1 Ensuring Product Safety and Quality

Prebiotics, probiotics, and synbiotics are generally safe for human consumption [48, 226]. The safety of these products is important, and the detection of safe products is required for health purposes [48]. The safety measures for synbiotics are similar to those for probiotics and prebiotics [48]. Many studies suggest that prebiotics, probiotics, and synbiotics supplementation may be beneficial in prevention and management of nutritional and health [268].

Here are some ways to ensure safety and quality:

1. Use high-quality ingredients: Probiotics, prebiotics, and synbiotics should be made from high-quality ingredients that are safe for human and animal health. The selection process for probiotic strains should meet both safety and functionality criteria [269].
2. Ensure proper storage: Probiotics, prebiotics, and synbiotics should be stored in a cool, dry place to maintain their potency and effectiveness [225].
3. Follow regulatory guidelines: Probiotics are subject to regulations contained in the general food law, and according to them, they should be safe for human and animal health [269]. Regulatory claims on probiotic-based foods and beverages must be formulated and updated with policies to protect consumers [270].
4. Conduct clinical trials: Clinical trials can help determine the efficacy and safety of the products. Synbiotics, for example, have demonstrated the potential in alleviating global IBS symptoms [271]

14.5.2 Probiotic Strain Identification and Authentication

Probiotic strain identification and authentication are important for confirming the presence of specific probiotic strains, determining the viable cell counts, and ensuring product authenticity and quality assurance. Several DNA-based methods are used for probiotic strain or species identification, including species-specific and strain-specific PCR. Establishing an unequivocal taxonomic identity of any probiotic organism is necessary, and strain-specificity makes it essential. Accurate identification at the strain level is essential for determining the potential health benefits of probiotics [272].

14.5.3 Labeling Requirements and Transparency for Consumers

Labeling requirements and transparency for consumers are important aspects of probiotics, prebiotics, and synbiotics. Probiotics are identified by their specific strain, which includes the genus, the species, the subspecies (if applicable), and an alphanumeric strain designation [273].

14.5.4 Regulatory Oversight and Monitoring of Products on the Market

Probiotics, prebiotics, and synbiotics are regulated by various regulatory authorities to ensure their safety and efficacy. The regulatory requirements for probiotics differ depending on their intended use, whether as a drug or a dietary supplement [91]. The International Scientific Association for Probiotics and Prebiotics (ISAPP) was proposed a scientific definition of the term synbiotic to aid regulatory oversight of products labeled as "synbiotic" [226]. The ingestion of probiotics has been shown to regulate the intestinal microbiota by promoting the balance of specific microbes in the gut [274].

14.6 FUTURE PERSPECTIVES AND CHALLENGES IN REGULATORY LANDSCAPE

14.4.6.1 Exploration of Ongoing Research Trends in Prebiotics, Probiotics, and Synbiotics

Currently, the relationship between human health and gut microbiota is well-established. Prebiotics tend to influence the microbiota in the gut of humans which are responsible for maintaining good health [275, 276]. The gut microbiota has a crucial role in promoting positive outcomes, particularly in relation to gastrointestinal function, appetite regulation, and immunological response. There is a substantial body of research supporting the study of probiotics in the context of gastrointestinal illnesses [277].

The following section discusses some of the ongoing research trends in prebiotics, probiotics, and synbiotics.

14.4.6.1.1 Prebiotics

Research on prebiotics has been conducted since the early 20th century. In 1995, the term "prebiotics" was developed to refer to oligosaccharides (NDO) and polysaccharides (non-digestible) that promote the growth of beneficial lactic acid bacteria and reduce the presence of harmful bacteria such as E. coli and Salmonella [278, 279].

By 2012, some prebiotics like Inulin, FOS, GOS, lactulose, and polydextrose were recognized as established prebiotics, whereas isomaltooligosaccharides (IMO), XOS, and lactitol are categorized as emerging prebiotics [279, 280]. To date, the most widely studied types of prebiotics are the FOS and GOS [281].

14.4.6.1.2 Food Additive and in Starter Cultures

Prebiotics have gained interest from researchers in the food and nutrition industry because they have bioactive properties and they can also be a formulating component for increasing bulk for example in infant formula [282]. Moreover, not only are prebiotic soluble fiber like inulin useful in confectionary for improvement in the dough of bread, but it is also very important in the production of quality skim milk fermented by pure culture of *L. acidophilus, L. rhamnosus*, *L. bulgaricus* and *B. lactis, Streptococcus thermophilus*, or a cocktail. By 2012, investigation on a formulation containing equal ratios of inulin and FOS improved quality and facilitated the production of cheese with a lower atherogenic index [279]. Supplemented cow milk with polydextrose was enriched with ileal lactobacilli in 24-hour-old piglets on 18 days of consumption. The formula was lower pH because of the presence of lactic acid propionic [279].

14.4.6.1.3 Maintenance of Gut Health and Prevention of, Colitis, and Constipation

Researchers in 2008 established that prebiotics positively affected GALT. Prebiotics are known to specifically modulate the GALT immune parameters [279, 281]. One of the common causes of infant morbidity and mortality is necrotizing clotis huma. *In vivo* experiments have shown that the use of prebiotics can help reduce the incidences of mortality associated with NEC through modulation of the bacterial community of intestine [279]. Prebiotics like FOS were employed in the management of constipation which is a common malady in modern societies caused by low dietary fibers in foods consumed, they are known to increase the fecal bolus and the frequency of deposition [279, 283]. FOS and XOS in combination with zinc were used in human studies for the fortification of ORS to manage dehydration diarrhea in children. The therapy improved water and electrolyte absorption across gut mucosa and inhibited the pathogens with an effect greater than conventional ORS [279].

14.4.6.1.4 Anticancer Agent and Immunopotentiator

Several studies have shown that prebiotics have immunomodulatory properties partly through their ability to influence the physiological properties of immune cells like those of B-lyphocyte, these have made them also useful in the fight against cancer [284, 285]. Also, arabinoxylan oligosaccharides (AXOS)-enriched diet has shown promising results in reducing colon cancer in rats treated with 1,2-dimethylhydrazine [279, 281]. This shows the potential of prebiotics being used in the prevention of colon cancer which is one of the known causes of cancer-associated death in humans. Also, epi lactose produced by cellobiose 2-epimerase from *Ruminococus albus* is a prebiotic that inhibits primary bile salts from converting into secondary bile acids which are promoters of colon cancer [279]. SCFAs formed from the fermentation of GOS also encourage programmed cell death a known body mechanism for the destruction of cancerous cells [279]. Propionate, butyrate, and acetate have been found to play an important role in the immunological response to cancer cells including inflammation, suppressing the expression of transcription factor NF-jB in HT-29 cell lines, increasing the peripheral blood antibody production and NK activity in cancer patients among others [279]. Evidence from different studies from as early as 2010 suggested that prebiotics played a significant role in immune modulation a pathway significant in the fight against carcinogenesis and progress [279].

14.4.6.1.5 Removal of Cholesterol, Reduction of Cardiovascular Disease, and Prevention of Obesity

Prebiotic consumption has been associated with the modification of the gut microbiome and researchers have employed it to improve the microbiota responsible for the production of effects of SCFAs which are responsible for a reduced risk of cardiovascular diseases when one takes prebiotics which is established to be due to the plasma increase in ferulic acid as a result of consumption of high dietary fiber foods. In addition, supplementation with dietary short-chain FOS induces satiety and prevents obesity [279, 281, 286]. Fortifying foods with prebiotics like soy-fortified prebiotics were shown results in improving the serum cholesterol profile, through the reduction of LDL and increasing HDL [279]. Researchers have also explored the use of prebiotics in the prevention and treatment of obesity. NDO like pectic oligosaccharides, FOS, XOS, isomalto-oligosaccharides, manno-oligosaccharides, and other oligosaccharides was assisted in reversing obesity by stimulating favorable microorganisms, reducing the pathogenic microorganisms, and improved glucose homeostasis and lipid metabolism [287].

14.4.6.1.6 Prebiotics and Reproductive Health

Research has established that the female reproductive tract has its microbiome which is up to the uterus whose dysregulation was associated with recurrent implantation failure among others and there is ongoing research to establish the use of prebiotics in their treatment [288, 289]. Research was also shown that the consumption of prebiotics with probiotics restored the normal flora of the vagina which is normally altered in postmenopausal women for example through the use of prebiotic formulations like encapsulation [279, 281].

14.4.6.1.7 Antibiotics Production

This area even though not intensively researched has seen some antibiotics like bacteriocin being produced, Prebiotics like sorbitol, raffinose lactulose, and inulin have been used to influence the production of bacteriocin from organisms like *L. paracasei* CMGB16 and *Pediococcus acidilactici* LAB 5 were purified from products of vacuum-packed fermented meat [279, 281].

14.4.6.1.8 Production of Prebiotics from Food Industry Wastes

Prebiotics were produced from rice husk, wheat bran, finger millet seed coat, rice bran, and tofu that contain NDOs fermentations that improve the absorption of minerals in caecum [279, 281]. Soy sauce saccharides were promoted growth in *L. bulgaricus* and *S. thermophilus* [279, 281]. Bengal wheat bran and gram husk are hydrolyzed disease-causing enzymes and help to extract prebiotic polysaccharides [279]. Hydrothermal treatment of solid wastes from barley processing including spent grain and grain fragments yields XOS which when further refined produces prebiotic formate, butyrate, succinate, propionate, acetate, and lactate [279]. Simultaneous saccharification and solid-state fermentation of apple pomace process potentially prebiotic pectic oligosaccharide. Studies have also shown that mung beans have the potential to improve communities of *L. paracei* [281]. Prebiotics were also produced from date seeds because they are a rich source of flavonoids and phenolic acids. They also possess a high source of insoluble and soluble fiber. Grape seed and mango seed among others are also areas of current research in exploring sources of prebiotics [279, 281]. Research has also explored the production of prebiotics from industrial waste like Brewers Spent grains (for AXOS), and coffee spent grounds (for prebiotic monoligosaccharides) [279, 281].

14.4.6.1.9 Prebiotics from New Novel Sources

Researchers have explored several sources of prebiotics most of these sources are of plant origin however some of these are animal based, for example based on chitin [290]. The root of *Smallanthus sonchifolius* (yacon) a source of traditional food for the Andean population of South America is said to possess prebiotic properties [279]. Yams possess diosgenin, a steroid sapogenin that studies have shown to possess prebiotic properties among other steroidal sapogenins in murine models exhibited properties of restoring fecal LAB associated with food allergic reactions. It hypothesized that blueberry extracts have the potential to improve git health by modifying the gut microbiota [279, 291]. Studies have also shown that bifidobacterial and Lactobacilli have a good response to Vermont peal extract containing pectic oligosaccharides. There have been successful attempts to isolate inulin-type prebiotics from the roots of *Morinda officinale* [279, 292].

Oligosaccharides from dragon fruits have also shown growth-stimulating properties on lactobacilli and bifidobacterial [279, 293]. Glycated pea proteins which are usually not digested by gut enzymes have shown usefulness in providing energy for gut lactobacilli and bifidobacterial this therefore provides a novel source of prebiotics for the improvement of these communities in the gut.

Studies have also found that Selenium-containing green tea contains phenolics and minerals that are prebiotic to specifically *L. rhamnosus* and *B. breve* when added to Mann Rogosa-Sharpe broth. Prebiotic properties of polysaccharides from seaweeds are also a subject of continuous study due to the increasing consumption of seaweeds [279, 294]. Also, sulfated heteropolysaccharide, ulvan from *Ulvan rigid* green algae h are resistant to both gut enzymes and colon bacteria providing an avenue for scientific questions of whether these can be employed as prebiotics [279]. Oligosaccharides from alginate stimulates the growth of *B. bifidum* ATCC 29521 and *B. longum* SMU 27001, decreasing the abundance of Enterobacteriaceae and enterococci [279].

There is also potential for seaweed *Gelidium* CC2253 to be a novel source of prebiotic agar and alginate having low molecular weight polysaccharides with specific positive growth stimulation on Bifidobacteria [279]. Hydrolysis of agarose also produces prebiotic Neoagaro-oligosaccharides (NAOS) which are resistant to upper gut enzymes yet significantly stimulatory to *Bifidobacteria* and *lactobacilli* [279] agave plant a common source of alcoholic beverage tequila is also a potential source of FOS prebiotics [279]. Water-soluble prebiotic compounds were successfully isolated from *Arthropodium cirratum* and *Cordyline australis* plants.

14.4.6.1.10 Prebiotic Supplementation in Food

Prebiotics have been highly researched in improving the quality of food and diet by incorporating them in manufactured food including packaging like edible food packages [295]. Because of the prebiotic importance of *Cyanobacteria Spirulina* sp. It is an important consideration to supplement milk with *Spirulina platensis* dry biomass due to its ability to stimulate the growth of *Lactococcus lactis*, by 27% in concentration of 6 mg/mL [279]. Fibers with elevated viscoelastic properties enhance the sensory appeal of bread, reduce the amount of starch that can be readily digested, and increase the presence of resistant starch, consequently lowering the anticipated glycemic index when assessed *in vitro*. During the bread-making process, researchers studied the on-site production of prebiotic arabinoxylan oligosaccharides (AXOS). Th xylanase from the fungus *Hypocrea jecorina* was used to hydrolyze cereal arabinoxylan which increased AXOS content up to 2.1%. The AXOS-rich rye or wheat bran dough was enhanced the quality of the bread [279]. Additionally, the researchers evaluated the prebiotic effect of fermented cashew apple juice, which contains oligosaccharides. They assessed its impact on the growth of *Lactobacillus johnsonii* B-2178. The study showed that the use of xylanase during bread-making could lead to the production of prebiotic AXOS and the incorporation of rye or wheat bran enhanced bread quality. Furthermore, the prebiotic potential of fermented cashew apple juice, with its oligosaccharide content, was examined in terms of its ability to promote the growth of *Lactobacillus johnsonii* B-2178 [279]. Incorporating prebiotic lactulose into skim milk had several beneficial effects on the fermentation process. Specifically, increased probiotic counts, enhanced acidification rate, higher lactic acid production, and reduced fermentation time [279]. Therefore, the incorporation of prebiotic lactulose into skim milk not only boosted probiotic counts, particularly *B. lactis*, but also accelerated the fermentation process by increasing the acidification rate and lactic acid production, ultimately leading to a shorter fermentation time. This could have practical advantages in the production of fermented dairy products.

Various dehydrated prebiotic fibers, e.g., oat bran, β-glucan, and green banana flour, provided a substrate for microbial adherence, with trehalose serving as a cell protectant to extend the viability of *L. casei* [296]. In sensory evaluations, consumers readily accepted a dairy fruit beverage enriched with prebiotic oat bran. Apple purees enriched with two commercial FOS prebiotics, namely, Beneo GR (inulin) and HSI, remained stable during 30 days of storage at 4°C [297]. However, it's worth noting that substantial quantities of prebiotics were required to achieve their intended prebiotic effects, and high hydrostatic pressure posed a risk of hydrolyzing certain prebiotics [279]. Additionally, a buckwheat-based diet was found to increase the content of aerobic mesophilic and lactic acid bacteria compared to a control diet. This diet also contained beneficial bacteria such as *L. plantarum*, *Bifidobacterium* species, and *B. lactis*, indicating its potential as a prebiotic product [279]

14.4.6.1.11 Prebiotic Production by Various Techniques

The technology for generating oligosaccharides included extraction from plant sources, acid or enzymatic breakdown of polysaccharides [298], or synthesis through transglycosylation reactions [299]. They are usually produced from foods like wheat, soybean, banana, chicory root, honey, Jerusalem artichoke tuber, garlic, onion, rye, asparagus, barley, sugarcane juice, lentils, and milk. However, research is very active in exploring new ways of being able to sustainably produce them [300].

Another approach involves producing prebiotic oligosaccharides through Leuconostoc fermentation, where the polymer size is controlled by adding maltose or galactose. Alternatively, sugar beet pectin can be enzymatically degraded and then fractionated into rhamnogalacturonide and homogalacturonide oligosaccharides by using ion exchange chromatography [279]. Beta-galactosidase sourced from *Aspergillus oryzae* has undergone various immobilization techniques to facilitate the synthesis of

GOS from lactose [301]. Under the most favorable conditions, the conversion rate reached 30%. During sequential batch production, a substantial yield of 8,500g of galactooligosaccharides was obtained per gram of enzyme preparation after ten batches. This yield was projected to rise further with the replacement of the biocatalyst [279].

Thermoanaerobacter ethanolicus JW200 is the source of recombinant alpha-glucosidase that was cloned in *E. coli* and exhibited significant transglycosylation activity in the presence of maltose. The transglucosylation products resulting from this activity were identified as prebiotic isomaltooligosaccharides [279]. The alpha-glucosidase was derived from Bacillus licheniformis TH4-2 and employed to produce trisaccharide oligosaccharide via glucosyl transfer reaction [279, 302]. Levan, a polysaccharide extracted from *Zymomonas mobilis,* was hydrolyzed in an oven and produced oligo-fructans that stimulated probiotic bacteria in the colon of the host [279, 303]. The boiling, roasting, and baking increased resistant starch, followed by shallow frying. In contrast, steaming and frying resulted in a reduction of resistant starch content. Additionally, the analysis of commercial cereal products such as puffed, flaked, and extruded varieties revealed very low levels of retained resistant starch [279].

14.4.6.1.12 Probiotics

14.4.6.1.12.1 Management of IBS and IBD

In as much as there are studies that concluded the use of probiotics in the management of IBD is not enough to make conclusions on the benefits and that more studies are required, there are trials that have proved that numerous products of probiotic strains are useful in the management of IBS. Moreover as recent as 2017, the National Institute for Health and Care Excellence (NICE) established evidence that combination (multi-strain) probiotics significantly improve global IBS symptoms, pain, and bloating compared with placebo [277].

14.4.6.1.12.2 Obesity

In the management of obesity, Randomized Clinical Trials have shown that probiotics as adjuncts to a healthy diet have the potential to reduce weight as a low-risk option compared to conventional drugs that pose significant side effects after long-term use as the course of therapy always requires.

14.4.6.1.12.3 Gut–Brain Axis

Gut–brain axis describes the relationship between the gut microbiota and neuropsychiatric conditions. Other terms like psychobiotics have also been coined to imply studies associated with the gut–brain axis [277, 304]. There is a bilateral communication system between the brain and the gut, that employs neurological, immunological, and hormonal signaling pathways. Research in the field on the gut–brain axis is in rapid evolution although human trials are still limited with only a few studies showing promising results in depression and anxiety [277, 304]. Studies have shown that probiotic supplementation can alter the gut microbiota to ameliorate anxiety-like and depressive-like behavior in mice while other studies have shown that feeding rodents on probiotics is associated with low levels of ACTH, corticosterone, and epinephrine via the hypothalamic-pituitary-adrenal axis which is implicated in stress [277]. 2016 human studies showed that 8 weeks treatment with probiotic *Lactobacillus acidophilus, L. casei,* and *B. bifidum* significant reduction in depressive symptom scores as measured by the Beck's Depression Inventory. Scientific data has put a relationship between migraine and other neurodegenerative and gastrointestinal conditions [304, 305]. These data have been further supported by studies that investigated the effects of a multispecies probiotic supplement on migraine patients where multispecies probiotics provided a statistically and clinically significant reduction in frequency and severity of migraine attacks and reduced weekly abortive drug usage [277]

14.4.6.1.13 Probiotic Strains and Formulations

Due to the health benefits associated with probiotics, researchers have also focused their attention on processing and storage techniques because these have a significant impact on the quality in terms of viability and stability of the probiotic formulation products [306]. Preservation activities in the production of probiotics include drying techniques which may either be spray drying, freeze drying, vacuum drying, or fluidized bed drying. However, at the small laboratory level, the most preferred method of preservation is cryopreservation [306].

Researchers are also studying auxiliary methods that improve the effectiveness of traditional drying methods like fluid bed coating [306]. In addition to the traditional methods above, researchers are also working to develop novel immobilization methods for the preservation of probiotics. Examples of these are the development of two types of electrospun nanofibers: monolithic poly(ethylene oxide) and composite poly(ethylene oxide)/cryoprotectant where *L. plantarum* cells were applied to these nanofibers and achieved high cell concentrations (up to 7.6 × 108 cfu/mg) with promising survival at 25°C, and 3D printing technology for formulating customized products where microcapsules got from traditional drying techniques are used as base for 3D printing with food 3D printer [306].

The development of new applications of probiotics has influenced current research trends. While traditionally dried tableted probiotics were believed to be sufficient for oral administration, applications such as nasal and dermal require specific formulations like creams, lotions with controlled release, and nasal sprays. Since probiotics are usually formulated organisms, researchers and manufacturers are still facing challenges associated with conditions that ensure the viability of the organs in the formulations. These conditions impact the production technology for manufacture and the performance of the probiotic [275].

14.4.6.1.14 Synbiotics

Synbiotics are products composed of both Probiotics and Prebiotics, research has shown that synbiotics were not common in the market about 10 years ago compared to currently. More than 1% of the U.S. population reported consuming non-food synbiotics compared to 5% and 2% probiotics and synbiotics [307, 308].

Soy milk enhanced with FOS and maltodextrin improved the α-galactosidase activity of probiotics like L. acidophilus FTDC 8033, L. acidophilus ATCC 4356, *L. casei* ATCC 393, Bifidobacterium FTDC8943, and *B. longum* FTDC 8643 [309]. By improving their fructose and glucose utilization and hydrolysis abilities [279]. Experiments on cholesterol-lowering properties of symbiotic treatment involving *P. acidilactici* LAB 5 with sorbitol in Swiss albino Wister rats showed cholesterol lowering [279]. Researchers have studied the use of synbiotics in the treatment of type 2 diabetes mellitus where they are associated with disease-modifying factors like weight loss, and insulin sensitivity among others through the regulation of gut microbiota [308].

14.4.6.1.15 Approaches for Symbiotic Formulations Design

Designing of symbiotic formulations has the main challenge of cost associated with clinical trials, preclinical approaches to design and test for potential desired action are always very important and it's a requirement that formulations are compliant with this definition however this has been a challenge because of a deficiency in systematic approaches in formulation definition compliant synbiotics and scientific basis for combining the active components of the formulation is not clear even in the literature [308].

Research in the formulation of synbiotics seeks to establish approaches to make complementary and synergistic prebiotics. These have different factors to consider for example in formulation of complimentary synbiotics depends on the targeted clinical endpoint and the capacity of those components to achieve that endpoint. On the other hand, research on synergistic synbiotics has focused mainly on the ability of the product to exhibit synergistic activity between the probiotic and the substrate through ways like conversion of substrate to useful metabolites that are then used by the probiotics and or commensals [308]. The preclinical approaches currently being used include:

***In vivo* selection (IVS)**, the *in vivo* approach involves the administration of substrate to human subjects to enrich particular bacteria which can then be isolated for culturing and further clinical trial studies [308]. In earlier human studies, GOS was administered to human subjects which enriched *B. adolescentis* IVS-1 by 3% in the colon, this provided a basis for the formulation of GOS-IVS1 symbiotic which studies revealed to possess the ability to improve the IVS1 population by 37 [308].

***In vitro* enrichment (IVE),** this approach employs *in vitro* fecal fermentation enriched with substrate to select bacteria that can be further studied with the respective substrate for culture scale-up. In research studies in 2019, XOS were added to fecal fermentation vessels, followed by daily stepwise dilutions to mimic gastrointestinal flux strains that were able to resist dilution pressure, grow rapidly, persist in the *in vitro* environment, and out-compete commensal microbes for the XOS substrate and further cultured and grown with the respective substrate [308].

Gene-trait matchmaking, which involves matching phenotypic and genotypic properties of putative probiotic strains. Research involved 77 *Lactiplantibacillus plantarum* screened for their ability to grow on a range of prebiotics, including GOS, FOS, inulin, isomaltooligosaccharides (IMO), AXOS, and fucoidan along with characterization of carbohydrate utilization patterns combining strains with specific carbohydrates they utilized suggested formulations for the symbiotic [308].

14.4.6.1.16 Innovative Symbiotic Formulations

Updates in the definition of synbiotics do require the components to completely comply with the definitions of prebiotics and probiotics providing for innovative, ecologically based substrate microbe combinations. Some of these include *L. rhamnosus* GG and arginine, Bifidobacterium longum subsp. *infantis*, plus four so-called next-generation probiotic bacteria, including *Akkermansia muciniphila*, *Clostridium beijerinckii*, *Clostridium butyricum*, and *Anaerobutyricum hallii* [308].

14.4.6.1.17 Conclusion

It is evident that there is significant ongoing research with a focus on the potential health benefits and applications of prebiotics, probiotics, and synbiotics across various fields. They have shown promise in improving gut health, preventing diseases, and even influencing factors like obesity and mental health. Additionally, the development and formulation of these products are continually evolving, with a focus on optimizing their effectiveness and stability.

REFERENCES

[1] F. Zakir, S. Mohapatra, U. Farooq, M. A. Mirza, and Z. Iqbal, "Introduction to metabolic disorders," in *Drug Delivery Systems for Metabolic Disorders*, Edited by Harish Dureja,S. Narasimha Murthy, Peter R. Wich, and Kamal Dua, Elsevier, 2022, pp. 1–20.

[2] S.-H. Ko and H.-S. Kim, "Menopause-associated lipid metabolic disorders and foods beneficial for postmenopausal women," *Nutrients*, vol. 12, no. 1, p. 202, 2020.

[3] M. Marhl, V. Grubelnik, M. Magdič, and R. Markovič, "Diabetes and metabolic syndrome as risk factors for COVID-19," *Diabetes Metab Syndr: Clin Res Rev*, vol. 14, no. 4, pp. 671–677, 2020.

[4] O. Aubi et al., "The Pah-R261Q mouse reveals oxidative stress associated with amyloid-like hepatic aggregation of mutant phenylalanine hydroxylase," *Nat Commun*, vol. 12, no. 1, p. 2073, 2021.

[5] N. A. Elhawary et al., "Genetic etiology and clinical challenges of phenylketonuria," *Hum Genomics*, vol. 16, no. 1, pp. 1–17, 2022.
[6] A. I. Coelho, M. E. Rubio-Gozalbo, J. B. Vicente, and I. Rivera, "Sweet and sour: An update on classic galactosemia," *J Inherit Metab Dis*, vol. 40, no. 3, pp. 325–342, 2017.
[7] I. Badiu Tişa, A. C. Achim, and A. Cozma-Petruţ, "The importance of neonatal screening for galactosemia," *Nutrients*, vol. 15, no. 1, p. 10, 2022.
[8] Y. Li, X. Liu, C.-F. Duan, X.-F. Song, and X.-H. Zhuang, "Brain magnetic resonance imaging findings and radiologic review of maple syrup urine disease: Report of three cases," *World J Clin Cases*, vol. 9, no. 8, p. 1844, 2021.
[9] A. Bharadwaj, N. Wahi, and A. Saxena, "Occurrence of inborn errors of metabolism in newborns, diagnosis and prophylaxis," *Endocrine Metab Immune Disord Drug Targets*, vol. 21, no. 4, pp. 592–616, 2021.
[10] V. Rambani, D. Hromnikova, D. Gasperikova, and M. Skopkova, "Mitochondria and mitochondrial disorders: An overview update," *Endocr Regul*, vol. 56, no. 3, pp. 232–248, 2022.
[11] T. Wong et al., "Mitochondrial diseases in Hong Kong: Prevalence, clinical characteristics and genetic landscape," *Orphanet J Rare Dis*, vol. 18, no. 1, pp. 1–11, 2023.
[12] A. Molares-Vila, A. Corbalán-Rivas, M. Carnero-Gregorio, J. L. González-Cespón, and C. Rodríguez-Cerdeira, "Biomarkers in glycogen storage diseases: An update," *Int J Mol Sci*, vol. 22, no. 9, p. 4381, 2021.
[13] S. B. Wortmann et al., "Treating neutropenia and neutrophil dysfunction in glycogen storage disease type Ib with an SGLT2 inhibitor," *Blood, J Am Soc Hematol*, vol. 136, no. 9, pp. 1033–1043, 2020.
[14] J. A. Bevilacqua et al., "The Latin American experience with a next generation sequencing genetic panel for recessive limb-girdle muscular weakness and Pompe disease," *Orphanet J Rare Dis*, vol. 15, no. 1, pp. 1–11, 2020.
[15] M. K. Pandey, "Exploring pro-inflammatory immunological mediators: Unraveling the mechanisms of neuroinflammation in lysosomal storage diseases," *Biomedicines*, vol. 11, no. 4, p. 1067, 2023.
[16] S. J. Chin and M. Fuller, "Prevalence of lysosomal storage disorders in Australia from 2009 to 2020," *Lancet Reg Health-Western Pacific*, vol. 19, 100344, 2022.
[17] S. Demir, P. P. Nawroth, S. Herzig, and B. Ekim Üstünel, "Emerging targets in type 2 diabetes and diabetic complications," *Adv Sci*, vol. 8, no. 18, p. 2100275, 2021.
[18] N. G. Al-Thobhani, H. Aotoban, K. Al-Handali, Z. Al-Sharafi, and Z. Al-Hamadi, "Design and implementation of a smart WBAN for diabetes management in healthcare," *EasyChair*, Vol. 2022, pp. 1–17, 2022.
[19] H. Sun et al., "IDF diabetes atlas: Global, regional and country-level diabetes prevalence estimates for 2021 and projections for 2045," *Diabetes Res Clin Pract*, vol. 183, p. 109119, 2022.
[20] J. Liu, J. Fu, Y. Jia, N. Yang, J. Li, and G. Wang, "Serum metabolomic patterns in patients with autoimmune thyroid disease," *Endocr Pract*, vol. 26, no. 1, pp. 82–96, 2020.
[21] A. S. Mahmood, A. R. Reyadh, B. Q. Shareef, A. H. Albu-Rghaif, H. A. Al-hussaniy, and M. A. Naji, "Increasing prevalence of congenital hypothyroidism in children with down syndrome who have a family history of thyroid disease," *Res J Pharm Technol*, vol. 16, no. 3, pp. 1327–1332, 2023.
[22] J. Francois et al., "Hypothyroidism and heart failure: Epidemiology, pathogenetic mechanisms & therapeutic rationale," *Int J Clin Res Trials*, vol. 5, no. 1, p. 146, 2020.
[23] E. Di Pierro and F. Granata, "Nutrients and porphyria: An intriguing crosstalk," *Int J Mol Sci*, vol. 21, no. 10, p. 3462, 2020.
[24] L. Diab and N. F. Krebs, "Nutritional disorders," *Dev Behav Pediatr, E-Book*, p. 344, 2022.
[25] C. Meschini et al., "Hip and knee replacement in patients with ochronosis: Clinical experience and literature review," *Orthop Rev (Pavia)*, vol. 12, no. Suppl 1, p. 1062, 2020.
[26] R. Khalil et al., "Variant analysis of alkaptonuria families with significant founder effect in Jordan," *Biomed Res Int*, vol. 2021, pp. 1–9, 2021.
[27] F. Zhang, D. Fan, J. Huang, and T. Zuo, "The gut microbiome: Linking dietary fiber to inflammatory diseases," *Med Microecol*, vol. 2014, p. 100070, 2022.
[28] J. He et al., "Short-chain fatty acids and their association with signalling pathways in inflammation, glucose and lipid metabolism," *Int J Mol Sci*, vol. 21, no. 17, p. 6356, 2020.
[29] H. Han et al., "From gut microbiota to host appetite: Gut microbiota-derived metabolites as key regulators," *Microbiome*, vol. 9, no. 1, pp. 1–16, 2021.
[30] B. Das and G. B. Nair, "Homeostasis and dysbiosis of the gut microbiome in health and disease," *J Biosci*, vol. 44, pp. 1–8, 2019.
[31] C. J. Lee, C. L. Sears, and N. Maruthur, "Gut microbiome and its role in obesity and insulin resistance," *Ann N Y Acad Sci*, vol. 1461, no. 1, pp. 37–52, 2020.
[32] M. Bhagyanathan, D. Dhayanithy, V. Parambath, and R. Bijayraj, "Acanthosis nigricans: A screening test for insulin resistance - An important risk factor for diabetes mellitus type-2," *J Family Med Prim Care*, vol. 6, no. 1, 2017, doi: 10.4103/2249-4863.214961.
[33] A. K. Sikalidis and A. Maykish, "The gut microbiome and type 2 diabetes mellitus: Discussing a complex relationship," *Biomedicines*, vol. 8, no. 1, p. 8, 2020.
[34] B. Allam-Ndoul, S. Castonguay-Paradis, and A. Veilleux, "Gut microbiota and intestinal trans-epithelial permeability," *Int J Mol Sci*, vol. 21, no. 17, p. 6402, 2020.
[35] M. S. Thomas, C. N. Blesso, M. C. Calle, O. K. Chun, M. Puglisi, and M. L. Fernandez, "Dietary influences on gut microbiota with a focus on metabolic syndrome," *Metab Syndr Relat Disord*, vol. 20, no. 8, pp. 429–439, 2022.
[36] T. Liu et al., "The gut microbiota at the intersection of bile acids and intestinal carcinogenesis: An old story, yet mesmerizing," *Int J Cancer*, vol. 146, no. 7, pp. 1780–1790, 2020.
[37] M. Li et al., "Gut microbiota dysbiosis involves in host non-alcoholic fatty liver disease upon pyrethroid pesticide exposure," *Environ Sci Ecotechnol*, vol. 11, p. 100185, 2022.
[38] W. M. de Vos, H. Tilg, M. Van Hul, and P. D. Cani, "Gut microbiome and health: Mechanistic insights," *Gut*, vol. 71, no. 5, pp. 1020–1032, 2022.
[39] S. Caporali et al., "Anti-inflammatory and active biological properties of the plant-derived bioactive compounds luteolin and luteolin 7-glucoside," *Nutrients*, vol. 14, no. 6, p. 1155, 2022.
[40] F. Amati, L. J. McCann, and T. D. Spector, "The gut microbiome, health and personalised nutrition," *Trends Urol Men's Health*, vol. 13, no. 3, pp. 22–25, 2022.
[41] A. R. Kansra, S. Lakkunarajah, and M. S. Jay, "Childhood and adolescent obesity: A review," *Front Pediatr*, vol. 8, p. 866, 2021.

[42] Y. Sarmiento-Andrade, R. Suárez, B. Quintero, K. Garrochamba, and S. P. Chapela, "Gut microbiota and obesity: New insights," *Front Nutr*, vol. 9, p. 1018212, 2022.
[43] A. P. Kaur et al., "Plant prebiotics and their role in the amelioration of diseases," *Biomolecules*, vol. 11, no. 3, p. 440, 2021.
[44] D. Dahiya and P. S. Nigam, "Probiotics, prebiotics, synbiotics, and fermented foods as potential biotics in nutrition improving health via microbiome-gut-brain axis," *Fermentation*, vol. 8, no. 7, p. 303, 2022.
[45] E. Kaewarsar, C. Chaiyasut, N. Lailerd, N. Makhamrueang, S. Peerajan, and S. Sirilun, "Optimization of mixed inulin, fructooligosaccharides, and galactooligosaccharides as prebiotics for stimulation of probiotics growth and function," *Foods*, vol. 12, no. 8, p. 1591, 2023.
[46] FAO/WHO, "Guidelines for the evaluation of probiotics in food: Report of a joint FAO/WHO working group on drafting guidelines for the evaluation of probiotics in food," *World Health Organization and Food and Agriculture Organization of the United Nations, Rome, Italy*, 2002.
[47] D. Kumar et al., "Functional fermented probiotics, prebiotics, and synbiotics from non-dairy products: A perspective from nutraceutical," *Mol Nutr Food Res*, vol. 66, no. 14, p. 2101059, 2022.
[48] M. Yadav et al., "Synbiotics as potent functional food: Recent updates on therapeutic potential and mechanistic insight," *J Food Sci Technol*, vol. 61, no. 1, pp. 1–15, 2022.
[49] G. R. Gibson and M. B. Roberfroid, "Dietary modulation of the human colonic microbiota: Introducing the concept of prebiotics," *J Nutr*, vol. 125, no. 6, pp. 1401–1412, 1995.
[50] M. Pineiro et al., "FAO technical meeting on prebiotics," *J Clin Gastroenterol*, vol. 42, pp. S156–S159, 2008.
[51] M. De Vrese and J. Schrezenmeir, "Probiotics, prebiotics, and synbiotics," *Food Biotechnol*, vol. 111, pp. 1–66, 2008.
[52] K. R. Pandey, S. R. Naik, and B. V Vakil, "Probiotics, prebiotics and synbiotics-a review," *J Food Sci Technol*, vol. 52, pp. 7577–7587, 2015.
[53] R. W. Hutkins et al., "Prebiotics: Why definitions matter," *Curr Opin Biotechnol*, vol. 37, pp. 1–7, 2016.
[54] L. Oliver, H. Rasmussen, M. B. Gregoire, and Y. Chen, "Health care provider's knowledge, perceptions, and use of probiotics and prebiotics," *Top Clin Nutr*, vol. 29, no. 2, pp. 139–149, 2014.
[55] M. Betz, A. Uzueta, H. Rasmussen, M. Gregoire, C. Vanderwall, and G. Witowich, "Knowledge, use and perceptions of probiotics and prebiotics in hospitalised patients," *Nutr Dietetics*, vol. 72, no. 3, pp. 261–266, Sep. 2015, doi: https://doi.org/10.1111/1747-0080.12177.
[56] G. R. Gibson et al., "Dietary prebiotics: Current status and new definition," *Food Sci Technol Bull Funct Foods*, vol. 7, no. 1, pp. 1–19, 2010.
[57] M. Wang and K.-L. Cheong, "Preparation, structural characterisation, and bioactivities of fructans: A review," *Molecules*, vol. 28, no. 4, p. 1613, 2023.
[58] D. Peshev and W. Van den Ende, "Fructans: Prebiotics and immunomodulators," *J Funct Foods*, vol. 8, pp. 348–357, 2014.
[59] E. R. Caleffi et al., "Isolation and prebiotic activity of inulin-type fructan extracted from Pfaffia glomerata (Spreng) Pedersen roots," *Int J Biol Macromol*, vol. 80, pp. 392–399, 2015.
[60] Z. Dai et al., "Immunomodulatory effects of enzymatic-synthesized α-galactooligosaccharides and evaluation of the structure-activity relationship," *J Agric Food Chem*, vol. 66, no. 34, pp. 9070–9079, 2018.
[61] Z. Mei, J. Yuan, and D. Li, "Biological activity of galacto-oligosaccharides: A review," *Front Microbiol*, vol. 13, p. 993052, 2022.
[62] M. J. G. Farthing, "Bugs and the gut: An unstable marriage," *Best Pract Res Clin Gastroenterol*, vol. 18, no. 2, pp. 233–239, 2004.
[63] M. M. R. Do Carmo et al., "Polydextrose: Physiological function, and effects on health," *Nutrients*, vol. 8, no. 9, p. 553, 2016.
[64] D. C. Hernot et al., "*In vitro* fermentation profiles, gas production rates, and microbiota modulation as affected by certain fructans, galactooligosaccharides, and polydextrose," *J Agric Food Chem*, vol. 57, no. 4, pp. 1354–1361, 2009.
[65] Z. Jie et al., "Studies on the effects of polydextrose intake on physiologic functions in Chinese people," *Am J Clin Nutr*, vol. 72, no. 6, pp. 1503–1509, 2000.
[66] D. Davani-Davari et al., "Prebiotics: Definition, types, sources, mechanisms, and clinical applications," *Foods*, vol. 8, no. 3, p. 92, 2019.
[67] B. Gullón, B. Gómez, M. Martínez-Sabajanes, R. Yáñez, J. C. Parajó, and J. L. Alonso, "Pectic oligosaccharides: Manufacture and functional properties," *Trends Food Sci Technol*, vol. 30, no. 2, pp. 153–161, 2013.
[68] G. T. C. Delgado, W. M. S. C. Tamashiro, and G. M. Pastore, "Immunomodulatory effects of fructans," *Food Res Int*, vol. 43, no. 5, pp. 1231–1236, 2010.
[69] A. P. Vos, L. M'rabet, B. Stahl, G. Boehm, and J. Garssen, "Immune-modulatory effects and potential working mechanisms of orally applied nondigestible carbohydrates," *Crit Rev Immunol*, vol. 27, no. 2, pp. 97–140, 2007.
[70] G. Harris, R. KuoLee, and W. Chen, "Role of toll-like receptors in health and diseases of gastrointestinal tract," *World J Gastroenterol*, vol. 12, no. 14, p. 2149, 2006.
[71] L. Vogt et al., "Immune modulation by different types of β2→ 1-fructans is toll-like receptor dependent," *PLoS One*, vol. 8, no. 7, p. e68367, 2013.
[72] M. Asadpoor, G.-N. Ithakisiou, P. A. J. Henricks, R. Pieters, G. Folkerts, and S. Braber, "Non-digestible oligosaccharides and short chain fatty acids as therapeutic targets against enterotoxin-producing bacteria and their toxins," *Toxins (Basel)*, vol. 13, no. 3, p. 175, 2021.
[73] K. Krumova and G. Cosa, "Overview of reactive oxygen species," in *Singlet Oxygen: Applications in Biosciences and Nanosciences*, Edited by Santi Nonell, Cristina Flors, Santi Nonell, and Cristina Flors, vol. 2016, pp. 3–22, 2016.
[74] F. Liu, M. Prabhakar, J. Ju, H. Long, and H. W. Zhou, "Effect of inulin-type fructans on blood lipid profile and glucose level: A systematic review and meta-analysis of randomized controlled trials," *Eur J Clin Nutr*, vol. 71, no. 1, pp. 9–20, 2017.
[75] K. Wang, F. Duan, T. Sun, Y. Zhang, and L. Lu, "Galactooligosaccharides: Synthesis, metabolism, bioactivities and food applications," *Crit Rev Food Sci Nutr*, vol. 12, pp. 1–17, 2023.
[76] J. Wan, L. An, Z. Ren, S. Wang, H. Yang, and J. Ma, "Effects of galactooligosaccharides on maternal gut microbiota, glucose metabolism, lipid metabolism and inflammation in pregnancy: A randomized controlled pilot study," *Front Endocrinol (Lausanne)*, vol. 14, p. 1034266, 2023.

[77] C. M. Whisner et al., "Galacto-oligosaccharides increase calcium absorption and gut bifidobacteria in young girls: A double-blind cross-over trial," *Br J Nutr*, vol. 110, no. 7, pp. 1292–1303, 2013.
[78] M. Ryan-Harshman and W. Aldoori, "Health benefits of selected minerals," *Can Family Physic*, vol. 51, no. 5, p. 673, 2005.
[79] G. Cormick and J. M. Belizán, "Calcium intake and health," *Nutrients*, vol. 11, no. 7, p. 1606, 2019.
[80] C. Gao et al., "Resistant starch ameliorated insulin resistant in patients of type 2 diabetes with obesity: A systematic review and meta-analysis," *Lipids Health Dis*, vol. 18, pp. 1–9, 2019.
[81] Raza, G.S., Putaala, H., Hibberd, A.A., Alhoniemi, E., Tiihonen, K., Mäkelä, K.A. and Herzig, K.H., 2017. Polydextrose changes the gut microbiome and attenuates fasting triglyceride and cholesterol levels in Western diet fed mice. Scientific reports, 7(1), p.5294.
[82] K. Tiihonen, N. Rautonen, E. Alhoniemi, M. Ahotupa, J. Stowell, and T. Vasankari, "Postprandial triglyceride response in normolipidemic, hyperlipidemic and obese subjects-the influence of polydextrose, a non-digestible carbohydrate," *Nutr J*, vol. 14, pp. 1–9, 2015.
[83] E. Konings, P. F. Schoffelen, J. Stegen, and E. E. Blaak, "Effect of polydextrose and soluble maize fibre on energy metabolism, metabolic profile and appetite control in overweight men and women," *Br J Nutr*, vol. 111, no. 1, pp. 111–121, 2014.
[84] A. Act, "Dietary Supplement Health and Education Act of 1994 Public Law 103-417 103rd Congress," *Public Law*, vol. 103, p. 417, 1994.
[85] C. Devine and M. Dikeman, *Encyclopedia of Meat Sciences*. Elsevier, 2014.
[86] T. Shibamoto, K. Kanazawa, F. Shahidi, and C.-T. Ho, "Functional food and health: An overview," vol. 993, pp. 1–6, 2008. https://pubs.acs.org/doi/abs/10.1021/bk-2008-0993.ch001
[87] V. Arwanto et al., "The state of plant-based food development and its prospects in the Indonesia market," *Heliyon*, vol. 8, no. 10, pp. e11062, 2022.
[88] E. C. Ale and A. G. Binetti, "Role of probiotics, prebiotics, and synbiotics in the elderly: Insights into their applications," *Front Microbiol*, vol. 12, p. 631254, 2021.
[89] D. Guidance, "Complementary and alternative medicine products and their regulation by the food and drug administration," 2006. https://www.regulations.gov/docket/FDA-2006-D-0102.
[90] G. Precup, C. B. Pocol, B.-E. Teleky, and D. C. Vodnar, "Awareness, knowledge, and interest about prebiotics-a study among Romanian consumers," Int J Environ Res Public Health, vol. 19, no. 3, p. 1208, 2022.
[91] V. Venugopalan, K. A. Shriner, and A. Wong-Beringer, "Regulatory oversight and safety of probiotic use," Emerg Infect Dis, vol. 16, no. 11, p. 1661, 2010.
[92] P. O. Lelia and R. Suharoschi, "Emerging food processing technologies: Probiotics and prebiotics," in Nutraceutical and Functional Food Components, Elsevier, 2022, pp. 509–536.
[93] A. Anadón, M. R. Martínez-Larrañaga, I. Ares, and M. A. Martínez, "Probiotics: Safety and toxicity considerations," *Nutraceuticals*, 2021, [Online]. Available: https://api.semanticscholar.org/CorpusID:235913433
[94] G. Reid et al., "New scientific paradigms for probiotics and prebiotics," *J Clin Gastroenterol*, vol. 37, no. 2, pp. 105–118, 2003.
[95] A. Hernandez Jerez and F. Gil, "Nutraceuticals and adverse outcome pathways," 2021, pp. 1159–1174. doi: 10.1016/B978-0-12-821038-3.00069-0.
[96] J. Gu and K. Roberts, "Probiotics and prebiotics," in Adult Short Bowel Syndrome, Elsevier, vol. 2019, pp. 67–80, 2019.
[97] R. R. Watson and V. R. Preedy, Bioactive *F*ood as *D*ietary *I*nterventions for *L*iver and *G*astrointestinal *D*isease*:* *B*ioactive *F*oods in *C*hronic *D*isease *S*tates. Academic Press, 2012.
[98] T. Karakan, M. Ergun, I. Dogan, M. Cindoruk, and S. Unal, "Comparison of early enteral nutrition in severe acute pancreatitis with prebiotic fiber supplementation versus standard enteral solution: A prospective randomized double-blind study," World J *Gastroenterol*, vol. 13, no. 19, p. 2733, 2007.
[99] C. A. Daubioul, Y. Horsmans, P. Lambert, E. Danse, and N. M. Delzenne, "Effects of oligofructose on glucose and lipid metabolism in patients with nonalcoholic steatohepatitis: Results of a pilot study," *Eur J Clin Nutr*, vol. 59, no. 5, pp. 723–726, 2005.
[100] G. Fanelli and A. Serretti, "Depression, antidepressants, and insulin resistance: Which link?," *Eur* Neuropsychopharmacol, vol. 60, pp. 4–6, 2022.
[101] P. S. Panesar, V. Bali, S. Kumari, N. Babbar, and H. S. Oberoi, "Prebiotics," in Biotransformation of *W*aste *B*iomass into *H*igh *V*alue *B*iochemicals, vol. 2013, pp. 237–259, Springer, New York, 2014.
[102] M. Roberfroid et al., "Prebiotic effects: Metabolic and health benefits," *Br J Nutr*, vol. 104, no. S2, pp. S1–S63, 2010.
[103] I. H. R. Paiva, E. Duarte-Silva, and C. A. Peixoto, "The role of prebiotics in cognition, anxiety, and depression," *Eur Neuropsychopharmacol*, vol. 34, pp. 1–18, 2020.
[104] A. A. Gadir, R. Dhir, and G. Reid, "Probiotics: Reiterating what they are and what they are not," *Front Microbiol*, vol. 10, March 2019.
[105] N. T. Williams, "Probiotics," Am *J Health-Sys Pharm*, vol. 67, no. 6, pp. 449–458, 2010.
[106] G. Friedman, "The role of probiotics in the prevention and treatment of antibiotic-associated diarrhea and Clostridium difficile colitis," *Gastroenterol Clinic*, vol. 41, no. 4, pp. 763–779, 2012.
[107] A. Staniszewski and M. Kordowska-Wiater, "Probiotic and potentially probiotic yeasts-characteristics and food application," *Foods*, vol. 10, no. 6, p. 1306, 2021.
[108] S. H. Downs and N. Black, "The feasibility of creating a checklist for the assessment of the methodological quality both of randomised and non-randomised studies of health care interventions," J Epidemiol Community Health (1978), vol. 52, no. 6, pp. 377–384, 1998.
[109] G. V. Zuccotti et al., "Probiotics in clinical practice: An overview," J *I*nt *M*ed *R*es, vol. 36, no. 1_suppl, pp. 1A–53A, 2008.
[110] S. J. Allen et al., "Lactobacilli and bifidobacteria in the prevention of antibiotic-associated diarrhoea and Clostridium difficile diarrhoea in older inpatients (PLACIDE): A randomised, double-blind, placebo-controlled, multicentre trial," *The Lancet*, vol. 382, no. 9900, pp. 1249–1257, 2013.
[111] J. Plaza-Diaz, F. J. Ruiz-Ojeda, M. Gil-Campos, and A. Gil, "Mechanisms of action of probiotics," Advances in *N*utr, vol. 10, no. suppl_1, pp. S49–S66, 2019.

[112] A. Hashemi, C. R. Villa, and E. M. Comelli, "Probiotics in early life: A preventative and treatment approach," *Food* Funct, vol. 7, no. 4, pp. 1752–1768, 2016.

[113] M. Olivares et al., "Oral administration of two probiotic strains, *Lactobacillus gasseri* CECT5714 and *Lactobacillus coryniformis* CECT5711, enhances the intestinal function of healthy adults," Int J Food Microbiol, vol. 107, no. 2, pp. 104–111, 2006.

[114] M. Bermudez-Brito, J. Plaza-Díaz, S. Muñoz-Quezada, C. Gómez-Llorente, and A. Gil, "Probiotic mechanisms of action," Ann Nutr Metab, vol. 61, no. 2, pp. 160–174, 2012.

[115] J. Plaza-Díaz, F. J. Ruiz-Ojeda, M. Gil-Campos, and A. Gil, "Immune-mediated mechanisms of action of probiotics and synbiotics in treating pediatric intestinal diseases," *Nutrients*, vol. 10, no. 1, p. 42, 2018.

[116] S. Munoz-Quezada et al., "Competitive inhibition of three novel bacteria isolated from faeces of breast milk-fed infants against selected enteropathogens," Br *J N*utr, vol. 109, no. S2, pp. S63–S69, 2013.

[117] M. Kumar et al., "Probiotic metabolites as epigenetic targets in the prevention of colon cancer," *Nutr Rev*, vol. 71, no. 1, pp. 23–34, 2013.

[118] L. Dicks and M. Botes, "Probiotic lactic acid bacteria in the gastro-intestinal tract: Health benefits, safety and mode of action," *Benef Microbes*, vol. 1, no. 1, pp. 11–29, 2010.

[119] C. Buss, C. Valle-Tovo, S. Miozzo, and A. A. de Mattos, "Probiotics and synbiotics may improve liver aminotransferases levels in non-alcoholic fatty liver disease patients," *Ann Hepatol*, vol. 13, no. 5, pp. 482–488, 2014.

[120] V. Castillo, F. Figueroa, K. González-Pizarro, P. Jopia, and C. Ibacache-Quiroga, "Probiotics and prebiotics as a strategy for non-alcoholic fatty liver disease, a narrative review," *Foods*, vol. 10, no. 8, p. 1719, 2021.

[121] W. Xing et al., "The effects of supplementation of probiotics, prebiotics, or synbiotics on patients with non-alcoholic fatty liver disease: A meta-analysis of randomized controlled trials," *Front Nutr*, vol. 9, p. 1024678, 2022.

[122] N. Pavlović, K. Stankov, and M. Mikov, "Probiotics-interactions with bile acids and impact on cholesterol metabolism," *Appl Biochem Biotechnol*, vol. 168, pp. 1880–1895, 2012.

[123] R. Kumar, S. Grover, and V. K. Batish, "Hypocholesterolaemic effect of dietary inclusion of two putative probiotic bile salt hydrolase-producing *Lactobacillus plantarum* strains in Sprague-Dawley rats," *Br J Nutr*, vol. 105, no. 4, pp. 561–573, 2011.

[124] P. Markowiak-Kopeć and K. Śliżewska, "The effect of probiotics on the production of short-chain fatty acids by human intestinal microbiome," *Nutrients*, vol. 12, no. 4, p. 1107, 2020.

[125] J. Eastwood et al., "The effect of probiotic bacteria on composition and metabolite production of faecal microbiota using *in vitro* batch cultures," *Nutrients*, vol. 15, no. 11, p. 2563, 2023.

[126] C. Ferrario et al., "Modulation of fecal *Clostridiales bacteria* and butyrate by probiotic intervention with *Lactobacillus paracasei* DG varies among healthy adults," *J Nutr*, vol. 144, no. 11, pp. 1787–1796, 2014.

[127] S. Sierra, F. Lara-Villoslada, L. Sempere, M. Olivares, J. Boza, and J. Xaus, "Intestinal and immunological effects of daily oral administration of *Lactobacillus salivarius* CECT5713 to healthy adults," *Anaerobe*, vol. 16, no. 3, pp. 195–200, 2010.

[128] S. Macfarlane, S. Cleary, B. Bahrami, N. Reynolds, and G. T. Macfarlane, "Synbiotic consumption changes the metabolism and composition of the gut microbiota in older people and modifies inflammatory processes: A randomised, double-blind, placebo-controlled crossover study," Aliment Pharmacol Ther, vol. 38, no. 7, pp. 804–816, 2013.

[129] S. Macfarlane and G. T. Macfarlane, "Regulation of short-chain fatty acid production," Proc *Nutr Soc*, vol. 62, no. 1, pp. 67–72, 2003.

[130] S. M. Schneider et al., "Effects of *Saccharomyces boulardii* on fecal short-chain fatty acids and microflora in patients on long-term total enteral nutrition," World *J G*astroenterol, vol. 11, no. 39, p. 6165, 2005.

[131] C. C. Butler et al., "Effect of probiotic use on antibiotic administration among care home residents: A randomized clinical trial," *JAMA*, vol. 324, no. 1, pp. 47–56, 2020.

[132] G. Riezzo et al., "Randomised clinical trial: Efficacy of *Lactobacillus paracasei*-enriched artichokes in the treatment of patients with functional constipation-a double-blind, controlled, crossover study," Aliment Pharmacol Ther, vol. 35, no. 4, pp. 441–450, 2012.

[133] M. J. Sáez-Lara, C. Robles-Sanchez, F. J. Ruiz-Ojeda, J. Plaza-Diaz, and A. Gil, "Effects of probiotics and synbiotics on obesity, insulin resistance syndrome, type 2 diabetes and non-alcoholic fatty liver disease: A review of human clinical trials," *Int J Mol Sci*, vol. 17, no. 6, p. 928, 2016.

[134] J. Maldonado et al., "Safety and tolerance of the human milk probiotic strain *Lactobacillus salivarius* CECT5713 in 6-month-old children," *Nutrition*, vol. 26, no. 11–12, pp. 1082–1087, 2010.

[135] M. A. Underwood et al., "A randomized placebo-controlled comparison of 2 prebiotic/probiotic combinations in preterm infants: Impact on weight gain, intestinal microbiota, and fecal short-chain fatty acids," J Pediatr Gastroenterol Nutr, vol. 48, no. 2, pp. 216–225, 2009.

[136] K. Nishiyama, M. Sugiyama, and T. Mukai, "Adhesion properties of lactic acid bacteria on intestinal mucin," *Microorganisms*, vol. 4, no. 3, p. 34, 2016.

[137] T. K. Das, S. Pradhan, S. Chakrabarti, K. C. Mondal, and K. Ghosh, "Current status of probiotic and related health benefits," *Applied Food Research*, p. 100185, 2022.

[138] H.-Z. Gou, Y.-L. Zhang, L.-F. Ren, Z.-J. Li, and L. Zhang, "How do intestinal probiotics restore the intestinal barrier?," *Front Microbiol*, vol. 13, p. 929346, 2022.

[139] J. Zheng et al., "*Lactobacillus rhamnosus* CY12 enhances intestinal barrier function by regulating tight junction protein expression, oxidative stress, and inflammation response in lipopolysaccharide-induced caco-2 cells," *Int J Mol Sci*, vol. 23, no. 19, p. 11162, 2022.

[140] Z. Mujagic et al., "The effects of *Lactobacillus plantarum* on small intestinal barrier function and mucosal gene transcription; a randomized double-blind placebo controlled trial," *Sci Rep*, vol. 7, no. 1, p. 40128, 2017.

[141] P. D'Amelio and F. Sassi, "Gut microbiota, immune system, and bone," Calcif Tissue Int, vol. 102, pp. 415–425, 2018.

[142] K. M. Maslowski and C. R. Mackay, "Diet, gut microbiota and immune responses," *Nat* Immunol, vol. 12, no. 1, pp. 5–9, 2011.

[143] C. Gómez-Llorente, S. Munoz, and A. Gil, "Role of Toll-like receptors in the development of immunotolerance mediated by probiotics," Proc *Nutr Soc*, vol. 69, no. 3, pp. 381–389, 2010.

[144] R. H. McCusker and K. W. Kelley, "Immune-neural connections: How the immune system's response to infectious agents influences behavior," J *Experiment Biol*, vol. 216, no. 1. 2013. doi: 10.1242/jeb.073411.

[145] A.-K. Claes, J. Y. Zhou, and D. J. Philpott, "NOD-like receptors: Guardians of intestinal mucosal barriers," *Physiology*, vol. 30, no. 3, pp. 241–250, 2015.

[146] A. Hevia, S. Delgado, B. Sánchez, and A. Margolles, "Molecular players involved in the interaction between beneficial bacteria and the immune system," *Front Microbiol*, vol. 6, p. 1285, 2015.

[147] G. Giorgetti et al., "Interactions between innate immunity, microbiota, and probiotics," *J Immunol Res*, vol. 2015, pp. 1–8, 2015.

[148] H. Wang et al., "*Lactobacillus rhamnosus* GG modulates innate signaling pathway and cytokine responses to rotavirus vaccine in intestinal mononuclear cells of gnotobiotic pigs transplanted with human gut microbiota," *BMC Microbiol*, vol. 16, no. 1, pp. 1–14, 2016.

[149] S.-H. Huang, L. He, Y. Zhou, C.-H. Wu, and A. Jong, "*Lactobacillus rhamnosus* GG suppresses meningitic *E. coli* K1 penetration across human intestinal epithelial cells *in vitro* and protects neonatal rats against experimental hematogenous meningitis," *Int* J Microbiol, vol. 2009, pp. 647862, 2009.

[150] L. S. Harbige, E. Pinto, J. Allgrove, and L. V Thomas, "Immune response of healthy adults to the ingested probiotic *Lactobacillus casei* Shirota," *Scand J Immunol*, vol. 84, no. 6, pp. 353–364, 2016.

[151] G. Garcia, C. Dogi, A. De Moreno de LeBlanc, C. Greco, and L. Cavaglieri, "Gut-borne Saccharomyces cerevisiae, a promising candidate for the formulation of feed additives, modulates immune system and gut microbiota," *Benef Microbes*, vol. 7, no. 5, pp. 659–668, 2016.

[152] J. Tung et al., "Social networks predict gut microbiome composition in wild baboons," *Elife*, vol. 4, p. e05224, 2015.

[153] K. Tillisch et al., "Consumption of fermented milk product with probiotic modulates brain activity," *Gastroenterology*, vol. 144, no. 7, pp. 1394–1401, 2013.

[154] X. Cong et al., "Focus: Microbiome: Gut microbiome and infant health: Brain-gut-microbiota axis and host genetic factors," Yale J Biol Med, vol. 89, no. 3, p. 299, 2016.

[155] S. Huang, C. P. Zhang, K. Wang, G. Q. Li, and F. L. Hu, "Recent advances in the chemical composition of propolis," *Molecules*, vol. 19, no. 12. MDPI AG, pp. 19610–19632, Dec. 01, 2014. doi: 10.3390/molecules191219610.

[156] G. Akarca, M. Kilinç, and A. J. Denizkara, "Quality specification of ice creams produced with different homofermentative lactic acid bacteria," Food Sci Nutr, vol. 12, no. 1, pp. 192–103, 2023.

[157] M. Youssef et al., "Probiotic supplements: Their strategies in the therapeutic and prophylactic of human life-threatening diseases," Int J Mol Sci, vol. 22, no. 20, p. 11290, 2021.

[158] A. Polo et al., "Novel fermented ice cream formulations with Improved antiradical and anti-inflammatory features," *Fermentation*, vol. 9, no. 2, p. 117, 2023.

[159] H. Goktas, "Enrichment of antioxidant activity of ıce cream samples with addition of rowanberry (*Sorbus aucuparia* L.) pulp and production of functional probiotic ice cream with using L. rhamnosus," Int J Food Sci Technol, vol. 58, pp. 2962–5971, 2023.

[160] C. H. Halsted, "Dietary supplements and functional foods: 2 sides of a coin?," Am J Clin Nutr, vol. 77, no. 4, pp. 1001S–1007S, 2003.

[161] H. Goktas, H. Dikmen, H. Bekiroglu, N. Cebi, E. Dertli, and O. Sagdic, "Characteristics of functional ice cream produced with probiotic *Saccharomyces boulardii* in combination with *Lactobacillus rhamnosus* GG," *Lwt*, vol. 153, p. 112489, 2022.

[162] A. Sadeghi, M. Ebrahimi, S. Shahryari, M. S. Kharazmi, and S. M. Jafari, "Food applications of probiotic yeasts; focusing on their techno-functional, postbiotic and protective capabilities," Trends Food Sci Technol, vol. 128, pp. 278–295, 2022.

[163] D. Kothari, S. Patel, and S.-K. Kim, "Probiotic supplements might not be universally-effective and safe: A review," *Biomed Pharmacother*, vol. 111, pp. 537–547, 2019.

[164] W. Fiore, S. Arioli, and S. Guglielmetti, "The neglected microbial components of commercial probiotic formulations," *Microorganisms*, vol. 8, no. 8, p. 1177, 2020.

[165] S. J. Lahtinen, R. J. Boyle, A. Margolles, R. Frias, and M. Gueimonde, "Safety assessment of probiotics," in Prebiotics and Probiotics Science and Technology, 2009, pp. 1193–1235, Springer, New York, 2009. https://doi.org/10.1007/978-0-387-79058-9_31

[166] J. Xiao et al., "Long-term probiotic intervention mitigates memory dysfunction through a novel H3K27me3-based mechanism in lead-exposed rats," *Transl Psychiatry*, vol. 10, no. 1, p. 25, 2020.

[167] A. L. Roe et al., "Considerations for determining safety of probiotics: A USP perspective," Regul *Toxicol Pharmacol*, vol. 136, p. 105266, 2022.

[168] G. Wang, Y. Chen, Y. Xia, X. Song, and L. Ai, "Characteristics of probiotic preparations and their applications," *Foods*, vol. 11, no. 16, p. 2472, 2022.

[169] K. Fenster, B. Freeburg, C. Hollard, C. Wong, R. Rønhave Laursen, and A. C. Ouwehand, "The production and delivery of probiotics: A review of a practical approach," *Microorganisms*, vol. 7, no. 3, p. 83, 2019.

[170] M. Arora and A. Baldi, "Regulatory categories of probiotics across the globe: A review representing existing and recommended categorization," Indian J Med Microbiol, vol. 33, pp. S2–S10, 2015.

[171] J. J. Faith et al., "The long-term stability of the human gut microbiota," *Science* (1979), vol. 341, no. 6141, p. 1237439, 2013.

[172] M. X. Maldonado-Gómez et al., "Stable engraftment of *Bifidobacterium longum* AH1206 in the human gut depends on individualized features of the resident microbiome," *Cell Host Microbe*, vol. 20, no. 4, pp. 515–526, 2016.

[173] Y. Xiao, J. Zhao, H. Zhang, Q. Zhai, and W. Chen, "Mining Lactobacillus and Bifidobacterium for organisms with long-term gut colonization potential," *Clin Nutr*, vol. 39, no. 5, pp. 1315–1323, 2020.

[174] K. Charteris and C. Morelli, "Development and application of an *in vitro* methodology to determine the transit tolerance of potentially probiotic *Lactobacillus* and *Bifidobacterium* species in the upper human gastrointestinal tract," J Appl Microbiol, vol. 84, no. 5, pp. 759–768, 1998.

[175] Y. Huang and M. C. Adams, "*In vitro* assessment of the upper gastrointestinal tolerance of potential probiotic dairy propionibacteria," Int J Food Microbiol, vol. 91, no. 3, pp. 253–260, 2004.

[176] G. Li et al., "The effects of probiotics supplementation on glycaemic control among adults with type 2 diabetes mellitus: A systematic review and meta-analysis of randomised clinical trials," *J Transl Med*, vol. 21, no. 1, p. 442, 2023.

[177] E. Razmpoosh, A. Javadi, H. S. Ejtahed, P. Mirmiran, M. Javadi, and A. Yousefinejad, "The effect of probiotic supplementation on glycemic control and lipid profile in

patients with type 2 diabetes: A randomized placebo controlled trial," Diabet *Metab Syndr: Clin Res Rev*, vol. 13, no. 1, pp. 175–182, 2019.
[178] S. Sabico et al., "Effects of a multi-strain probiotic supplement for 12 weeks in circulating endotoxin levels and cardiometabolic profiles of medication naïve T2DM patients: A randomized clinical trial," *J Transl Med*, vol. 15, no. 1, pp. 1–9, 2017.
[179] S. Sabico et al., "Effects of a 6-month multi-strain probiotics supplementation in endotoxemic, inflammatory and cardiometabolic status of T2DM patients: A randomized, double-blind, placebo-controlled trial," *Clin Nutr*, vol. 38, no. 4, pp. 1561–1569, 2019.
[180] M.-C. Hsieh et al., "The beneficial effects of *Lactobacillus reuteri* ADR-1 or ADR-3 consumption on type 2 diabetes mellitus: A randomized, double-blinded, placebo-controlled trial," *Sci Rep*, vol. 8, no. 1, p. 16791, 2018.
[181] N. Kobyliak, T. Falalyeyeva, N. Boyko, O. Tsyryuk, T. Beregova, and L. Ostapchenko, "Probiotics and nutraceuticals as a new frontier in obesity prevention and management," Diabetes Res Clin Pract, vol. 141, pp. 190–199, 2018.
[182] B. Abbasi, R. Ghiasvand, and M. Mirlohi, "Kidney function improvement by soy milk containing *Lactobacillus plantarum* A7 in type 2 diabetic patients with nephropathy: A double-blinded randomized controlled trial," Iran J Kidney Dis, vol. 11, no. 1, pp. 36–43, 2017.
[183] Z. S. Ebrahimi, E. Nasli-Esfahani, A. Nadjarzade, and H. Mozaffari-Khosravi, "Effect of symbiotic supplementation on glycemic control, lipid profiles and microalbuminuria in patients with non-obese type 2 diabetes: A randomized, double-blind, clinical trial," J Diabetes Metab Disord, vol. 16, pp. 1–10, 2017.
[184] S. Firouzi, H. A. Majid, A. Ismail, N. A. Kamaruddin, and M.-Y. Barakatun-Nisak, "Effect of multi-strain probiotics (multi-strain microbial cell preparation) on glycemic control and other diabetes-related outcomes in people with type 2 diabetes: A randomized controlled trial," *Eur* J Nutr, vol. 56, pp. 1535–1550, 2017.
[185] R. Mobini et al., "Metabolic effects of *Lactobacillus reuteri* DSM 17938 in people with type 2 diabetes: A randomized controlled trial," Diabetes Obes Metab, vol. 19, no. 4, pp. 579–589, 2017.
[186] J. Sato et al., "Probiotic reduces bacterial translocation in type 2 diabetes mellitus: A randomised controlled study," *Sci Rep*, vol. 7, no. 1, p. 12115, 2017.
[187] L. B. Tonucci, K. M. O. Dos Santos, L. L. de Oliveira, S. M. R. Ribeiro, and H. S. D. Martino, "Clinical application of probiotics in type 2 diabetes mellitus: A randomized, double-blind, placebo-controlled study," *Clin Nutr*, vol. 36, no. 1, pp. 85–92, 2017.
[188] M. Rezaei, A. Sanagoo, L. Jouybari, N. Behnampoo, and A. Kavosi, "The effect of probiotic yogurt on blood glucose and cardiovascular biomarkers in patients with type II diabetes: A randomized controlled trial," *Evidence Based Care*, vol. 6, no. 4, pp. 26–35, 2017.
[189] Z. Asemi, S. Bahmani, H. Shakeri, A. Jamal, and A.-M. Faraji, "Effect of multispecies probiotic supplements on serum minerals, liver enzymes and blood pressure in patients with type 2 diabetes," Int J Diabetes Dev Ctries, vol. 35, pp. 90–95, 2015.
[190] Z. Asemi, Z. Zare, H. Shakeri, S. Sabihi, and A. Esmaillzadeh, "Effect of multispecies probiotic supplements on metabolic profiles, hs-CRP, and oxidative stress in patients with type 2 diabetes," Ann Nutr Metab, vol. 63, no. 1–2, pp. 1–9, 2013.
[191] Z. Asemi, A. Khorrami-Rad, S.-A. Alizadeh, H. Shakeri, and A. Esmaillzadeh, "Effects of synbiotic food consumption on metabolic status of diabetic patients: A double-blind randomized cross-over controlled clinical trial," *Clin Nutr*, vol. 33, no. 2, pp. 198–203, 2014.
[192] M. S. Alokail et al., "Effects of probiotics in patients with diabetes mellitus type 2: Study protocol for a randomized, double-blind, placebo-controlled trial," *Trials*, vol. 14, pp. 1–8, 2013.
[193] H. S. Ejtahed et al., "Effect of probiotic yogurt containing *Lactobacillus acidophilus* and *Bifidobacterium lactis* on lipid profile in individuals with type 2 diabetes mellitus," *J Dairy Sci*, vol. 94, no. 7, pp. 3288–3294, 2011.
[194] H. S. Ejtahed, J. Mohtadi-Nia, A. Homayouni-Rad, M. Niafar, M. Asghari-Jafarabadi, and V. Mofid, "Probiotic yogurt improves antioxidant status in type 2 diabetic patients," *Nutrition*, vol. 28, no. 5, pp. 539–543, 2012.
[195] C. Moroti, L. F. Souza Magri, M. de Rezende Costa, D. C. U. Cavallini, and K. Sivieri, "Effect of the consumption of a new symbiotic shake on glycemia and cholesterol levels in elderly people with type 2 diabetes mellitus," Lipids Health Dis, vol. 11, pp. 1–8, 2012.
[196] N. Kobyliak et al., "Probiotics in prevention and treatment of obesity: A critical view," Nutr Metab (Lond*)*, vol. 13, no. 1, pp. 1–13, 2016.
[197] M. Wiciński, J. Gębalski, J. Gołębiewski, and B. Malinowski, "Probiotics for the treatment of overweight and obesity in humans-a review of clinical trials," *Microorganisms*, vol. 8, no. 8, p. 1148, 2020.
[198] A. Alisi et al., "Randomised clinical trial: The beneficial effects of VSL# 3 in obese children with non-alcoholic steatohepatitis," Aliment Pharmacol Ther, vol. 39, no. 11, pp. 1276–1285, 2014.
[199] F. Famouri, Z. Shariat, M. Hashemipour, M. Keikha, and R. Kelishadi, "Effects of probiotics on nonalcoholic fatty liver disease in obese children and adolescents," J Pediatr Gastroenterol Nutr, vol. 64, no. 3, pp. 413–417, 2017.
[200] J. Sanchis-Chordà, E. M. G. Del Pulgar, J. Carrasco-Luna, A. Benítez-Páez, Y. Sanz, and P. Codoñer-Franch, "*Bifidobacterium pseudocatenulatum* CECT 7765 supplementation improves inflammatory status in insulin-resistant obese children," *Eur J Nutr*, vol. 58, pp. 2789–2800, 2019.
[201] A. C. Gomes, R. G. M. de Sousa, P. B. Botelho, T. L. N. Gomes, P. O. Prada, and J. F. Mota, "The additional effects of a probiotic mix on abdominal adiposity and antioxidant Status: A double-blind, randomized trial," *Obesity*, vol. 25, no. 1, pp. 30–38, 2017.
[202] F. Higashikawa et al., "Antiobesity effect of *Pediococcus pentosaceus* LP28 on overweight subjects: A randomized, double-blind, placebo-controlled clinical trial," Eur J Clin Nutr, vol. 70, no. 5, pp. 582–587, 2016.
[203] S. Jung et al., "Supplementation with two probiotic strains, *Lactobacillus curvatus* HY7601 and *Lactobacillus plantarum* KY1032, reduced body adiposity and Lp-PLA2 activity in overweight subjects," *J Funct Foods*, vol. 19, pp. 744–752, 2015.
[204] S.-P. Jung et al., "Effect of *Lactobacillus gasseri* BNR17 on overweight and obese adults: A randomized, double-blind clinical trial," Korean J Fam Med, vol. 34, no. 2, p. 80, 2013.
[205] J. Minami et al., "Effects of *Bifidobacterium breve* B-3 on body fat reductions in pre-obese adults: A randomized, double-blind, placebo-controlled trial," Biosci Microbiota Food Health, vol. 37, no. 3, pp. 67–75, 2018.

[206] A. Pedret et al., "Effects of daily consumption of the probiotic *Bifidobacterium animalis* subsp. lactis CECT 8145 on anthropometric adiposity biomarkers in abdominally obese subjects: A randomized controlled trial," *Int J Obes*, vol. 43, no. 9, pp. 1863–1868, 2019.
[207] M. Sanchez et al., "Effects of a diet-based weight-reducing program with probiotic supplementation on satiety efficiency, eating behaviour traits, and psychosocial behaviours in obese individuals," *Nutrients*, vol. 9, no. 3, p. 284, 2017.
[208] M. Szulińska, I. Łoniewski, S. Van Hemert, M. Sobieska, and P. Bogdański, "Dose-dependent effects of multispecies probiotic supplementation on the lipopolysaccharide (LPS) level and cardiometabolic profile in obese postmenopausal women: A 12-week randomized clinical trial," *Nutrients*, vol. 10, no. 6, p. 773, 2018.
[209] H.-S. Ejtahed et al., "Probiotics supplementation for the obesity management; A systematic review of animal studies and clinical trials," *J Funct Foods*, vol. 52, pp. 228–242, 2019.
[210] S. Nagata, Y. Chiba, C. Wang, and Y. Yamashiro, "The effects of the *Lactobacillus casei* strain on obesity in children: A pilot study," *Benef Microbes*, vol. 8, no. 4, pp. 535–543, 2017.
[211] M. Safavi, S. Farajian, R. Kelishadi, M. Mirlohi, and M. Hashemipour, "The effects of synbiotic supplementation on some cardio-metabolic risk factors in overweight and obese children: A randomized triple-masked controlled trial," Int J Food Sci Nutr, vol. 64, no. 6, pp. 687–693, 2013.
[212] Z.-B. Wang et al., "The potential role of probiotics in controlling overweight/obesity and associated metabolic parameters in adults: A systematic review and meta-analysis," Evidence-Based Complementary Altern Med, vol. 2019, pp. 3862971, 2019.
[213] Z. Karbaschian et al., "Probiotic supplementation in morbid obese patients undergoing one anastomosis gastric bypass-mini gastric bypass (OAGB-MGB) surgery: A randomized, double-blind, placebo-controlled, clinical trial," *Obes Surg*, vol. 28, pp. 2874–2885, 2018.
[214] R. Kelishadi, S. Farajian, M. Safavi, M. Mirlohi, and M. Hashemipour, "A randomized triple-masked controlled trial on the effects of synbiotics on inflammation markers in overweight children," J Pediatr (Rio J), vol. 90, pp. 161–167, 2014.
[215] J. Ilmonen, E. Isolauri, T. Poussa, and K. Laitinen, "Impact of dietary counselling and probiotic intervention on maternal anthropometric measurements during and after pregnancy: A randomized placebo-controlled trial," *Clin Nutr*, vol. 30, no. 2, pp. 156–164, 2011.
[216] R. Luoto, K. Laitinen, M. Nermes, and E. Isolauri, "Impact of maternal probiotic-supplemented dietary counselling on pregnancy outcome and prenatal and postnatal growth: A double-blind, placebo-controlled study," Br *J N*utr, vol. 103, no. 12, pp. 1792–1799, 2010.
[217] K. Śliżewska, P. Markowiak-Kopeć, and W. Śliżewska, "The role of probiotics in cancer prevention," *Cancers (*Basel*)*, vol. 13, no. 1, p. 20, 2021.
[218] C. Quin, M. Estaki, D. M. Vollman, J. A. Barnett, S. K. Gill, and D. L. Gibson, "Probiotic supplementation and associated infant gut microbiome and health: A cautionary retrospective clinical comparison," *Sci Rep*, vol. 8, no. 1, p. 8283, 2018.
[219] K. Lu, S. Dong, X. Wu, R. Jin, and H. Chen, "Probiotics in cancer," *Front Oncol*, vol. 11, p. 638148, 2021.
[220] E. L. Ma, Y. J. Choi, J. Choi, C. Pothoulakis, S. H. Rhee, and E. Im, "The anticancer effect of probiotic *Bacillus polyfermenticus* on human colon cancer cells is mediated through ErbB2 and ErbB3 inhibition," *Int J Cancer*, vol. 127, no. 4, pp. 780–790, 2010.
[221] M. Wada et al., "Effects of the enteral administration of *Bifidobacterium breve* on patients undergoing chemotherapy for pediatric malignancies," Supportive Care Cancer, vol. 18, pp. 751–759, 2010.
[222] M. Toi et al., "Probiotic beverage with soy isoflavone consumption for breast cancer prevention: A case-control study," Curr Nutr Food Sci, vol. 9, no. 3, pp. 194–200, 2013.
[223] Y. Ohashi et al., "Habitual intake of lactic acid bacteria and risk reduction of bladder cancer," *Urol Int*, vol. 68, no. 4, pp. 273–280, 2002.
[224] H. S. El-Nezami et al., "Probiotic supplementation reduces a biomarker for increased risk of liver cancer in young men from Southern China," Am J Clin Nutr, vol. 83, no. 5, pp. 1199–1203, 2006.
[225] K. R. Pandey, S. R. Naik, and B. V Vakil, "Probiotics, prebiotics and synbiotics-a review," J Food Sci Technol, vol. 52, pp. 7577–7587, 2015.
[226] K. S. Swanson et al., "The International Scientific Association for Probiotics and Prebiotics (ISAPP) consensus statement on the definition and scope of synbiotics," *Nat Rev Gastroenterol Hepatol*, vol. 17, no. 11, pp. 687–701, 2020.
[227] M. Mounir, A. Ibijbijen, K. Farih, H. N. Rabetafika, and H. L. Razafindralambo, "Synbiotics and their antioxidant properties, mechanisms, and benefits on human and animal health: A narrative review," *Biomolecules*, vol. 12, no. 10, p. 1443, 2022.
[228] A. A. Mohammed, S. Jiang, J. A. Jacobs, and H. W. Cheng, "Effect of a synbiotic supplement on cecal microbial ecology, antioxidant status, and immune response of broiler chickens reared under heat stress," *Poult Sci*, vol. 98, no. 10, pp. 4408–4415, 2019.
[229] H. J. Zheng et al., "The effect of probiotic and synbiotic supplementation on biomarkers of inflammation and oxidative stress in diabetic patients: A systematic review and meta-analysis of randomized controlled trials," *Pharmacol Res*, vol. 142, pp. 303–313, 2019.
[230] J. Pizzorno, "Glutathione!," Int *Med* Clinician *J*, vol. 13, no. 1, p. 8, 2014.
[231] A. Ghiselli, M. Serafini, F. Natella, and C. Scaccini, "Total antioxidant capacity as a tool to assess redox status: Critical view and experimental data," Free Radic Biol Med, vol. 29, no. 11, pp. 1106–1114, 2000.
[232] P. Kleniewska and R. Pawliczak, "Influence of synbiotics on selected oxidative stress parameters," Oxid Med Cell Longev, vol. 2017, 2017.
[233] P. Kleniewska, A. Hoffmann, E. Pniewska, and R. Pawliczak, "The influence of probiotic Lactobacillus casei in combination with prebiotic inulin on the antioxidant capacity of human plasma," Oxid Med Cell Longev, vol. 2016, pp. 1340903, 2016.
[234] H. Roshan et al., "Effects of probiotics and synbiotic supplementation on antioxidant status: A meta-analysis of randomized clinical trials," Clin Nutr ESPEN, vol. 30, pp. 81–88, 2019.
[235] F. Bahmani et al., "The consumption of synbiotic bread containing *Lactobacillus sporogenes* and inulin affects nitric oxide and malondialdehyde in patients with type 2 diabetes mellitus: Randomized, double-blind, placebo-controlled trial," J Am Coll Nutr, vol. 35, no. 6, pp. 506–513, 2016.

[236] A. Ghavami, F. Khorvash, S. Khalesi, Z. Heidari, and G. Askari, "The effects of synbiotic supplementation on oxidative stress and clinical symptoms in women with migraine: A double-blind, placebo-controlled, randomized trial," *J Funct Foods*, vol. 86, p. 104738, 2021.

[237] M. Saracila, A. E. Untea, and T. D. Panaite, "Evaluation of the effect of synbiotic in Piglets' diet on the nutritional quality of pork," *Archiva Zootechnica*, vol. 24, no. 2, pp. 67–75, 2021.

[238] Nurliyani Nurliyani, Eni Harmayani, Sunarti Sunarti et al. Synbiotic Goat Milk Kefir Lowered Peroxisome Proliferator Activated Receptor Gamma (PPARγ) Gene Expression in Rat Adipose and Liver Tissue, 11 February 2021, PREPRINT (Version 1) available at Research Square [https://doi.org/10.21203/rs.3.rs-159681/v1]

[239] I. Cornejo-Pareja, A. Munoz-Garach, M. Clemente-Postigo, and F. J. Tinahones, "Importance of gut microbiota in obesity," Eur J Clin Nutr, vol. 72, no. Suppl 1, pp. 26–37, 2019.

[240] J. Alard et al., "Beneficial metabolic effects of selected probiotics on diet-induced obesity and insulin resistance in mice are associated with improvement of dysbiotic gut microbiota," *Environ Microbiol*, vol. 18, no. 5, pp. 1484–1497, 2016.

[241] Y. Zhong, C. Zheng, J. H. Zheng, and S. C. Xu, "The relationship between intestinal flora changes and osteoporosis in rats with inflammatory bowel disease and the improvement effect of probiotics," *Eur Rev Med Pharmacol Sci*, vol. 24, pp. 5697–5702, 2020.

[242] T. P. M. Scheithauer et al., "Gut microbiota as a trigger for metabolic inflammation in obesity and type 2 diabetes," *Front Immunol*, vol. 11, p. 571731, 2020.

[243] C.-N. Hsu, C.-Y. Hou, J. Y. H. Chan, C.-T. Lee, and Y.-L. Tain, "Hypertension programmed by perinatal high-fat diet: Effect of maternal gut microbiota-targeted therapy," *Nutrients*, vol. 11, no. 12, p. 2908, 2019.

[244] S. Garg, T. P. Singh, and R. K. Malik, "In vivo implications of potential probiotic *Lactobacillus reuteri* lr6 on the gut and immunological parameters as an adjuvant against protein energy malnutrition," Probiotics Antimicrob Proteins, vol. 12, pp. 517–534, 2020.

[245] Y. Li et al., "Oral supplements of combined *Bacillus licheniformis* Zhengchangsheng(r) and xylooligosaccharides improve high-fat diet-induced obesity and modulate the gut microbiota in rats," *Biomed Res Int*, vol. 2020, 2020. https://link.gale.com/apps/doc/A635579983/HRCA?u=anon~337678f3&sid=googleScholar&xid=e64f58a2.

[246] Y. J. Oh, H. J. Kim, T. S. Kim, I. H. Yeo, and G. E. Ji, "Effects of *Lactobacillus plantarum* PMO 08 alone and combined with chia seeds on metabolic syndrome and parameters related to gut health in high-fat diet-induced obese mice," *J Med Food*, vol. 22, no. 12, pp. 1199–1207, 2019.

[247] H. B. Overby and J. F. Ferguson, "Gut microbiota-derived short-chain fatty acids facilitate microbiota: Host cross talk and modulate obesity and hypertension," Curr Hypertens Rep, vol. 23, pp. 1–10, 2021.

[248] J. Alard et al., "Multiple selection criteria for probiotic strains with high potential for obesity management," *Nutrients*, vol. 13, no. 3, p. 713, 2021.

[249] D.-E. Kim, J.-K. Kim, S.-K. Han, S.-E. Jang, M. J. Han, and D.-H. Kim, "*Lactobacillus plantarum* NK3 and *Bifidobacterium longum* NK49 alleviate bacterial vaginosis and osteoporosis in mice by suppressing NF-κ B-Linked TNF-α expression," *J Med Food*, vol. 22, no. 10, pp. 1022–1031, 2019.

[250] Z. Liu et al., "High-dietary fiber intake alleviates antenatal obesity-induced postpartum depression: Roles of gut microbiota and microbial metabolite short-chain fatty acid involved," J Agric Food Chem, vol. 68, no. 47, pp. 13697–13710, 2020.

[251] Z. M. Kundi et al., "Dietary fiber from oat and rye brans ameliorate Western diet-induced body weight gain and hepatic inflammation by the modulation of short-chain fatty acids, bile acids, and tryptophan metabolism," Mol Nutr Food Res, vol. 65, no. 1, p. 1900580, 2021.

[252] J. Lee et al., "Oral intake of *Lactobacillus plantarum* L-14 extract alleviates TLR2-and AMPK-mediated obesity-associated disorders in high-fat-diet-induced obese C57BL/6J mice," *Cell* Prolif, vol. 54, no. 6, p. e13039, 2021.

[253] S. Isozaki et al., "Probiotic-derived polyphosphate accelerates intestinal epithelia wound healing through inducing platelet-derived mediators," *Mediators Inflamm*, vol. 2021, pp. 1-14, 2021.

[254] J. F. Cavallari et al., "Muramyl dipeptide-based postbiotics mitigate obesity-induced insulin resistance via IRF4," *Cell* Metab, vol. 25, no. 5, pp. 1063–1074, 2017.

[255] J. F. Cavallari et al., "Postbiotics for NOD2 require nonhematopoietic RIPK2 to improve blood glucose and metabolic inflammation in mice," Am *J Physiol-Endocrinol Metabol*, vol. 318, no. 4, pp. E579–E585, 2020.

[256] M. Mounir, A. Ibijbijen, K. Farih, H. N. Rabetafika, and H. L. Razafindralambo, "Synbiotics and their antioxidant properties, mechanisms, and benefits on human and animal health: A narrative review," *Biomolecules*, vol. 12, no. 10, p. 1443, 2022.

[257] T. Levkovich et al., "Probiotic bacteria induce a 'glow of health,'" *PLoS One*, vol. 8, no. 1, p. e53867, 2013.

[258] D. R. Whitlock, "Compositions including ammonia oxidizing bacteria to increase production of nitric oxide and nitric oxide precursors and methods of using same." *Google Patents*, Oct. 26, 2010.

[259] J. M. Yano et al., "Indigenous bacteria from the gut microbiota regulate host serotonin biosynthesis," *Cell*, vol. 161, no. 2, pp. 264–276, 2015.

[260] Y.-G. Kim et al., "Neonatal acquisition of Clostridia species protects against colonization by bacterial pathogens," *Science (1979)*, vol. 356, no. 6335, pp. 315–319, 2017.

[261] J. A. Krumbeck et al., "In vivo selection to identify bacterial strains with enhanced ecological performance in synbiotic applications," Appl Environ Microbiol, vol. 81, no. 7, pp. 2455–2465, 2015.

[262] S. M. Kearney and S. M. Gibbons, "Designing synbiotics for improved human health," *Microb* Biotechnol, vol. 11, no. 1, p. 141, 2018.

[263] M. X. Maldonado-Gómez et al., "Stable engraftment of *Bifidobacterium longum* AH1206 in the human gut depends on individualized features of the resident microbiome," *Cell Host Microbe*, vol. 20, no. 4, pp. 515–526, 2016.

[264] S. Devkota et al., "Dietary-fat-induced taurocholic acid promotes pathobiont expansion and colitis in Il10–/– mice," *Nature*, vol. 487, no. 7405, pp. 104–108, 2012.

[265] P. Panigrahi et al., "A randomized synbiotic trial to prevent sepsis among infants in rural India," *Nature*, vol. 548, no. 7668, pp. 407–412, 2017.

[266] F. Mofidi et al., "Synbiotic supplementation in lean patients with non-alcoholic fatty liver disease: A pilot, randomised, double-blind, placebo-controlled, clinical trial," *Br J Nutr*, vol. 117, no. 5, pp. 662–668, 2017.

[267] A. Zepeda-Hernández, L. E. Garcia-Amezquita, T. Requena, and T. García-Cayuela, "Probiotics, prebiotics, and synbiotics added to dairy products: Uses and applications to manage type 2 diabetes," *Food Res Int*, vol. 142, p. 110208, 2021.

[268] N.-M. Maftei, "Probiotic, prebiotic and synbiotic products in human health," in *Frontiers and New Trends in the Science of Fermented Food and Beverages*, IntechOpen, 2019. doi: 10.5772/intechopen.81553.

[269] P. Markowiak and K. Śliżewska, "The role of probiotics, prebiotics and synbiotics in animal nutrition," *Gut Pathog*, vol. 10, no. 1, pp. 1–20, 2018.

[270] S. Koirala, S. P. Thapa, and A. K. Anal, "Overall safety considerations and regulatory oversight for probiotics-based foods and beverages," in Probiotics, *P*rebiotics and *S*ynbiotics*:* Technological *A*dvancements *T*owards *S*afety and *I*ndustrial *A*pplications, vol. 2022, pp. 441–461, 2022. Wiley. https://doi.org/10.1002/9781119702160.ch18

[271] M. Z. Asha and S. F. H. Khalil, "Efficacy and safety of probiotics, prebiotics and synbiotics in the treatment of irritable bowel syndrome: A systematic review and meta-analysis," Sultan Qaboos Univ Med J, vol. 20, no. 1, p. e13, 2020.

[272] H. R. Shehata and S. G. Newmaster, "The power of DNA based methods in probiotic authentication," *Front Microbiol*, vol. 14, p. 1158440, 2023.

[273] M. E. Sanders and D. D. Levy, "The science and regulations of probiotic food and supplement product labeling," *Ann* N Y Acad Sci, vol. 1219, no. Suppl. 1, 2011, doi: 10.1111/j.1749-6632.2010.05956.x.

[274] C. Li et al., "Probiotics, prebiotics, and synbiotics regulate the intestinal microbiota differentially and restore the relative abundance of specific gut microorganisms," *J Dairy Sci*, vol. 103, no. 7, pp. 5816–5829, 2020.

[275] R. El Hage, E. Hernandez-Sanabria, and T. Van de Wiele, "Emerging trends in 'smart probiotics': Functional consideration for the development of novel health and industrial applications," *Front* Microbiol, vol. 8, no. SEP., Frontiers Media S.A., Sep. 29, 2017. doi: 10.3389/fmicb.2017.01889.

[276] I. Khangwal and P. Shukla, "Potential prebiotics and their transmission mechanisms: Recent approaches," J *Food* Drug Anal, vol. 27, no. 3. Elsevier Taiwan LLC, pp. 649–656, Jul. 01, 2019. doi: 10.1016/j.jfda.2019.02.003.

[277] R. L. J. Day, A. J. Harper, R. M. Woods, O. G. Davies, and L. M. Heaney, "Probiotics: Current landscape and future horizons," Future Sci *OA*, vol. 5, no. 4. Future Medicine Ltd., Apr. 01, 2019. doi: 10.4155/fsoa-2019-0004.

[278] M. Hegarty, "The history of prebiotics," *prebiofibres.co.uk*, Accessed: Sep. 28, 2023. [Online]. Available: https://www.prebiofibres.co.uk/insights/history-of-prebiotics

[279] S. Patel and A. Goyal, "The current trends and future perspectives of prebiotics research: A review," 3 Biotech, vol. 2, no. 2, pp. 115–125, Jun. 2012, doi: 10.1007/s13205-012-0044-x.

[280] M. Cunningham et al., "Shaping the future of probiotics and prebiotics," *Trends* Microbiol, vol. 29, no. 8. Elsevier Ltd., pp. 667–685, Aug. 01, 2021. doi: 10.1016/j.tim.2021.01.003.

[281] G. B. Bamigbade, A. J. Subhash, A. Kamal-Eldin, L. Nyström, and M. Ayyash, "An updated review on prebiotics: Insights on potentials of food seeds waste as source of potential prebiotics," *Molecules*, vol. 27, no. 18, p. 5947, Sep. 2022, doi: 10.3390/molecules27185947.

[282] V. Ambrogi, F. Bottacini, L. Cao, B. Kuipers, M. Schoterman, and D. van Sinderen, "Galacto-oligosaccharides as infant prebiotics: Production, application, bioactive activities and future perspectives," Crit Rev Food Sci Nutr, vol. 63, no. 6, pp. 753–766, Feb. 2023, doi: 10.1080/10408398.2021.1953437.

[283] A. Pandey, A. Mazumder, and S. Das, "A critical evaluation of beneficial gut flora: Probiotics, prebiotics, postbiotics and synbiotics to treat constipation and haemorrhoids," *Allelopathy J*, vol. 59, no. 2, 2023.

[284] A. Rousseaux, C. Brosseau, and M. Bodinier, "Immunomodulation of B Lymphocytes by prebiotics, probiotics and synbiotics: Application in pathologies," *Nutrients*, vol. 15, no. 2, p. 269, Jan. 2023, doi: 10.3390/nu15020269.

[285] P. Mishra et al., "Prebiotics: Ignored player in the fight against cancer," Cancer Rep, Jul. 2023, doi: 10.1002/cnr2.1870.

[286] V. Vu, Y. M. Kim, and M. Cho, "Effects of SCFAs and TMAO on non-alcoholic fatty liver disease indicating the therapeutic benefits of plant-based diet, and supplemental prebiotics, probiotics and synbiotics," Appl Biol Chem, vol. 66, no. 1, p. 11, Feb. 2023, doi: 10.1186/s13765-022-00755-1.

[287] G. Divyashri et al., "Non-digestible oligosaccharides-based prebiotics to ameliorate obesity: Overview of experimental evidence and future perspectives," *Food Sci Biotechnol*, Aug. 2023, doi: 10.1007/s10068-023-01381-3.

[288] A. Sola Leyva, "Microbial landscape in female reproductive health: Unravelling its composition and host-microbe interactions," pp. 1–174, 2023.

[289] K. Rani, G. Kaur, and S. A. Ali, "Probiotic-prebiotic therapeutic potential: A new horizon of microbial biotherapy to reduce female reproductive complications," *PharmaNutrition*, vol. 24, p. 100342, Jun. 2023, doi: 10.1016/j.phanu.2023.100342.

[290] A. Lopez-Santamarina, A. del C. Mondragon, A. Lamas, J. M. Miranda, C. M. Franco, and A. Cepeda, "Animal-origin prebiotics based on chitin: An alternative for the future? a critical review," *Foods*, vol. 9, no. 6, p. 782, 2020.

[291] X. Jiao et al., "Blueberry polyphenols extract as a potential prebiotic with anti-obesity effects on C57BL/6J mice by modulating the gut microbiota," *J Nutr Biochem*, vol. 64, pp. 88–100, 2019.

[292] D. Chen et al., "Prebiotic effect of fructooligosaccharides from *Morinda officinalis* on Alzheimer's disease in rodent models by targeting the microbiota-gut-brain axis," *Front Aging Neurosci*, vol. 9, p. 403, 2017.

[293] N. Pansai, K. Chakree, C. Takahashi Yupanqui, P. Raungrut, N. Yanyiam, and S. Wichienchot, "Gut microbiota modulation and immune boosting properties of prebiotic dragon fruit oligosaccharides," Int J Food Sci Technol, vol. 55, no. 1, pp. 55–64, 2020.

[294] P. Cherry et al., "Prebiotics from seaweeds: An ocean of opportunity?," *Mar Drugs*, vol. 17, no. 6, p. 327, 2019.

[295] H. G. Ceylan and A. F. Atasoy, "New bioactive edible packing systems: Synbiotic edible films/coatings as carries of probiotics and prebiotics," Food Bioproc Tech, vol. 16, no. 7, pp. 1413–1428, Jul. 2023, doi: 10.1007/s11947-022-02983-1.

[296] M. Y. Mohamed Imran, N. Reehana, G. Muralitharan, N. Thajuddin, and D. Dhanasekaran, "New formulations and products in prebiotic food," *Advance in Probiotics*, Elsevier, 2021, pp. 437–447. doi: 10.1016/b978-0-12-822909-5.00026-5.

[297] Lacombe, A. and Wu, V.C., 2022. "Dietary Modulation of the Gut Microbiota by Prebiotics and Other Dietary Nutrients and Relevant Health Effect (s)," In The Gut Microbiome, pp. 157-179. CRC Press.
[298] C. Vera, A. Illanes, and C. Guerrero, "Enzymatic production of prebiotic oligosaccharides," Curr *Opin Food Sci*, vol. 37, pp. 1–178, 2021. doi: 10.1016/j.cofs.2020.10.013.
[299] С. Н. Туровская, "The synthesis of galactooligosaccharides is a promising direction of the bioconversion of lactose-containing milk systems," *Food Process Ind*, no. 3, pp. 15–19, 2022, doi: 10.52653/ppi.2022.3.3.004.
[300] A. R. Chavan et al., "Recent trends in the biotechnology of functional non-digestible oligosaccharides with prebiotic potential," Biotechnol Genet Eng Rev, pp. 1–46, Jan 30. 2023, doi: 10.1080/02648725.2022.2152627.
[301] A. Shafi, M. Khan, and Q. Husain, "Nanosupport immobilized β-galactosidases, their stabilization, and applications," in Nanomaterials for Biocatalysis, Edited by Guillermo Raul Castro, Ashok Kumar Nadda, Tuan Anh Nguyen, Xianghui Qi, and Ghulam Yasin, Elsevier,. 2021. doi: 10.1016/B978-0-12-824436-4.00023-X.
[302] P. Nimpiboon, S. Nakapong, R. Pichyangkura, K. Ito, and P. Pongsawasdi, "Synthesis of a novel prebiotic trisaccharide by a type I α-glucosidase from B. licheniformis strain TH4-2," *Process Biochem*, vol. 46, no. 2, pp. 448–457, Feb. 2011, doi: 10.1016/j.procbio.2010.09.018.
[303] V. C. de Paula, I. O. Pinheiro, C. E. Lopes, and G. M. T. Calazans, "Microwave-assisted hydrolysis of *Zymomonas mobilis* levan envisaging oligofructan production," *Bioresour Technol*, vol. 99, no. 7, pp. 2466–2470, May 2008, doi: 10.1016/j.biortech.2007.04.062.
[304] N. Kim, M. Yun, Y. J. Oh, and H.-J. Choi, "Mind-altering with the gut: Modulation of the gut-brain axis with probiotics," *J Microbiol*, vol. 56, no. 3, pp. 172–182, Mar. 2018, doi: 10.1007/s12275-018-8032-4.
[305] S. Westfall, N. Lomis, I. Kahouli, S. Y. Dia, S. P. Singh, and S. Prakash, "Microbiome, probiotics and neurodegenerative diseases: Deciphering the gut brain axis," Cell Mol Life Sci, vol. 74, pp. 3769–3787, 2017.
[306] J. Kiepś and R. Dembczyński, "Current trends in the production of probiotic formulations," *Foods*, vol. 11, no. 15. MDPI, Aug. 01, 2022. doi: 10.3390/foods11152330.
[307] D. F. Gomez Quintero, C. R. Kok, and R. Hutkins, "The future of synbiotics: Rational formulation and design," *Front* Microbiol, vol. 13, p. 919725, 2022, doi: 10.3389/fmicb.2022.919725.
[308] H. Jiang, M. Cai, B. Shen, Q. Wang, T. Zhang, and X. Zhou, "Synbiotics and gut microbiota: New perspectives in the treatment of type 2 diabetes mellitus," *Foods*, vol. 11, no. 16. MDPI, Aug. 01, 2022. doi: 10.3390/foods11162438.
[309] S. K. Yeo and M. T. Liong, "Effect of prebiotics on viability and growth characteristics of probiotics in soymilk," J Sci Food Agric, vol. 90, no. 2, 2010, doi: 10.1002/jsfa.3808.

15 Synbiotics

Present Status and Future Prospectives to Control Metabolic Disorders

Sanzia Mehjabin, Md. Khokon Miah Akanda, A. H. M. Nazmul Hasan, and G. M. Masud Parvez

15.1 INTRODUCTION

The increased prevalence of metabolic disorders, including type 2 diabetes mellitus (T2DM) and cardiovascular disease (CVD) in industrialized and developing nations concerns society. Substantial changes in dietary intake and lifestyle choices are mainly responsible for the noticeable increase in metabolic disease incidence in recent years. The observed tendency is linked to the widespread adoption of harmful lifestyle choices. Recently, nutritionists and researchers have become more interested in the idea that changes in the makeup of intestinal microbiota may lead to metabolic disorders (Kasubuchi et al., 2015; Nagatomo et al., 2015; Haque et al., 2016). Bacteroidetes and Firmicutes comprise more than 90% of all intestines or stomach bacteria (Afroja et al., 2017). These taxa are essential for the formation of xenobiotic metabolism, nutritional mucosal barrier fortification, absorption, angiogenesis, and gut function after birth. The composition of intestinal microbiota is significantly influenced by individuals' dietary decisions, which subsequently play a role in the pathogenesis of metabolic diseases (Ley et al., 2006; Parvez and Akanda, 2019). Prebiotics and probiotics are regarded as alternative supplements for addressing metabolic problems due to their hypothesized mechanism of action, which primarily involves modulating the makeup and function of the intestinal microbiota. The preventive potential of probiotics and prebiotics against CVD and T2DM has been demonstrated in various studies (Calcinaro et al., 2005).

Several researchers have conducted studies to explore the possibilities of utilizing food-grade bacteria for the treatment and prevention of diabetes. The research findings suggest that specific probiotics, such as *L. lactis* and bifidobacteria, have the ability to produce a substance similar to insulin. This substance has been observed to have the anticipated physiological impact on adipocytes, both in human and animal models (Ejtahed et al., 2011). An increasing amount of scientific literature suggests that probiotic and prebiotic administration may have therapeutic and preventative effects on CVD. Their ability to decrease inflammation, total blood cholesterol, and low-density lipoprotein (LDL) cholesterol is the primary cause of this occurrence (Sun and Buys, 2015; Roller et al., 2004).

15.2 SYNBIOTICS

The term "synbiotics" pertains to dietary components or nutritional additives that demonstrate a synergistic amalgamation of probiotic and prebiotic properties (Figure 15.1) (Pandey et al., 2015). The synbiotic concept was originally postulated as a combination of probiotics and prebiotics, which bolstered the host's ability to sustain and promote the proliferation of living microbial dietary supplements in the intestines. The favorable results observed can be attributed to the synbiotic concept. This outcome is attained by intentionally promoting advantageous microorganisms' proliferation and metabolic activity, thereby ultimately aiding in enhancing the individual's overall health and welfare (Gibson and Roberfroid, 1995). Complementary synbiotics are formulations where the inclusion of each component is determined by its unique capacity to impact the host's health. On the other hand, synergistic synbiotics refer to combinations where the selection of prebiotic components is intentional with the purpose of enhancing the effectiveness of the probiotic (Rijkers et al., 2011). The term "probiotic" derives from the Greek word "for life". Probiotics are defined as "live microbial feed supplements that improve the intestinal equilibrium of the host animal" (Fuller, 1989).

Conversely, probiotics are a class of live bacteria that dwell in the digestive tract and can provide a host with a number of health benefits, such as improved digestion and reduced weight. Postbiotics, on the other hand, are thought to be a result of bacterial fermentation in the intestines (Gibson and Roberfroid, 1995). Probiotics (especially bifidobacterial and lactic acid bacteria [LAB]) and prebiotics have long been consumed by humans, where they can be found in fermented foods or as natural dietary ingredients. In the year 76 B.C., the Roman historian Plinius advised a patient who was suffering from gastroenteritis the advice to consume fermented milk products (Cruchet et al., 2015). Utilizing probiotics and prebiotics saw a sharp increase in popularity in the latter half of the 19TH and early 20TH centuries. Subsequently, Metchnikoff noted that the alteration of the microbial equilibrium in the intestines had a beneficial impact on health. He developed a theory in which the ingestion of yogurt containing *Lactobacillus* would result in a reduction in the number of bacteria in

DOI: 10.1201/9781032702438-15

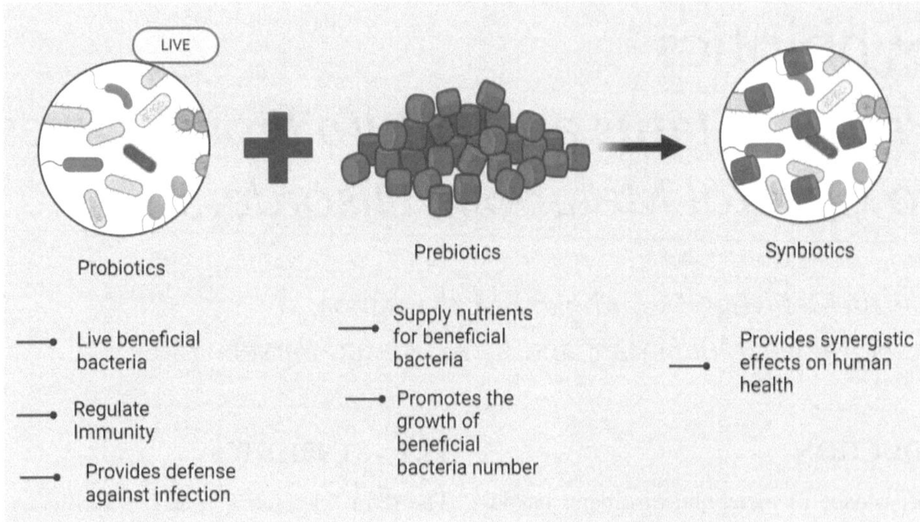

FIGURE 15.1 Definition of synbiotics.

the digestive system that create toxins and an increase in the length of time an organism might survive. This theory was based on the idea that eating of yogurt would also enhance the amount of time an organism might live. Later on, the findings of additional researchers lent credence to Metchnikoff's concept (Verna and Lucak, 2010). In the year 1900, Tissier made a recommendation about the inclusion of bifidobacteria in the dietary regimen of children afflicted with diarrhea. Tissier asserted that bifidobacteria possessed superior qualities compared to putrefactive bacteria, which were identified as the causative agents of this particular ailment (Lee et al., 2010).

15.3 PRESENT STATUS TO CONTROL METABOLIC DISORDERS

15.3.1 Support Digestive Health

Synbiotics provide a dual benefit to gut health by delivering a continuous supply of both prebiotics and probiotics to the human body. Probiotics refer to a category of advantageous microorganisms that play a role in facilitating optimal digestive processes. An increasing amount of evidence backs up the claims made about the beneficial effects of probiotics. It improved gastrointestinal health, immune system support, cancer prevention potential, and decreased blood cholesterol levels. Probiotics are supported by a considerable body of evidence for their ability to prevent antibiotic-induced diarrhea, treat acute diarrheal diseases, and enhance lactose metabolism. However, the available evidence is inadequate to support for their application in other therapeutic contexts (Kechagia et al., 2013). Probiotics have the potential to improve several aspects of digestive health, including the treatment of ulcerative colitis and irritable bowel syndrome (IBS). Comparable in effectiveness and tolerability to the gold standard mesalazine, the probiotic drug *E. coli* Nissle 1917 maintains remission in patients with ulcerative colitis (Kruis et al., 2004). Individuals who provide a binary result for the presence of IBS symptoms. Probiotics substantially alleviated the IBS symptoms (Moayyedi et al., 2010). Prebiotics are able to improve digestive health because they feed the good bacteria already present in the gut. Subsequently, additional butyric acid and short-chain fatty acids are generated. Numerous scientific investigations have provided evidence that butyric acid has the potential to alleviate symptoms associated with inflammatory bowel disease (IBD) and IBS, in addition to supporting regularity. Both of these conditions affect the digestive tract. A study evaluated butyric acid's effectiveness for IBS. There are two types of IBS patients: those who have constipation (IBS-C) and those who have diarrhea (IBS-D). Each category received enteric-coated tablets containing butyric acid at a dose of 1 g/day. At the beginning and end of the trial, the IBS form and the intensity of symptoms were noted. In total, 71% of IBS-D patients and 16% of IBS-C patients reported a reduction or normalization of symptoms after receiving butyric acid treatment (Scarpellini et al., 2007).

15.3.2 Enhance Immune Function

According to research, gut health and immunological function are inextricably related. Approximately 70%–80% of the body's immune cells are found in the gastrointestinal system of the human body, according to numerous studies. The immune system's location has been connected to this dispersion of immune cells. Utilization of synbiotics has been shown to potentially augment immune function through the promotion of beneficial gut flora and the concurrent reduction of inflammation. Numerous studies have shown that taking probiotic supplements as a dietary supplement may improve immune function (Furness et al., 1999; Uzzaman et al., 2018). According to a Finnish study, drinking milk that has been supplemented with probiotics can reduce children's respiratory illness frequency and severity by about 17% effects of the probiotic strain *Lactobacillus GG* were observed (Hatakka et al., 2001). Studies have shown that premenopausal women who take probiotics have around a 50% lower risk of developing urinary tract infections (UTIs) than women who have not yet reached menopause. One hundred young women with a history of recurring UTIs were randomly assigned to receive Lactin-V (*Lactobacillus crispatus* intravaginal suppository probiotic) once daily for 5 days and once weekly for 10 weeks after antibiotics were administered to treat an acute UTI. This regimen was followed by the administration of antibiotics to treat the acute UTI. Following the intervention, participants were checked for UTIs and at 1-week and 10-week intervals. The patient's urine and vaginal samples contained detectable amounts of *L. crispatus* via the culture process's real-time quantitative 16's ribosomal RNA gene polymerase chain reaction. The study found that 15% of women who were administered Lactin-V exhibited the desired outcome, whereas 27% of women who were given a placebo demonstrated the same outcome. The study observed a consistent association between the presence of a significant quantity of *Lactobacillus crispatus* in the vaginal region over time and a noteworthy reduction in the frequency of recurrent UTIs. This association was specifically observed in relation to the utilization of Lactin-V (Stapleton et al., 2011).

15.3.3 Improve Mental Health

Our mental health includes not only our emotional and psychological well-being but also our social well-being as well. Think, feel, and behave differently as a result of this. In addition, it influences how we cope with stress, how well we get along with other people, and how well we make decisions. The usage of drugs to improve mental health is going up day by day (Parvez et al., 2018; Sultana et al., 2017). The inclusion of synbiotics in a person's diet has the potential to enhance cognitive function and safeguard mental well-being through the simultaneous provision of substantial quantities of probiotics and prebiotics in each consumption. Previous research has shown that particular bacteria strains, specifically *Bifidobacterium* and *Lactobacillus* and, exhibit the capacity to augment memory function and ameliorate symptoms associated with anxiety, depression, obsessive-compulsive disorder (OCD), and autism spectrum disorder (ASD). The doses of *Bifidobacterium* species such as *B. longum*, *B. infantis*, and *B. breve* as well as *Lactobacillus* species such as *L. rhamnosus* and *L. helveticus* were varied and ranged from 10^9 to 10^{10} colony-forming units (CFUs). For animals, the intervention lasted for 2 weeks; for humans, it lasted for 4 weeks. Studies demonstrated that these probiotics can help people with anxiety, sadness, ASD, and OCD. They can also improve memory, both spatial and non-spatial (Wang et al., 2016). The results of another study done in Iran showed that taking probiotic supplements for 8 weeks significantly reduced depressive symptoms in comparison to a control group (Akkasheh et al., 2015). However, it has been shown that taking probiotics can assist enhance other elements of mental health, specifically by reducing the symptoms of stress and anxiety. In petrochemical workers, the use of probiotic yogurt or a multispecies probiotic medication was found to have favorable impacts on mental health measures (Mohammadi et al., 2016).

15.3.4 Boost Weight Loose

Synbiotics have many great health advantages, but one of the most impressive is their ability to speed up fat burning and accelerate weight loss. For example, probiotics may help prevent the absorption of fat, which in turn reduces calorie consumption. In humans, *Lactobacillus gasseri* promotes fecal fat excretion and inhibits lipase-mediated fat hydrolysis, both of which are advantageous metabolic effects (Ogawa et al., 2015). In fact, after just 12 weeks of use, taking *Lactobacillus gasseri* as a dietary supplement led to an 8.5% reduction in belly fat. This reduction occurred despite the fact that the supplement was taken for the same amount of time as a placebo (Kadooka et al., 2013). Conversely, prebiotics are typically found in foods high in fiber and have been linked to a decrease in body fat as well as a lower body weight. The amount of fiber taken at all fat intake levels is inversely linked with the body mass index, even after controlling for confounding variables. Intervention study results are less consistent, but adding dietary fiber usually reduces food consumption and, consequently, body weight (Slavin, 2005). Additionally, prebiotic meals have been demonstrated to assist in tests on animals, which may help enhance sensations of fullness to aid in weight loss (Parnell and Reimer, 2012).

15.3.5 Promote Cardiac Health

CVD is a significant issue in every region of the world. Based on certain projections, it is anticipated that by the year 2030, a substantial proportion of the US population, specifically over 44%, will be afflicted with one or more manifestations of CVD. By reducing several of the risk factors linked to heart disease, synbiotics can help maintain a strong and healthy heart. People who had been diagnosed with diabetes and coronary heart disease (CHD) were included in a study that was carried out in 2017, and it was found that individuals who were given synbiotics for a period of time totaling 12 weeks were able to experience improvements in insulin metabolism as well as high amounts of HDL cholesterol, which is also known as "good" cholesterol. A total of 60 individuals diagnosed with both CHD and diabetes were administered synbiotic supplements for a duration of 12 weeks. Three probiotic bacterial strains were combined in these supplements: *Bifidobacterium bifidum*, *Lactobacillus acidophilus*, and *Lactobacillus casei*. Patients who took a synbiotic capsule for the full course of treatment experienced significant improvements in their serum insulin concentrations, HLDL cholesterol, fasting plasma glucose levels (Tajabadi-Ebrahimi et al., 2017). HDL cholesterol is carried through the bloodstream, where it helps prevent the accumulation of fatty plaque and contributes to the clearness of the arteries. Furthermore, several investigations have discovered evidence that probiotics may assist in lowering blood pressure, which is advantageous for heart health. Consuming probiotics can lower blood pressure a little bit. However, if baseline blood pressure is high, multiple probiotic species are consumed, the intervention lasts longer than 8 weeks, or the daily ingestion dose exceeds ten CFUs, there may be a more notable impact (Khalesi et al., 2014). According to Nguyen et al., *Lactobacillus plantarum* significantly decreased the levels of triglycerides and total serum cholesterol in hypercholesterolemic mice (Nguyen et al., 2007). In addition, compared to the control group, milk yogurt and buffalo soymilk yogurt containing *Bifidobacterium longum* Bb-46 or *Bifidobacterium lactis* Bb-12 significantly reduced LDL-cholesterol concentrations by 56.3%, triglycerides by 51.2%, and total cholesterol by 50.3% (Abd El-Gawad et al., 2005). In a related trial, also used a probiotic, but it was *Lactobacillus acidophilus* L1. When compared to the outcomes of the control group, which was given a placebo, the study's findings provided evidence to support the researcher's conclusion that regular consumption of 200 grams of yogurt containing *Lactobacillus acidophilus* after the evening meal resulted in a significant drop in serum cholesterol levels (Anderson and Gilliland, 1999). According to the findings of another study, the combination of bacteria strains was superior than individual bacteria strains in terms of their ability to reduce liver and total cholesterol. The liver cholesterol concentrations of the given mixed bacteria and *Lactobacillus acidophilus* were shown to be reduced by 23%–57%. Furthermore, compared to the groups supplemented with individual bacteria, the group supplemented with mixed bacteria had a lower concentration of cholesterol (Fukushima et al., 1999). There are two potential pathways that prebiotics can use to bring about hypocholesterolemia. First, increased elimination of cholesterol through stools results in decreased absorption of cholesterol. The other mechanism is the selective fermentation of gut bacterial microflora, which produces SCFAs (Kim and Shin, 1998). Causey et al. looked into the consequences of consuming 20 g of inulin daily in their study. Prebiotics with longer chains, such as inulin, ferment more slowly and have between 9 and 64 links per saccharide molecule. Researchers discovered that the inulin-consuming group's blood triglyceride levels significantly decreased. They also found that when inulin was given, serum HDL cholesterol rose and serum LDL-cholesterol decreased in contrast to the control group (Causey et al., 2000). A separate investigation revealed that individuals with normolipidemia who consumed a daily dosage of 18% inulin, without adhering to any supplementary dietary limitations, experienced reductions in triacylglycerols and total plasma cholesterol levels by 5.4%, 7.9%, 7.8%, and 21.2%, respectively. Inulin significantly increased fecal *Lactobacillus-lactate* concentration and breath H_2 excretion (placebo 78 ± 26 ppm × h; IAUC test 280 ± 40) according to glucose tolerance tests (Brighenti et al., 1999). Therefore, inulin may be able to decrease cholesterol in individuals with normolipidemia, perhaps through mechanisms connected to colonic fermentation. Rats fed inulin-containing diets had higher levels of cholesterol and lipids excreted in their stools than rats fed a control group diet. The primary cause for the heightened excretion levels can be linked to a decrease in cholesterol absorption (Dikeman et al., 2006).

15.3.6 Decrease Inflammation

Acute inflammation contributes to the body's defense against illness and infection and is a normal and essential part of that response. Conversely, persistent inflammation is thought to be essential to both health and disease. Furthermore, it might have a role in the progression of long-term illnesses like diabetes, cancer, and heart disease (Hunter, 2012; Akanda and Hasan, 2021). A concentrated dose of probiotics and prebiotics, both of which enhance gut health and reduce inflammation, can be delivered via synbiotics. For instance, research demonstrated that probiotics can assist in modulating the immune response of individuals afflicted with milk allergies. In milk-sensitive individuals, exposure to milk consumption has considerably grown the expression of FcgammaRI, FcalphaR, and CR1 in neutrophils, and FcalphaR, CR3, and CR1 in monocytes. The presence of *Lactobacillus GG* in milk effectively inhibited the upregulation of receptor expression (Pelto et al., 1998). Another study documented a comparable result, whereby participants who had been diagnosed with severe depressive disorder demonstrated decreased concentrations of C-reactive protein (CRP) after receiving probiotics. CRP functions as a fundamental biomarker of inflammation within the body (Akkasheh et al., 2016). One study found that children who ate *B. lactis* and *L. acidophilus* had less severe and shorter-lasting cold and flu-like symptoms. These symptoms included fever, coughing, runny nose, and fever (Leyer et al., 2009). The presence of *Lactobacillus rhamnosus* in yogurt was linked to a decreased risk of upper respiratory tract infections (URI), such as tonsillitis and pharyngitis (Villena et al., 2012). Nishihira et al. (2018) have noted that probiotics represent a viable strategy for the prevention of influenza virus infection, among other potential possibilities. Additional research indicated that regular intake of a fermented dairy product with a particular strain of *L. casei* showed promise in lowering the incidence of common illnesses like respiratory and gastrointestinal infections (Guillemard et al., 2010). The incidence, severity, and duration of URTI symptoms in patients were significantly reduced who took a combination of probiotics (*L. rhamnosus*, *B. lactis*, and *L. plantarum*) with either galacto-oligosaccharide (GOS) or fructo-oligosaccharide (FOS) prebiotics over the course of a multi-year clinical research (Pregliasco et al., 2008).

15.3.7 Control Type 2 Diabetes

Probiotics like *Bifidobacterium animalis* subsp. lactis 420 have been shown by Amar et al. to be effective in reversing the low-grade inflammatory response. The goal can be achieved through the translocation of gram-negative *Enterobacteriaceae* bacteria and reduced adhesion of these bacteria to mucosal surfaces. As a consequence of this phenomena, probiotics have the ability to reduce inflammation in adipose tissue, in addition to other symptoms linked with T2DM (Amar et al., 2011). Asemi et al. investigated how probiotic oral supplements affected metabolic profiles, oxidative stress, and hs-CRP in individuals with T2DM. The goal of this research was to investigate the effects of an orally taken supplement that contained seven different live and freeze-dried strains by employing a design that was randomized, controlled by a placebo, and parallel. These strains include *Bifidobacterium breve* and *Bifidobacterium longum* in addition to *Streptococcus thermophilus*, *Lactobacillus bulgaricus*, *Lactobacillus casei*, *Lactobacillus rhamnosus,* and *Lactobacillus acidophilus.* During the course of the study, the participants took the nutritional supplement on a daily basis. Comparing the multi-probiotic group's fasting plasma glucose levels to those of the placebo-treated control group, the study's findings showed a significant reduction in this parameter. Even if the active ingredient was administered in the identical quantity to each group, this was nevertheless the case. The fact that the individuals' blood glucose levels were substantially lower during their fasting periods served as evidence for this (Asemi et al., 2013). Additionally, probiotic therapy has been proposed as a potential means of improving antioxidative processes in people with T2DM. The probiotic yogurt supplementation group showed higher levels of total antioxidants, erythrocyte superoxide dismutase, and glutathione peroxidase activity (Ejtahed et al., 2012). Combining *Lactobacillus casei* and *Lactobacillus acidophilus* with dahi, a yogurt that is traditionally consumed in the Indian subcontinent. By preventing the synthesis of lipid nitric oxide and peroxidation, the drug administration successfully reduced the oxidative damage brought on by streptozotocin (STZ) in the pancreatic tissues (Yadav et al., 2008). Furthermore, Yadav et al. found that incorporating the probiotic dahi into one's diet significantly postponed the development of dyslipidemia, hyperinsulinemia, hyperglycemia, and glucose intolerance. It also reduced oxidative stress in patients with high fructose-induced diabetes. These findings were based on research conducted on patients who had developed diabetes as a result of eating a diet rich in fructose (Yadav et al., 2007).

15.3.8 Combat Antibiotic Resistance

The human digestive system is home to billions of different bacteria that live in harmony with one another. This community is known as the gut microbiome. Numerous health advantages of these microbes for humans include enhanced immunity, better digestion, healthier skin, and more vitality. The beneficial and more hazardous microorganisms that naturally colonize the gut need to coexist in a healthy balance for the gut to function properly. A number of lifestyle choices, including eating a diet low in fiber, traveling frequently, or getting sick, can upset this balance. A person's digestive system may suffer as a result of taking antibiotics. While antibiotics are effective at eradicating bad bacteria, they are essentially non-selective and can reduce good bacteria in the stomach. Probiotic supplementation helps to rebalance the gut microbiota. The NHS has acknowledged the health benefits of probiotic supplements (Zhang et al., 2015). The frequency of antibiotic-associated diarrhea (ADD), a typical side effect of antibiotics, ranges from 5% to 35% based on the antibiotic type. By comparing and merging data from different trials, a meta-analysis of 23 studies from the prestigious Cochrane Collaboration conducted in 2012 discovered that probiotics can cut the risk of antibiotic-associated adverse effects by 64%. The infection caused by *Clostridium difficile* is one type of autoimmune bowel disease (AAD), and its symptoms include colitis, chronic diarrhea, and in more severe cases. This phenomenon poses a specific area of apprehension among the aged population, as it has the potential to occasionally lead to mortality. The available evidence indicates that probiotics exhibit a favorable safety profile and demonstrate efficacy in promoting the well-being of the gut microbiota and alleviating gastrointestinal disturbances associated with *Clostridium difficile*-associated diarrhea. A comprehensive review with a total of 4213 participants provides the basis of this evidence (Goldenberg et al., 2017; Akter et al., 2020). In a recent meta-analysis, researchers at the University of Toronto examined data from 16 different trials involving 3,403 patients in total who were getting antibiotic therapy. According to the findings, individuals who took probiotics alongside their antibiotic treatment had a much lower risk of having ADD or *C. difficile* infection (Videlock and Cremonini, 2012). As antibiotic-resistant bacteria proliferate, probiotics are being used more and more by the medical community and the cattle agriculture industry as an alternative to antibiotic treatment. Probiotic consumption may slow the emergence of antibiotic-resistant strains caused by extensive and excessive antibiotic use by reducing the use of antibiotics (Verraes et al., 2013).

15.4 WAY TO FIND THE BEST SYNBIOTIC

Both food and supplement forms of synbiotics are available for use in enhancing gut flora and overall well-being (Pandey et al., 2015). Synbiotic food are created by combining prebiotic-rich foods with a variety of probiotic-rich foods to provide a concentrated dose of both to the diet. Chicory root, green bananas, oats, onions, garlic, asparagus, and acacia gum are all examples of foods that contain prebiotics. In the meanwhile, natto, tempeh, kimchi, sauerkraut, and kefir kombucha are some examples of fermented foods that contain probiotics (Artiss et al., 2006).

If a person decides to take a synbiotic supplement instead of a probiotic supplement, they should be sure to get one that is of a high quality and comes from a well-known and respected company. When seeking optimal synbiotic supplements, it is advisable to prioritize products exhibiting a substantial CFU count, containing live and active cultures, and demonstrating a commendable level of diversity in probiotic strains. Additionally, products must to incorporate healthy plant-based sources of fiber in order to deliver an adequate quantity of prebiotics (Fotiadis et al., 2008).

In order for a product to be considered a true synbiotic, it must contain live and active bacterial cultures, and the packaging must clearly state this information. The quantity of bacterial cells present in a single treatment can be expressed as CFUs, which must be carefully monitored. It is commonly recommended to select probiotic products that possess a minimum of 1 billion CFUs and encompass the genera *Lactobacillus*, *Bifidobacterium*, *Bacillus*, *Saccharomyces boulardii*. These are some of the probiotics that have received the most study attention (Hardy et al., 2013). In addition to this, it is essential to read the label carefully and pay attention to the proper storage methods for synbiotics. Any person wants to keep them cooled and make sure the seller does too. Incorrect storage of probiotics might result in the microorganisms in the product being destroyed by heat. It is also very important to pay strict attention to the expiration date, as the number of CFUs tends to decrease with time, making the product less useful. Because probiotics are offered as supplements, they are not regulated by the FDA. This means that corporations can basically put whatever they want in a supplement and call it a probiotic. Maintaining a close eye on the label and reading up on scientific studies and research papers to learn which probiotics have made beneficial impacts on specific conditions will help it stay safe and ensure desired probiotics (García-Núñez et al., 2022). Avoid using probiotic supplements and eating probiotic foods if any person has an impaired or weakened immune system, such as in the case of someone who is undergoing chemotherapy treatments, has a serious illness, or has recently undergone surgery. In some instances, anyone could develop an allergic reaction, so it is essential to always read the label of probiotic products carefully (Arab et al., 2022).

15.5 FUTURE PERSPECTIVE TO CONTROL METABOLIC DISORDERS

15.5.1 Identify Specific Strain

Future research may identify specific symbiotic strains that have more pronounced effects on metabolic health. Identifying and isolating these strains could lead to the development of highly specialized synbiotic products. Researchers have discovered that the administration of various probiotic strains is associated with diverse categories of advantages, including enhancements in digestive and immune system functioning. However, the task of locating a specific strain and understanding its effects on health in order to validate theories regarding the health advantages of a different strain is a challenge. This is due to the fact that different synbiotic strains each exhibit their own set of unique qualities. These characteristics may have an impact on the suitability of the strain as well as its advantages, safety, and effectiveness. Additionally, strains are crucial to survivability in both production processes and reaching the stomach safely. So, a product's amount of CFUs does not necessarily mean you're getting the benefit you want if the strain you are taking in hasn't been studied and shown to support that benefit at that serving size (Walden et al., 2022). A study was done to see how the probiotic *Bacillus coagulans* GBI-30, 6086 affected the IBS symptoms. Patients who suffer from IBS may find that the patented probiotic known as *B. coagulans* GBI-30, 6086 is an alternative that is both safe and helpful for the treatment of abdominal pain and bloating. In order to stop digestive symptoms from developing in those who are sensitive to lactose and fructose, research has been done on the potential role that GanedenBC30 (strains of *Bacillus coagulans*) may have in the digestion of these carbohydrates. If a higher proportion of *Bacillus coagulans* cells had undergone germination, it is likely that there would have been a more significant impact on the digestion of proteins and carbohydrates (Maathuis et al., 2010). Some research suggests that a certain strain of *Lactobacillus casei* can influence the immune system when consumed in fermented dairy products, leading to an augmented antibody response to the influenza vaccine. Moreover, it has been observed that this particular product increases the velocity of seroconversion and seroprotection (Boge et al., 2009). According to a study, a particular strain of *Lactobacillus casei* can regulate the immune response in the upper and systemic airways of runners. Furthermore, middle-aged, healthy office workers, elderly day care center residents, and athletes have shown that this strain can reduce the frequency and duration of URTIs (Vaisberg et al., 2019; Shida et al., 2017; Fujita et al., 2013; Gleeson et al., 2011).

15.5.2 Clinical Trial to Improve Safety and Efficacy

Confirmation of synbiotics' efficacy and safety in metabolic diseases requires extensive, long-term clinical trials, and investigations. These studies can provide more robust evidence and guidelines for their use. There have been several in vivo, in vitro studies conducted that have utilized a broad range of probiotics and/or prebiotics. Safety and effectiveness are two of the most important concerns in this area. At now, certain strains of probiotics, namely, *Bifidobacterium, Lactobacillus*, as well as specific types of prebiotics, such as *inulin* and *oligofructose*, do not necessitate regulatory clearance from the FDA and are commonly found in our everyday dietary consumption. While probiotics, prebiotics, and synbiotics for food application have received safety confirmation from various legal authorities globally, limited research has been undertaken on the occurrence of flatulence, excessive osmotic pressure, bloating. These factors can potentially result in gastrointestinal discomfort (Williams, 1999). In addition, the effects could be different from one person to the next as well as depending on the kind of food that the prebiotics or probiotics are found in. It is generally accepted that synbiotics can be used orally without the risk of experiencing any detrimental effects due to their limited potential for doing so. Presently, there is a lack of established safety protocols for the oral administration of prebiotics and probiotics in human subjects. Hence, it is imperative to assess the potential adverse responses of individual prebiotics and probiotics at specific dosages. Even though BSH has been demonstrated to have advantages, using it may cause the enterohepatic circulation to contain more potentially hazardous secondary bile acids. Consequently, this could potentially enhance the susceptibility to colorectal cancer or cholestasis (Tan et al., 2007). The studies conducted by Beilke et al. demonstrated that giving animals lithocholic acid (LCA) and its conjugates can result in the development of intrahepatic cholestasis. Patients with cystic fibrosis or chronic cholestatic liver disease exhibit aberrant bile acid composition, namely, an elevated presence of LCA, in the human body (Beilke et al., 2008).

15.5.3 Reduce Genetic Interaction between Ingested Probiotic and Native Intestinal Microbe

The investigation of genetic connections between orally consumed probiotics and the endogenous gut microbiota has been a topic of significant scholarly interest. There are three primary techniques that can be used to transfer genetic material, and they are called transduction, conjugation, and transformation. The DNA-induced alterations to the gut microbiota that occur when bacteria are eaten may worsen and lead to chromosomal rearrangements. Furthermore, the transfer of antibiotic-resistant genes between commensal bacteria, pathogenic microorganisms may be linked to the intricate microbial community residing in the gastrointestinal tract. The transmission of genetic material can subsequently result in the development of probiotics that are resistant to antibiotics, hence increasing the likelihood of the establishment of infections that are also resistant to these drugs (Deichelbohrer et al., 1985). The phenomenon of antibiotic resistance poses a substantial threat and leads to considerable harm for numerous individuals afflicted with prevalent bacterial diseases that were previously manageable by antibiotic treatment. For a number of decades, the species that are therapeutically relevant have been the primary focus of study on the selection and propagation of antibiotic resistance. This is because these species are more likely to develop resistance. Researchers are becoming increasingly concerned in the modern era about commensal bacteria—specifically, LAB carrying antibiotic-resistance genes that are genetically identical to those found in human illnesses. This concern is particularly prevalent in the case of LAB. The primary concern linked with these bacteria is in their ability to horizontally transfer resistance genes to dangerous bacteria. Recent research has identified and analyzed genetic components that confer resistance to erythromycin, vancomycin, and tetracycline in *Enterococci, Lactococcus lactis*, and, more recently, *Lactobacillus species* collected from meat products and fermented milk. In recent times, numerous organizations worldwide have undertaken a range of activities aimed at addressing the biosafety considerations associated with starter cultures and probiotic bacteria (Mathur and Singh, 2005).

15.5.4 Quality Assurance Development

There exists a growing need for the integration of probiotics and prebiotics that are resistant to changes in temperature and moisture, into innovative food products and dietary supplements. This demand is characterized by a desire for higher concentrations and intricate blends of these components. The progress in establishing quality assurance systems to ensure the stability, durability, uniformity across batches, and functional validity of these bioactive compounds has been impeded by this inclination (Feng and Wang, 2020). Over the course of time, a multitude of research endeavors has raised concerns regarding the quality and reliability of probiotic products available in the commercial market. Consequently, there have been appeals for the development of standardized evaluation and certification mechanisms in order to enhance confidence among consumers and other relevant parties. Similar principles can be extended to the domains of prebiotics, probiotics, and synbiotics (Jackson et al., 2019). When identifying a probiotic strain correctly, one must use the current nomenclature (which has recently changed in the case of lactobacilli) to determine the species, genus, subspecies, or strain to which it belongs. This will be the case if the probiotic strain has been correctly identified. In commercial quality control laboratories, the identification of probiotics is typically carried out using phenotypic techniques. These methods provide limited resolution, frequently only to the genus level, and are hence not preferred (Huys et al., 2013). The widespread application of whole-genome sequencing (WGS) and next-generation sequencing (NGS) technology has had a substantial impact on the discipline of study pertaining to microbial communities. These advanced techniques have become standard tools in assessing food quality and safety. Although these methods can help accurately identify probiotics in complex mixtures with several strains and identify potential contaminants, they are not widely used in quality control labs at the moment. This is despite the fact that they can also detect possible contaminants and have the potential to be used (Quigley et al., 2013). The assessment of microbial viability is traditionally conducted by evaluating culturability, specifically by counting CFUs. Nevertheless, this approach has notable constraints, such as the incapacity to quantify organisms that are viable but unable to form colonies, sometimes referred to as the viable but nonculturable state (Davis, 2014). Laboratories are presently in pursuit of expedited, cost-effective, less labor-intensive, and highly dependable methodologies that may be used to diverse matrices and developing genera. Flow cytometry is a method that can be employed to assess the viability of certain species of LAB. When combined with polyclonal antibodies, this technique exhibits potential for accurately quantifying multistrain mixtures (Chiron et al., 2018). In the future, research will continue to prioritize finding ways to improve the stability of living cells in a variety of product formats across the course of their shelf lives. The utilization of large-scale data and machine-learning techniques in the study of strain phenomics and fluxomics has the potential to enhance our comprehension of product efficacy and stability across different applications (Kiekens et al., 2019).

15.5.5 Implementation into Policy and Practice

Although there exists persuasive evidence supporting the efficacy of certain prebiotics and probiotics in many health contexts, their widespread integration into dietary and healthcare practices remains constrained. Both professionals in the medical field and average consumers frequently display a certain degree of skepticism when it comes to the possible efficacy of synbiotics as well as the quality of the clinical evidence supporting their usage (Mercer et al., 2012). The regulatory framework exerts a substantial influence on the capacity to disseminate information pertaining to prebiotics and probiotics to key stakeholders. The regulatory status of probiotics and prebiotics varies across different nations and regions, resulting in differences in how they are used in product formulations, health claims, labeling, and other forms of communication with end-users. Numerous nations have effectively established distinct regulatory frameworks and granted approval for probiotic and prebiotic claims based on evidence. However, in certain jurisdictions, the number of allowed claims is limited, resulting in a constrained dissemination of information regarding health benefits in the market. The European framework holds substantial significance in shaping the trajectory of industry-driven research on probiotics, prebiotics, and synbiotics, owing to its rigorous standards and considerable market scale. The global landscape of scientific and technical prerequisites for product development and marketing, particularly in the realm of food and dietary supplements, exhibits significant diversity. Stakeholders operating within separate countries are obligated to adhere to these varying frameworks, which may entail differing scientific criteria for identical concepts (Dronkers et al., 2018). It is imperative to promote both existing and emerging initiatives aimed at advancing worldwide harmonization. One of the most significant issues that will arise during the implementation of future prebiotics, probiotics, and synbiotics will be working toward convergent frameworks while simultaneously adapting these to forthcoming scientific and technological discoveries (Morris et al., 2011). The primary objective of the All-Party Parliamentary Group (APPG) on the Human Gut Microbiome is to provide comprehensive information and exert influence on key stakeholders, including politicians, with the aim of integrating the understanding of the gut microbiome's significance into legislative frameworks. The APPG is comprised of political activists and scientists working in the field of microbiome research. The utilization of a fact-based narrative approach serves to elucidate the scientific concepts within the complex domain of prebiotic, probiotic, and synbiotic science. This process of "decoding" scientific data improves accessibility, relevance, and understanding while raising the likelihood of participation and action. For the full potential of prebiotics and probiotics in healthcare to be realized, there needs to be an increase in recognition at all levels, including among prescribers, consumers, governments, then there needs to be an integration of these concepts into policy, practice, and lifestyle (Dahlstrom, 2014).

15.6 CONCLUSION

In conclusion, the present and future status of synbiotics in controlling metabolic disorders represents a dynamic and promising field of research and application. Prebiotics and probiotics together have been shown in the scientific literature to have synbiotic properties that can significantly influence metabolic health. By focusing on the gut microbiota, which is essential to metabolic processes, they provide hope to those who are battling diseases including obesity, type 2 diabetes, heart health, antibiotic resistance, and metabolic syndrome. As time goes on, the role that synbiotics will play in managing metabolic disorders seems to be getting better. The complex interplay between gut microbiota and metabolic health is being better understood via research, which will help create more individualized and targeted synbiotic therapies. With improved control over their diseases, people with metabolic disorders may be able to minimize their need for medicine and the negative consequences that come with it. Furthermore, technological developments like NGS, the ability to identify particular strains, the development of quality assurance, the application of policy and practice, and improved analytics will make it possible to comprehend the function of the microbiome in metabolic disorders on a deeper level. This understanding will enable the development of synbiotic formulations that are exceptionally precise and customized to the unique characteristics of each patient, thereby optimizing their efficacy. Nevertheless, it is critical to recognize that despite the encouraging potential of synbiotics, there remain obstacles that must be surmounted. Standardization of synbiotic products, safety evaluations, and regulatory considerations are among these. Furthermore, because metabolic problems are complicated and multifaceted, a comprehensive strategy combining dietary and lifestyle changes with synbiotic therapies is required. In conclusion, the current and future status of synbiotics in metabolic disorders control gives considerable optimism for improved patient outcomes and a reduction in the worldwide burden of these ailments. Assuming ongoing investigation, cooperation, and invention, synbiotics are expected to be pivotal in the integrative treatment of metabolic diseases. In the end, this would contribute to increased health and well-being for people all around the world.

15.7 ABBREVIATION

IBS "Irritable bowel syndrome"; IBD "Inflammatory bowel disease"; T2DM "Type 2 diabetes mellitus"; CVD "Cardiovascular diseases"; IBS-C "IBS with constipation"; IBS-D "IBS with diarrhea"; UTI "Urinary tract infection", RNA "Ribonucleic acid"; OCD "Obsessive-compulsive disorder"; ASD "Autism spectrum disorder"; HDL "High-density lipoprotein"; CHD "Coronary heart disease"; SCFA "Short-chain fatty acids" CRP "C-reactive protein", URI "Upper respiratory tract infections"; GOS "Galacto-oligosaccharide"; FOS "Fructo-oligosaccharide"; hs-CRP "High sensitivity C-reactive protein"; STZ "Streptozotocin"; ADD "Antibiotic-associated diarrhea"; CFU "Colony-forming units"; FDA "Food and Drug Administration"; LCA "Lithocholic acid"; DNA "Deoxyribonucleic acid"; LAB "Lactic acid bacteria"; WGS "Whole-genome sequencing"; NGS "Next-generation sequencing"; APPG "All-Party Parliamentary Group".

REFERENCES

Abd El-Gawad, I. A.; El-Sayed, E. M.; Hafez, S. A.; El-Zeini, H. M.; Saleh, F. A. The Hypocholesterolaemic Effect of Milk Yoghurt and Soy-Yoghurt Containing Bifidobacteria in Rats Fed on a Cholesterol-Enriched Diet. *Int. Dairy J.* **2005**, *15* (1), 37–44. https://doi.org/10.1016/j.idairyj.2004.06.001.

Afroja, S.; Falgunee, F. N.; Jahan, M. M.; Akanda, K. M.; Mehjabin, S.; Parvez, M. Antibacterial Activity of Different Citrus Fruits. *Spec. J. Med. Res. Health Sci.* **2017**, *2* (1), 25–32.

Akanda, K. M.; Hasan, A. H. M. N. Characterization of Pharmacological Properties of Methanolic Seed and Stem Bark Extracts of Ziziphus mauritiana (BAU Kul) Using in-vitro and in-vivo Animal (Swiss Albino Male Mice) Model. *Clin. Phytosci.* **2021**, *7* (8), 1–13. https://doi.org/10.1186/s40816-020-00246-0

Akkasheh, G.; Kashani-Poor, Z.; Tajabadi-Ebrahimi, M.; Jafari, P.; Akbari, H.; Taghizadeh, M.; Memarzadeh, M. R.; Asemi, Z.; Esmaillzadeh, A. Clinical and Metabolic Response to Probiotic Administration in Patients with Major Depressive Disorder: A Randomized, Double-Blind, Placebo-Controlled Trial. *Nutrition* **2016**, *32* (3), 315–320. https://doi.org/10.1016/j.nut.2015.09.003.

Akter, R.; Akanda, K. M.; Islam, S.; Rana, M. Assessment of Drug Utilization Pattern among Outpatients in the Orthopedic Department of Several Private Clinics in Rajshahi City, Bangladesh. *Int. J. Pharmaceutic. Sci. Res.* **2020**, *5* (4), 13–16.

Amar, J.; Chabo, C.; Waget, A.; Klopp, P.; Vachoux, C.; Bermúdez-Humarán, L. G.; Smirnova, N.; Bergé, M.; Sulpice, T.; Lahtinen, S.; Ouwehand, A.; Langella, P.; Rautonen, N.; Sansonetti, P. J.; Burcelin, R. Intestinal Mucosal Adherence and Translocation of Commensal Bacteria at the Early Onset of Type 2 Diabetes: Molecular Mechanisms and Probiotic Treatment. *EMBO Mol. Med.* **2011**, *3* (9), 559–572. https://doi.org/10.1002/emmm.201100159.

Anderson, J. W.; Gilliland, S. E. Effect of Fermented Milk (Yogurt) Containing *Lactobacillus acidophilus* L1 on Serum Cholesterol in Hypercholesterolemic Humans. *J. Am. Coll. Nutr.* **1999**, *18* (1), 43–50. https://doi.org/10.1080/07315724.1999.10718826.

Arab, A.; Karimi, E.; Bagherniya, M.; Sathyapalan, T.; Sahebkar, A. The Effect of Probiotic and Synbiotic Consumption on the Most Prevalent Chemotherapy-Related Complications: A Systematic Review of Current Literature. *Curr. Med. Chem.* **2022**, *29* (33), 5462–5473. https://doi.org/10.2174/0929867329666220415114343.

Artiss, J. D.; Brogan, K.; Brucal, M.; Moghaddam, M.; Jen, K.-L. C. The Effects of a New Soluble Dietary Fiber on Weight Gain and Selected Blood Parameters in Rats. Metabolism **2006**, 55 (2), 195–202. https://doi.org/10.1016/j.metabol.2005.08.012.

Asemi, Z.; Zare, Z.; Shakeri, H.; Sabihi, S.; Esmaillzadeh, A. Effect of Multispecies Probiotic Supplements on Metabolic Profiles, Hs-CRP, and Oxidative Stress in Patients with Type 2 Diabetes. *Ann. Nutr. Metab.*, **2013**, 63 (*1–2*), 1–9. https://doi.org/10.1159/000349922.

Beilke, L. D.; Besselsen, D. G.; Cheng, Q.; Kulkarni, S.; Slitt, A. L.; Cherrington, N. J. Minimal Role of Hepatic Transporters in the Hepatoprotection against LCA-Induced Intrahepatic Cholestasis. *Toxicol. Sci.* **2008**, *102* (1), 196–204. https://doi.org/10.1093/toxsci/kfm287.

Boge, T.; Rémigy, M.; Vaudaine, S.; Tanguy, J.; Bourdet-Sicard, R.; van der Werf, S. A Probiotic Fermented Dairy Drink Improves Antibody Response to Influenza Vaccination in the Elderly in Two Randomized Controlled Trials. Vaccine **2009**, 27 (41), 5677–5684. https://doi.org/10.1016/j.vaccine.2009.06.094.

Brighenti, F.; Casiraghi, M. C.; Canzi, E.; Ferrari, A. Effect of Consumption of a Ready-to-Eat Breakfast Cereal Containing Inulin on the Intestinal Milieu and Blood Lipids in Healthy Male Volunteers. *Eur. J. Clin. Nutr.* **1999**, *53* (9), 726–733. https://doi.org/10.1038/sj.ejcn.1600841.

Calcinaro, F.; Dionisi, S.; Marinaro, M.; Candeloro, P.; Bonato, V.; Marzotti, S.; Corneli, R. B.; Ferretti, E.; Gulino, A.; Grasso, F.; De Simone, C.; Di Mario, U.; Falorni, A.; Boirivant, M.; Dotta, F. Oral Probiotic Administration Induces Interleukin-10 Production and Prevents Spontaneous Autoimmune Diabetes in the Non-Obese Diabetic Mouse. *Diabetologia* **2005**, *48* (8), 1565–1575. https://doi.org/10.1007/s00125-005-1831-2.

Causey, J. L.; Feirtag, J. M.; Gallaher, D. D.; Tungland, B. C.; Slavin, J. L. Effects of Dietary Inulin on Serum Lipids, Blood Glucose and the Gastrointestinal Environment in Hypercholesterolemic Men. *Nutr. Res.* **2000**, *20* (2), 191–201. https://doi.org/10.1016/s0271-5317(99)00152-9.

Chiron, C.; Tompkins, T. A.; Burguière, P. Flow Cytometry: A Versatile Technology for Specific Quantification and Viability Assessment of Micro-Organisms in Multistrain Probiotic Products. *J. Appl. Microbiol.* **2018**, *124* (2), 572–584. https://doi.org/10.1111/jam.13666.

Cruchet, S.; Furnes, R.; Maruy, A.; Hebel, E.; Palacios, J.; Medina, F.; Ramirez, N.; Orsi, M.; Rondon, L.; Sdepanian, V.; Xóchihua, L.; Ybarra, M.; Zablah, R. A. The Use of Probiotics in Pediatric Gastroenterology: A Review of the Literature and Recommendations by Latin-American Experts. Paediatr. Drugs **2015**, *17* (3), 199–216. https://doi.org/10.1007/s40272-015-0124-6.

Dahlstrom, M. F. Using Narratives and Storytelling to Communicate Science with Nonexpert Audiences. *Proc. Natl. Acad. Sci. U. S. A.* **2014**, *111* (supplement_4), 13614–13620. https://doi.org/10.1073/pnas.1320645111.

Davis, C. Enumeration of Probiotic Strains: Review of Culture-Dependent and Alternative Techniques to Quantify Viable Bacteria. *J. Microbiol. Methods* **2014**, *103*, 9–17. https://doi.org/10.1016/j.mimet.2014.04.012.

Deichelbohrer, I.; Alonso, J. C.; Lüder, G.; Trautner, T. A. Plasmid Transduction by *Bacillus subtilis* Bacteriophage SPP1: Effects of DNA Homology between Plasmid and Bacteriophage. *J. Bacteriol.* **1985**, *162* (3), 1238–1243. https://doi.org/10.1128/jb.162.3.1238-1243.1985.

Dikeman, C. L.; Murphy, M. R.; Fahey, G. C., Jr. Dietary Fibers Affect Viscosity of Solutions and Simulated Human Gastric and Small Intestinal Digesta. *J. Nutr.* **2006**, *136* (4), 913–919. https://doi.org/10.1093/jn/136.4.913.

Dronkers, T. M. G.; Krist, L.; Van Overveld, F. J.; Rijkers, G. T. The Ascent of the Blessed: Regulatory Issues on Health Effects and Health Claims for Probiotics in Europe and the Rest of the World. *Benef. Microbes* **2018**, *9* (5), 717–723. https://doi.org/10.3920/bm2017.0196.

Ejtahed, H. S.; Mohtadi-Nia, J.; Homayouni-Rad, A.; Niafar, M.; Asghari-Jafarabadi, M.; Mofid, V. Probiotic Yogurt Improves Antioxidant Status in Type 2 Diabetic Patients. *Nutrition* **2012**, *28* (5), 539–543. https://doi.org/10.1016/j.nut.2011.08.013.

Ejtahed, H. S.; Mohtadi-Nia, J.; Homayouni-Rad, A.; Niafar, M.; Asghari-Jafarabadi, M.; Mofid, V.; Akbarian-Moghari, A. Effect of Probiotic Yogurt Containing *Lactobacillus acidophilus* and *Bifidobacterium lactis* on Lipid Profile in Individuals with Type 2 Diabetes Mellitus. *J. Dairy Sci.* **2011**, *94* (7), 3288–3294. https://doi.org/10.3168/jds.2010-4128.

Feng, T.; Wang, J. Oxidative Stress Tolerance and Antioxidant Capacity of Lactic Acid Bacteria as Probiotic: A Systematic Review. *Gut Microbes* **2020**, *12* (1), 1801944. https://doi.org/10.1080/19490976.2020.1801944.

Fotiadis, C.-I.; Stoidis, C.-N.; Spyropoulos, B.-G.; Zografos, E.-D. Role of Probiotics, Prebiotics and Synbiotics in Chemoprevention for Colorectal Cancer. *World J. Gastroenterol.* **2008**, *14* (42), 6453–6457. https://doi.org/10.3748/wjg.14.6453.

Fujita, R.; Iimuro, S.; Shinozaki, T.; Sakamaki, K.; Uemura, Y.; Takeuchi, A.; Matsuyama, Y.; Ohashi, Y. Decreased Duration of Acute Upper Respiratory Tract Infections with Daily Intake of Fermented Milk: A Multicenter, Double-Blinded, Randomized Comparative Study in Users of Day Care Facilities for the Elderly Population. *Am. J. Infect. Control* **2013**, *41* (12), 1231–1235. https://doi.org/10.1016/j.ajic.2013.04.005.

Fukushima, M.; Yamada, A.; Endo, T.; Nakano, M. Effects of a Mixture of Organisms, *Lactobacillus acidophilus* or *Streptococcus faecalis* on Delta6-Desaturase Activity in the Livers of Rats Fed a Fat- and Cholesterol-Enriched Diet. *Nutrition* **1999**, *15* (5), 373–378. https://doi.org/10.1016/s0899-9007(99)00030-1.

Fuller, R. Probiotics in Man and Animals. *J. Appl. Bacteriol.* **1989**, *66* (5), 365–378. https://doi.org/10.1111/j.1365-2672.1989.tb05105.x.

Furness, J. B.; Kunze, W. A.; Clerc, N. Nutrient Tasting and Signaling Mechanisms in the Gut. II. The Intestine as a Sensory Organ: Neural, Endocrine, and Immune Responses. *Am. J. Physiol.* **1999**, *277* (5 Pt. 1), G922–G928. https://doi.org/10.1152/ajpgi.1999.277.5.G922.

García-Núñez, I. M.; Santacruz, A.; Serna-Saldívar, S. O.; Hernandez, S. L. C.; Amaya Guerra, C. A. Assessment of Potential Probiotic and Synbiotic Properties of Lactic Acid Bacteria Grown in Vitro with Starch-Based Soluble Corn Fiber or Inulin. Foods **2022**, 11 (24), 4020. https://doi.org/10.3390/foods11244020.

Gibson, G. R.; Roberfroid, M. B. Dietary Modulation of the Human Colonic Microbiota: Introducing the Concept of Prebiotics. *J. Nutr.* **1995**, *125* (6), 1401–1412. https://doi.org/10.1093/jn/125.6.1401.

Gleeson, M.; Bishop, N. C.; Oliveira, M.; Tauler, P. Daily Probiotic's (*Lactobacillus casei* Shirota) Reduction of Infection Incidence in Athletes. *Int. J. Sport Nutr. Exerc. Metab.* **2011**, *21* (1), 55–64. https://doi.org/10.1123/ijsnem.21.1.55.

Goldenberg, J. Z.; Yap, C.; Lytvyn, L.; Lo, C. K.-F.; Beardsley, J.; Mertz, D.; Johnston, B. C. Probiotics for the Prevention of Clostridium Difficile-Associated Diarrhea in Adults and Children. *Cochrane Libr.* **2017**, *2017* (12). https://doi.org/10.1002/14651858.cd006095.pub4.

Guillemard, E.; Tanguy, J.; Flavigny, A.; de la Motte, S.; Schrezenmeir, J. Effects of Consumption of a Fermented Dairy Product Containing the Probiotic *Lactobacillus casei* DN-114 001 on Common Respiratory and Gastrointestinal Infections in Shift Workers in a Randomized Controlled Trial. *J. Am. Coll. Nutr.* **2010**, *29* (5), 455–468. https://doi.org/10.1080/07315724.2010.10719882.

Haque, M. U.; Ahmmed, S. B.; Akanda, M. K. M.; Hasan, M. T.; Mou, S. A.; Sajon, S. R.; Islam, M. A. U. Prevalence and Risk Factors of Obesity and Hypertension among University Students in Rajshahi City, Bangladesh. *Bangladesh Pharmaceutic. J.* **2016**, *19* (2), 179–184. https://doi.org/10.3329/bpj.v19i2.29277

Hardy, H.; Harris, J.; Lyon, E.; Beal, J.; Foey, A. D. Probiotics, Prebiotics and Immunomodulation of Gut Mucosal Defences: Homeostasis and Immunopathology. *Nutrients* **2013**, *5* (6), 1869–1912. https://doi.org/10.3390/nu5061869.

Hatakka, K.; Savilahti, E.; Pönkä, A.; Meurman, J. H.; Poussa, T.; Näse, L.; Saxelin, M.; Korpela, R. Effect of Long Term Consumption of Probiotic Milk on Infections in Children Attending Day Care Centres: Double Blind, Randomised Trial. *BMJ* **2001**, *322* (7298), 1327. https://doi.org/10.1136/bmj.322.7298.1327.

Hunter, P. The Inflammation Theory of Disease: The Growing Realization That Chronic Inflammation Is Crucial in Many Diseases Opens New Avenues for Treatment. *EMBO Rep* **2012**, *13* (11), 968–970. https://doi.org/10.1038/embor.2012.142.

Huys, G.; Botteldoorn, N.; Delvigne, F.; De Vuyst, L.; Heyndrickx, M.; Pot, B.; Dubois, J.-J.; Daube, G. Microbial Characterization of Probiotics-Advisory Report of the Working Group "8651 Probiotics" of the Belgian Superior Health Council (SHC). *Mol. Nutr. Food Res.* **2013**, *57* (8), 1479–1504. https://doi.org/10.1002/mnfr.201300065.

Jackson, S. A.; Schoeni, J. L.; Vegge, C.; Pane, M.; Stahl, B.; Bradley, M.; Goldman, V. S.; Burguière, P.; Atwater, J. B.; Sanders, M. E. Improving End-User Trust in the Quality of Commercial Probiotic Products. *Front. Microbiol.* **2019**, *10*, 739. https://doi.org/10.3389/fmicb.2019.00739.

Kadooka, Y.; Sato, M.; Ogawa, A.; Miyoshi, M.; Uenishi, H.; Ogawa, H.; Ikuyama, K.; Kagoshima, M.; Tsuchida, T. Effect of *Lactobacillus gasseri* SBT2055 in Fermented Milk on Abdominal Adiposity in Adults in a Randomised Controlled Trial. *Br. J. Nutr.* **2013**, *110* (9), 1696–1703. https://doi.org/10.1017/S0007114513001037.

Kasubuchi, M.; Hasegawa, S.; Hiramatsu, T.; Ichimura, A.; Kimura, I. Dietary Gut Microbial Metabolites, Short-Chain Fatty Acids, and Host Metabolic Regulation. *Nutrients* **2015**, 7 (4), 2839–2849. https://doi.org/10.3390/nu7042839.

Kechagia, M.; Basoulis, D.; Konstantopoulou, S.; Dimitriadi, D.; Gyftopoulou, K.; Skarmoutsou, N.; Fakiri, E. M. Health Benefits of Probiotics: A Review. *ISRN Nutr.* **2013**, *2013*, 481651. https://doi.org/10.5402/2013/481651.

Khalesi, S.; Sun, J.; Buys, N.; Jayasinghe, R. Effect of Probiotics on Blood Pressure: A Systematic Review and Meta-Analysis of Randomized, Controlled Trials. *Hypertension* **2014**, *64* (4), 897–903. https://doi.org/10.1161/hypertensionaha.114.03469.

Kiekens, S.; Vandenheuvel, D.; Broeckx, G.; Claes, I.; Allonsius, C.; De Boeck, I.; Thys, S.; Timmermans, J.-P.; Kiekens, F.; Lebeer, S. Impact of Spray-Drying on the Pili of Lactobacillus rhamnosus GG. *Microb. Biotechnol.* **2019**, *12* (5), 849–855. https://doi.org/10.1111/1751-7915.13426.

Kim, M.; Shin, H. K. The Water-Soluble Extract of Chicory Influences Serum and Liver Lipid Concentrations, Cecal Short-Chain Fatty Acid Concentrations and Fecal Lipid Excretion in Rats. *J. Nutr.* **1998**, *128* (10), 1731–1736. https://doi.org/10.1093/jn/128.10.1731.

Kruis, W.; Fric, P.; Pokrotnieks, J.; Lukás, M.; Fixa, B.; Kascák, M.; Kamm, M. A.; Weismueller, J.; Beglinger, C.; Stolte, M.; Wolff, C.; Schulze, J. Maintaining Remission of Ulcerative Colitis with the Probiotic Escherichia Coli Nissle 1917 Is as Effective as with Standard Mesalazine. *Gut* **2004**, *53* (11), 1617–1623. https://doi.org/10.1136/gut.2003.037747.

Lee, J.-H.; O'Sullivan, D. J. Genomic Insights into Bifidobacteria. *Microbiol. Mol. Biol. Rev.* **2010**, *74* (3), 378–416. https://doi.org/10.1128/mmbr.00004-10.

Ley, R. E.; Turnbaugh, P. J.; Klein, S.; Gordon, J. I. Microbial Ecology: Human Gut Microbes Associated with Obesity. *Nature* **2006**, *444* (7122), 1022–1023. https://doi.org/10.1038/4441022a.

Leyer, G. J.; Li, S.; Mubasher, M. E.; Reifer, C.; Ouwehand, A. C. Probiotic Effects on Cold and Influenza-Like Symptom Incidence and Duration in Children. *Pediatrics* **2009**, *124* (2), e172– e179. https://doi.org/10.1542/peds.2008-2666.

Maathuis, A.; Keller, D.; Farmer, S. Survival and Metabolic Activity of the GanedenBC30 Strain of *Bacillus Coagulans* in a Dynamic *in Vitro* Model of the Stomach and Small Intestine. *Benef. Microbes* **2010**, *1* (1), 31–36. https://doi.org/10.3920/bm2009.0009.

Mathur, S.; Singh, R. Antibiotic Resistance in Food Lactic Acid Bacteria–a Review. *Int. J. Food Microbiol.* **2005**, *105* (3), 281–295. https://doi.org/10.1016/j.ijfoodmicro.2005.03.008.

Mercer, M.; Brinich, M. A.; Geller, G.; Harrison, K.; Highland, J.; James, K.; Marshall, P.; McCormick, J. B.; Tilburt, J.; Achkar, J.-P.; Farrell, R. M.; Sharp, R. R. How Patients View Probiotics: Findings from a Multicenter Study of Patients with Inflammatory Bowel Disease and Irritable Bowel Syndrome. *J. Clin. Gastroenterol.* **2012**, *46* (2), 138–144. https://doi.org/10.1097/MCG.0b013e318225f545.

Moayyedi, P.; Ford, A. C.; Talley, N. J.; Cremonini, F.; Foxx-Orenstein, A. E.; Brandt, L. J.; Quigley, E. M. M. The Efficacy of Probiotics in the Treatment of Irritable Bowel Syndrome: A Systematic Review. *Gut* **2010**, *59* (3), 325–332. https://doi.org/10.1136/gut.2008.167270.

Mohammadi, A. A.; Jazayeri, S.; Khosravi-Darani, K.; Solati, Z.; Mohammadpour, N.; Asemi, Z.; Adab, Z.; Djalali, M.; Tehrani-Doost, M.; Hosseini, M.; Eghtesadi, S. The Effects of Probiotics on Mental Health and Hypothalamic-Pituitary-Adrenal Axis: A Randomized, Double-Blind, Placebo-Controlled Trial in Petrochemical Workers. *Nutr. Neurosci.* **2016**, *19* (9), 387–395. https://doi.org/10.1179/1476830515y.0000000023.

Morris, Z. S.; Wooding, S.; Grant, J. The Answer Is 17 Years, What Is the Question: Understanding Time Lags in Translational Research. *J. R. Soc. Med.* **2011**, *104* (12), 510–520. https://doi.org/10.1258/jrsm.2011.110180.

Nagatomo, Y.; Tang, W. H. W. Intersections between Microbiome and Heart Failure: Revisiting the Gut Hypothesis. *J. Card. Fail.* **2015**, *21* (12), 973–980. https://doi.org/10.1016/j.cardfail.2015.09.017.

Nguyen, T. D. T.; Kang, J. H.; Lee, M. S. Characterization of *Lactobacillus plantarum* PH04, a Potential Probiotic Bacterium with Cholesterol-Lowering Effects. *Int. J. Food Microbiol.* **2007**, *113* (3), 358–361. https://doi.org/10.1016/j.ijfoodmicro.2006.08.015.

Nishihira, J.; Nishimura, M.; Moriya, T.; Sakai, F.; Kabuki, T.; Kawasaki, Y. Lactobacillus Gasseri Potentiates Immune Response Against Influenza Virus Infection. In *Immunity and Inflammation in Health and Disease*; Chatterjee, S., Jungraithmayr, W., Bagchi, D., Eds.; Elsevier, **2018**; pp. 249–255.

Ogawa, A.; Kobayashi, T.; Sakai, F.; Kadooka, Y.; Kawasaki, Y. *Lactobacillus gasseri* SBT2055 Suppresses Fatty Acid Release through Enlargement of Fat Emulsion Size in Vitro and Promotes Fecal Fat Excretion in Healthy Japanese Subjects. *Lipids Health Dis.* **2015**, *14* (1). https://doi.org/10.1186/s12944-015-0019-0.

Pandey, K. R.; Naik, S. R.; Vakil, B. V. Probiotics, Prebiotics and Synbiotics-a Review. *J. Food Sci. Technol.* **2015**, *52* (12), 7577–7587. https://doi.org/10.1007/s13197-015-1921-1.

Parnell, J. A.; Reimer, R. A. Prebiotic Fibres Dose-Dependently Increase Satiety Hormones and Alter Bacteroidetes and Firmicutes in Lean and Obese JCR:LA-Cp Rats. *Br. J. Nutr.* **2012**, *107* (4), 601–613. https://doi.org/10.1017/S0007114511003163.

Parvez, M.; Akanda, K. M. Foods and Arthritis: An Overview. In *Bioactive Food as Dietary Interventions for Arthritis and Related Inflammatory Diseases*; Second Edition; Watson, R. R., Preedy, V. R., Eds.; Academic Press, Elsevier, **2019**; pp. 3–22. https://doi.org/10.1016/B978-0-12-813820-5.00001-5

Parvez, M.; Sultana, R.; Akanda, K. M.; Mehjabin, S.; Mosaddik, A. Nature and Cause of Taking Psychotropic Drugs: A Cross-sectional Health Survey in Northern Regions of Bangladesh. *Int. J Pharm. Sci. Res.* **2018**, *9* (1), 361–368. https://dx. doi.org/10.13040/IJPSR.0975-8232.9(1).361-68

Pelto, L.; Isolauri, E.; Lilius, E. M.; Nuutila, J.; Salminen, S. Probiotic Bacteria Down-Regulate the Milk-Induced Inflammatory Response in Milk-Hypersensitive Subjects but Have an Immunostimulatory Effect in Healthy Subjects: Immunomodulation by Probiotic Bacteria. *Clin. Exp. Allergy* **1998**, *28* (12), 1474–1479. https://doi.org/10.1046/j.1365-2222.1998.00449.x.

Pregliasco, F.; Anselmi, G.; Fonte, L.; Giussani, F.; Schieppati, S.; Soletti, L. A New Chance of Preventing Winter Diseases by the Administration of Synbiotic Formulations. *J. Clin. Gastroenterol.* **2008**, *42* (Supplement 3), S224–S233. https://doi.org/10.1097/mcg.0b013e31817e1c91.

Quigley, L.; McCarthy, R.; O'Sullivan, O.; Beresford, T. P.; Fitzgerald, G. F.; Ross, R. P.; Stanton, C.; Cotter, P. D. The Microbial Content of Raw and Pasteurized Cow Milk as Determined by Molecular Approaches. *J. Dairy Sci.* **2013**, *96* (8), 4928–4937. https://doi.org/10.3168/jds.2013-6688.

Rijkers, G. T.; de Vos, W. M.; Brummer, R.-J.; Morelli, L.; Corthier, G.; Marteau, P. Health Benefits and Health Claims of Probiotics: Bridging Science and Marketing. *Br. J. Nutr.* **2011**, *106* (9), 1291–1296. https://doi.org/10.1017/S000711451100287X.

Roller, M.; Rechkemmer, G.; Watzl, B. Prebiotic Inulin Enriched with Oligofructose in Combination with the Probiotics *Lactobacillus rhamnosus* and *Bifidobacterium lactis* Modulates Intestinal Immune Functions in Rats. *J. Nutr.* **2004**, *134* (1), 153–156. https://doi.org/10.1093/jn/134.1.153.

Scarpellini, E.; Lauritano, E. C.; Lupascu, A.; Petruzzellis, C.; Novi, M. L.; Roccarina, D.; Gabrielli, M.; Serricchio, M.; Gasbarrini, G.; Gasbarrini, A. Efficacy of Butyrate in the Treatment of Diarrhoea-Predominant Irritable Bowel Syndrome. *Dig. Liver Dis. Suppl.* **2007**, *1* (1), 19–22. https://doi.org/10.1016/s1594-5804(08)60006-6.

Shida, K.; Sato, T.; Iizuka, R.; Hoshi, R.; Watanabe, O.; Igarashi, T.; Miyazaki, K.; Nanno, M.; Ishikawa, F. Daily Intake of Fermented Milk with *Lactobacillus casei* Strain Shirota Reduces the Incidence and Duration of Upper Respiratory Tract Infections in Healthy Middle-Aged Office Workers. *Eur. J. Nutr.* **2017**, *56* (1), 45–53. https://doi.org/10.1007/s00394-015-1056-1.

Slavin, J. L. Dietary Fiber and Body Weight. *Nutrition* **2005**, *21* (3), 411–418. https://doi.org/10.1016/j.nut.2004.08.018.

Stapleton, A. E.; Au-Yeung, M.; Hooton, T. M.; Fredricks, D. N.; Roberts, P. L.; Czaja, C. A.; Yarova-Yarovaya, Y.; Fiedler, T.; Cox, M.; Stamm, W. E. Randomized, Placebo-Controlled Phase 2 Trial of a *Lactobacillus crispatus* Probiotic Given Intravaginally for Prevention of Recurrent Urinary Tract Infection. *Clin. Infect. Dis.* **2011**, *52* (10), 1212–1217. https://doi.org/10.1093/cid/cir183.

Sultana, R.; Akanda, K. M.; Mehjabin, S.; Parvez, M. Prescribing Trends of Psychotropic Drugs in Northern Bangladesh. *Spec. J. Med. Res. Health Sci.* **2017**, *2* (2), 17–25.

Sun, J.; Buys, N. Effects of Probiotics Consumption on Lowering Lipids and CVD Risk Factors: A Systematic Review and Meta-Analysis of Randomized Controlled Trials. *Ann. Med.* **2015**, *47* (6), 430–440. https://doi.org/10.3109/07853890.2015.1071872.

Tajabadi-Ebrahimi, M.; Sharifi, N.; Farrokhian, A.; Raygan, F.; Karamali, F.; Razzaghi, R.; Taheri, S.; Asemi, Z. A Randomized Controlled Clinical Trial Investigating the Effect of Synbiotic Administration on Markers of Insulin Metabolism and Lipid Profiles in Overweight Type 2 Diabetic Patients with Coronary Heart Disease. *Exp. Clin. Endocrinol. Diabetes* **2017**, *125* (1), 21–27. https://doi.org/10.1055/s-0042-105441.

Tan, K. P.; Yang, M.; Ito, S. Activation of Nuclear Factor (Erythroid-2 like) Factor 2 by Toxic Bile Acids Provokes Adaptive Defense Responses to Enhance Cell Survival at the Emergence of Oxidative Stress. *Mol. Pharmacol.* **2007**, *72* (5), 1380–1390. https://doi.org/10.1124/mol.107.039370.

Uzzaman, S.; Akanda, K. M.; Mehjabin, S.; Parvez, M. A Short Review on a Nutritional Fruit: Guava. *Opn Acc Tox & Res.* **2018**, *1* (1), 1–8.

Vaisberg, M.; Paixão, V.; Almeida, E. B.; Santos, J. M. B.; Foster, R.; Rossi, M.; Pithon-Curi, T. C.; Gorjão, R.; Momesso, C. M.; Andrade, M. S.; Araujo, J. R.; Garcia, M. C.; Cohen, M.; Perez, E. C.; Santos-Dias, A.; Vieira, R. P.; Bachi, A. L. L. Daily Intake of Fermented Milk Containing *Lactobacillus casei* Shirota (LcS) Modulates Systemic and Upper Airways Immune/Inflammatory Responses in Marathon Runners. *Nutrients* **2019**, *11* (7), 1678. https://doi.org/10.3390/nu11071678.

Verna, E. C.; Lucak, S. Use of Probiotics in Gastrointestinal Disorders: What to Recommend? *Therap. Adv. Gastroenterol.* **2010**, *3* (5), 307–319. https://doi.org/10.1177/1756283x10373814.

Verraes, C.; Van Boxstael, S.; Van Meervenne, E.; Van Coillie, E.; Butaye, P.; Catry, B.; de Schaetzen, M.-A.; Van Huffel, X.; Imberechts, H.; Dierick, K.; Daube, G.; Saegerman, C.; De Block, J.; Dewulf, J.; Herman, L. Antimicrobial Resistance in the Food Chain: A Review. *Int. J. Environ. Res. Public Health* **2013**, *10* (7), 2643–2669. https://doi.org/10.3390/ijerph10072643.

Videlock, E. J.; Cremonini, F. Meta-Analysis: Probiotics in Antibiotic-Associated Diarrhoea. *Aliment. Pharmacol. Ther.* **2012**, *35* (12), 1355–1369. https://doi.org/10.1111/j.1365-2036.2012.05104.x.

Villena, J.; Salva, S.; Núñez, M.; Corzo, J.; Tolaba, R.; Faedda, J.; Font, G.; Alvarez, S. Probiotics for Everyone! The Novel Immunobiotic *Lactobacillus rhamnosus* CRL1505 and the Beginning of Social Probiotic Programs in Argentina. *Int. J. Biotechnol. Wellness Indust.* **2012**, *1*, 189–198. https://dx.doi.org/10.6000/1927-3037/2012.01.03.05

Walden, K. E.; Hagele, A. M.; Orr, L. S.; Gross, K. N.; Krieger, J. M.; Jäger, R.; Kerksick, C. M. Probiotic BC30 Improves Amino Acid Absorption from Plant Protein Concentrate in Older Women. *Probiotics Antimicrob. Proteins* **2022**. https://doi.org/10.1007/s12602-022-10028-4.

Wang, H.; Lee, I.-S.; Braun, C.; Enck, P. Effect of Probiotics on Central Nervous System Functions in Animals and Humans: A Systematic Review. *J. Neurogastroenterol. Motil.* **2016**, *22* (4), 589–605. https://doi.org/10.5056/jnm16018.

Williams, C. M. Effects of Inulin on Lipid Parameters in Humans. *J. Nutr.* **1999**, *129* (7 Suppl), 1471S–1473S. https://doi.org/10.1093/jn/129.7.1471S.

Yadav, H.; Jain, S.; Sinha, P. R. Antidiabetic Effect of Probiotic Dahi Containing *Lactobacillus acidophilus* and *Lactobacillus casei* in High Fructose Fed Rats. *Nutrition* **2007**, *23* (1), 62–68. https://doi.org/10.1016/j.nut.2006.09.002.

Yadav, H.; Jain, S.; Sinha, P. R. Oral Administration of Dahi Containing Probiotic *Lactobacillus acidophilus* and *Lactobacillus casei* Delayed the Progression of Streptozotocin-Induced Diabetes in Rats. *J. Dairy Res.* **2008**, *75* (2), 189–195. https://doi.org/10.1017/S0022029908003129.

Zhang, Y.-J.; Li, S.; Gan, R.-Y.; Zhou, T.; Xu, D.-P.; Li, H.-B. Impacts of Gut Bacteria on Human Health and Diseases. *Int. J. Mol. Sci.* **2015**, *16* (4), 7493–7519. https://doi.org/10.3390/ijms16047493.

Index

Note: **Bold** page numbers refer to tables and *italic* page numbers refer to figures.